5.1.2.1.1 Ineffective Family Coping: Disabling

5.1.2.1.2 Ineffective Family Coping: Compromised

5.1.3.1 Potential for Enhanced Community Coping

5.1.3.2 Ineffective Community Coping

5.1.2.2 Family Coping: Potential for Growth

5.2.1 Ineffective Management of Therapeutic Regimen (individuals)

5.2.1.1 Noncompliance (Specify)

5.2.2 Ineffective Management of Therapeutic Regimen: Families

5.2.3 Ineffective Management of Therapeutic Regimen:Community

5.2.4 Ineffective Management of Therapeutic Regimen: Individual

5.3.1.1 Decisional Conflict (Specify)

5.4 Health Seeking Behaviors (Specify)

PATTERN 6 MOVING

6.1.1.1 Impaired Physical Mobility

6.1.1.1.1 Risk for Peripheral Neurovascular Dysfunction

6.1.1.1.2 Risk for Perioperative Positioning Injury

6.1.1.2 Activity Intolerance

6.1.1.2.1 Fatigue

6.1.1.3 Risk for Activity Intolerance

6.2.1 Sleep Pattern Disturbance

6.3.1.1 Diversional Activity Deficit

6.4.1.1 Impaired Home Maintenance Management

6.4.2 Altered Health Maintenance

6.5.1 Feeding Self Care Deficit

6.5.1.1 Impaired Swallowing

6.5.1.2 Ineffective Breastfeeding

6.5.1.2.1 Interrupted Breastfeeding

6.5.1.3 Effective Breastfeeding

6.5.1.4 Ineffective Infant Feeding Pattern

6.5.2 Bathing/Hygiene Self Care Deficit

6.5.3 Dressing/Grooming Self Care Deficit

6.5.4 Toileting Self Care Deficit

6.6 Altered Growth and Development

6.7 Relocation Stress Syndrome

6.8.1 Risk for Disorganized Infant Behavior

6.8.2 Disorganized Infant Behavior

6.8.3 Potential for Enhanced Organized Infant Behavior

PATTERN 7 PERCEIVING

7.1.1 Body Image Disturbance

7.1.2 Self Esteem Disturbance

7.1.2.1 Chronic Low Self Esteem

7.1.2.2 Situational Low Self Esteem

7.1.3 Personal Identity Disturbance

7.2 Sensory/Perceptual Alterations (Specify) (Visual, auditory, kinesthetic, gustatory, tactile, olfactory)

7.2.1.1 Unilateral Neglect

7.3.1 Hopelessness

7.3.2 Powerlessness

PATTERN 8 KNOWING

8.1.1 Knowledge Deficit (Specify)

8.2.1 Impaired Environmental Interpretation Syndrome

8.2.2 Acute Confusion

8.2.3 Chronic Confusion

8.3 Altered Thought Processes

8.3.1 Impaired Memory

PATTERN 9 FEELING

9.1.1 Pain

9.1.1.1 Chronic Pain

9.2.1.1 Dysfunctional Grieving

9.2.1.2 Anticipatory Grieving

9.2.2 Risk for Violence: Self-directed or directed at others

9.2.2.1 Risk for Self-Mutilation

9.2.3 Post-Trauma Response

9.2.3.1 Rape-Trauma Syndrome

9.2.3.1.1 Rape-Trauma Syndrome: Compound Reaction

9.2.3.1.2 Rape-Trauma Syndrome: Silent Reaction

9.3.1 Anxiety

9.3.2 Fear

PRIORITIES IN

Critical Care Nursing

PRIORITIES IN

Critical Care Nursing

SECOND EDITION

LINDA D. URDEN, DNSc, RN, CNA

Administrative Director, Nursing Services, Quality, Education, and Research
Butterworth Hospital, Grand Rapids, Michigan

MARY E. LOUGH, MS, RN, CCRN

Critical Care Cardiovascular Clinical Nurse Specialist
Sequoia Hospital, Redwood City, California
Assistant Clinical Professor, University of California at San Francisco

KATHLEEN M. STACY, MS, RN, CCRN

Critical Care Clinical Specialist
Tri-City Medical Center, Oceanside, California

with 143 illustrations

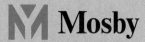

Mosby

St. Louis Baltimore Boston Carlsbad Chicago Naples New York Philadelphia Portland
London Madrid Mexico City Singapore Sydney Tokyo Toronto Wiesbaden

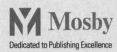

Mosby
Dedicated to Publishing Excellence

A Times Mirror
Company

Acquisition Editor: **Robin Carter**
Developmental Editor: **Jolynn Gower**
Editorial Assistant: **Kristin Geen**
Project Manager: **Linda McKinley**
Production Editor: **René Spencer**
Designer: **Liz Fett**
Manufacturing Manager: **Theresa Fuchs**

Second edition

Copyright © 1996 by Mosby–Year Book, Inc.

Previous edition copyrighted 1992

Printed in the United States of America.

Composition by Clarinda Company
Printing/binding by Rand McNally, Inc.

Mosby-Year Book, Inc.
11830 Westline Industrial Drive
St. Louis, MO 63146

Library of Congress Cataloging in Publication Data

Priorities in critical care nursing / [edited by] Linda D. Urden, Mary
E. Lough, Kathleen M. Stacy. — 2nd ed.
    p.   cm.
    Rev. ed. of: Essentials of critical care nursing / Linda Diann
Urden, Joseph Kevin Davie, Lynne Ann Thelan. c1992.
    Includes bibliographical references and index.
    ISBN 0-8151-8947-8
    1. Intensive care nursing.   I. Urden, Linda Diann.   II. Lough,
Mary E.   III. Stacy, Kathleen M.   IV. Urden, Linda Diann.
Essentials of critical care nursing.
    [DNLM: 1. Critical Care—nurses' instruction.   2. Nursing Care.
WY 154 P958 1995]
RT 120.I5E83 1995
610.73'61—dc20
DNLM/DLC
for Library of Congress   95-20589
                                                           CIP

96 97 98 99 00 / 9 8 7 6 5 4 3 2 1

Contributors & Consultants

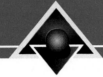

CONTRIBUTORS

JENNIFER BLOOMQUIST,
MN, RN

Cardiac Rehabilitation Clinical Nurse
Specialist
Naval Medical Center
San Diego, California

WENDY BODWELL,
MSN, RN, C, CNAA

Assistant Director of Nursing
Life Care Center of Aurora
Aurora, Colorado

LOIS CATTS, MS, RN, CCRN

Critical Care Clinical Nurse Specialist
St. Elizabeth Medical Center
Yakima, Washington

JOANN M. CLARK,
MSN, RN, CFNP

Assistant Clinical Professor
School of Medicine, Nursing Division
University of California-San Diego
La Jolla, California

JONI DIRKS, MS, RN, CCRN

Clinical Nurse Specialist, SICU
Department of Veterans Affairs Medical
Center
Palo Alto, California

LORRAINE FITZSIMMONS,
DNS, RN

Associate Professor and Chair, Critical
Care Nurse Specialist Concentration
San Diego State University School of
Nursing
San Diego, California

KATHERINE FORTINASH,
MSN, RN, CS

Clinical Nurse Specialist
Grossmont Hospital and Cabrillo
Hospital Behavioral Health Services
Sharp Healthcare
San Diego, California

KAREN JOHNSON,
MSN, RN, CCRN

Doctoral Student
University of Kentucky
Lexington, Kentucky

JACQUELINE KARTMAN,
MS, RN, CS, CCRN

Nurse Practitioner-Cardiothoracic
Surgery
Lutheran Hospital-LaCrosse
LaCrosse, Wisconsin

MARTHA LOVE, MN, RN

Cardiovascular Clinical Nurse Specialist
Department of Veterans Affairs Medical
Center
San Diego, California

KATHLEEN A. MENDEZ,
MS, RN, CCRN, CNS

Assistant Unit Manager, Adult Critical
Care Unit
Tri-City Medical Center
Oceanside, California

MARY COURTNEY MOORE,
PhD, RN, RD

Associate Professor
Austin Peay State University School of
Nursing
Clarksville, Tennessee

COLLEEN O'DONNELL,
MS, RN, CCRN

Nurse Manager, ICU
Montrose Memorial Hospital
Montrose, Canada

MIMI O'DONNELL, MS, RN, CS

Cardiovascular Clinical Nurse Specialist
Massachusetts General Hospital
Boston, Massachusetts

MARIANN REBENSON-PIANO,
PhD, RN

Assistant Professor
University of Illinois-Chicago
Chicago, Illinois

LINDA VALENTINO, BSN, RN

Nurse Educator
Beth Israel Medical Center
New York City, New York

CONSULTANTS

**SHEANA WHELAN
FUNKHOUSER, DNSc, RN**

Research and Education Consultant
Palo Alto, California

CATHY R. KESSENICH, RNC, MS

Husson College/EMMC
Bangor, Maine

KAY E. McCASH, MSN, RNC

University of New Mexico College of
   Nursing
Albuquerque, New Mexico

MARY REDMON, MSN, RN

Lorain County Community College
Brooklyn, Ohio

**DEBRA SIELA,
MN, RN, CCRN, RRT**

Ball State University
Muncie, Indiana

To Lynne A. Thelan
for her inspiration, encouragement,
and continuing friendship

LDU

To my wonderful family
Jim, Michael, and Madeleine

MEL

To my husband, James,
and my daughter, Sherrie-Anne,
whose love and encouragement
keep me moving forward

KMS

To the memory of Joseph K. Davie
for his commitment
to nursing education excellence

LDU   MEL   KMS

Preface

We are grateful to the many students and nurses who made the first edition of *Essentials of Critical Care Nursing* successful. We actively solicited input from users of the first edition and incorporated their comments and suggestions regarding format, content, and organization for this edition. The emphasis for the second edition is on priorities for the critical care nurse. We believe that prioritizing conditions and issues will assist critical care nurses in quickly assessing and intervening in the most efficient and effective manner. Consistent with this shift of emphasis, the book title was changed to *Priorities in Critical Care Nursing*

Organization

The book is again organized around alterations in dimensions of human functioning that span biopsychosocial realms. We have gone beyond the traditional physiologic focus of critical care and incorporated chapters on the following subjects:

Nursing Process
Ethical and Legal Issues
Patient and Family Education
Psychosocial Alterations
Sleep Alterations
Nutritional Alterations
Gerontologic Alterations

Organizationally the book comprises ten major units. The chapter content of Unit I, *Foundations of Critical Care Nursing Practice*, forms the basis of practice regardless of the physiologic alterations of the critically ill patient. Although chapters in this book may be studied in any sequence, we recommend that Chapter 1, *The Nursing Process*, be studied first because it clarifies the major assumptions on which the book is based.

Unit II, *Common Problems in Critical Care*, examines perennial critical care practice problems and is divided into four chapters: *Psychosocial Alterations, Sleep Alterations, Nutritional Alterations,* and *Gerontologic Alterations.*

Unit III, *Cardiovascular Alterations,* Unit IV, *Pulmonary Alterations,* and Unit V, *Neurologic Alterations,* are each structured by the following chapters:

Assessment and Diagnostic Procedures
Disorders
Therapeutic Management

The organization permits easy retrieval of information for students and clinicians and provides flexibility for the instructor to individualize teaching methods by assigning chapters that best suit student needs.

Unit VI, *Renal Alterations,* Unit VII, *Gastrointestinal Alterations,* and Unit VIII, *Endocrine Alterations,* are each organized by the following two chapters:

Assessment and Diagnostic Procedures
Disorders and Therapeutic Management

Unit IX, *Multisystem Alterations,* addresses disorders that affect multiple body systems and necessitate discussion as a separate category. Unit IX includes three chapters:

Trauma
Burns
Shock and Multiple Organ Dysfunction Syndrome (MODS)

Unit X, *Nursing Management,* contains the core of critical care nursing practice in nursing process format: signs and symptoms, nursing diagnosis, outcome criteria, and interventions. The Nursing Management plans are referenced throughout the book with "Nursing Diagnosis Priorities" boxes.

Finally, two appendixes are included that contain useful information for all students and practitioners of critical care. Appendix A, *Advanced Cardiac Life Support (ACLS) Guidelines,* presents selected decision trees from the American Heart Association for use in treating life-threatening emergencies. Appendix B, *Physiologic Formulas for Critical Care,* features commonly encountered hemodynamic and oxygenation formulas and other calculations presented in easily understood terms.

Nursing Diagnosis and Management

The power of research-based critical care practice has been incorporated into nursing interventions. To foster critical thinking and decision-making, a boxed "menu" of nursing diagnoses complete with specific etiologic or related factors accompanies each medical disorder and major medical treatment discussion and directs the learner to the section of the book where appropriate nursing management is detailed. In keeping with the emphasis on priorities in critical care, "Nursing Diagnosis Priorities" boxes list the most urgent potential nursing diagnoses to be addressed. To facilitate student learning, the nursing management plans incorporate nursing diagnosis, etiologic or related factors, clinical manifestations, and interventions with rationale. The nursing management plans are liberally cross-referenced throughout the book for easy retrieval by the reader.

New to Edition

New to this second edition are the following chapters:

Gerontologic Alterations
Burns
Shock and Multiple Organ Dysfunction Syndrome

Also new to this edition are discussions of critical care pharmacologic interventions related to cardiovascular, pulmonary, neurologic, renal, gastrointestinal, and endocrine alterations. Action priorities for nursing interventions appear in color.

To accompany the *Priorities in Critical Care Nursing* textbook, a comprehensive Instructor's Resource Manual is available, featuring the following elements: chapter issues, adapted course outlines, student worksheets: text and answers, a test bank with answers, student worksheets: videos, student worksheets: interactive video discs with answers, and a section on integrating multimedia in the class.

In addition, an eight-part *Critical Care Nursing Video* series exists, containing the following videos: *Introduction to Critical Care, Mechanical Ventilation: Concepts, Mechanical Ventilation: Nursing Management, Oxygenation, Hemodynamic Pressure Monitoring: Concepts, Hemodynamic Pressure Monitoring: Nursing Management, Intracranial Pressure Monitoring,* and *Ethical Issues in Critical Care Nursing.* These videos address both basic critical care skills and current issues in a creative yet easily understood manner.

Also unique is the four-part *IVD Critical Care Nursing Critical Thinking* series developed in conjunction with FITNE, which features the following titles: *Orientation to Critical Care Nursing, Cardiovascular Care, Pulmonary Care,* and *Neurologic Care.* Using this series as part of a critical care learning package provides "layers" of learning, exposing students to both visual and auditory instruction.

These interactive programs supplement *Priorities in Critical Care Nursing,* simulating the critical care environment and promoting invaluable critical thinking skills in nursing students. By combining current technology with accurate and clear content, these multimedia supplements make teaching *and* learning interesting and more effective. The variety of mediums available addresses different learning styles and facilitates teaching in different settings and to varying levels of students.

Acknowledgments

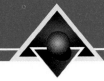

The talent, hard work, and inspiration of many people have produced *Priorities in Critical Care Nursing*. We appreciate the assistance of our Acquisitions Editors, Tim Griswold, Robin Carter, and Barry Bowlus; Developmental Editor Jolynn Gower; and Editorial Assistant Kristin Geen. We are also grateful to our Production Editor, René Spencer, for her scrupulous attention to detail, and to Linda McKinley, Liz Fett, and Theresa Fuchs.

We would also like to acknowledge contributors to the second edition of *Critical Care Nursing: Diagnosis and Management:* Karen Brasfield, Dorothy Brundage, Jeannine Forrest, Susan Frye, Sheana Funkhouser, Angela Palomo, Jeanne Raimond, and Helen Vos. In addition, we extend appreciation to those who also contributed to the first edition of *Essentials of Critical Care Nursing:* Joy Boarini, Ruth Bryant, Kathleen Crocker, Jane Frein, Judith Heggie, Cristine Kennedy-Caldwell, Gere Lane, Thomas Oertel, Judith Hartman-Ruekberg, Lynne Thelan, David Unkle, and Evelyn Wasli. Their earlier work contributed to the evolution of our current book.

Contents

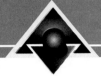

Detailed Contents

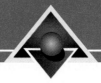

UNIT THREE
Cardiovascular Alterations

UNIT FOUR
Pulmonary Alterations

UNIT SIX
Renal Alterations

UNIT TEN
Nursing Management Plans of Care

APPENDIXES

Foundations of Critical Care Nursing Practice

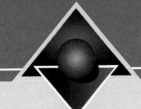

1

The Nursing Process

LINDA D. URDEN

CHAPTER OBJECTIVES

- Define nursing diagnosis.
- Differentiate the methods of stating actual and risk nursing diagnoses.

- Formulate nursing diagnosis statements from the North American Nursing Diagnosis Association's taxonomy of approved diagnoses, etiologic/related factors, and defining characteristics.

KEY TERMS

etiologies, p. 5
inference, p. 4

nursing diagnosis, p. 4

nursing process, p. 3

The **nursing process** is a method for making clinical decisions. It is a way of thinking and acting in relation to the clinical phenomena of concern to nurses. Traditionally the nursing process comprises five phases or dimensions: assessment, nursing diagnosis, planning, implementation, and evaluation. The nursing process is a systematic decision-making model that is cyclic, not linear (Fig. 1-1). By virtue of its evaluation phase the nursing process incorporates a feedback loop that maintains quality control of its decision-making outputs.

The nursing process, however, is not merely a problem-solving method. As with a problem-solving method the nursing process offers an organized, systematic approach to clinical problems, but unlike most problem-solving methods, the nursing process is continuous, not episodic. The five phases constitute a continuous cycle throughout the nurse's moment-to-moment data interpretation and management of patient care. Kritek[1] describes the phases of the nursing process as being not only continuous but "interactive"; each phase operates and influences the others and the patient simultaneously.

Why a nursing process? Why a systematic method for approaching, analyzing, and managing clinical problems?

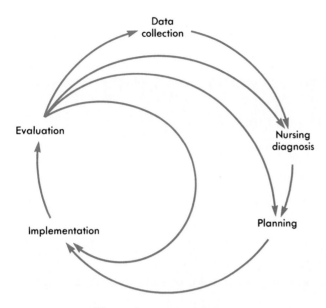

FIG. 1-1 The cyclic nature of the nursing process.

The reasons are that it yields sound decisions and grooms the novice critical care practitioner for expert practice by necessitating organized thinking and maximizing the nurse's analytic skills.

Nursing Diagnosis

Nursing diagnosis, a process whereby nurses interpret assessment data and apply standardized labels to human responses they identify and anticipate treating, is rapidly evolving in clinical and educational settings. Not coincidentally, this evolution is taking place alongside the professionalization of nursing.[2] Critical attention is being focused on aspects of nursing practice and education that either foster or inhibit the establishment of nursing.

A traditional reliance on the language and therapeutics of other sciences is inhibiting nursing as a freestanding profession. Efforts to identify and name the conditions that nurses study and treat, on the other hand, foster nursing's professional identity by clarifying its distinct services to society and providing a vehicle for the building of its science.

An approved nursing diagnosis is one accepted by the North American Nursing Diagnosis Association (NANDA) as having been refined to the point of clinical usefulness and approved for clinical validation through formal research methods. Practitioners using approved nursing diagnoses, etiologies, and defining characteristics are participating in the preliminary testing of the diagnoses as related to the health states described by the diagnostic labels. NANDA seeks input from practicing nurses regarding the development and refinement of nursing diagnoses. The association publishes guidelines for submitting new diagnoses to its Diagnosis Review Committee, and direct input into the proceedings of the biennial conferences is possible through membership and participation in NANDA and any of its regional associations.

Definition of Nursing Diagnosis

At its Ninth Conference in 1990, NANDA endorsed the following definition of nursing diagnosis[3]:

> A nursing diagnosis is a clinical judgment about individual, family or community responses to actual or potential health problems/life processes. Nursing diagnoses provide the basis for selection of nursing interventions to achieve outcomes for which the nurse is accountable.

Another term useful in defining nursing diagnosis is **inference,** which emphasizes the tentative and assumptive nature of diagnoses. *Webster's New Collegiate Dictionary* defines *inference* as the "process of arriving at a conclusion by reasoning from evidence" and warns that "if the evidence is slight the term comes close to *surmise.*"[4] Recognition that elements of judgment and inference are part of nursing diagnosis facilitates appreciation of the need to limit the influence of bias in diagnosing so that the conclusion is as logical and factual as possible.

The human response to health challenges encountered in birth, illness, wellness, growth and development, and death constitutes the focus of concern to nurses and is the object of nurses' diagnostic activities. In 1980 the American Nurses Association (ANA) issued *Nursing: A Social Policy Statement*, which defined the nature and scope of the profession as follows: "Nursing is the diagnosis and treatment of human responses to actual or potential health problems."[5]

The most essential and distinguishing purpose of any nursing diagnosis is to describe a human response *primarily resolved* by nursing interventions or therapies. There is, however, some difficulty in applying this criterion to the broad spectrum of human responses nurses identify and treat. The boundaries of nursing, particularly those that it shares with other health professions, are dynamic and not easily delineated.[5]

Formulating Nursing Diagnosis Statements

Guidelines for use of the taxonomy of approved nursing diagnoses

Classification of the phenomena to which a profession addresses itself is a sizable and ongoing task.[6-8] Several diagnoses have etiologies and defining characteristics yet to be developed, making clinical use difficult and frustrating. Other diagnoses may be deleted from the approved list at various conferences. Such changes are necessary and usual in the process of taxonomy development.

Guidelines for diagnostic labels

DEFINITIONS OF HEALTH PROBLEMS. Nearly all approved diagnoses have definitions to better explain the human responses they represent. These definitions are important because they clarify more about the health state than is apparent from the label alone. For example, the definitions accompanying the diagnoses *Fear* and *Anxiety* draw a particularly useful distinction between the two problems: Fear is an emotion that has an identifiable source or object that the patient validates, whereas *Anxiety* is an emotion that has a nonspecific or unknown source.[9] Other good examples of such definitions accompany the diagnoses *Social Isolation, Powerlessness, Altered Parenting,* and *Caregiver Role Strain.*

Until definitions accompany all approved diagnoses, nurses collaborating in care should establish consensus about the meaning and scope of the health problems stated.

MAKING DIAGNOSTIC LABELS SPECIFIC. Some nursing diagnoses require specifiers based on the characteristics of the human response as it manifests itself in a particular patient. For example, *Fear* requires specification as to its object, such as death, pain, disfigurement, or malignancy. Similarly, *Knowledge Deficit* requires specification about its content, such as use of an incentive spirometer, counting of the pulse rate, or implementation of respiratory muscle strengthening exercise. Following is a list of nursing diagnoses requiring specification, each with an example of a particular circumstance:

Fear: Postoperative Pain
Knowledge Deficit: Self-Monitoring of Oral Anticoagulation Therapy
Altered Peripheral Tissue Perfusion
Altered Nutrition: Less than Body Potassium Requirements

Guidelines for etiologic/related factors

MAKING ETIOLOGIES SPECIFIC. In many instances, **etiologies** devised by NANDA are broad categories or examples requiring specification based on characteristics of the health state and the patient being treated. For example, one of several possible etiologies for the diagnosis *Fluid Volume Excess* is *compromised regulatory mechanism.* Considering compromised regulatory mechanism to be the cause of the fluid excess in a particular patient, nurses should specify which regulatory mechanism is in question and in what way it is compromised (for example, inappropriate antidiuretic hormone [ADH] secretion by the neurohypophysis) before the diagnosis can be formally stated (disregarding the question of whether this problem is treatable by nurses or requires referral).

NURSING DIAGNOSES AS ETIOLOGIES. Nursing diagnostic labels may serve as etiologies for other diagnoses. Examples are *Anxiety* R/T* knowledge deficit and *Activity Intolerance R/T* decreased cardiac output.

ETIOLOGIES AS THE FOCUS OF TREATMENT. The treatment plan for a diagnosis must include interventions aimed at resolution or management of the etiologic factors and the human response. In fact, in some instances, nursing treatment is directed exclusively at the etiology of a diagnosis with the logical expectation that if the

causative factors are reduced, the problem should begin to resolve itself. This situation is especially true in instances in which a nursing diagnosis has another nursing diagnosis as its etiology. One example is treatment approaches to the diagnosis *Ineffective Breathing Pattern R/T* high abdominal incision pain. Predictably, little effectiveness is shown if the interventions are focused solely on reviewing the rationale for slow, deep, symmetrical breathing; demonstrating the technique; and encouraging the patient in performance of interventions without some plan for manipulation of the pain variable.

Guidelines for defining characteristics

MAKING DEFINING CHARACTERISTICS SPECIFIC. As with diagnostic labels and statements of etiology, defining characteristics of diagnoses are nonspecific and often require modification to reflect the particular situation of the patient being examined. For example, the diagnosis *Impaired Gas Exchange* has as one of its possible defining characteristics abnormal blood gases. In the nurse's formulation of this diagnostic statement for clinical use the specific blood gas value used to diagnose the problem should be cited in the statement (e.g., P_{O_2}: 54 mm Hg and/or P_{CO_2}: 50 mm Hg) versus the nonspecific sign category, abnormal blood gases.

Several defining characteristics are cited as follows in nonspecific form with examples of proper specification:

◆ Respiratory depth changes (hypoventilation)
◆ Blood pressure changes (hypotension)
◆ Autonomic responses (dilated pupils, tachycardia)
◆ Altered electrolytes (hypokalemia)
◆ Change in mental state (confusion, obtundation, apprehension)

MAJOR OR CRITICAL DEFINING CHARACTERISTICS. Major or critical defining characteristics are designated signs and/or symptoms that *must be present* for the health problem *to be considered present.* Major defining characteristics, when applicable, must be present in the nurse's assessment profile to diagnose the corresponding human response with any degree of certainty. For example, the diagnosis *Unilateral Neglect* has as its major defining characteristic consistent inattention to stimuli on affected side. It is essential, then, that this characteristic be present in the patient's situation (perhaps in addition to several other noncritical signs) for the diagnosis of this problem. The assignment of major or critical status to a defining characteristic is based on research or extensive clinical experience in which the signs and symptoms of a health problem are tested to predict reliably the presence of the diagnosis and are to be used with confidence by the nurse diagnostician.

Guidelines for diagnosing risk states

DETERMINING A RISK DIAGNOSIS. Predicting a potential health problem in a patient involves an estimation of probability. The potential for an event or a pattern of re-

---

*R/T, Related to.

sponse to occur can exist in almost any situation. To state each diagnosis on a treatment plan without regard for probabilities and develop desired patient outcomes and interventions for each is pointless.

An appraisal should be made of the patients' health status and identification of factors that place them at an increased vulnerability than the general population for the human response. For example, all persons recovering from abdominal surgery have the potential for *constipation* because of the effects of general anesthesia and narcotic analgesics, manipulation of abdominal viscera, and postoperative immobility. All nurses have a tacit understanding of this risk, and monitoring and intervention are carried out as part of routine nursing care to avert the problem; hence there is no need to state the problem.* A patient is at higher risk than the general population of postoperative patients if, for example, a history of dependence on laxatives, fluid volume deficit, prolonged immobility, or noncompliance with nursing prescriptions for ambulation exists. The diagnosis indicating this potential and its risk factors is stated so that additional and/or more intensified interventions can be planned.

STATING RISK DIAGNOSES. Potential nursing diagnoses are composed of two parts: the health problems at risk and the risk factors.[10] An example of a health problem at risk is ineffective individual coping; examples of risk factors are malignant biopsy results, absence of interpersonal support system, and history of alcohol abuse. Other such diagnoses include the following:

Risk for Aspiration
Risk for Infection
Risk for Impaired Skin Integrity
Risk for Injury

Planning

In the planning phase of the nursing process the following are accomplished: (1) patient *outcome criteria* are established, and (2) *nursing interventions* are selected.

Outcome Criteria

Outcome statements consist of highly specific indicators that will be used by the nurse in the evaluation phase as criteria showing that either (1) the actual diagnosis has been resolved or reduced or (2) the risk diagnosis has not occurred. An outcome statement is a projection of the expected influence that the nursing intervention will have on the patient in relation to the identified diagnosis and its etiology. Though often confused, statements of ex-

pected patient outcome are *not* patient goals or nursing goals, nor should they describe nursing interventions.

Outcome criteria for an *actual* diagnosis are developed from the signs and symptoms (defining characteristics) of the nursing diagnosis. In other words, the assessment findings that were used to certify the existence of a diagnosis should also be used to establish its resolution or improvement. The following is an example:

NURSING DIAGNOSIS	OUTCOME CRITERIA
Ineffective breathing pattern R/T respiratory muscle fatigue AEB*: $Pco_2 = 52$ RR = 28	$Pco_2 \leq 45$ RR ≤ 20 at rest

Outcome criteria for a *risk* diagnosis differ only in that being a two-part statement, clinical manifestations are absent from the diagnostic statement:

NURSING DIAGNOSIS	OUTCOME CRITERIA
Risk for Aspiration	Lungs clear to auscultation
RISK FACTORS Endotracheal tube Continuous intraenteral feedings Decreased level of consciousness	Absence of blue tinge to tracheal aspirate Afebrile $Svo_2 \geq 94\%$

Outcome criteria should be measurable, desirable, and attainable.

Measurable outcome criteria consist of patient behaviors, statements, and/or physiologic parameters that are recognizable at their occurrence. Many phenomena that critical care nurses diagnose and treat are readily measurable, such as adequacy of spontaneous ventilation, cardiac output, and tissue perfusion. Many phenomena, however, are not readily measurable and thus present a challenging task to care planning in general and outcome criteria development specifically. Phenomena such as *Anxiety, Powerlessness, Disturbed Body Image, and Ineffective Coping* involve the patient's subjective perception and, as such, resist the nurse's quantification. Outcome statements such as "less anxiety," "perceives personal power," or "copes effectively" represent favorable goals for nursing interventions but offer little in the way of criteria against which successful patient attainment can be measured. Again, nurses should consider the signs and symptoms of the response being treated and modify them to reflect a situation in which the response is absent or reduced. Several examples follow:

---

*No need to state the problem on an individualized nursing care plan; however, this risk diagnosis should be on record in a standards-of-care manual or standardized care plan.

---

*AEB, As evidenced by.

TABLE 1-1

CORRECT AND INCORRECT OUTCOME CRITERIA STATEMENTS

NURSING DIAGNOSIS	INCORRECT OUTCOME	CORRECT OUTCOME
Fluid volume deficit	Improved hydration will occur Patient will be offered 100 ml fluid q 2 hr	Systolic blood pressure $\geq$ 100 mm Hg 24-hr fluid intake $\geq$ body surface area fluid requirements Skin turgor $\leq$ 3 s
Decreased cardiac output Risk for disuse syndrome	Hemodynamic stability will be achieved Patient will be taught active leg exercises Patient will perform active leg exercises 10 times q 1 hr	Cardiac index 2.5-4.0 No calf tenderness No ankle swelling
Pain Powerlessness	Patient will have a reduction in pain Patient will perceive greater control over situation	Pain $\leq$ "4/10" 10 min after IV narcotic Formulation by patient of five decisions regarding care

CLINICAL MANIFESTATIONS	OUTCOME CRITERIA
Asks, "Why do I have no say in any of this?"	Patient makes five decisions regarding care
Appears distracted, preoccupied	Patient maintains eye contact throughout interactions
Looks away during stoma care	Patient visually regards stoma

Outcome statements are made more measurable by indicating the date and time of anticipated attainment. Projecting outcome attainment sometimes seems to be an arbitrary exercise, such as in the prediction of the date or hour for the return of clear lung fields. However, the importance of this aspect of outcome criteria development is that a specific deadline for evaluation of outcome attainment has been designated. Evaluating attainment of the outcome at designated intervals ensures that certain problems do not persist beyond acceptable time periods and that modification of the treatment approach occurs regularly. The outcome criteria applied throughout this text purposefully do not include date and time projection for attainment because this criteria should be a reflection of actual, not hypothetical, patient characteristics.

The desirability and attainability of patient outcome criteria are important aspects of planning nursing management. Individual patient baseline, patterns, and nurse and patient resources are the dominant considerations to a projection of desired outcome versus normative values. An example of an undesirable outcome is "RR < 16 at rest" for a patient with an unmodifiable chest wall restriction. "Absence of pain" in a patient with a sternotomy incision is also an undesirable target for early postoperative intervention. Examples of outcome criteria that are unattainable (and therefore undesirable) are "P_{CO_2} < 40" in a patient who chronically retains carbon dioxide and "no anxiety" in a patient preoperatively for open heart surgery. (Table 1-1 shows examples of correct and incorrect outcome criteria statements for assorted nursing diagnoses.)

Developing outcome criteria statements has particular relevance to critical care nurses because the statements describe in measurable terms the effects or results of critical care nursing practice. Also, the statements communicate the influence nursing intervention has in preventing, resolving, or improving various human responses and provide a basis for justifying the allocation and reimbursement of professional nursing resources.

Nursing Intervention

The power of nursing intervention

Interventions are the power of nursing and a distinct strength of this text. Also known as *nursing orders* or *nursing prescriptions*, interventions constitute the treatment approach to an identified health alteration and are selected to satisfy the outcome criteria and prevent or resolve the nursing diagnosis.

A common shortcoming of nursing interventions, as much in the literature as in individual practice, is the prescription of vague, weak, nonsubstantive nursing actions. By definition, a *nursing diagnosis* is a human response that nurses treat. *Treatment* implies producing a change in a situation, not merely maintaining equilibrium, and *prescribe* connotes recommending a course of action, not simply supporting an existing regimen. Intervention strategies that consist solely of monitoring, measuring, checking, obtaining physician orders, documenting, reporting, and notifying do not fulfill criteria for the treatment of a problem. Nursing intervention for nursing diagnoses should designate therapeutic activity that assists the patient in moving from one state of health to another. The growing body of research-based, independent nursing therapies should be liberally applied to treatment plans for nursing diagnoses in critical care. Exciting advances in nurse management of phenomena, such as ventilation-perfusion inequalities, excessive preload and afterload, increased intracranial pressure, and sensory-perceptual alterations, associated with critical illness, afford the critical care nurse the opportunity to incorporate potency into treatment plans.

Focus for interventions

As discussed earlier, interventions have the greatest impact when they are directed at the etiologic/related factors of the diagnosis or, in the case of a risk diagnosis, the risk factors. This point stipulates that the etiologic factors of a problem be modifiable by nursing. For the most favorable patient outcome to be achieved, the multiple etiologic factors of a problem should be studied carefully and interventions selected to modify them.

Specificity of interventions

Planned interventions should provide clarity, specificity, and direction to the spectrum of nurses implementing care for a patient. Statements such as "check vital signs" and "measure I&O" provide no real direction to nursing care and are therefore useless. Instead, "monitor for heart rate elevations 30 beats/min over baseline" and "look for 24-hr positive fluid balances" are preferable.

A brief rationale as part of the intervention statement should be included where it would enhance understanding of the treatment maneuver. The following is an example of such a statement: "Change position dynamically q 2 hr, to *match ventilation with perfusion*." (Rationales are italicized.)

Medically delegated actions, such as administering medications and initiating ventilator setting changes, should be included in the interventions but with the emphasis placed squarely on the assessments and judgments nurses make in evaluating their effectiveness, patient tolerance, safety, dosage, titration, and discontinuance. For example, statements such as "administer nitroprusside as ordered" do not exist in critical care. Adequate specificity of nursing orders has been achieved when nurses unfamiliar with patients can review management plans and implement the kind of care intended by primary nurses or case managers.

Implementation

Implementation is the action component of planning, the phase of the nursing process in which the treatment plan is implemented. Data collection and evaluation are continuous throughout this phase.

Evaluation

Evaluation of attainment of the expected patient outcomes occurs formally at intervals designated in the outcome criteria. (Informal evaluation occurs continuously.) Evaluation is conducted in relation to the outcome criteria for actual and risk diagnoses, respectively.

Two components to the evaluation phase of the nursing process exist. First, nurses should compare patients' current state with that described by the outcome criteria and query: "Are breath sounds clear and equal bilaterally? Is the tidal volume of spontaneous respirations > 500 ml, as projected to be by this time?" An evaluation of nursing effectiveness is completed by commenting on the extent to which a predicted outcome has been attained.

Second, nurses should query, "If not, why not? Is it too soon to evaluate? Should the plan be continued for 24 hours and then reevaluated? Should the interventions be intensified, perhaps increasing the frequency of respiratory muscle strengthening exercises? Are the outcome criteria impractical for this patient? Is the validity of the nursing diagnosis questionable? Are more data needed?" Specific recommendations are then proposed that include either continuing implementation as outlined or returning to the data collection, nursing diagnosis, planning, or implementation phase of the process.

The evaluation phase and the activities that take place within it are perhaps the most important dimensions of the nursing process (Fig. 1-1). Evaluation of patient progress against a standard of nursing care incorporates accountability into the process—accountability to the standard of care. Lack of progress in outcome attainment or problem solving is readily identified and kept in check, and alternative solutions can then be proposed.

References

1. Kritek PB: Generation and classification of nursing diagnoses: toward a theory of nursing, *Image J Nurs Sch* 10:33, 1978.
2. Mitchell GJ: Nursing diagnosis: an ethical analysis, *Image J Nurs Sch* 23(2):99-103, 1991.
3. Carroll-Johnson RM: *Classification of nursing diagnoses: proceedings of the Ninth Annual Conference*, Philadelphia, 1991, JB Lippincott.
4. *Webster's New Collegiate Dictionary*, ed 9, Springfield, Mass, 1986, Merriam-Webster.
5. American Nurses Association: *Nursing: a social policy statement*, Kansas City, Mo, 1980, The Association.
6. Doughterty CM, Jankin JK, Lunney MR, and others: Conceptual and research-based validation of nursing diagnoses: 1950-1993, *Nursing Diagnosis* 4(4):156-165, 1993.
7. Jankin J: Research validation of nursing diagnoses: how much progress? *Nursing Diagnosis* 5(1):46, 1994.
8. Sparks SM, Lien-Gieschen T: Modification of the diagnostic content validity model, *Nursing Diagnosis* 5(1):31-35, 1994.
9. Whitley GG: Concept analysis of anxiety, *Nursing Diagnosis* 3(3):78, 1992.
10. Gordon M: *Nursing diagnosis: process and application*, ed 3, St Louis, 1994, Mosby.

2

Ethical and Legal Issues

LINDA D. URDEN

CHAPTER OBJECTIVES

- Differentiate between morals and ethics.
- Discuss ethical principles as they relate to critical care patients.
- Discuss the concept of medical futility.
- Describe what constitutes an ethical dilemma.
- List steps for making ethical decisions.

- Delineate strategies for ethical decision making in critical care.
- Identify legal and professional obligations of critical care nurses.
- Describe the elements of certain torts that may result from critical care nursing practice.
- Identify and discuss specific legal issues in critical care nursing practice.

KEY TERMS

abandonment, p. 15

autonomy, p. 10

breach of duty, p. 15

chemical impairment, p. 17

ethics, p. 10

false imprisonment, p. 14

malpractice, p. 15

morals, p. 10

negligence, p. 15

nonmaleficence, p. 10

paternalism, p. 10

unintentional tort, p. 15

veracity, p. 11

Morals and Ethics

Morals Defined

The word *moral* is derived from the Latin *moralis,* which is defined as "good or right in conduct or character . . . making the distinction between right and wrong . . . principles of right and wrong based on custom."[1] Closely related to sexual mores and behaviors in Western society, **morals** are the "shoulds," "should nots," "oughts," and "ought nots" of actions and behaviors. Religious and cultural values and beliefs largely mold moral thoughts and actions. Morals form the basis for action and provide a framework for evaluation of behavior.

Ethics Defined

The word ***ethics*** is derived from the Greek *ethos,* which is defined as "the system or code of morals of a particular person, religion, group, or profession . . . the study of standards of conduct and moral judgment."[1] The term *ethics* is sometimes used interchangeably with the word *morals.* However, ethics is more concerned with the "why" of the action rather than with whether the action is right or wrong, good or bad.[2] *Ethics* implies that an evaluation is being made that is theoretically based on or derived from a set of standards. Normative ethics is the division of ethics that focuses on "norms or standards of behavior and value and their ultimate application to daily life,"[3] with an emphasis on evaluation for purposes of guiding moral action. Bioethics incorporates all aspects of life but most frequently refers to health care ethics and the application of ethical principles to individual cases.

Ethical Principles

Certain ethical principles derived from classic ethical theories are used in health care decision making.[4] Principles are general guidelines that govern conduct, provide a basis for reasoning, and direct actions.[5] The five ethical principles discussed in this chapter are autonomy, beneficence, nonmaleficence, veracity, and fidelity.

Autonomy

The concept of autonomy appears in all ancient writings and early Greek philosophy. Immanuel Kant described an ethical person as one who is guided and motivated in response to one's own inward obedience, free from coercion, desire, or fear of future consequences.[6] Persons are not to be treated as a means to an end but rather as an end themselves.[7] In health care, **autonomy** can be viewed as the freedom to make decisions about one's own body without the coercion or interference of others. A basic human right, autonomy is a freedom of choice or self-determination that can be experienced in all human life events.

Critical care nurses are often "caught in the middle" in ethical situations, and promoting autonomous decision making is one of those situations. As nurses work closely with patients and families to promote autonomous decision making, another crucial element becomes clear. Patients and families must have all the information about a certain situation to make the decision that is best for them. They should not only be given all the information and facts but also have a clear understanding of what was presented. This is where nurses become the most important members of the health care team—that is, as patient advocates, providing more information, clarifying points, reinforcing information, and providing support during the process.[8]

Beneficence

The concept of doing good and preventing harm to patients is a *sine qua non* for the nursing profession. However, the ethical principle of beneficence—which requires that one promote the well-being of patients—points to the importance of this duty for the health care professional. According to Davis and Aroskar,[5] the principle of beneficence presupposes that harms and benefits are balanced, leading to positive or beneficial outcomes.

Beneficence frequently seems to be at odds with another principle, autonomy. **Paternalism** exists when nurses or physicians make decisions for patients without consulting or including them in the decision process. Paternalism is "making people do what is good for them" and "preventing people from doing what is bad for them."[6] Jameton[6] described two types of paternalists: strong paternalists who make decisions for obviously competent persons and weak paternalists who make decisions for persons who are mentally or physically unable to make their own decisions.

Nonmaleficence

The ethical principle of **nonmaleficence,** which dictates that one prevent harm and remove harmful situations, is a *prima facie* duty for nurses. Thoughtfulness and care are necessary, as is balancing risks and benefits as discussed earlier. Beneficence and nonmaleficence are on two ends of a continuum and are often carried out differently, depending on the views of practitioners. Practitioners using a utilitarian approach consider long-term consequences and the good to society as a whole. Practitioners operating from a deontologic basis consider the principle and its effect on the individual in the situation.

Complex issues such as quality of life versus sanctity of life are always difficult to analyze in both critical care and non–critical care settings. Flynn described decisions such as withholding and withdrawing treatments as being based on not one ethical principle alone but rather on a balance of all ethical principles so that the most appropriate moral decision can be made.[10] Nonmaleficence should serve as the guide for practice of health care professionals.[4]

Veracity

Veracity, or truth telling, is an important ethical principle that underlies the nurse-patient relationship. Veracity is important in soliciting informed consent and in ensuring that the patient is aware of all potential risks and benefits from specific treatments or their alternatives. However, the critical care nurse may not be aware of all the facts and information about a particular treatment option. Sometimes information is accurate but has been delivered with bias or in a misleading way. In these instances the ethical principle of autonomy has been violated.[12]

Fidelity

Fidelity is another ethical principle closely related to autonomy and veracity. Fidelity, or faithfulness and promise keeping to patients, is a *sine qua non* for nursing and the basis of all relationships, both professional and personal. Regardless of the amount of autonomy that patients have in the critical care areas, they still depend on nurses for physical care and emotional support. Positive for all involved,[13] a trusting relationship establishes and maintains an open atmosphere.

As do all the other principles, fidelity extends to families of critical care patients. After promising families that they will be called if an emergency arises or that they will be informed of other special events, nurses should make every effort to follow through on the promise. These efforts will not only uphold fidelity in this particular relationship but also reflect positively on the institution and nursing profession as a whole.

An element of fidelity, confidentiality is based on traditional health care professional ethics. According to Veatch and Fry,[14] the nursing and medical professions have established ethical codes that allow no patient-centered reasons for breaking the principle of confidentiality. *Confidentiality* is described as a right whereby patient information can be shared only with those involved in the care of the patient. An exception to this guideline might be when the welfare of others is at risk by keeping patient information confidential. In this situation nurses must balance ethical principles and weigh risks with benefits. Special circumstances, such as mandatory reporting laws, will often guide nurses.

Privacy is described as another element inherent in the principle of fidelity. It may be closely aligned with confidentiality of patient information and patients' rights to privacy of their person, such as maintaining privacy for patients by pulling the curtains around beds or making sure that they are adequately covered.[15,16]

Allocation of Scarce Resources in Critical Care

Engelhardt and Rie[17] described critical care units as providing optimal care to all who require it. Yet those responsible for the costs of critical care can no longer afford to pay for the advanced treatments and technologies that have been developed and refined and made available.

Limitations of resources force society and critical care health professionals to reexamine the goals of critical care for patients.[18] Once considered experimental, coronary artery bypass surgery, magnetic resonance imaging, kidney dialysis, and heart transplantation are now widely accepted and funded by payers. Because the possibilities and number of organ transplants are increasing, there are not enough available organs. To increase the availability of donated organs, most states have enacted "required request" laws, which mandate that families must be approached about donation of organs on the death of their loved ones.[19-21] Procurement of organs has posed new ethical dilemmas for health care professionals, who must now act in accordance with state laws.

When examining the use of technologies, health care professionals should consider quality of life. It is an area that is personal, value laden, conditional, and different for all involved.[22,23] Quality of life has dual dimensions of objectivity and subjectivity. An objective perspective examines the person's functionability, whereas a subjective approach concentrates on the patient's psychosocial state. Only after patients receive the technology and "live" that "new" life can the quality of their lives be evaluated.[24] Critical care nurses face rationing of critical care beds and nursing staff daily. Strengths and weaknesses of the staff must be balanced with the needs of patients. Orientation and other special circumstances—such as designation for charge nurse, trauma nurse, and code nurse—must be considered when scheduling staff and making assignments. Any inexperienced staff, float staff, or registry staff must receive appropriate orientation and backup during the shift.

A triage system for critical care units is frequently used when there are more admissions than available beds. Critical care nurses are instrumental in helping medical directors to determine patient selection for transfer, if appropriate. Some hospitals use a set of standards, criteria, or guidelines for determining patient admission and transfer to and from critical care areas.

Medical Futility

The concept of medical futility has been discussed recently in terms of definition and ethical implications.[25-28] *Medical futility* has both a qualitative and quantitative basis and can be defined as "any effort to achieve a result that is possible but that reasoning or experience suggests is highly improbable and that cannot be systematically reproduced."[28]

Therapy or treatment that achieves its predictable outcome and desired effect is, by definition, effective. However, effect must be distinguished from benefit. If that predictable and desired effect is of no benefit to patients, it is nonetheless futile. Some experts suggest that when physicians conclude from personal or colleague experiences or empiric data that a particular treatment has been useless in the most recent 100 cases in which it has been used, the treatment should be considered futile.[28] Physicians should always make optimal use of health-related resources in a technically appropriate and effective manner. In this era of escalating health care costs and limited resources, physicians have a particular responsibility to avoid futile treatment.[28]

Ethics as a Foundation for Nursing Practice

Traditional theories of professions include a code of ethics as the basis for the practice of professionals. Various authors identify the unique relationship of professional nurses with patients, a relationship that establishes care and trust, as the moral foundation of nursing.[29-31] By adhering to a code of ethics, professionals fulfill a societal obligation for high-quality practice.

Nursing Code of Ethics

The American Nurses Association (ANA) provides the major source of ethical guidance for the nursing profession.[32,33] According to the preamble of the *Code for Nurses*, "when individuals become nurses, they make a moral commitment to uphold the values and special moral obligations expressed in their code."[34] The 11 statements of the code are found in Box 2-1. They are based on the underlying assumption that nursing is concerned with protection, promotion, and restoration of health; prevention of illness; and the alleviation of suffering of patients.[34]

The *Code for Nurses* was adopted by the ANA in 1950 and has undergone revisions. It provides a framework for nurses in ethical decision making and provides society with a set of expectations for the profession. The code is "not open to negotiation in employment settings, nor is it permissible for individuals or groups of nurses to adapt or change the language of this code" according to the ANA.[34] The ANA also suggests that although the requirements of the code may not be in concert with the law, nurses are nevertheless obliged to uphold the code because of the societal commitment that is inherent in nursing.

BOX 2-1

CODE OF ETHICS FOR NURSES

1. The nurse provides services with respect for human dignity and the uniqueness of the client, unrestricted by considerations of social or economic status, personal attributes, or the nature of health problems.
2. The nurse safeguards the client's right to privacy by judiciously protecting information of a confidential nature.
3. The nurse acts to safeguard the client and the public when health care and safety are affected by the incompetent, unethical, or illegal practice of any person.
4. The nurse assumes responsibility and accountability for individual nursing judgments and actions.
5. The nurse maintains competence in nursing.
6. The nurse exercises informed judgment and uses individual competence and qualifications as criteria in seeking consultation, accepting responsibilities, and delegating nursing activities to others.
7. The nurse participates in activities that contribute to the ongoing development of the profession's body of knowledge.
8. The nurse participates in the profession's efforts to implement and improve standards of nursing.
9. The nurse participates in the profession's efforts to establish and maintain conditions of employment conducive to high-quality nursing care.
10. The nurse participates in the profession's effort to protect the public from misinformation and misrepresentation and to maintain the integrity of nursing.
11. The nurse collaborates with members of the health professions and other citizens in promoting community and national efforts to meet the health needs of the public.

From American Nurses Association: *Code for nurses with interpretive statements,* Kansas City, Mo, 1985, The Association.

Ethical Decision Making in Critical Care
The Nurse's Role

As discussed earlier in this chapter, critical care nurses confront ethical issues daily. Although nurses may feel powerless to influence ethical decisions,[35] this need not be the case. Because nurses are on the "front line" with such issues as do-not-resuscitate (DNR) orders, response to treatments, and application of new technologies and protocols, they may be the ones who best know patients' and/or families' wishes about treatment prolongation or cessation. Therefore nurses should be included as part of the health care team determining the ethical resolution of dilemmas.[36-38]

What Is an Ethical Dilemma?

In general, ethical cases are not clear-cut but are fraught with innumerable side issues and distractions.[39-40] The most common ethical dilemmas in critical care involve forgoing treatment and allocating the scarce resource of critical care. How do health care professionals know that a true ethical dilemma exists?

Before applying any decision model, nurses must decide whether a true ethical dilemma exists. Thompson and Thompson[2] delineated the following criteria for defining moral and ethical dilemmas in clinical practice:

1. Awareness of different options
2. An issue with different options
3. Two or more options with true or "good" aspects, with the choice of one compromising the option not chosen

Krekeler asserted that ethical conflicts arise when "the moral decision of one person conflicts with the moral decision of another. Both decisions may be good for each individual in question and undoubtedly are made according to their traditional values."[4] What complicates this process is the involvement of a third person, as is the case in most treatment care decisions in the critical care areas.

Steps in Ethical Decision Making

To facilitate the ethical decision process, professionals must use a model or framework so that all involved will consistently examine the multiple ethical issues that arise in critical care. Steps in ethical decision making are listed in Box 2-2.

Step one. The major aspects of the medical and health problem must be identified. In other words the scientific basis of the problem, potential sequelae, prognosis, and all data relevant to the health status must be examined.

Step two. The ethical problem must be clearly delineated from other types of problems. Systems problems—that is, those resulting from failures and inadequacies in the organization and operation of the health care facility and the health care system as a whole—are often misidentified as ethical issues. Occasionally a social problem that stems from conditions existing in the community, state, or country is also confused with an ethical issue. Social problems can lead to a systemic problem, which can constrain responses to ethical problems.

Step three. Although categories of necessary additional information vary, whatever is missing in the initial problem presentation should be obtained. If not already known, the health prognosis and potential sequelae should be clarified. Usual demographic data—such as age, ethnicity, religious preferences, and educational and economic status—may be considered in the decision process. In addition to the perspective of family, extended

---

BOX 2-2

STEPS IN ETHICAL DECISION MAKING

1. Identify the health problem.
2. Define the ethical issue.
3. Gather additional information.
4. Delineate the decision maker.
5. Examine ethical and moral principles.
6. Explore alternative options.
7. Implement decisions.
8. Evaluate and modify actions.

---

family, and other support systems, any desires that patients may have expressed in writing or in conversation about treatment decisions are essential to consider.

Step four. Patients are the primary decision makers and autonomously make these decisions after receiving information about the alternatives and sequelae of treatments. However, in many ethical dilemmas patients are comatose or otherwise physically or mentally unable to make a decision. Because the urgency of the situation requires a quick decision, surrogates are designated or court appointed in these situations. Although the decision process and ultimate decision are more important than who makes the decision, delineating the decision maker is an important step in the process.[2]

Others involved in decisions should also be identified at this time, such as families, nurses, physicians, social workers, clergy, and any other members of disciplines having close contact with the patient. The role of nurses should be examined. Nurses may not need to make decisions; nurses may instead provide additional information and support to decision makers.

Step five. All involved in the decision process must make known their personal values, beliefs, and moral convictions. Whether achieved through a group meeting or through personal introspection, values clarification facilitates the decision process. Professional ethical codes of nurses and physicians serve as a foundation for future decisions. Legal constraints or previous legal decisions also need to be assessed.

General ethical principles need to be examined in relation to the case at hand. For instance, are veracity, informed consent, and autonomy promoted? Beneficence and nonmaleficence should be analyzed as they relate to the conditions and desires of patients. Close examination of these principles reveals any compromise of ethical or moral principles for either patients or health care providers and assists in decision making.

Step six. After identifying alternative options, decision makers should predict the outcome of each action. This analysis helps them to select the option with the best "fit" for the specific situation or problem. Decision makers should also examine short- and long-range consequences of each action and encourage new or creative actions. The "no action" option also merits consideration.[2]

Step seven. Even after much thought and consideration, rarely do all interested persons completely agree on a decision.[2] Krekeler described following the action until the actual results of the decision can be seen.[4] Fowler stated that the decision may need to be modified to meet legal or policy requirements.[41]

Step eight. Evaluating an ethical decision serves to assess the decision at hand and its potential use as a precedent for future ethical decisions. If outcomes are not as predicted, modifying the plan or using an alternative one are possibilities.

Legal Issues in Critical Care

Legal Relationships

When nurses begin employment in a critical care unit and assume the care of patients, a relationship forms between patients and nurses and between employers and nurses. Every state has a law mandating entry-level educational requirements for the license to practice nursing; thus the act of licensing creates a legal relationship between nurses and the state.

These relationships impose legal obligations. For example, nurses owe patients reasonable and prudent care under the circumstances. Nurses owe employers competency and the ability to follow policies and procedures, as well as other contractual duties that may exist. Nurses owe the state and public the duty of safe, competent practice as legally defined by practice standards.

Because these duties are enforceable by law, critical care nurses can be held accountable for breach or violation through several laws and legal processes. Nurses, hospitals, patients, and other health care providers are involved in a variety of legal disputes, including negligence and professional malpractice, incompetence, unauthorized practice, unprofessional or illegal conduct, workers' compensation, and contract and labor disputes.[42]

The scope of legal issues in nursing is broad. For example, in the past two decades, health law as a specialty has evolved, embracing more than 60 subspecialty areas of practice.[43] Nurses should seek their own legal advice and counsel for any questions and concerns and not rely on the overview of material provided in this chapter.

Tort Liability

The area of civil law is divided into many categories, two of which are contracts and torts. The law of contracts contains a set of rules governing the creation and enforcement of an agreement between two or more parties (en-

---

BOX 2-3

CLASSIFICATION OF TORTS

INTENTIONAL TORTS

Assault
Battery
False imprisonment
Trespass
Infliction of emotional distress

SPECIFIC TORTS

Defamation
  Slander
  Libel
Invasion of privacy

UNINTENTIONAL TORTS

Negligence
Medical/nursing treatment torts
  Professional malpractice
Abandonment

STRICT LIABILITY

Products liability

---

tities or individuals). A tort is a type of civil wrong, meaning that a dispute occurred between the parties.

Tort law is generally divided into intentional and unintentional torts, strict liability, and specific torts. Box 2-3 classifies torts and lists examples within each category.

Intentional torts involve (1) intent and (2) an act. Intent exists when the actor plans to achieve a particular outcome and consequence. Assault, battery, false imprisonment, trespass, and infliction of emotional distress are examples of intentional torts. These torts require a specific act and intentional interference with the person or property.

In assault, the act is behavior that places the plaintiff (the one being wronged who later sues) in fear or apprehension of offensive physical contact. The person being sued for wronging another in civil law is referred to as the *defendant*. *Battery* is the unlawful or offensive touching of, or contact with, the plaintiff or something attached to the plaintiff. **False imprisonment** is detaining, confining, or restraining another against the person's will.

There are two types of trespass: one type involves a person's land, and the other involves personal property. These acts are defined as unauthorized entry onto another's land or unauthorized handling of another's personal property. In addition, the law protects a person's interest in peace of mind through the tort claim of *infliction of mental or emotional distress*. The act, however, must be one of extreme misconduct or outrageous behavior.

Unintentional torts involve failures or breach of nursing duties that lead to harm, including negligence, malpractice, and abandonment. **Negligence** is the failure to meet an ordinary standard of care, resulting in injury to the patient or plaintiff. **Malpractice** is a type of professional liability based on negligence and includes professional misconduct, breach of a duty or standard of care, illegal or immoral conduct, or failure to exercise reasonable skill, all of which lead to harm. A more complete outline of the elements of these torts will follow. **Abandonment** is a type of negligence in which a duty to give care exists, is ignored, and results in harm to a patient.

Specific torts involve privacy interests and interests in a person's reputation. Invasion of privacy and defamation are examples of such torts. Defamation is composed of two torts, *slander* (oral defamation) and *libel* (written defamation). Defamation is not the mere statement or writing of words that injure another person's reputation or good name. The words must be communicated to someone else, and if the words are true, this may provide a defense against a defamation claim. Invasion of privacy involves the violation of a person's right to privacy. Nurses can invade patients' privacy by revealing confidential information without authorization or by failing to follow patients' health care decisions.

Administrative Law and Licensing Statutes

A second type of law and legal process involving nurses is administrative law and the regulatory process. This area of law governs nurses' relationship with the government, either state or federal. Administrative law concerns the rules of the government's activities in regulating health care delivery and practice. Several government health care agencies are involved in such regulation.

Because the state is responsible for the health, safety, and welfare of its citizens, it has the power to regulate nursing. Therefore establishing minimal entry-level requirements, standards of nursing practice, and educational requirements is an acceptable state action. The state legislatures create laws (generally termed *nurse practice acts*) governing nursing practice, and a unit of the state government within the executive branch of government is responsible for the enforcement of nursing laws. This unit is often called the *State Board of Nursing or Board of Nurse Examiners*. Because the laws of states vary, however, nurses must seek advice from counsel licensed to practice law within their own states. In administrative law the rules of investigation, procedure, and evidence differ from those of civil and criminal law.

Negligence and Malpractice

As defined earlier, negligence is an unintentional tort involving a breach of duty or failure (through an act or omission) to meet a standard of care causing patient harm. Malpractice is a type of professional liability based on negligence in which the defendant is held accountable for breach of a duty of care involving special knowledge and skill. These torts have several elements, all of which the plaintiff has the burden of proving.

Definition of elements

The law recognizes the following four elements of negligence and malpractice:

- ◆ Duty and standard of care
- ◆ Breach of duty
- ◆ Causation
- ◆ Injury or damages

A duty, or legal obligation, must be one recognized by law requiring the actor to conform to a certain standard of conduct for the protection of others against unreasonable risks.[44] The legal duty of critical care nurses is to act in a reasonable and prudent manner, as all other critical care nurses would act under similar circumstances. The standard is that of a critical care nurse, one with special knowledge and skill in critical care. The standard is one that is owed at the time the incident or injury occurred, not at the time of litigation. In most jurisdictions the standard of care is a national standard as opposed to a local, community standard.

Breach of duty involves a failure on the actor's part to conform to the standard required. Causation, the third element, requires proof that the actor's breach was reasonably close or causally connected to the resulting injury. This is also referred to as *proximate cause.*

The fourth element, injury, must involve an actual loss or damage to the plaintiff or the plaintiff's interest. Plaintiffs may claim different types of damages, such as compensatory or punitive. Patient injuries range in value. Plaintiffs must produce evidence of the damages and their value. If nurses breach a standard of care that leads to injury, plaintiffs must show what amount of money will compensate for their injuries. The goal of compensation is to provide the amount of money that will return plaintiffs to the same position as before the injury occurred.

Res ipsa loquitur is a rule of evidence used by plaintiffs in negligence or malpractice litigation and literally means "the thing speaks for itself." It is a rebuttable presumption or inference of negligence by the defendant, which arises on plaintiff's proof that (1) the injury does not ordinarily happen in the absence of negligence and (2) the instrumentality causing the injury was in the defendant's exclusive management and control. The burden then shifts to the defendant, who must prove absence of negligence. For example, negligence can be inferred when muscle ischemia and necrosis occur as a result of improper body positioning and the application of splints or restraints. Negligence can also be inferred from a foreign object left in a patient's body cavity after surgery.

Because critical care nurses deal with life-threatening situations, patient injury is potentially severe and may result in death. Should death occur as a result of negligence, nurses may be held liable for the patients' deaths

---

BOX 2-4

Examples of Critical Care Nursing Actions Involved in Negligence Suits

GENERAL

- Failure to advise physician and/or supervisor of change in patient's health status
- Failure to monitor patients at requisite intervals
- Failure to adhere to established institutional protocols
- Failure to adequately assess clinical status
- Failure to respond to alarms
- Failure to maintain accurate, timely, and complete medical records
- Failure to properly carry out treatment and evaluate results of treatment
- Failure to use safe, functional equipment

SPECIFIC

- Failure to provide supplemental oxygen when the ventilator cannot be promptly reattached
- Failure to properly use intravenous infusion equipment, causing extensive extravasation of fluid
- Failure to monitor intravenous infusions, recognize infiltration, and discontinue intravenous therapy
- Failure to recognize signs of intracranial bleeding
- Failure to investigate patient's complaint of pain and discover hematoma under blood pressure cuff

---

and resulting losses to surviving family members. All states have wrongful death acts, and a number of states have both death acts and survival acts, which are prosecuted concurrently. With the two causes of action, compensation for expenses, pain and suffering and the decedent's loss of earnings up to the time of death is allocated to the survival action and the loss of benefits of the survivors is allocated to the wrongful death action.

Box 2-4 illustrates specific examples of actions by critical care nurses that have resulted in litigation. In cases such as these, the nurse's action is central to the lawsuit. However, nurses are named as sole or codefendants in a comparatively small percentage of cases. Although this pattern is changing, physicians and hospitals are generally named as defendants.

Typically, nursing negligence cases involve breach or failure in six general categories. The first category includes the use of defective equipment or the failure to perform safety and maintenance assessments. Nurses commonly make errors in drug identification, administration, and dosages. Nurses have failed to make timely reports to physicians after changes in patient status and have also failed to inform supervisors of physicians' failures to respond to the nurses' communication. Failure to supervise and assist patients who subsequently fall is also a source of nursing negligence. Improper wound care

with resulting infection, and incorrect instrument and sponge counts in the surgical setting are areas of practice that have led to patient injury and lawsuits.

Legal doctrines and theories of liability

In tort law, there are several theories of liability whereby nurses' actions may be examined and legal duties defined:

- ◆ Personal
- ◆ Vicarious: *respondeat superior*
- ◆ Corporate
- ◆ Other doctrines, such as temporary or borrowed servant and captain of the ship

Under the theory of personal liability, individuals are responsible for their own actions. This theory includes critical care nurses, supervisors, physicians, hospitals, and patients, each of whom has unique responsibilities. In contrast to personal liability, nurses may be afforded the protection of personal immunity. In certain health care situations, the U.S. Congress or state legislatures have determined that nurses do not have personal liability and are therefore immune from liability. Again, seeking advice to determine what employment settings and laws apply to a particular situation is appropriate.

As a general rule in most jurisdictions, mandatory reporting statutes include personal immunity provisions. For example, child abuse and dependent adult abuse statutes provide that nurses who make good faith reports will not be liable for making those reports or for the consequences of those reports. Similarly, physicians, nurses, and hospitals that are mandated to report communicable and infectious diseases to state or federal authorities are immune from liability for good faith reporting in a confidential manner. Also, nurses who in good faith render voluntary emergency care in the field to a stranger are immune from liability for negligence under state good samaritan laws. Finally, federally employed nurses are protected by immunity provisions under the Federal Tort Claims Act.[45] However, immunity at state and local levels may be greatly restricted. Certain personal immunities are not a guarantee against lawsuits; rather, they are potential defenses.

Vicarious liability is indirect responsibility—for example, the liability of an employer for the acts of the employee. Under the doctrine of *respondeat superior*, a master is liable for certain wrongful acts of a servant, as is a principal for those of an agent. An employer may be liable for an employee's acts when they are performed within the legitimate scope of employment. In critical care, nurses are typically employees of the hospital. However, nurses may be independent contractors with the hospital through critical care nursing agencies or businesses. In the latter case, nurses are not employees of the hospital and the hospital is not vicariously liable for their actions.

Critical care nurses who are hospital employees receive work assignments and equipment to perform those assignments by the employer's agent, a supervisor. As a general rule, the hospital is responsible for the patient census, staffing on the critical care unit, and clinical orientation of the staff. Because of these responsibilities, the hospital employer is generally responsible for employees' performances within parameters determined by the employer. Although holding nurses solely responsible for errors created at the administrative level (such as patient care assignments and staffing patterns) appears unjust, this does occur in some cases.

Corporate liability, for example, attaches to the corporate entity (the hospital, for example) as a result of its corporate activities and decisions.

Other doctrines, such as temporary or borrowed servant and captain of the ship, may apply to critical care nurses and critical care units. These doctrines are used when the plaintiff argues that the physician is responsible for the nurse's actions, even though the nurse is an employee of the hospital and not the physician. If it can be shown that the nurse acted under the direction and control of the physician, the physician may be accountable for the nurse's actions. However, these doctrines are becoming increasingly uncommon. What viability remains is typically found in cases involving nurse anesthetists and operating room nurses.

Nurse Practice Acts

The practice of nursing is regulated by the state. As a general rule the state's police power to regulate prevails as long as the state's actions are not arbitrary or capricious. All nurses must be licensed to practice under their individual state's licensure statutes. Licensure authorizes (1) the right to practice and (2) access to employment. Therefore licensure is a property right that is constitutionally protected.[46] Every state has legislation defining the legal scope of nursing practice and unprofessional and illegal conduct that may lead to investigation and disciplinary action by the state and sanctions on the right to practice. The state nurse practice act establishes entry requirements, definitions of practice, and criteria for discipline. Although licensure is mandatory for registered nurses, statutory content varies among the states.

Generally, state law contains two definitions of nursing: one for the registered (or professional) nurse and one for the licensed practical (or vocational or technical) nurse. These definitions determine titles that may be used by nurses, the scope of nursing practice, and requirements for entering the nursing profession. In some states, advanced registered nursing practice, prescriptive authority for certain nurses, and third-party reimbursement are also defined by statute.[47] Mandatory continuing education requirements are also defined by statute in most states. The state authorizes the board of nursing to monitor practice, implement standards of care, enforce rules and regulations, and issue sanctions. Sanctions include additional education, restricted practice, supervised practice, license suspension, and license revocation. Some form of

disciplinary action generally occurs as a result of unauthorized practice, negligence or malpractice, incompetence, chemical or other impairment, criminal acts, or violations of specific nurse practice act provisions.

Because it is afforded constitutional protection, the right to practice cannot be violated without due process of the law. The amount of due process in administrative law differs from other legal processes. Due process involves notifying nurses that a complaint has been filed (voluntarily or by mandate); notices are written and contain the charges. Nurses in this situation should seek independent legal counsel immediately; the state will not provide it. Nurses have the right to be heard, often in more than one forum, and the right to present their own evidence.

Chemical impairment is a common reason for disciplinary action. In some states impaired nurses may avoid serious sanctions by voluntarily suspending practice and entering a rehabilitation program. This should be done with the advice of counsel (the nurse's own lawyer). Generally this option is available provided that no patient has been harmed because of the nurse's impairment.

Specific Patient Care Issues

Myriad legal issues and controversies exist in the field of critical care. Concerns frequently arise in the areas of (1) informed consent and authorization for treatment and (2) the right of patients to accept or refuse medical treatment.

Informed consent and authorization for treatment

The common law right not to be touched without giving consent has existed since the early eighteenth century. In the 1914 case of *Schloendorff v. Society of New York Hospital*, a court held that all adults of sound mind have the right to determine what shall be done with their own bodies, including the right to give and refuse consent to treatment.[48] Most states now have informed consent statutes, and the body of case law on this subject has developed impressively since the early days of *Schloendorff.*

Intrinsic to the doctrine of informed consent is the legal duty of physicians to disclose certain information to patients and the legal right of patients to informed consent to accept or refuse medical treatment. The extent to which nurses are involved in obtaining consent is an issue central to critical care nursing. As a general rule, physicians cannot delegate this function entirely to registered nurses, and nurses' exposure to liability increases if nurses accept full responsibility for obtaining patient consent. It is common practice for nurses to witness and document the procedure and to obtain signatures from patients after physicians have disclosed the required information. However, nurses should be thoroughly familiar with the state's informed consent statute and the individual institution's policy and procedure for obtaining informed consent. Because nurse anesthetists, nurse midwives, and nurse researchers are held to higher standards than other nurses, they may have increased responsibility in obtaining consent.[49]

There are two types of consent: express and implied. Express consent may be written or verbal and is given specifically for nonroutine procedures. Implied consent may be implied in fact, an assumption based on patient behavior (e.g., patients extending their arms for venipuncture or nodding approval), or implied in law (e.g., unconscious, hemorrhaging patients in the emergency department).

The following discussion summarizes the elements of valid informed consent, the adequacy of consent and negligent nondisclosure, and exceptions to consent requirements and the duty to disclose.

Valid consent must be (1) voluntary, (2) obtained, and (3) informed. Although consent can be verbal or written, most hospital policies require that informed, voluntary consent to nonroutine procedures be obtained and confirmed in writing, signed and dated by the patient, physician, and witness (if required). Most informed consent statutes provide that a written consent to a medical or surgical procedure meeting the consent and disclosure requirements of the statute creates the legal presumption of informed consent being given.

In the vast majority of jurisdictions the decision maker (the one giving the consent) must be a legally competent adult (that is, a person who has reached majority or, in most states, the age of 18 years). Competence is a legal judgment, and as a general rule, there is a legal presumption of patient competence.[50] A person is mentally incompetent (thereby rendering a consent invalid) if adjudicated incompetent. A person must likewise have the capacity (a medical and nursing judgment) to give consent: patients must be oriented and must understand information being given; medications patients are taking must be documented. For those adults legally adjudicated incompetent, guardians may give consent if invested with this authority.

Minors are legally incompetent, and consent is obtained from parents or guardians. However, in many jurisdictions, there are two important exceptions to this rule: (1) mature minors may consent to treatment for substance abuse, sexually transmitted disease, and matters involving contraception and reproduction; and (2) emancipated minors may consent to treatment in general: minors are considered emancipated if married or divorced before the age of majority, serving in the military, or living independently with parental consent.

Consent must be informed and timely. Physicians have the duty to disclose the following: diagnosis, condition, prognosis, material risks and benefits associated with the treatment or procedure; explanation of the treatment; providers of the treatment (who is performing, supervising, and/or assisting in the procedure); material risks and benefits of alternative therapy; and the probable outcome (including material risks and benefits) if patients refuse the treatment or procedure. Failure to disclose such information or inadequate disclosure with resultant injury may constitute negligence and give rise to tort claims of malpractice, battery, negligent nondisclosure, and abandonment. Consent is generally valid for 7 to 30 days; the time at which consent expires must be explicitly stated in the institutional policy and procedure manual.

There are many exceptions to consent requirements and the duty to disclose, and clearly the exceptions vary according to jurisdiction. Emergencies constitute one exception, unless patients refuse treatment or have previously made a competent and informed refusal. States vary significantly in the following treatment situations: endangered fetal viability, alcohol or other drug detoxification, emergency blood transfusions, cesarean sections, and substance abuse during pregnancy. Jurisdictions also vary on the issue of sources of consent (informal directives) for incompetent patients or patients in an emergency who have no legal guardians. Alternatives include consensus from as many next of kin as possible, with evidence that (1) the treatment is reasonable and necessary and (2) the family's decision would not be contrary to the patient's wishes. (This is known as *substituted judgment* made by a surrogate decision maker.) Another alternative is court order for treatment. In the absence of substituted judgment, many courts use what is known as the *best interests standard.*

Lawsuits involving informed consent and the duty to disclose generally require three elements: (1) proof that the health care provider failed to disclose an existing material risk unknown to the patient or alternatives to the proposed treatment, (2) proof that the patient would not have consented if the risk had been disclosed (in other words, that disclosure of the risk would have led a reasonable patient in the plaintiff's position to refuse the procedure or choose a different course of treatment), and (3) proof of injury occurring as a result of the failure to disclose.[49,51]

The right to accept or refuse medical treatment and the law of advance directives

THE COMPETENT PATIENT'S RIGHT TO REFUSE TREATMENT. The right to consent and informed consent includes the right to refuse treatment. In most cases a competent adult's decision to refuse even life-sustaining treatment is honored.[52-56] The underlying rationale is that the state's interest in preserving life does not outweigh the right of patients to withdraw from or refuse treatment.

In some situations the right to refuse treatment is not honored. These include but are not limited to the following situations:

◆ The treatment relates to a contagious illness that threatens the health of the public (e.g., immuniza-

tions are required, even over religious objections, if there is substantial danger to the community).
◆ Innocent third parties will suffer (e.g., a parent's wish to refuse a blood transfusion most likely would be overruled to save the life of a child; these cases are often decided case by case, and legal counsel should always be sought).
◆ The refusal violates ethical standards. For example, a Massachusetts court held that a hospital was not required to compromise its ethical principles by following a patient's decision but must cooperate in the transfer of the patient to a hospital willing to cooperate.[57] However, a New Jersey court ruled to the contrary. A patient indicated that she did not want to be fed if she became incapacitated; the hospital opposed this. The court upheld the patient's right and refused to order her transfer.[58] Again, obtaining legal counsel in these instances is strongly advised.
◆ Treatment must be instituted to prevent suicide and to preserve life (courts have clearly indicated, however, that terminally ill and/or comatose patients with no hope of recovery do not intend suicide when refusing treatment).

When patients refuse treatment, complex ethical, legal, and practical problems arise. Hospitals should have specific policies to guide nurses in these areas, and nurses' participation in hospital ethics committees or institutional ethics committees is strongly advised.

WITHHOLDING AND WITHDRAWING TREATMENT. As indicated earlier, adults have the right to refuse treatment, even treatment that sustains life.[59-61] This right means that critical care nurses may participate in the withholding or withdrawing of treatment. Historically, the distinction between withholding and withdrawing treatments was considered the issue of importance, but that is no longer the case. Health care decisions become most complex when patients lose competency and capacity to make their own decisions.

ORDERS NOT TO RESUSCITATE AND OTHER ORDERS. All critical care units should have written policies that address orders to withhold or withdraw treatment. For example, DNR orders should be governed by written policies including but not limited to the following:

◆ DNR orders should be entered in the patient's record with full documentation by the responsible physician regarding the patient's prognosis, the patient's agreement (if capable), or alternatively the family's consensus.
◆ DNR orders should have the concurrence of another physician, designated in the policy.
◆ Policies should specify that orders be reviewed periodically (some policies require daily review).
◆ Patients with capacity must give their informed consent.

◆ For patients without capacity, that incapacity must be thoroughly documented, along with the diagnosis, prognosis, and family consensus.
◆ Judicial intervention before writing a DNR order is usually indicated when patients families do not agree or there is uncertainty or disagreement about patients' prognoses or mental statuses. As a general rule, however, in the absence of conflict or disagreement, DNR orders are legal in a majority of jurisdictions if executed clearly and properly.
◆ Policies should specify who is to be notified within the hospital administration.

Other orders to withhold or withdraw treatment may involve mechanical ventilation,[62-64] dialysis, nutritional support, hydration, and medications such as antibiotics. Health care providers must consider carefully the legal and ethical implications of these orders for each patient. Policies must cover the way decisions will be made: who will decide and what the roles of patient, family, health care providers, and the institution will be. Policies must be developed in the context of state laws and judicial opinions.

ADVANCE DIRECTIVES AND THE PATIENT SELF-DETERMINATION ACT (OBRA 1990). Rarely has a case so galvanized public opinion as the case of Nancy Cruzan.[65,66] The tragic experience and hardships of Nancy Cruzan and her family left an indelible mark in American jurisprudence, legislation, and health care.

In *Cruzan* the issue before the U.S. Supreme Court was to consider whether Cruzan had a federal constitutional right that would require the hospital to withdraw life-sustaining treatment from her under the circumstances. The court rejected the request for authority to withdraw artificial nutrition and hydration and held that the U.S. Constitution did not prohibit the state of Missouri from requiring clear and convincing evidence of Cruzan's wishes before treatment withdrawal.

The court stated that when a person is incompetent and unable to exercise the right to refuse treatment and a surrogate must act on the person's behalf, the state may institute procedural safeguards to ensure that the surrogate honors the wishes expressed by the person while competent. The court also held that the U.S. Constitution does not require a state to accept the substituted judgment of the family; the state may recognize only a personal right to make such health care decisions. Rather than relying on the family's decision, a state may choose to defer only to the person's express wishes.

Perhaps more important, the court also held that competent adults have the federal constitutional right to refuse medical treatment, including life-sustaining hydration and nutrition. This right falls under the Fourteenth Amendment due process clause and is not a fundamental privacy right under the First Amendment.

The Cruzan decision quickly mobilized the U.S. Congress to pass landmark legislation known as the *Patient Self-Determination Act/Omnibus Budget Reconciliation Act of 1990.*[67-76] The statute requires that all adults receive written information on their rights under state law to make medical decisions, including the right to refuse treatment and the right to formulate advance directives.

The act mandates that providers of health care services under Medicare and Medicaid must comply with requirements relating to patient advance directives, written instructions recognized under state law for provisions of care when persons are incapacitated. Providers may not be reimbursed for the care they provide unless they meet the requirements of this provision.

Providers must have written policies and procedures to (1) inform all adult patients at the time treatment is initiated of their right to execute an advance directive and of the provider's policies on the implementation of that right, (2) document in medical records where patients have executed advance directives, (3) not condition care and treatment or otherwise discriminate on the basis of whether patients have executed advance directives, (4) comply with state laws on advance directives, and (5) provide information and education to staff and the community on advance directives. The provisions became effective in December 1991.

Patients themselves can provide clear direction by specifying their wishes in advanced directives.[77-79] These written documents include the living will and durable power of attorney for health care. To be effective in a jurisdiction, both directives must be statutorily or judicially recognized. The living will specifies that if certain circumstances such as terminal illness occur patients will decline specific treatment, such as cardiopulmonary resuscitation and mechanical ventilation.[80-82] The living will does not cover all treatment. For example, in some states, nutritional support may not be declined through a living will. The durable power of attorney for health care is a directive whereby patients designate agents who will make decisions if patients become unable to do so. Critical care nurses whose patients have executed advance directives must follow state law provisions and the hospital's policies.

Some states have also passed laws providing that a county, municipality, region, or medical center may establish a substitute medical decision-making board composed of health care professionals and lay persons. The board acts as a substitute decision maker if patients do not already have their own surrogates. The critical care staff should always consult with hospital legal counsel if patients have designated surrogates or have executed one or more advance directives and also have had court-appointed guardians. Various statutory provisions in the context of guardianship are incongruous with many of the new laws relating to surrogate or substitute decision making and the laws of advance directives. The staff must know without question who has primary legal authority for patients, and this information must be documented unambiguously.

References

1. Guralnik D, editor: *Webster's new world dictionary of the American language,* New York, 1981, Simon & Schuster.
2. Thompson J, Thompson H: *Bioethical decision-making for nurses,* Norwalk, Conn, 1985, Appleton-Century-Crofts.
3. Fowler M: Introduction to ethics and ethical theory: a road map to the discipline. In Fowler M, Levine-Ariff J, editors: *Ethics at the bedside,* Philadelphia, 1987, JB Lippincott.
4. Krekeler K: Critical care nursing and moral development, *Crit Care Nurs* 10(2):1, 1987.
5. Davis A, Aroskar M: *Ethical dilemmas and nursing practice,* Norwalk, Conn, 1983, Appleton-Century-Crofts.
6. Jameton A: Duties to self: professional nursing in the critical care unit. In Fowler M, Levine-Ariff J, editors: *Ethics at the bedside,* Philadelphia, 1987, JB Lippincott.
7. Fry S: Autonomy, advocacy, and accountability: ethics at the bedside. In Fowler M, Levine-Ariff J, editors: *Ethics at the bedside,* Philadelphia, 1987, JB Lippincott.
8. Singleton KA, Dever R: The challenge of autonomy: respecting the patient's wishes, *DCCN* 10(3):160, 1991.
9. Reference deleted in proofs.
10. Flynn P: Questions of risk, duty, and paternalism: problems in beneficence. In Fowler M, Levine-Ariff, editors: *Ethics at the bedside,* Philadelphia, 1987, JB Lippincott.
11. Reference deleted in proofs.
12. Aroskar M: Fidelity and veracity: questions of promise keeping, truth telling and loyalty. In Fowler M, Levine-Ariff J, editors: *Ethics at the bedside,* Philadelphia, 1987, JB Lippincott.
13. Washington G: Trust: a critical element in critical care nursing, *Focus Crit Care* 17(5):418, 1990.
14. Yeatch R, Fry S: *Case studies in nursing ethics,* Philadelphia, 1987, JB Lippincott.
15. Curtain L: Privacy: belonging to one's self, *Nursing Management* 23(4):7, 1992.
16. Milholland DK: Privacy and confidentiality of patient information: challenges for nursing, *JONA* 24(2):19, 1994.
17. Englehardt T, Rie M: Intensive care units, scarce resources, and conflicting principles of justice, *JAMA* 255:1159, 1986.
18. White J: Rationing health care resources, *Nursing Connections* 4(1):22, 1991.
19. DeYoung S, Temmler L, Adama EF, and others: Brief: organ referrals—would nurses do more if they knew more? *J Continuing Ed Nur* 22(5):219, 1994.
20. Rushton CH: Organ donation: it begins with you! *Focus on Critical Care* 18(4):269, 1991.
21. Stoeckle ML: Issues of transplantation: ethics of potential legislative changes, *DCCN* 12(3):158, 1993.
22. Oleson M: Subjectively perceived quality of life, *Image J Nurs Sch* 22(3):187, 1990.
23. Kleinpell RM: Concept analysis of quality of life, *DCCN* 10(4):223, 1991.
24. O'Mara R: Dilemmas in cardiac surgery: artificial heart and left ventricular assist device, *Crit Care Nurs* 10:48, 1987.
25. Daly BJ: Futility, *AACN Clinical Issues* 5(1):77, 1994.
26. DeWolf Bosek MS, Lowry E: When care is futile, *MedSurg Nursing* 3(3):225, 1994.
27. Hudson T: Are futile-care policies the answer? *Hosp Health Netw* Feb 20, 1994, p 26.
28. Schneiderman LJ, Jecker NS, Jonsen AR: Medical futility: its meaning and ethical implications, *Ann Intern Med* 112(12):949, 1990.
29. Dallery A: Professional loyalties, *Holistic Nurs Prac* 1:64, 1986.

30. Packard J, Ferrara M: In search of the moral foundation of nursing, *Adv Nurs Sci* 10:60, 1988.
31. Yarling R, McElmurry B: The moral foundation of nursing, *Adv Nurs Sci* 8:63, 1986.
32. Cianci M: The code of ethics and the role of nurses: an historical perspective, *Nurs Connect* 5(1):37, 1992.
33. Miller BK, Beck L, Adams D: Nurses' knowledge of the code for nurses, *J Contin Educ Nurs* 22(5):198, 1991.
34. American Nurses Association: *Code for nurses with interpretive statements,* Kansas City, Mo, 1985, The Association.
35. Erlen JA, Frost B: Nurses' perceptions of powerlessness in influencing ethical decisions, *West J Nurs Res* 13(3):397, 1991.
36. Baggs JG: Collaborative interdisciplinary bioethical decision making in intensive care units, *Nurs Outlook* 41(3):108, 1993.
37. Corley MC, Selig P, Ferguson C: Critical care nurse participation in ethical and work decision, *Critical Care Nurse* Jun 1993, p 120.
38. Dunn DG: Bioethics and nursing, *Nurs Connect* 7(3):43, 1994.
39. Broom C: Conflict resolution strategies: when ethical dilemmas evolve into conflict, *DCCN* 10(6):354, 1991.
40. Wicclair MR: Differentiating ethical decisions from clinical standards, *DCCN* 10(5):280, 1991.
41. Fowler M: Piecing together the ethical puzzle: operationalizing nursing's ethics in critical care. In Fowler M, Levine-Ariff J, editors: *Ethics at the bedside,* Philadelphia, 1987, JB Lippincott.
42. Northrop CE, Kelly ME: *Legal issues in nursing,* St Louis, 1987, Mosby.
43. Christoffel T: *Health and the law: a handbook for health professionals,* New York, Free Press; London, 1982 Collier Macmillan.
44. Prosser WL, Keeton WP, Dobbs DB, and others: *The law of torts,* ed 5, St Paul, Minn, 1988, West.
45. 28 U.S.C. Secs. 2671-80 (1986).
46. Walker DJ: Nursing 1980: new responsibility, new liability, *Trial* 16(12):43, 1980.
47. Hoffman NA: Nursing and the future of health care: the independent practice imperative, *Specialty L Dig: Health Care* 160:7, 1992.
48. *Schloendorff v. Soc'y of N.Y. Hosp.,* 105 N.E. 92 (1914), *overruled on other grounds.*
49. Murphy EK: Informed consent doctrine: little danger of liability for nurses, *Nurs Outlook* 39(1):48, 1991.
50. Northrop CE: Nursing practice and the legal presumption of competency, *Nurs Outlook* 36(2):112, 1988.
51. *Pauscher v. Iowa Methodist Med. Center,* 408 N.W.2d 355 (Iowa 1987).
52. *Bouvia v. Superior Court,* 225 Cal. Rptr. 297; 179 C.A.3d 1127, *review denied* (Cal. App. 1986).
53. *In Re Farrell,* 529 A.2d 404 (N.J. 1987).
54. *McKay v. Bergstedt,* 801 P.2d 617 (Nev. 1990).
55. *State v. McAfee,* 385 S.E.2d 651 (Ga. 1989).
56. Wilson-Clayton ML, Clayton MA: Two steps forward, one step back: *McKay v. Bergstedt, Whittier L Rev* 12:439, 1991.
57. *Brophy v. New England Sinai Hosp.,* 497 N.E.2d 626 (Mass. 1986).
58. *In Re Requena,* 517 A.2d 869 (N.J. App. Div. 1986).
59. Curtain L: Ethical concerns of nutritional support, *Nurs Manage* 25(4):14, 1994.
60. Miedema F: Withdrawing treatment from the hopelessly ill, *DCCN* 12(1):40, 1993.
61. Smejkal CM, Hill FJ: Life-sustaining treatment: a legal-ethical dilemma, *JONA* 20(7/8):49, 1990.
62. Campbell ML, Carlson RW: Terminal weaning from mechanical ventilation: ethical and practical considerations for patient management, *Am J Crit Care* 1(3):52, 1992.
63. Clarke DE, Vaughn L, Raffin TA: Noninvasive positive pressure ventilation for patients with terminal respiratory failure: the ethical and economic costs of delaying the inevitable are too great, *Am J Crit Care* 3(1):4, 1994.
64. Daly BJ, Newton B, Montenegro HD, and others: Withdrawal of mechanical ventilation: ethical principles and guidelines for terminal weaning, *Am J Crit Care* 2(3):217, 1993.
65. Flarey FL: Advanced directives: in search of self-determination, *JONA* 21(11):16, 1991.
66. Flarey DL: Ethical decisions: what we learned from Cruzan about the right to die, *Nurs Admin Q* 15(4):13, 1991.
67. *Advance directives for health care: deciding today about your care in the future,* Iowa Hospital Association, Iowa Medical Society, Iowa State Bar Association, 1991.
68. American Hospital Association: *Put it in writing: a guide to promoting advance directives,* Chicago, 1992 The Association.
69. Cate FH, Gill BA: *The Patient Self-Determination Act: implementation issues and opportunities,* Washington, DC, 1991, The Annenberg Washington Program.
70. Choice in Dying: *Advance directive protocols and the Patient Self-Determination Act: a resource manual for the development of institutional protocols,* New York, 1991, Choice in Dying.
71. Emanuel L, Emanuel E: The medical directive: a new comprehensive advance care document, *JAMA* 261(22):3, 288, 1989.
72. Iowa Hospital Association: *The Patient Self-Determination Act of 1990: implementation in Iowa Hospitals,* Des Moines, 1991, Iowa Hospital Association.
73. National Hospice Organization: *Advance medical directives,* Arlington, Va, 1991, National Hospice Organization.
74. National Health Lawyers Association: *The patient self-determination directory and resources guide,* Washington, 1991, The Association.
75. Patient Self-Determination Act/Omnibus Budget Reconciliation Act of 1990, Pub L No 101-508, Sec. 4206; 42 U.S.C. Sec. 1395cc(a)(1) (1990).
76. Unisys Corp: *Advance directives,* Des Moines, 1991 (brochure).
77. Campbell ML, Hoyt JW, Nelson LJ: Healthcare ethics forum '94: Perspectives on withholding and withdrawal of life-support, *AACN Clinical Issues* 5(3):353, 1994.
78. Hudson T: Advance directives: still problematic for providers, *Hosp Health Net,* March 20, 1994, p 46.
79. Reigle J: Preserving patient self-determination through advance directives, *Heart Lung* 21(2):196, 1992.
80. Dooley J, Marsden C: Healthcare ethics forum '94: advance directives: the critical challenges, *AACN Clinical Issues* 5(3):340, 1994.
81. Quigley FM: Why have a living will? *Focus on Critical Care* 18(1):30, 1991.
82. Singleton KA, Dever R, Donner TA: Durable power of attorney: nursing implications, *DCCN* 11(1):41, 1992.

3

Patient and Family Education

COLLEEN O'DONNELL

CHAPTER OBJECTIVES

- Adapt and apply teaching-learning theory to the critical care setting.
- Describe the stages of adaptation to illness and the implications of each for the patient teaching plan.
- Perform a learning needs assessment.

- Construct a teaching plan for patients in the critical care unit.
- Discuss four methods of instruction and the appropriateness of each to the critical care setting.
- Describe informational needs of families of critically ill patients.

KEY TERMS

This chapter explores educational theories and techniques and delineates the teaching-learning process. In addition, informational needs of family members are described to provide a holistic approach to education.

Patient and Family Education

Educating patients and their families is an important nursing function in all settings of practice. Because the critical care unit often appears foreign and threatening to patients and their families, this setting presents additional challenges. Nurses have a legal and ethical responsibility to meet standards of care related to patient education. These standards include identifying the learning needs of patients and their families, assessing their readiness to learn, teaching the appropriate content, documenting the teaching plan, and evaluating and documenting the results of the patient teaching.[1] Standards for patient and family education have been published by professional organizations such as the American Association of Critical Care Nurses and the American Nurses Association, as well as by regulatory agencies such as the Joint Commission on Accreditation of Health Care Organizations.

The belief that patients and families have the right to information about diagnosis, treatment, and prognosis in terms that are understandable to them serves as the basis for all educational activities.[2] Nurses should acknowledge that each patient is unique, with individual learning methods, skills, and motivation. These differences in individuals account for varied responses to the same teaching strategies.

Coupled with patients' right to know is their right not to know in some cases. The right not to know must be respected when patients prefer not to learn about their illnesses. Simple, basic information about monitors and unit policy, for example, usually suffices in these cases. Indeed, receiving more information than they can process and integrate can greatly increase anxiety and may result in slower recovery for some patients.[3,4] Individuals have the right to accept, adopt, or reject the information provided in educational encounters, however frustrating this may be to the nurse.[3]

Adult Learning Theory

Incorporating the principles of adult learning theory is central to the successful implementation of an educational plan in the critical care and telemetry environment. An educational plan that considers the uniqueness of the adult population can fail, however. Nurses should understand this theory before planning or implementing the educational plan of care. Unfortunately, more is known about how animals and children learn than adults. Nonetheless, Knowles[5] described several elements of **adult learning theory** that suggest adults learn differently than children. Adults must be ready to learn, having moved from one developmental or educational task to the next. Before they can actually learn something, they need to know why it is important. Inherent in their attitudes is the sense that they are responsible for their own decisions. Consequently, they may resent attempts by others to force different beliefs on them. Educational techniques should recognize and promote contributions that adults, with their wealth of experience, can bring to the learning environment. Because adults' orientation to learning is life centered, teachers should focus on current problem resolution. Internal pressures such as self-esteem and quality of life also motivate the adult learner.

Teaching-Learning Process

The **teaching-learning process** used in the health care setting incorporates the dynamics of adult learning theory. This process can be defined as a set of activities organized and structured to maximize the results for pa-

---

B O X   3 - 1

THE TEACHING-LEARNING PROCESS

1. Assessment of the need to learn
2. Assessment of readiness to learn
3. Setting of objectives
4. Teaching-learning activities
5. Evaluation and reteaching (if necessary)

---

tients and to minimize the amount of time and effort on the part of health care practitioners.[6] It can be divided into the five steps summarized in Box 3-1. These steps can be closely related to the nursing process. Table 3-1 shows the application of the nursing process to the teaching-learning process in the care of critically ill patients.

Assessment

The assessment step, a vital part of any successful educational plan, involves gathering data to assist nurses in meeting the learning needs of patients and their families.[6] Components of this assessment in the critical care unit include identification of the various physiologic, psychologic, environmental, and sociocultural stressors present; patients' responses to these stressors; adaptation to illness; and an examination of motivation and readiness to learn. In reality, these issues are often related to one another and cannot be assessed as separate entities.

MOTIVATION AND READINESS TO LEARN. Assessment of **motivation and readiness to learn** are important parts of the teaching-learning process.[7] This assessment incorporates an analysis of multiple factors that have previously been discussed, including an appreciation of multiple stressors and their response and the stage of adaptation to illness. In addition, familiarity with motivation theory is helpful. One well-known and important theory describing human behavior motivation is Maslow's hierarchy of needs, which provides background for the discussion of motivation to learn.

According to Maslow's theory, human beings have a number of interrelated and hierarchic needs that motivate all behavior. Lower-level needs must be met before higher-level needs can emerge and be satisfied. The basic needs are physiologic: safety, belongingness, love, esteem, and self-actualization. The need to know and understand is one of the highest-level needs. During critical illness, lower-level physiologic and safety needs often consume patients' energy and make learning impossible. Attempting to teach patients who fear for their lives and safety is of little use unless they are being taught that they are in no immediate danger of dying. Once their lower-level needs are met and patients feel that they are out of danger, they will be more ready to focus on higher-level needs. Therefore if the assessment discloses significant needs in lower areas, nurses should address those

TABLE 3-1
APPLICATION OF THE NURSING PROCESS TO THE TEACHING-LEARNING PROCESS

NURSING PROCESS	TEACHING-LEARNING PROCESS
Assessment	Physiologic
	Psychologic
	Environmental
	Sociocultural
	Stress response
	Physiologic
	Heart rate
	Blood pressure
	Peristalsis
	Mental acuity
	Blood glucose
	Dilated pupils
	Psychologic
	Anxiety
	Depression
	Panic
	Withdrawal
	Denial
	Hostility
	Regression
	Frustration
	Readiness to learn
Nursing diagnosis and plan	Identification of specific knowledge deficit
	Identification of causes and associated factors
	Identification of expected outcomes and behavioral objectives
	Development of teaching plan
Nursing intervention	Teaching-learning activities and experience
Evaluation	Evaluation and documentation of effectiveness of teaching-learning process
	Measurement of knowledge gain
	Measurement of behavior changes

needs before attempting to teach. Once met, these needs cease to be the primary motivators of behavior, and patients can attend to learning and other higher-level needs.

Nursing diagnosis and plan

Assessment assists critical care nurses in the establishment of an adequate data base from which to formulate nursing diagnoses and devise an educational plan of care.

In this plan of care, expected outcomes and behavioral objectives are identified. Nursing management plans for *Knowledge Deficit* can be found in Unit X.

TEACHING CONTENT. The content of teaching material presented in the critical care unit varies depending on each patient's clinical and emotional status. As soon as possible, nurses should set learning priorities based on the assessment. However, an acute event sometimes precludes full assessment at the time of admission. In this case, behavior crucial to patients' treatment and participation in care can be taught as soon as appropriate. Teaching should be guided by patients and their families—that is, nurses should teach what they want to know when they want to know it. If patients' questions and concerns are left unanswered during this time of high anxiety, their unmet needs will distract them and block further communication.

Although specific content varies, certain areas should be covered with all conscious patients. Environmental factors in a critical care unit can frighten patients and should be explained as soon as possible. Unless their purpose or function is understood, cardiac monitors, oxygen equipment, indwelling lines and catheters, frequent laboratory tests, and vital signs checks may cause the patient undue anxiety. Nurses should also explain briefly the reason for procedures as well as their associated sensations or discomfort. This information may require several repetitions, but it will decrease anxiety and provide a sense of control for the moment.

Giving information about the illness or diagnosis in the critical phase of care is usually appropriate. Nurses must often interpret and explain information provided by physicians. Despite the denial often present, some patients want to know about their illness, prognosis, complications, and reason for admission to the critical care unit. Patients may ask whether they are going to die, a traumatic question for patients and nurses. Questions should be answered as honestly, compassionately, and sensitively as possible and should be followed by supportive care as necessary.

Patients in critical care units experience many stressful medical and nursing procedures during the course of their care, including radiologic procedures, placement of vascular access or monitoring devices, intubation, suctioning, and spinal taps. Educational and psychologic preparation for these procedures can decrease anxiety and increase cooperation with care. Nurses can offer two types of information to patients in preparation for these procedures. *Procedural information* refers to what will be done, when and where it will happen, and who will provide the service. *Sensory information* refers to what patients should expect to feel during and after the procedure.[8] When time permits, allowing patients to ask questions, see equipment that will be used, and practice movements or body positions that will be required can help to reduce anxiety. In addition, teaching basic relaxation techniques, such as deep breathing or guided imagery, can be effective in helping patients relax during a stressful or uncomfortable procedure.[8,9] When these procedures must occur on an emergent basis without time for patient preparation, nurses should explain what happened and why as soon as patients stabilize and are able to understand the information.

Another important educational consideration in the critical care environment is that patients learn not only by what is said directly but also by inadvertent comments or nonverbal cues. Nurses should be especially attuned to staff or physician discussions at patients' bedsides, where information heard by patients can be misinterpreted and possibly lead to increased anxiety and misinformation. In addition, if nurses give nonverbal cues that do not coincide with the reality of the situation or the severity of patients' conditions, mistrust can ensue and alter the nurse-patient therapeutic relationship. These dynamics can also affect educational efforts with families.

OBJECTIVES. Inherent in any educational plan of care is the careful consideration of desired objectives. Objectives state the desired behaviors expected from the implementation of the plan.[2] Based on the learning needs of patients, they serve as a guide for the teaching-learning process. Objectives are written in measurable behavioral terms and should correspond with what patients are to learn rather than what nurses are to teach. Terms such as *to know, understand, be familiar with, realize,* and *appreciate* are difficult to measure and subject to many interpretations. Active verbs such as to *identify, state, list, describe,* and *demonstrate* should be used instead because they are readily understood and conducive to evaluation.

Both long- and short-term objectives are appropriate, although in many cases it takes days, weeks, or even months of repetition and practice to master a new skill. Indeed, constraints of time in the critical care and telemetry units may necessitate a consideration of only realistic and important needs, with follow-up education after discharge.[10]

Decreasing lengths of stay and the policy of admitting patients on the same day as their scheduled procedure or surgery require the implementation of creative and innovative teaching approaches.[11] However, nurses in the critical care setting should not hesitate to identify goals that surpass the critical care phase because the educational plan of care continues as patients improve and are transferred to the telemetry unit. Generalized objectives have been developed for programs in which large numbers of patients are taught, such as cardiac teaching plans for patients recovering from myocardial infarctions. Standardized plans can be useful resource materials in developing a teaching plan but must not take the place of individualized, specific objectives designed for each patient. Box 3-2 provides a sample educational plan for patients undergoing coronary artery bypass surgery.

Nursing intervention

THE TEACHING-LEARNING EXPERIENCE. Patients in the critical care environment are educated in many informal interactions with nurses, and the knowledge they gain fosters their understanding and well-being. Various nursing care activities, such as bathing and administration of medication, present educational opportunities. Each encounter with the patient and family should also be viewed as a teaching opportunity. There are times during the hospitalization, however, when more formal or structured educational experiences are in order. Structured educational approaches have been found to help patients gain knowledge immediately.[12] Included in this discussion are techniques in creating a learning environment and various teaching activities or methods that can be used to accomplish the desired outcomes based on patients' individual learning objectives.

CREATING A LEARNING ENVIRONMENT. Barriers to learning related to motivational factors have been discussed. To structure a successful teaching-learning experience in a critical care area, nurses must also carefully assess environmental and iatrogenic factors that affect interactions. Bright lights, unpleasant odors, unfamiliar noises, and untidy surroundings can distract patients and add to their cognitive impairment. Controlling these factors can facilitate the learning process. When they cannot be controlled, they should be explained to patients to alleviate anxiety and facilitate a trusting relationship.

Nurses should examine barriers to learning that they may bring to the interaction. Nurses have been found to set up these barriers both consciously and unconsciously.[13] The use of medical terms and other language that may be unfamiliar to patients may adversely affect the teaching-learning process.[14] Nurses may also fail to set aside time just for teaching, resulting in hurried and fragmented sessions. Nonverbal cues from nurses, such as glancing at the clock or breaking eye contact, may interrupt patient interactions. The plan and execution of teaching sessions can have as important an effect on patient learning as the material itself.

TEACHING METHODS. The three basic methods of teaching are lecture, discussion, and demonstration.[3] The choice of method depends on the material to be taught.

LECTURE. Lecture is the presentation of information in a highly structured format to a group. In this method, teachers present a great deal of material but may not provide ample opportunities for teacher-learner interaction. This style of teaching is inappropriate for acutely ill individuals in the critical care unit. However, it may be useful in the telemetry unit. Optimally the group size should be arranged to enable learners to ask questions.

DISCUSSION. Less structured than lecture, discussion allows an exchange and feedback between teachers and learners. Teachers can adapt material to meet the needs of the individual or group. The discussion approach is probably most useful when learning should result in behavior change or development of an attitude.[3] Hospitalized patients with similar problems and at similar stages of adaptation can benefit from discussion groups. Individual discussion with patients and families is appropriate and valuable during the acute phase of illness because it allows them to express their feelings and interpretations. This individual approach is ideal for teaching about sensitive issues, such as resuming sexual activity after myocardial infarction.[3]

TEACHING PLAN FOR THE PATIENT UNDERGOING CORONARY ARTERY BYPASS SURGERY

PREOPERATIVE PHASE

During preoperative educational interactions, the nurse should assess the patient's and family's levels of anxiety and their effect on the ability or desire to learn. Preoperative education should be individualized to prepare the patient appropriately for the surgery, to provide education about postoperative care, and to minimize anxiety. Before the teaching-learning experience, the nurse should do the following:

- Assess the patient's level of anxiety and desire to learn about the upcoming surgery
- Individualize the preoperative teaching plan based on assessment findings

The following content may be included in the preoperative teaching session:

- Review of the coronary artery bypass graft (CABG) procedure
- Time leaving room for surgery, length of surgery
- Location of family waiting area
- Surgical preparation and shave
- Nothing by mouth after midnight
- What to expect when awakening from anesthesia
- Sights and sounds of the recovery room and/or critical care unit
- Tubes and drains: chest tubes, hemodynamic monitoring lines, Foley catheter, intravenous lines, pacemaker wires (if appropriate), endotracheal tube
- Inability to speak with endotracheal tube in place
- Discomfort to expect from incisions, availability of pain medication
- Coughing and deep breathing practice
- Use of incentive spirometer
- When family can visit, how long, how often
- Usual length of critical care unit stay

In addition to this content, the nurse needs to do the following:

- Reassure patient that many staff members and much activity around bedside is normal and does not indicate complications
- Elicit and answer any specific questions the patient and family have at that time
- Determine specific needs and desires for day of surgery (e.g., patient needs hearing aid or glasses as soon as possible)
- Meet with the family alone to offer support and address concerns they may not wish to voice to the patient

CRITICAL CARE UNIT PHASE

During the critical care unit phase, patient and family education is designed to meet immediate needs and reduce anxiety. The following are examples of content appropriate for this time:

- Basic explanation of bedside equipment
- Review of tubes and drains
- Turning, coughing, deep breathing
- Use of incentive spirometer
- Use of oxygen equipment

- Orientation to time, place, situation
- Explanation of procedures
- Basic purpose of medications
- Explanation of normal progression in early postoperative period
- Basic range-of-motion exercises (e.g., ankle circles, point and flex)

During this phase, the nurse also does the following:

- Reassures patient and family of normal progression
- Repeats and reinforces information as necessary
- Answers questions as they arise
- Begins early to prepare patient for transfer to prevent transfer anxiety
- Determines family learning needs and addresses them together with patient or in separate teaching sessions as appropriate

STEP-DOWN UNIT PHASE

After transfer from the critical care unit, the patient's and family's educational needs increase. Short daily educational sessions should be planned to cover the following content:

- Basic pathophysiology of coronary artery disease
- Review of surgical procedure
- Risk factors for coronary artery disease
- Upper-extremity range-of-motion exercises
- Dietary recommendations (salt- and fat/cholesterol-modified diet)
- Taking of own pulse
- Recognition and treatment of angina (use of nitroglycerin)

During this phase, the nurse also does the following:

- Uses audiovisual materials in teaching sessions or as reinforcement of content
- Provides printed take-home materials outlining important content
- Answers questions as they arise

DISCHARGE TEACHING

Before discharge, the following content should be covered with the patient and family:

- Activity guidelines
- Lifting restrictions
- Incision care
- Possibility of patient being extremely fatigued or depressed after discharge
- Guidelines for return to work, driving, sexual activity
- Medication safety and administration

Before discharge, the nurse also does the following:

- Reassures patient that ups and downs are normal
- If necessary, reassures patient and family that likelihood of cardiac emergencies at home is small
- Provides printed material for further study by patient and family
- Answers questions as they arise
- Provides phone number for patient or family to call when further questions arise

DEMONSTRATION. Demonstration involves acting out a procedure while giving appropriate explanation so that learners understand how to perform their tasks. Patients can then practice skills and receive feedback about their performances. This method is often used in the acute care setting, such as when teaching patients coughing, deep breathing, and taking their own pulse.

OTHER METHODS OF INSTRUCTION. In addition to the three basic methods just presented, several other approaches to delivering or augmenting information in a patient teaching program are available. They include commercially prepared or custom-designed printed materials, bedside videotape programs, and computer-assisted patient education programs. Computer programs, relatively new to health education, have been used in community-based education programs, hospital waiting rooms, designated teaching rooms, and in some cases, at the bedside with microcomputers on transportable carts.[15] These programs allow learners to set the pace of the program and are generally presented in an attractive, colorful format.[16]

Written materials are also useful tools in patient and family education, allowing repetition and reinforcement of content and providing basic information in printed form for future reference. To be useful, however, the content must be accurate, current, and comprehensible to patients and their families. Research links the varied comprehensibility of instructions to compliance with medical regimens.[17]

The median literacy level of the U.S. population is estimated to be at the tenth grade level, with about 20% of the population at the fifth grade level or lower.[2] Other research indicates that approximately 50% of health care patients have serious difficulty reading instructional materials written at the fifth grade level.[18] Most patient education materials are written at or above the eighth grade level.[19] To ensure that patients receive educational materials at the appropriate reading level, nurses should question patients about the last grade level completed in school. Because this level may not represent actual reading ability, nurses should select written material two to four grade levels below the level indicated.[20] Box 3-3 depicts examples of an instruction written at various reading levels.

In recent years the use of educational videotapes at the bedside or in group settings has become increasingly popular. A recent review of literature on the use of videotapes verifies that the medium can address the basic and repetitive aspects of patient education and that it is effective for gaining short-term knowledge.[21] The use of videotapes, however, should not be considered a substitute for individualized patient teaching; it is most effective when promoted by staff as reinforcement for other educational activities.[21,22] Before showing tapes to patients, staff members should preview them to ensure the accuracy and appropriateness of the content and to assess the best way to introduce and reinforce the material. Again, it is essential that nurses realize audiovisual accessories are an adjunct to teaching, not a replacement

---

BOX 3-3

SAMPLES OF DIFFERENT READING LEVELS

COLLEGE READING LEVEL

Consult your physician immediately with the onset of chest discomfort, shortness of breath, or increased perspiration.

TWELFTH GRADE READING LEVEL

Call your physician immediately if you experience chest discomfort, shortness of breath, or increased sweatiness.

EIGHTH GRADE READING LEVEL

Call your doctor immediately if you start having chest pain or shortness of breath or feel sweaty.

FOURTH GRADE READING LEVEL

Call your doctor right away if you start having chest pain, can't breathe, or feel sweaty.

---

for the central role of nurses in objective accomplishment. Indeed, discrepancies between the videotapes and information that is reinforced can seriously affect the credibility of nurses and educational care plans.

Teaching critically ill patients may require modification of traditional teaching methods and strategies. In critical care units, patient goals are generally short-term and objectives are concrete. Teaching should be done briefly and in terms that patients can understand. The many stressors of illness and critical care and the effects of sedation and other drugs may cause patients to require frequent repetitions and reinforcement of information. This is to be expected with critically ill persons and should not be considered as a failure of the teaching experience. Each educational interaction between patients and nurses is valuable, even when it does not result in long-term behavioral change. Nurses should remember that family members are also stressed and may forget pertinent information about visiting hours, unit policies, and how to contact staff members. It is helpful to provide them with written information to supplement and reinforce verbal instructions.[23,24]

Evaluation

Evaluation of the educational plan of care focuses on the plan's ability to accomplish the objectives and outcomes developed in the planning phase. Evaluation should include documentation of the effectiveness of the teaching-learning process, with measurement of the knowledge gain and behavior changes identified.

In addition to the traditional evaluation of the educational plan based on objectives, other subtle effects of patient education can be identified. If nurses in the critical care setting limit measurement of teaching effectiveness to long-term behavior changes, they will judge as failures many critical educational activities necessary for the well-being of patients. If the teaching meets a momentary need, the effect is no less valuable and successful. Less concrete but equally valuable outcomes, such as signs of relaxation or greater participation in self-care, also document beneficial effects of the educational plan. Recognizing these subtle effects does not negate the necessity and usefulness of written, measurable objectives, but it does mean that they should not be the sole measures of educational success.[25] For example, in teaching the reason for and function of the cardiac monitor when patients are admitted to the critical care unit, nurses not only increase patients' knowledge about cardiac monitoring but may also decrease their anxiety about the critical care setting and thereby promote rest and healing.

Informational Needs of Families in Critical Care

Family members and significant others of critically ill patients are integral to the recovery of their loved ones. When planning for the overall care of patients, nurses and other caregivers should consider the informational and emotional support needs of this important group.[26-28] According to Henneman et al,[29] families of critically ill patients report that their greatest need is for information. Flexible visiting hours and informational booklets regarding the critical care experience were recommended as ways to meet this need. Important specific information for families delineated by Miracle and Hovenkamp[28] are listed in Box 3-4.

> **BOX 3-4**
>
> *IMPORTANT INFORMATIONAL NEEDS OF FAMILIES*
>
> - To have questions answered honestly
> - To know the facts about the prognosis
> - To know the results of the procedure as soon as they are available
> - To have a staff member inform them of the patient's progress
> - To know why things are being done
> - To know about possible complications
> - To have explanations that can be understood
> - To know exactly what is being done
> - To know about the staff providing care
> - To have directions about what to do during the procedure

References

1. Smith E: Patient teaching—it's the law, *Nursing '87* 17(7):67, 1987.
2. Redman BK: *The process of patient teaching in nursing,* ed 7, St Louis, 1993, Mosby.
3. Burke LE, Scalzi CC: *Education of the patient and family.* In Underhill S and others, editors: *Cardiac nursing,* Philadelphia, 1982, JB Lippincott.
4. Storlie F: *Patient teaching in critical care,* New York, 1975, Appleton-Century-Crofts.
5. Knowles M: *The adult learner: a neglected species,* ed 3, Houston, 1990, Gulf Publishing.
6. Billie DA: The teaching-learning process. In Billie DA: *Practical approaches of patient teaching,* Boston, 1981, Little, Brown.
7. Rega MD: A model approach for patient education, *Med Surg Nurs* 2(6):477, 1993.
8. Williams CL, Kendall PC: Psychological aspects of education for stressful medical procedures, *Health Educ Q* 12(3):135, 1985.
9. Frenn M, Fehring R, Kartes S: Reducing the stress of cardiac catheterization by teaching relaxation, *Dimens Crit Care Nurs* 5(2):108, 1986.
10. Chan V: Content cardiac teaching: patient's perceptions of the importance of teaching content after myocardial infarction, *J Adv Nurs* 15(10):1139, 1990.
11. Recker D: Patient perception of preoperative cardiac surgical teaching done pre- and postadmission, *Crit Care Nurse* 14(4):52, 1994.
12. Davis TMA and others: Preparing patients for cardiac catheterization: Informational treatment and coping style interactions, *Heart Lung* 23(2):130, 1994.
13. Nite G, Willis F: *The coronary patient: hospital care and rehabilitation,* New York, 1979, Macmillan.
14. Eaton S, Davis G, Brenner P: Discussion stoppers in teaching, *Nurs Outlook* 25(9):578, 1977.
15. Bell JA: The role of microcomputers in patient education, *Comput Nurs* 4(6):255, 1986.
16. Dobberstein K: Computer-assisted patient education, *Am J Nurs* 87(5):697, 1987.
17. Ley P and others: Improving doctor-patient communication in general practice, *J Royal Coll Gen Practitioners* 25:558, 1975.
18. Doak L, Doak C: Patient comprehension profiles: recent findings and strategies, *Patient Couns Health Educ* 3:101, 1980.
19. Streiff LD: Can clients understand our instructions? *Image J Nurs Sch* 18(2):48, 1986.
20. Boyd MD: A guide to writing effective patient education materials, *Nurs Manage* 18(7):56, 1987.
21. Neilsen E, Sheppard MA: Television as a patient education tool: a review of its effectiveness, *Patient Educ Couns* 11:3, 1988.
22. Durand RP, Counts CS: Developing audio-visual programs for patient education, *Am Neph Nurs Assoc* 13(3):158, 1986.
23. Burke LE: Learning and retention in the acute care setting, *Crit Care Q* 4:3, 1981.
24. Foster DS: Written reinforcement for teaching, *MCN* 11(5):347, 1986.
25. Billie DA: Process oriented patient education, *Dimens Crit Care Nurs* 2:2, 1983.
26. Gaw-Ens BA: Informational support for families immediately after CABG surgery, *Crit Care Nurse* 14(2):41, 1994.
27. Long CO, Greeneich DS: Family satisfaction techniques: meeting family expectations, *DCCN* 13(2):104, 1994.
28. Miracle VA, Hovenkamp G: Needs of families of patients undergoing invasive cardiac procedures, *Am J Crit Care* 3(3):155, 1994.
29. Henneman EA, McKenzie JB, Dewa CS: An evaluation of interventions for meeting the information needs of families of critically ill patients, *Am J Crit Care* 1(3):85, 1993.

UNIT TWO

Common Problems in Critical Care

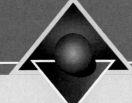

4

Psychosocial Alterations

KATHERINE FORTINASH

CHAPTER OBJECTIVES

- Explain the following coping strategies as they relate to critically ill patients: regression, suppression, denial, trust, religious beliefs, and family support.
- Describe the needs and coping mechanisms of families of critically ill patients.
- Explain interventions and nursing management for patients with coping alterations.

- Identify situations that increase the risk of disturbances of self-concept.
- Match relevant interventions with expected outcomes in a situation in which patients experience self-concept alterations.

KEY TERMS

body image, p. 32   powerlessness, p. 34   self-esteem, p. 33

denial, p. 35

Patients requiring critical care must cope with a variety of stressors (Box 4-1). Patients' responses to these stressors depend on individual differences, such as age, gender, social supports, medical diagnosis, cultural background, current hospital course, and prognosis. Nurses' knowledge of assessment, diagnosis, and intervention in effective coping also affects how well patients cope. Nurs-

ing management plans for psychological alterations can be found in Unit X.

Self-Concept Alterations

Self-concept is a relatively stable, yet modifiable construct useful for understanding individuals and their be-

STRESSORS IN THE CRITICAL CARE SETTING

Patients' experience of critical illness and care will vary. However, each patient must cope with at least some of the following stressors:

- Threat of death
- Threat of survival, with significant residual problems related to the illness or injury
- Pain or discomfort
- Lack of sleep
- Loss of autonomy over most aspects of life and daily functioning
- Loss of control over environment, including loss of privacy and exposure to light, noise, and general activity of the critical care unit, including the care of other patients
- Loss of usual role and arena in which usual coping mechanisms serve the patient
- Separation from family and friends
- Loss of dignity
- Boredom broken only by brief visits, threatening stimuli, and frightening thoughts
- Loss of ability to express self verbally when undergoing intubation

havior. It influences how people react to and manage problems in daily life. Self-concept is a major concern for nurses who care for patients because nursing interventions that do not consider the whole individual—including the self-concept—are probably ineffective.

Two major subcomponents of the self-concept are discussed in this chapter: body image and self-esteem. Pertinent to these diagnoses are the following key factors that affect self-concept[1]:

1. Previous perception of appraisals about self from significant others
2. Experience with developmental and situational crises and how they were managed
3. Experiences with success and failure and current expectations of self
4. Positive and negative feelings of self-worth from interpersonal experiences
5. Level of physiologic functioning

Assessment of the Self-Concept

The self-concept is what individuals believe about themselves; the self-report is what individuals are willing to share about themselves. Lee's phases of response to illness or injury[2] are useful in assessing the self-concept of critically ill patients. She identified four phases: impact, retreat, acknowledgment, and reconstruction.

Patients in critical care units are primarily in the first two phases. During phase one—impact—signs of de-

spair, discouragement, passive acceptance, anger, and hostility may be present. Shock, anxiety, numbness, and unreality may be the immediate responses. During the retreat phase, patients may try to avoid reality; denial is common. Patients are not ready to consider the meaning or implications of the situation and may repress or suppress reality. When repression or suppression of reality is no longer possible, patients may become intensely angry. Patients are usually transferred to an intermediate unit before the acknowledgment phase occurs. This phase is marked by the conflicting emotions associated with recognition of the changes or losses that have occurred or will occur. The final phase is reconstruction. In this phase, patients attempt a new approach to life.

Body Image Disturbance

Based on past and present perceptions, **body image** is the mental picture, including attitudes and feelings, that individuals have of their bodies and physical functioning. The body image develops from internal-sensation postural changes, contact with people and objects in the environment, emotional experiences, and fantasies.[3] Although it is a stable part of the self-concept, body image changes over time and is influenced by cognitive growth and physical changes in the body. Fisher[4] suggested that body experiences can be minimized, or magnified to the point at which they are the center of attention. He also described the *body boundary*, the demarcation between the self and the environment and the pattern of body awareness. The pattern of body awareness refers to the variation in attention given to parts of the body; more attention is given to the parts that have symbolic significance or are being threatened.

A change in the body's appearance, structure, and/or function necessitates a change in the body image. Such changes may be caused by disease, trauma, or surgery. The cause of *Body Image Disturbance* may be biophysical, cognitive perceptual, psychosocial, cultural, or spiritual. *Body Image Disturbances* arise when disruption exists in the way individuals perceive their bodies. In these instances, people fail to perceive or adapt to the changed body (Table 4-1). Such disturbances are manifested by verbal or nonverbal responses to the actual or perceived change in appearance, structure, or function.[5]

Some patients must extend their body images to incorporate environmental objects.[6] Patients temporarily requiring assisted respirations must extend their body images to include the ventilator and its accessories. Explanations to patients and their families are helpful in this situation. Patients admitted to a surgical critical care unit after a traumatic amputation may awake to find a leg missing with no prior knowledge of the loss. Reliving the accident and receiving explanations about the need for the amputation are priorities for such patients. Critical care nurses must begin the process of helping patients live with this permanent alteration. Interventions by nurses and others on the health team focus on helping

TABLE 4 - 1 BODY IMAGE PROBLEMS			
STRUCTURE	**ALTERED BY**	**TREATMENT**	**ALTERATION**
Skin	Burns	Grafts	Scars
	Lacerations	Sutures	Contractures
			Change in skin color, texture
Teeth	Automobile accident	Dentures	Altered speech, eating habits
Leg	Traumatic amputation	Artificial limb	Altered gait
Heart	Myocardial infarction with abnormal rhythms	Automatic implantable cardio-defibrillators	Dependence on equipment
Spinal cord	Diving accident	Rehabilitation	Altered mobility
Kidney	Renal failure	Hemodialysis	Dependence on equipment
		Peritoneal dialysis	
		Renal transplant	Acceptance of a donated organ

patients manage the physical and psychosocial changes. Helping patients recognize, accept, and live with the change requires recognition that self-esteem and role performance may also be affected.

Body image has received considerable attention in nursing literature.[6-11] This body of knowledge forms the basis for interventions with patients experiencing losses associated with altered body image. Body image may also be altered by the need to incorporate a prosthetic device or donated body part.

Self-Esteem Disturbance

Self-esteem develops as a part of self-concept through the reflected appraisals of significant others. The interpretation of such information is probably more important than the content. Self-esteem, which is a section of the hierarchy of human needs postulated by Maslow,[11] is only partly related to material, economic, or social conditions. Having high self-esteem helps individuals deal with the environment and face the maturational and situational crises of life. A low self-regard impairs the ability to adapt. Overall, the goal is for individuals to maintain a high regard for themselves in the midst of ever-changing views. When met, this goal contributes to the quality of life for individuals. People with well-developed self-esteem are at less risk for such disturbances than those with poorly developed self-esteem.

Self-Esteem Disturbances arise when individuals experience a decrease in self-worth, self-respect, self-approval, or self-confidence. Causes of the decrease include repeated negative interactions with significant others and cognitive-perceptual difficulties.

Self-esteem, which has been studied frequently in a variety of contexts,[12-18] is an important concept for nurses and other health professionals, who have a significant impact on patients. When the illness is critical, the self-esteem level of patients may be imperiled. Perhaps patients caused the accident that injured themselves and others, including family members. Perhaps the patients were under the influence of alcohol or drugs. Perhaps they will be subject to arrest. Perhaps they will lose their jobs or be unable to return to work. Nurses tend to avoid topics that make them uncomfortable, and patients and families can easily get the message not to discuss those issues. Nurses who express negative reactions to patients, either openly or covertly, reinforce patients' low self-esteem.

Older people face loss of autonomy that may lower self-esteem, and changes in the expectations of others for behavior and capacity may occur. Losses related to aging, dependency, retirement, and deaths of friends and family may also affect self-esteem. If nurses are impatient with performance deficits, patients may feel inadequate and guilty. If patients are treated as children, they may consider themselves burdens and react with resentment. Failure to include patients in decision making may cause them to feel useless and rejected. On the other hand, individuals with a strong sense of self-worth are likely to be adjusted, confident, and competent.

The level of self-esteem is an important factor in the response to a critical illness, and lowered self-esteem may negatively affect behavior during illness. Patients with severe burns may interpret the avoidance behavior of nurses and family who are appalled by the patients' appearance and the odor in their rooms as a devaluation of themselves. Patients may refuse to cooperate with the treatment regimen and may judge themselves failures. They may be unable to see their future productivity. Anticipatory interventions that assist the staff and family members in their care of patients help to avoid such a situation. Nurses should communicate acceptance, genuine interest, and concern and should avoid being judgmental.

Powerlessness

Powerlessness may be defined as the perceived inability to influence or control an outcome. *Powerlessness* as a nursing diagnosis is defined as the perception of individuals that their own actions will not significantly affect an outcome.[5]

Most people expect to have the power to participate in making decisions that affect them. When they feel their choices are limited, patients may act against their own best interests.[19] Given enough frustration, any exercise of control—even one with negative outcomes, such as signing out of the hospital against medical advice (AMA)—can become attractive.

Individuals vary in the amount of control they prefer.[20] Patients may feel power but may not desire it. Important variables in this regard are the illness; values, traits, attitudes, and experiences; hospital setting; and social displacement. Personality, age, religion, occupation, income, residence, and race may all be pertinent factors. Apparently an increase exists in variability in the amount of control preferred as people age. Rodin[20] pointed out that giving individuals more control than desired may result in negative outcomes: stress, worry, and self-blame. The critical care unit routines may oppose or preclude any control by patients. Persons to whom control is important should be encouraged to continue to control as many areas of their lives as possible. On the other hand, patients must be given the opportunity to choose not to control.[21]

One explanation of this variable interest in control is the concept of locus of control. This idea of expectancy of control developed by Rotter[22] has been particularly helpful in explaining the variability of responses of individuals to similar situations. The locus of control is a personality characteristic, a relatively stable tendency for people to perceive events and outcomes as within or outside their control regardless of the situation.

People with an internal locus of control tend to believe that events are under their control. People with an external locus of control, however, tend to believe that events are related to chance, fate, or others. Situations exist in which people with an internal locus of control have made serial lifestyle changes based on medical advice and then have experienced a major illness, typically a myocardial infarction. This experience forces them to believe that their own actions will not (because they have not) significantly affect the outcome. Repeated or significant experiences with illness may reinforce belief in an external locus of control for people who originally possessed an internal locus of control. Nursing interventions that support the power or influence individuals wield help prevent an all-encompassing sense of *Powerlessness*.

In the critical care unit, threats to patients' control include the unusual signs and symptoms of the illness and inadequate knowledge about the situation.[23] The disease process and the personal, psychologic, and social situation interact to affect patients' perception of control or lack of control. If *control* is defined as the ability to determine the use of time, space, and resources, admission to a critical care unit curtails control to varying extents. Patients can no longer decide about physical care, socializing, or privacy. They are under the close scrutiny of the nurses and physicians and have decreased physical strength.

The extent of *Powerlessness* is determined by the situation. Critically ill patients generally have experienced a rapid onset of illness without time to acquire the illness role. A sense of *Powerlessness* in such situations is not unexpected. Poor interactions with health care providers may make the situation worse. Patients may react aggressively, try bargaining, or refuse to comply with diagnostic and treatment regimens. Nurses have a primary role in preventing and alleviating the perception of personal *Powerlessness* in patients and families.

Coping Alterations

According to White,[24] coping is an adaption strategy. People use coping when faced with serious problems that they cannot master with familiar behaviors. Uncomfortable affects such as anxiety and grief accompany coping.[25,26] Age and gender affect coping and necessitate different social supports.

When patients cope effectively, what they are doing to cope often goes unnoticed. Emotionally, patients seem relatively comfortable, cooperating with care and exhibiting nonproblematic behavior. Such patients are using appropriate, possibly multiple, coping or defense mechanisms without interfering with care.

Coping Mechanisms

Regression

Regression is an unconscious defense mechanism that involves a retreat in the face of stress to behavior characteristic of an earlier developmental level.[27] Regression allows patients to give up their usual roles, autonomy, and privacy to become passive recipients of medical and nursing care. Patients who do not regress jeopardize their own care. For example, patients may insist on conducting business from the bedside or demand bathroom privileges when getting out of bed would be unsafe. Conversely, patients who become too regressed present another problem. They may become childlike in interactions with staff, whining, clinging to staff, and attempting to keep nurses at the bedside constantly.

Although the behavior of these patients can be extremely provocative, avoiding confrontations or reprimands is advisable. Negative responses from staff may only worsen a situation in which patients are already struggling with issues of dependence and autonomy.

Suppression

Suppression is a conscious, intentional process in which patients push ideas, problems, or desires out of their conscious thoughts.[27] Patients often use suppression when they are in no position to resolve overwhelming problems. Weissman[28] describes strategic suppression as a conscious attempt to focus only on the problems patients can solve in the present. For example, a patient who has lost a job before emergency coronary artery bypass surgery uses suppression appropriately by postponing worry about employment until after recovery from surgery.

Denial

Denial is an unconscious defense mechanism that reduces anxiety by eliminating or reducing the seriousness of the perceived threat. According to NANDA,[29] *denial* includes conscious and unconscious attempts to disavow knowledge or the meaning of an event.[29] In this text the psychoanalytic definition is used rather than the nursing diagnosis to allow for the distinction between denial and suppression. When used by a critically ill patient, denial reduces the anxiety and the threat of the illness.[30] The degree to which denial is used varies among patients and may vary in the same patient at different times.

Other Factors

Trust

Trust manifests itself in critical care patients as the belief that the staff will get them through the illness, managing any untoward event that might occur. Trust is an unconscious process in which patients transfer the trust learned in early significant relationships onto caregivers in the present.[31] Trust not only reduces fear of death but also allows patients to put themselves "in your hands," thereby fostering compliance with all aspects of care.

Hope

Although hope has long been recognized as a significant factor in patient recovery and survival, the phenomenon receives little attention until patients become hopeless. Hope, which can exist even in grim circumstances, is the expectation that a desire will be fulfilled.[32] Hope supports patients and helps them endure the physical and psychologic insults that are part of daily experience.

Religious beliefs and practices

Religious beliefs and practices may provide patients with some acceptance of an illness, a sense of mastery and control, a source of hope and trust beyond the limits the staff can provide, and the strength to endure stress. Patients may discuss religious beliefs and concerns openly or view the subject as a private matter. Patients who rely on religious beliefs benefit from nurses who respect those beliefs and who remain sensitive to patients' willingness or reluctance to discuss these beliefs.[33]

Use of family support

Patients can use the presence of a supportive family to cope with critical illness.[34,35] Patients with a supportive family know that family members share with them a past and hope for a future. Supportive families also love the

patients as individuals and members of the family and know the patients in ways the staff cannot. With a supportive family, patients may know that their experience is truly understood, even when little is said. Family members can also attend to the practical problems patients cannot, such as managing finances.

Sharing concerns

Sharing concerns with caring and understanding listeners can relieve some of patients' emotional distress. Patients may share concerns and are consoled knowing that they are not alone in the experience.[28] However, patients may be reluctant to upset loved ones further or may have a family in which such communication is not the norm. Patients who rely on this coping mechanism benefit from nurses who recognize when patients need to talk and who know how to listen.

Family Member Support

By showing support to family members at the bedside, nurses enhance the value of the visits for patients.[35-38] Patients often look to family for love, understanding, support, and care of matters to which they cannot attend themselves. Although nurses cannot perform full family assessment and give ongoing support to all family members, critical care nurses can observe the quality of the patient-family interaction and formulate interventions that will aid families in supporting patients. (Specific nursing interventions to support family members are listed in Box 4-2)

Assessment of Ineffective Coping

Patients may indicate *Ineffective Coping* through behaviors. Overt hostility, severe regression, or noncompliance with treatment may also suggest *Ineffective Coping*. Patients may report such problems as severe *anxiety* or despondence. Nurses who suspect that coping is ineffective should consider a number of factors before questioning patients directly.

Witnessing problematic behavior can be extremely uncomfortable for nurses, especially when that behavior is directed at them. Nurses can examine their own feelings by asking, Have I taken the behavior personally? Do I find the behavior particularly distasteful? Can I proceed with objectivity to serve patients' needs, or should I consult with others?

Whether coping is truly ineffective and whether intervention is indicated is not always clear. Nurses might ask whether patients' *Ineffective Coping* will jeopardize their care or the care of others and whether staff have anything to offer patients that will help them cope more effectively.

Clinical examples

One aspect of critical care nursing is knowing what emotional and behavioral responses should be expected in a

BOX 4 - 2

NURSING INTERVENTIONS TO SUPPORT FAMILY MEMBERS

- If family members are at a loss for what to say or do, nurses might offer a suggestion and find some words to put family members at ease. For example, nurses who observe family members staring helplessly at a confused patient experiencing intubation might say, "You can take his hand and tell him you are here."
- If family members are so upset that they completely lose composure, a brief attempt at supporting them away from the bedside may be adequate. In doing so, nurses may determine that family members need a consistent outside source of support and may make a referral according to department guidelines.
- If family members become more focused on the technical aspects of care than on patients, nurses can gently redirect the family members to the patients with the assurance that the staff will attend to the technical care.
- If family members are angry, hostile, cold, or aloof during visits, nurses may reflect those observations back to family members. For example, nurses may say, "I've been noticing an angry tone in your voice during visits with your wife." If this approach does not result in some resolution or explanation of the problem, a referral for family evaluation may be indicated.
- If family members seem unattuned to patients' experiences, nurses could try to convey what patients are experiencing and how best to provide support.

given patient care situation and recognizing atypical responses. When such responses are observed, careful assessment of underlying causes for *Anxiety* and appropriate interventions are essential.

When patients are restless or agitated, and nurses have ruled out physical causes such as hypoxia, other evidence of *Anxiety* should be sought. Are patients hypervigilant? Do they report *Fear* or *Anxiety?* If nursing measures do not reduce patients' *Anxiety* nurses might recommend evaluation for an anxiolytic medication or consider consultation with a psychiatric clinical nurse specialist.

When a patient overtly express distress about issues of autonomy and control as evidenced by unreasonable demands for attention or privileges in the critical care unit, a unified, consistent plan is essential. All staff members should agree to the plan, which is then written in the patient's record and presented to the patient in a caring and supportive manner. The plan should consider the patient's feeling of *Powerlessness* and make certain the limits on unreasonable behavior are clear to the patient.

Whenever possible, the staff should attempt to give the patient any control, autonomy, or privilege that is reasonable in the critical care setting.

When patients are so mistrustful of staff that their questions seem like interrogation, nurses should recognize that mistrust has a number of possible sources. Nurses may learn from family members that a patient has a lifelong history of being mistrustful or that the mistrust stems from experience with medical or nursing care that did not meet expectations or resulted in a negative outcome. In either case the staff should continue to work conscientiously and competently with the patient to build trust. However, if direct questioning reveals paranoid ideation or delusional thinking, nurses should recommend a psychiatric evaluation.

References

1. Driever MJ: *Theory of self-concept.* In Roy C, Sr, editor: *Introduction to nursing: an adaptation model,* Englewood Cliffs, NJ, 1976, Prentice-Hall.
2. Lee JM: Emotional reactions to trauma, *Nurs Clin North Am* 5(4):577, 1970.
3. Salkin J: *Body ego technique,* Springfield, Ill, 1973, Charles C Thomas.
4. Fisher S: *Body experience in fantasy and behavior,* New York, 1970, Appleton-Century-Crofts.
5. Kim M and others: *Pocket guide to nursing diagnosis,* ed 5, St Louis, 1993, Mosby.
6. Smith S: Extended body image in the ventilated patient, *Intensive Care Nurs* 5(1):31, 1989.
7. Baxley KO and others: Alopecia: effect on cancer patient's body image, *Cancer Nurs* 7(6):499, 1984.
8. Brundage DJ, Broadwell DC: *Altered body image.* In Phipps WJ, Long BC, Woods NF, editors: *Medical-surgical nursing: clinical concepts and practice,* ed 4, St Louis, 1991, Mosby.
9. Champion VL, Austin JK, Tzeng O: Assessment of relationships between self-concept and body image using multivariate techniques, *Issues Ment Health Nurs* 4(4):299, 1982.
10. Price B: A model for body-image care, *J Adv Nurs* 15:585, 1990.
11. Maslow AH: *Motivation and personality,* New York, 1954, Harper & Row.
12. Antonucci TC, Jackson JS: Physical health and self-esteem, *Fam Community Health* 6(4):1, 1983.
13. Cormack D: *Geriatric nursing: a conceptual approach,* Oxford, 1985, Blackwell Scientific Publications.
14. Hirst SP, Metcalf BJ: Promoting self-esteem, *J Gerontol Nurs* 10(2):72, 1984.
15. Meisenhelder JB: Self-esteem: a closer look at clinical interventions, *Int J Nurs Stud* 22(2):127, 1985.
16. Meisenhelder JB: Self-esteem in women: the influence of employment and perception of husband's appraisals, *Image J Nurs Sch* 18(1):8, 1986.
17. Norris J, Kunes-Connell M: Self-esteem disturbance, *Nurs Clin North Am* 20(4):745, 1985.
18. Stanwyck DJ: Self-esteem through the life span, *Fam Community Health* 6(4):11, 1983.
19. Janis IL, Rodin J: *Attribution, control, and decision-making: social psychology and health care.* In Stone GC, Adler NC, editors: *Health psychology—a handbook,* San Francisco, 1979, Jossey-Bass.
20. Rodin J: Aging and health: effects of the sense of control, *Science* 233:1271, 1986.

21. Roberts SL, White BS: Powerlessness and personal control model applied to the myocardial infarction patient, *Prog Cardiovasc Nurs* 5(3):84, 1990.

22. Rotter JB: Generalized expectancies for internal versus external control of reinforcement, *Psychol Monogr* 80(609):1, 1966.

23. Roberts SL: *Behavioral concepts and the critically ill patient,* ed 2, Norwalk, Conn, 1986, Appleton-Century-Crofts.

24. White RW: *Strategies of adaption: an attempt at systematic description.* In Monat A, Lazarus RS, editors: *Stress and coping: an anthology,* ed 2, New York, 1985, Columbia University Press.

25. Friedman M: Social support sources and psychological well-being in older women with heart disease, *Res Nurs Health* 16(4):405, 1993.

26. Webb M, Riggin O: A comparison of anxiety levels of female and male patients with myocardial infarction, *Crit Care Nurs* 17(2):118, 1994.

27. Stuart GW, Sundeen SJ, editors: *Principles and practice of psychiatric nursing,* ed 5, St Louis, 1995, Mosby.

28. Weissman AD: *The coping capacity,* New York, 1984, Human Sciences Press.

29. North American Nursing Diagnosis Association: *Taxonomy I Revised,* St Louis, 1990, The Association.

30. Robinson K: Developing a scale to measure denial levels of clients with actual or potential myocardial infarctions, *Heart Lung* 23(1):36, 1994.

31. Relling-Garskof K: Transferring the past to the present, *Am J Nurs* 87:476, 1987.

32. *Webster's ninth new collegiate dictionary,* Springfield, Mass, 1991, G & C Merriam.

33. Shaffer JL: Spiritual distress and critical illness, *Crit Care Nurs* 2:42, 1991.

34. Artinian N: Spouses' perceptions of readiness for discharge after cardiac surgery, *Appl Nurs Res* 6(2):80, 1993.

35. Halm M, Alpen M: The impact of technology on patients and families, *Nurs Clin North Am* 28(2):443, 1993.

36. Halm M, Alpern M: Support groups: an annotated bibliography for critical care nurses, *Crit Care Nurs* 17(6):118, 1994.

37. Kleiber C and others: Emotional responses of family members during critical care hospitalization, *Am J Crit Care* 3(1):70, 1994.

38. Warren N: Perceived needs of the family members in the critical care waiting room, *Crit Care Nurs Q* 16(3):56, 1993.

5

Sleep Alterations

JACQUELINE KARTMAN

CHAPTER OBJECTIVES

- State the stages of sleep.
- Explain three physiologic effects that occur during rapid eye movement (REM) sleep.
- Describe circadian desynchronization and its primary effects.
- Describe the changes in sleep resulting from the aging process.

- Define *dysfunctional sleep.*
- Name three commonly prescribed critical care medications that decrease REM sleep.
- Describe common symptoms of sleep deprivation.

KEY TERMS

circadian desynchronization, p. 42

NREM sleep, p. 39

REM rebound, p. 44

REM sleep, p. 40

sleep deprivation, p. 43

Because critical illness requires frequent treatments and 24-hour intensive monitoring, patients admitted to critical care units often suffer an altered sleep pattern. The inability to rest and sleep is one of the causes as well as one of the outcomes accompanying critical illness. A lack of sleep can have disastrous results for patients who are critically ill. Critical care nurses can promote recovery and healing through facilitating sleep for patients.[1] The purpose of this chapter is to familiarize critical care nurses with the phenomenon of sleep and the various types of sleep pattern disturbances that may occur in the critical care environment and to describe the assessment of sleep pattern disturbances in patients who are critically ill.

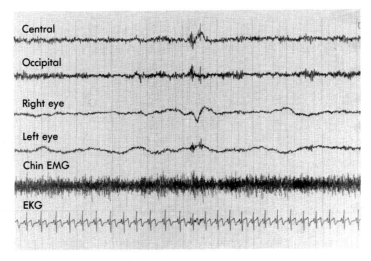

FIG. 5-1 Awake.

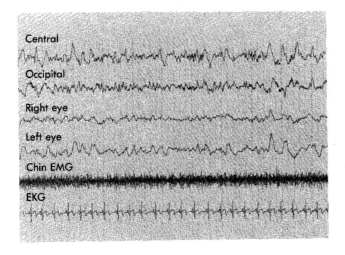

FIG. 5-2 Delta sleep NREM stage 4.

Physiology of Sleep

Sleep has been defined as "a state of unconsciousness from which a person can be aroused by appropriate sensory or other stimuli."[2] Adults normally spend approximately one third of their lives asleep. Research involving the simultaneous monitoring of the electroencephalogram (EEG), electrooculogram (EOG), and electromyogram (EMG) has shown that there are two distinct stages of sleep: rapid eye movement (REM) and non–rapid eye movement (NREM).

NREM Sleep

NREM sleep is divided into four stages (NREM 1 through 4), which are associated with progressive relaxation. NREM stage 1 is a transitional state, with the EEG being similar to that seen in the awake stage (Fig. 5-1). Stage 1 is the lightest level of sleep, lasting only 1 to 2 minutes. This stage is characterized by aimless thoughts, a feeling of drifting, and frequently, myoclonic jerks of the face, hands, and feet. People awaken easily during this stage.

NREM stage 2 differs from stage 1 in that the background wave frequency on the EEG is slower, with sleep spindles (characteristic waveforms) superimposed and high voltage spikes known as *K-complexes*.[3] This stage lasts from 5 to 15 minutes, during which time people become more relaxed but still awaken easily. Stages 1 and 2 in average young adults constitute 50% to 60% of the total sleep time.

Characterized by large, slow-frequency delta waves on the EEG, stages 3 and 4 are primarily differentiated by the relative percentage of these waves (Fig. 5-2). Random stimuli do not arouse individuals from these deepest levels of sleep. The time spent in stages 3 and 4 varies from 15 to 30 minutes and constitutes approximately 20% of the total sleep time. During NREM sleep the EOG gradually slows and eye movements cease. The EMG also declines, indicating profound muscle relaxation; however, it does not reach the low levels that it does in REM sleep. The parasympathetic nervous system predominates during NREM sleep. The cardiac and respiratory rates, the metabolic rate, and the blood pressure decrease to basal levels. Thus the supply/demand ratio of coronary blood flow is likely to improve.[4] NREM sleep may in fact have antidysrhythmic properties.

In addition, during slow wave sleep the anterior pituitary gland secretes growth hormone (GH), which functions to promote protein synthesis while sparing catabolic breakdown. Elevated GH and other anabolic hormones, such as prolactin and testosterone, imply that anabolism is taking place during NREM stage 4, particularly in tissues with a high protein content. Thus activities associated with NREM stage 4 include protein synthesis and tissue repair, such as the repair of epithelial and specialized cells of the brain, skin, bone marrow, and gastric mucosa.[5] NREM dreams are often realistic and thoughtlike,

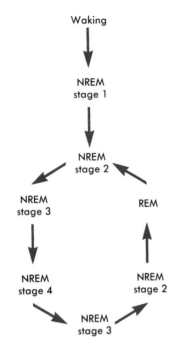

FIG. 5-3 The cyclic nature of sleep.

rarely in color, and often similar to a recent activity. These dreams are generally more difficult to remember than REM dreams. NREM sleep, then, is a time of energy conservation and renewal.

REM Sleep

REM, or paradoxical, **sleep** constitutes 20% to 25% of the total sleep time in young adults. This type of sleep is paradoxical in that some areas of the brain are quite active during REM sleep while other areas are suppressed. During REM sleep the EOG displays bursts of eye movements often associated with periods of dreaming. The EMG becomes essentially flat, indicating immobility and functional paralysis of the skeletal muscles. The cerebral cortical activity increases during REM, so the EEG resembles one taken during the waking state. It is more difficult to awaken from REM sleep than from any other stage of sleep.[3] In this regard, REM sleep can be considered a "dissociative state."

The sympathetic nervous system predominates during REM sleep. Oxygen consumption increases, and cardiac output, blood pressure, heart rate, and respiratory rate may become erratic. An increase in premature ventricular contractions (PVCs) and tachydysrhythmias associated with respiratory pauses may occur during REM sleep.[4] Evidence suggests that the adrenalin surge that more than doubles during REM sleep may be responsible for episodes of ischemia, sudden cardiac death, and strokes in the early morning hours.[6] Serum cholesterol and antidiuretic hormone levels increase, and perfusion to the gray matter in the brain doubles. The dreams of REM sleep tend to be colorful, vivid, and implausible,

often containing an element of paralysis. REM sleep filters information stored from the day's activities, sifting the important from the trivial, helping psychologically to integrate activities such as problem solving. REM sleep seems to facilitate emotional adaptation to the physical and psychologic environment and is needed in large quantities after periods of stress or learning. The adequacy of sleep is judged by the relative periods spent in each of the stages of sleep.[7]

REM sleep, like the other stages of sleep, is essential to physiologic and psychologic well-being. REM sleep is of great importance to nurses because as patients enter this stage of sleep, nurses may be concerned by changes in vital signs. If nurses increase the monitoring of patients, adjust drips, and measure vital signs in response to this perceived change in condition, patients may awaken before getting sufficient sleep. Further research must address the ways in which nurses can assess sleep and all of its stages without unnecessarily disrupting patients from their much-needed sleep. An accurate knowledge of sleep will assist nurses in monitoring patients safely while ensuring that they achieve optimal quality of sleep.

Cyclic Aspects of Sleep

At the onset of sleep, people normally progress through repetitive cycles, beginning with NREM stages 1 through 4 and then back again to stage 2. From stage 2, they enter REM. Stage 2 is then reentered, and the cycle repeats (Fig. 5-3). These cycles occur at approximately 90-minute intervals, so four or five cycles are normally completed in the sleep period. Early in the sleep period, NREM predominates. During the end of the sleep period, REM periods tend to be longer than those of NREM sleep.

The rhythmic nature of sleep is not unique. The body experiences rhythms in temperature, blood pressure, heart rate, respiratory rate, and hormone secretion. This cyclic 24-hour rhythm has been termed the *circadian rhythm.* Within the central nervous system the bilaterally paired suprachiasmatic nuclei are the major endogenous pacemaker for the circadian rhythms.[8] Sleep normally occupies the low phase of the circadian rhythm, whereas wakefulness and activity normally occupy the higher phase. Although regular nighttime sleep is synchronized with other circadian rhythms, such as hormone levels, temperature, and metabolic rate, the major determinants of human sleep are external time cues such as light and dark changes and particular social events such as meal times.[9]

The cyclic nature of sleep and wakefulness is thought to be regulated by complex neurochemical reactions arising in the tissues of the brain stem known as the *reticular formation.* The sleep-wakefulness cycles as well as the REM/nonREM cycle are thought to be mediated by the neurotransmitters *serotonin, dopamine, norepinephrine,* and *epinephrine.* Research suggests that the control of sleep is a complex process not confined to one localized part of the brain.[10]

The sleep-wake cycle follows the circadian rhythm in a 24-hour cycle synchronized with other biologic rhythms. Nighttime sleep is the normal pattern for most adults. Serotonin, for example, is usually released around 8 PM to prepare the body for sleep. Conversely, adreno-corticotropic hormone (ACTH), corticotropin-releasing hormone (CRH), and cortisol all normally peak in the early morning hours to prepare individuals for the day's stresses. If people are deprived of sleep, especially the deeper stages, these hormones will still be released but at times that may or may not coordinate appropriately with the stresses that must be faced. Thus an abnormal sleep pattern compromises patients' ability to cope with the stress of critical illness, thereby complicating their recovery. When sleep occurs during the low phase of the circadian rhythm, circadian synchronization is present. Sleep that occurs during normal waking hours is out of phase or desynchronized (Fig. 5-4). Desynchronized sleep is rated as poor quality and causes a decreased arousal threshold; therefore frequent awakenings are more likely. Irritability, restlessness, depression, anxiety, and decreased accuracy in task performance are characteristic effects of desynchronized sleep. Resynchronization with the circadian rhythm must occur whenever sleep has become desynchronized for individuals to establish a normal sleep-activity pattern. Although variable among individuals, the resynchronization process is thought to require a minimum of 3 days with a consistent sleep-wake schedule. Persons experiencing resynchronization often feel fatigued and unable to perform all their daily activities.

Sleep Changes with Age

As the biologic systems change during the normal aging process, stress is placed on the human system and the delicate mechanism of sleep is altered.[11] Hayter,[7] in a study of 212 healthy, noninstitutionalized older adults ages 65 to 93, found extreme variability in the sleep behaviors of different subjects within age groups. Sleep behaviors between men and women had few differences, although women did report more difficulty getting to sleep and more frequent use of sleep aids than men. The number of daytime naps and nighttime awakenings and variability in sleep behaviors increased with age. By age 75, the number of naps and length of naptime increased, resulting in a gradual increase in the total sleep time. Therefore both the time needed to fall asleep and the amount of time spent in bed increased with age.

The number of awakenings increases significantly, from one or two to as many as six per night; thus older persons experience an increase in the total duration of NREM stage 1 sleep and an increase in the number of shifts into stage 1. The duration of NREM stage 2 sleep changes very little; however, awakenings from NREM stage 2 sleep become more frequent. NREM stage 3

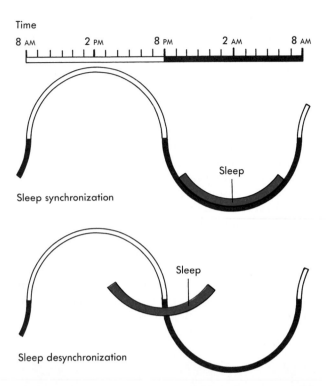

FIG. 5-4 Sleep synchronization and desynchronization with circadian rhythm.

tends to be normal. The duration of NREM stage 4, however, declines rapidly; by age 50, it is reduced by 50%. Little or no stage 4 sleep may be found in 25% of the population in the sixth decade of life. Stage 4 sleep is virtually absent in old age, with REM sleep remaining stable but more equally distributed through the night. These changes—along with more fragmentation, increased sleep-onset problems, and frequent long periods of wakefulness at night—cause older persons to perceive an impairment in their quality of sleep. In caring for older persons, nurses must remember that individuals differ widely in terms of both the age of onset of these changes and individual adaptations.

Dysfunctional Sleep

In acutely ill patients the amount, quality, and consistency of sleep may all decrease. Total sleep deprivation rarely occurs outside the experimental setting; however, in the critical care unit, sleep is often interrupted or fragmented, which alters the normal stages and cycles and produces dysfunctional sleep.[12] With frequent interruptions in sleep, patients spend a larger proportion of time in the transitional stages (NREM stages 1 and 2) and less time in the deeper stages of sleep (NREM stages 3 and 4 and REM). Thus patients may suffer a decrease in total sleep time (TST) if they do not receive their usual amount of sleep and may also experience selective deprivation of the deeper stages of sleep.[13,14]

Circadian Desynchronization

Circadian desynchronization is another form of sleep pattern disturbance that may affect critically ill patients. The loss of rhythmicity that may result from external stressors then alters the timing relationships of neural, hormonal, and cellular systems. Animals and humans respond to stressors such as surgery, immobilization, and pain with increased levels and altered timing of adrenal and other hormones. Farr and others[15] reported that circadian levels; the timing of temperature, blood pressure, and heart rate; and urinary excretion of catecholamines, sodium, and potassium were altered after surgery in hospitalized patients. Nurses should closely observe patients for clinical manifestations of such alterations and anticipate such problems as poor responses to physiologic challenges, disruption of sleep, gastrointestinal disturbances, decreased vigilance and attention span, and malaise. Nursing interventions that maintain normal rhythmicity of the day-night cycle—opening window blinds, placing clocks and calendars within the view of patients, allow-

ing patients to retire and rise at familiar times and following individual sleep-related rituals—should be encouraged. Nurses should also minimize disruption during rest periods.[15]

Pharmacology and Sleep

Patients hospitalized in critical care units often receive pharmacologic therapy, which may affect their quality of sleep and compound sleep disturbances. Critical care nurses should be aware of the effects that commonly used drugs have on sleep. In fact, hypnotic drugs have been found to promote the lighter stages of sleep (e.g., NREM stage 2) and may, paradoxically, be the cause of night terrors, hallucinations, and agitation in older patients.[15]

Barbiturates and sedative-hypnotic and analgesic medications may compound sleep disorders by further decreasing NREM stages 3 and 4 and REM sleep. Amobarbital, secobarbital, and pentobarbital reduce REM and increase NREM stage 2 sleep. Phenobarbital decreases

TABLE 5-1

COMMON DRUGS THAT AFFECT SLEEP

DRUG	EFFECT ON SLEEP	COMMENTS
BARBITURATES		
Amobarbital	Increases NREM 2	These are not considered drugs of choice because of toxicity and long-lasting effects.
Pentobarbital	Suppresses REM	
Secobarbital		Often patients experience rebound insomnia, restless sleep, and frequent dreaming and nightmares when drugs are discontinued.
BENZODIAZEPINES		
Diazepam	Increases NREM 1	NREM suppression is not dose related.
	Decreases NREM 3 and 4	REM suppression is dose related.
	Decreases REM	Drug may increase sleep apneic episodes.
Flurazepam	Increases total sleep time	There are conflicting reports about effects on sleep.
	Decreases NREM 2, 3, and 4	
	Decreases REM	Long half-life may produce daytime drowsiness.
Midazolam hydrochloride	No reports available	
Triazolam	Decreases sleep latency (time it takes to get to sleep)	Drug has a short half-life.
		Should not be used for a prolonged time because of decreased effectiveness.
	Decreases awakenings	
	Increases total sleep time	Nurses should use decreased doses with older patients.
MISCELLANEOUS		
Chloral hydrate	Thought to be an effective sedative that does not disrupt sleep	Drug has a short half-life, and some reports of nightmares exist.
		Increased daytime drowsiness occurs.
Chlordiazepoxide	Minimally disrupts sleep	
Methaqualone		
Morphine sulfate	Decreases NREM 3 and 4	Drug results in increased spontaneous arousals and overall lighter sleep.
	Decreases REM	

REM sleep in doses greater than 200 mg. REM rebound (discussed later in this chapter) has been documented after withdrawal from phenobarbital therapy.[13]

Diazepam increases NREM stage 1 and reduces both NREM stages 3 and 4 and REM. REM suppression depends on the dose, with larger doses leading to greater suppression. Flurazepam hydrochloride may be an effective hypnotic if administered in dosages equaling less than 60 mg/day. However, the long half-life of flurazepam may lead to morning drowsiness and may increase sleep apneic episodes in susceptible persons. Chloral hydrate has been shown to be an effective sedative that does not simultaneously disrupt sleep. Chlordiazepoxide and methaqualone also minimally disrupt sleep. Triazolam is effective for short-term use in increasing the total sleep time and decreasing the number of nocturnal awakenings, although it decreases REM sleep during the first 6 hours of sleep. These REM changes have been predominantly noted in young adults. An early morning "hangover" may occur with triazolam, and rebound insomnia may occur in the first two nights after discontinuation of the drug.[16] Morphine increases spontaneous arousals during sleep and shortens the sleep time by reducing both REM and NREM stages 3 and 4, resulting in overall lighter sleep.[17]

The prolonged half-life of medications, coupled with altered metabolism or decreased excretion of the drug resulting from renal or liver disease that may occur in older persons, can cause the effects of sedatives to continue into the daytime, leading to confusion and sluggishness. Adequate pain management facilitates sleep and rest. A low-dose narcotic analgesic, administered continuously at night and set for patient control during the day, allows for relief without causing patients to awaken and request pain medication.[18] Sedative and analgesic medications should not be withheld, but rather, drugs that minimally disrupt sleep should be used to complement comfort measures, with dosages reduced gradually as the medication is no longer necessary. Critical care nurses must assess the need for sedative and analgesic medications, administer them in the most effective manner to promote sleep, and monitor their effectiveness (Table 5-1).

Sleep Deprivation

Much of what is known about the function of sleep has been learned from observations made when people are deprived of sleep in the laboratory setting. Both physiologic and psychologic symptoms of **sleep deprivation** have been reported[16,19] (Box 5-1). These symptoms may be but are not always associated with the length of sleep deprivation. The symptoms vary among individuals with such factors as age, premorbid personality, motivation, and environmental factors.[20]

Selective REM Deprivation

Selective REM deprivation leads to irritability, apathy, decreased alertness, and increased sensitivity to pain.

Continued loss of REM sleep may lead to perceptual distortion and significant disturbance in mental-emotional function, often within 72 hours of REM deprivation. Manifestations of sleep deprivation range from disorientation and restlessness to frank auditory and visual hallucinations, with personality changes such as withdrawal and paranoia.[20]

Selective NREM Deprivation

Selective NREM deprivation is less well studied, but it appears to result primarily in fatigue.[17] Because of the renewal, repair, and conservation functions of NREM sleep, deprivation may impair the immune system and depress the body's defenses, making patients vulnerable to disease.

The critical care environment affects both the quantity and quality of sleep critically ill patients receive.[21] Patients admitted to the critical care unit are bombarded with combined sensory overload and deprivation and unfamiliar sights, sounds, people, and perceptions. The critical care unit affords little time for sleep; noise, lights, and patient care activities interfere with sleep patterns.[22,23] Such environmental conditions have been shown to be of primary importance in sleep deprivation in the critical care unit. Dlin and others[24] showed that the chief deterrents to sleep in the critical care unit were, in order of importance (1) activity and noise, (2) pain and physical condition, (3) nursing procedures, (4) lights, (5) vapor tents, and (6) hypothermia. Woods and Falk[25] found that 10% to 17% of noises in the critical care unit were of a level capable of arousing patients from sleep (greater than 70 decibels).

Psychologic stresses and fear associated with the critical care environment and the critical illness make it difficult for patients to relax and fall asleep. Fear and stress precipitate sympathetic nervous system stimulation, which decreases the arousal threshold and results in frequent awakenings and sleep stage transitions.[11]

The relationship between sleep deprivation and de-

B O X   5 - 1

Effects of Selective Sleep Deprivation

SYMPTOMS OF NREM SLEEP DEPRIVATION

Fatigue
Anxiety
Increased illness

SYMPTOMS OF REM SLEEP DEPRIVATION

Restlessness
Disorientation
Combativeness
Delusions/illusions
Hallucinations

lirium in the critical care unit is significant.[26] Helton and others[26] correlated mental status alterations (disorientation, combativeness, hallucinations, paranoia, and delusions) and sleep deprivation. A 33% increase in mental status alterations was found in severely sleep-deprived patients, defined as those who received less than 50% of their normal sleep time. Shaver, in a review of sleep research, notes that sleep deprivation is considered to be a contributing factor in postoperative psychosis.[27]

Mortality is higher in critical care patients who exhibit symptoms of psychosis or delirium.[28] Perhaps persons experiencing hallucinations and paranoia (the most severe consequences of sleep deprivation and critical care unit psychosis) are in fact dreaming in the awake state. This hypothesis remains to be verified by research; however, caution needs to be taken in diagnosing previously nonconfused elderly patients as having organic mental disorder (OMD) until the possibility of sleep deprivation has been ruled out.

Recovery Sleep

The changes in physiologic and psychologic performance resulting from sleep deprivation can be reversed through recovery sleep. Rosa and others[29] found that recall returned to baseline with 4 to 8 hours of recovery sleep after 40 to 64 hours of total sleep deprivation.

Deprivation of REM and NREM stage 4 results in rebounds in an attempt to compensate for "debts." The phenomenon of **REM rebound** occurs after selective REM deprivation. In an attempt to make up for lost REM and NREM stage 4 sleep, REM and NREM stage 4 periods quantitatively increase in the sleep periods after the deprivation. NREM stage 4 sleep is preferentially restored first, presumably because of its anabolic function. Because REM sleep is replenished last, it is more likely that REM debts will occur. REM rebound can exacerbate angina, dysrhythmias, duodenal ulcer pain, or sleep apneic episodes.[11] When patients exhibit any of these symptoms and have had periods of sleep deprivation, nurses should consider REM rebound when determining the cause. Although the symptoms of angina, dysrhythmias, duodenal ulcer pain, and sleep apnea are treated as usual, further REM deprivation should be avoided.

Assessment and Intervention of Sleep Pattern Disturbance

Assessment of patients on admission to the critical care unit should include a description of the normal sleep pattern, including awakenings, naps, normal bedtime and waking time, and customary habits that enhance sleep; any recent changes in patients' normal pattern resulting from the acute illness; recent and more distant history of sleep disturbances; the severity, duration, and frequency of the problem; and history of chronic illnesses and physical conditions that may disturb sleep, such as pain, chronic obstructive pulmonary disease, bronchial asthma, bronchitis, arthritis, nocturnal angina, hyperthyroidism, hypertension, duodenal ulcer, or reflux esophagitis and nocturia. The patient's response to the critical care environment should be assessed, along with the noise level in the patient's immediate environment.

For patients most at risk for a *Sleep Pattern Disturbance* (e.g., patients with invasive monitoring, those requiring hourly or more frequent assessments and interventions, patients whose illness will require an extended stay in critical care, patients in pain, and patients exhibiting initial signs of sleep deprivation), keeping a sleep chart for 48 to 72 hours may help nurses assess actual quantity of sleep and necessary and unnecessary wakenings.[30] Sleep charts should include the date and time, whether patients were awake or asleep, and any procedures for which it was necessary to awaken them. A 24-hour flow sheet, common in critical care units, could include an area for documentation of sleep. Just as nurses document other data relevant to recovery, sleep periods of more than 90 minutes in duration, number and length of awakenings, and total possible sleep time should be recorded and evaluated. Nursing interventions specific to sleep pattern disturbances are found in Unit X.

References

1. Richards K: Sleep promotion in the critical care unit, *AACN Clin Iss* 5(2):152, 1994.
2. Guyton AC: *Medical physiology,* ed 8, Philadelphia, 1991, WB Saunders.
3. Rechtschaffen A, Kales A: *A manual of standardized terminology, techniques and scoring systems for sleep stages of human subjects,* 1968, US Department of Health, Education and Welfare.
4. Verrier RL, Kirby DA: Sleep and cardiac arrhythmias, *Ann N Y Acad Sci* 533:238, 1988.
5. Closs SJ: Assessment of sleep in hospitalized patients: a review of methods, *J Adv Nurs* 13:501, 1988.
6. Somers VL and others: Sympathetic/nerve activity during sleep in normal subjects, *N Engl J Med* 328(5):303, 1993.
7. Hayter J: Sleep behaviors of older persons, *Nurs Res* 32(4):242, 1983.
8. Brock MA: Chronobiology and aging, *J Am Geriatr Soc* 39(1):74, 1991.
9. Hodgson L: Why do we need sleep: relating theory to nursing practice, *J Advanced Nurs* 16:1503, 1991.
10. Fordham M. *Patient problems.* In Wilson Bennett J, Butemp L, editors: *A research base for nursing care,* London, 1988, Scutain Press.
11. Wilse WB: Age related changes in sleep, *Clin Geriatr Med* 5(2):275, 1989.
12. Fontaine D: Measurement of nocturnal sleep patterns in trauma patients, *Heart Lung* 18(4):402-410, 1989.
13. Sanford S: Sleep and the cardiac patient, *Cardiovasc Nurs* 19(5):19, 1983.
14. Topf M, Davis J: Critical care unit noise and rapid eye movement sleep, *Heart Lung* 22:252-258, 1993.
15. Farr LA, Campbell-Grossman C, Mack JM: Circadian disruption and surgical recovery, *Nurs Res* 37(3):170, 1988.
16. Brewer MJ: To sleep or not to sleep: the consequences of sleep deprivation, *Crit Care Nurse* 5(6):35, 1985.

17. Wotring K: Using research in practice, *Focus Crit Care* 9(5):34, 1982.
18. *Acute pain management guideline,* AHCPR publication no 92-0021, US Department of Health and Human Services, Feb 1992.
19. Baker C and others: The effect of environmental sound and communication on CCU patients' heart rate and blood pressure, *Res Nurs Health* 16:415, 1993.
20. Freemon F: *Sleep research,* Springfield, Ill, 1972, Charles C Thomas.
21. Hilton B: Quantity and quality of patient's sleep and sleep disturbing factors in a respiratory intensive care unit *Adv Nurs* 1:453, 1976.
22. Kido L: Sleep deprivation and intensive care unit psychosis, *Emphasis: Nurs* 4(1):23, 1991.
23. Spenceley S: Sleep inquiry: a look with fresh eyes, *Image J Nurs Sch* 25(3):249, 1993.
24. Dlin B, Rosen H, Dickstein K: The problems of sleep and rest in the intensive care unit, *Psychosomatics* 12:155, 1971.
25. Woods N, Falk S: Noise stimuli in the acute care area, *Nurs Res* 23:144, 1974.
26. Helton M, Gordon S, Nunnery S: The correlation between sleep deprivation and ICU syndrome, *Heart Lung* 9(3):464, 1980.
27. Shaver JL, Giblin EC: Sleep, *Annu Rev Nurs Res* 4:71-93, 1989.
28. Noble M: Communication in the ICU: therapeutic or disturbing, *Nurs Outlook* 27:195, 1979.
29. Rosa R, Bonnet M, Warm J: Recovery of performance during sleep following sleep deprivation, *Psychophysiology* 20:152, 1983.
30. Edwards G, Schuring L: Pilot study: validating staff nurses' observations of sleep and wake states among critically ill patients using polysomnography, *Am J Crit Care* 2(2):125-131, 1993.

6

Nutritional Alterations

MARY COURTNEY MOORE

CHAPTER OBJECTIVES

- Describe the adverse effects of nutritional impairments on critically ill patients.
- Assess the nutritional status of critically ill patients with cardiovascular, pulmonary, neurologic, renal, gastrointestinal, and endocrine alterations.
- Recognize nutritional alterations commonly associated with cardiovascular, pulmonary, neurologic, renal, gastrointestinal, and endocrine systems.

- Collaborate with a multidisciplinary team in designing a nutrition program for critically ill patients.
- Identify complications of nutrition support and nursing interventions for prevention and management of these complications.

KEY TERMS

kwashiorkor, p. 48
marasmus, p. 48

protein-calorie malnutrition
  (PCM), p. 48

total parenteral nutrition (TPN),
  p. 64

Metabolic Response to Undernutrition and Stress

Physiologic stress resulting from injury, trauma, major surgery, and/or sepsis makes patients vulnerable to malnutrition.[1-4] This physiologic stress results in profound metabolic alterations that persist from the time of the stressful event until the completion of wound healing and recovery. Stress normally causes an increased metabolic rate (hypermetabolism) that necessitates a rise in oxygen consumption and energy expenditure.[1]

The hypermetabolic process begins with hormonal changes triggered by the stressful event. With stimulation of the sympathetic nervous system, the adrenal medulla releases catecholamines (epinephrine and norepinephrine),[5] which stimulate the body's metabolic re-

46

sponse to stress. Also released in response to stress are adrenocorticotropic hormone (ACTH) and antidiuretic hormone (ADH) as well as glucocorticoids and mineralocorticoids.[5] Insulin resistance caused by the release of glucagon allows nutrient substrates, primarily amino acids, to move from peripheral tissues (e.g., skeletal muscle) to the liver for gluconeogenesis.[1]

This hypermetabolic process is the body's effort to mobilize the supply of circulating nutrient substrates such as glucose and amino acids. Unfortunately, this mobilization occurs at the expense of body tissue and function at a time when the needs for protein synthesis (e.g., for wound healing and acute phase proteins) also are high. Hyperglycemia prevails as the effects of increased catecholamines, glucocorticoids, and glucagon diminish the effects of insulin and the release of free fatty acids. Again the body relies on its protein stores to provide substrates for gluconeogenesis because glucose now becomes the major fuel source. Loss of protein results in a negative nitrogen balance and weight loss. The classic response to metabolic stress is the use of protein for fuel. Box 6-1 describes metabolic responses during stress.

B O X   6 - 1

METABOLIC RESPONSE TO STRESS

"EBB" PHASE (FIRST 24 TO 48 HOURS)
↓Metabolic rate
↓Body temperature
↓Blood insulin levels
↑Blood glucose levels
↑Blood lactate levels
↑Blood fatty acid levels

"FLOW" PHASE (FOLLOWS THE EBB PHASE)
Catabolic subphase

↑Metabolic rate
↑Body temperature
↑Heart rate
↑Blood glucose levels
↑Urinary nitrogen losses (resulting from decreased protein synthesis, increased protein degradation, or both)

Turning point subphase

Normalization of blood glucose
↓Urinary nitrogen excretion

Anabolic subphase

↓Protein synthesis

Resolution subphase

Return to normal metabolism

Modified from Moore F, Brennan M: *Surgical injury: body composition, protein metabolism, and neuroendocrinology,* In Ballinger WE, editor: *Manual of surgical nutrition,* Philadelphia, 1975, WB Saunders.

Implications of Undernutrition for the Sick or Stressed Patient

When protein and calorie intake are inadequate for more than a few hours, existing body proteins will be broken down to meet the body's needs. Even when people have large fat reserves, catabolism of body proteins will occur. Unlike fat, proteins can provide a significant source of glucose and the amino acids needed for tissue synthesis and repair. Well-nourished people tolerate a few days of starvation when not exposed to stress, but undernourished people with trauma, surgery, burns, or infection will have accelerated catabolism. Already undernourished patients exposed to stress (e.g., cancer patients with anorexia and weight loss who undergo surgery) are especially vulnerable.

Malnutrition in very ill patients is an ominous finding. Compared with well-nourished patients, undernourished patients are more likely to have major surgical complications. Wound dehiscence, decubitus ulcers, sepsis, and pulmonary infections are more common among undernourished patients. Malnourished patients also have longer hospital stays than well-nourished patients.[6]

Assessing Nutritional Status

Nutritional assessment is a multistep process involving the collection and evaluation of pertinent information from the patient's diet and medical history, physical examination, and laboratory values. The assessment can be performed by a designated member of the health care team, such as the dietitian or the nurse, or it can be a team effort.

History

Information about dietary intake and significant variations in weight is a vital part of patients' histories. A change of 10% or more in body weight during the past year or 5% to 6% during the past 3 months is usually considered significant. Significant findings from the nutrition history are delineated in Table 6-1.

Physical Examination

A thorough physical examination is an essential part of nutritional assessment. Checking for signs of muscle wasting, loss of subcutaneous fat, changes in skin or hair, and impairment of wound healing is especially important.

Laboratory Data

A wide range of diagnostic tests can provide information about nutritional status. Those most often used in the clinical setting are described in Table 6-2. As the table suggests, no diagnostic tests for evaluation of nu-

TABLE 6 - 1
NUTRITION HISTORY INFORMATION

AREA OF CONCERN	SIGNIFICANT FINDINGS	NUTRIENTS OF SPECIAL CONCERN
Inadequate intake of nutrients	Avoidance of specific food groups because of poverty or poor dentition	Protein, iron
	Alcohol abuse	Protein, vitamin B_1, niacin, folate
	Anorexia, nausea, vomiting	Most nutrients, particularly protein, electrolytes
	Confusion, coma	All nutrients
Inadequate absorption of nutrients	Previous GI surgeries:	
	Gastrectomy	Vitamin B_{12}, minerals, calories (if the patient experiences dumping syndrome)
	Ileal resection	Vitamins B_{12}, A, E; minerals; calories (in extensive small bowel resection)
	Certain medications:	
	Antacids, cimetidine (reduce upper duodenal acidity)	Minerals
	Cholestyramine (binds fat-soluble nutrients)	Vitamins A, D, E, K
	Corticosteroids	Protein
	Anticonvulsants	Calcium
Increased nutrient losses	Chronic or acute blood loss	Iron
	Severe diarrhea	Fluid, electrolytes
	Fistulas, draining abscesses, wounds	Protein, zinc
	Nephrotic syndrome	Protein, zinc
	Peritoneal dialysis or hemodialysis	Protein, zinc, water-soluble vitamins
Increased nutrient requirements	Fever*	Calories
	Surgery, trauma, burns, infection	Calories, protein, zinc, vitamin C
	Neoplasms (some types)	Calories, protein
	Physiologic demands (pregnancy, lactation, growth)	Calories, protein, iron

*Each 1° C (1.8° F) elevation in temperature increases caloric needs by approximately 13%.

trition are perfect; care must be taken in interpreting the results of the tests.

Evaluating Nutritional Assessment Findings and Determining Nutritional Needs

Patients rarely lack only one nutrient. Usually nutritional deficiencies are combined, with the patient lacking adequate amounts of protein, calories, and possibly vitamins and minerals. A common form of combined nutritional deficit among hospitalized patients is **protein-calorie malnutrition (PCM).** Two types of PCM are kwashiorkor and marasmus. **Kwashiorkor** is evidenced by low levels of the serum proteins albumin, transferrin, and prealbumin; low total lymphocyte count; impaired immunity; loss of hair or hair pigment; edema; and an enlarged, fatty liver. **Marasmus** is recognizable by weight loss, a decrease in skinfold measurements, loss of subcutaneous fat, muscle wasting, and low levels of creatinine excretion. Because PCM weakens musculature, increases vulnerability to infection, and sometimes prolongs hospital stays, the health

care team should diagnose this serious disorder as quickly as possible so that appropriate nutritional intervention can be implemented.

Nutritional Management by Systems

Nutrition and Cardiovascular Alterations

Diet and cardiovascular disease may interact in a variety of ways. In one situation, excessive nutrient intake—manifested by overweight or obesity and a diet rich in cholesterol and saturated fat—is a risk factor for development of arteriosclerotic heart disease. Conversely, the consequences of chronic myocardial insufficiency can include malnutrition.

Nutritional assessment in cardiovascular alterations

Nutritional assessments provide the information nurses and other members of the health care team need in planning patients' nutrition care and education. Table 6-3 summarizes key points of the nutrition assessment of cardiovascular patients. The major nutritional concerns relate to appropriateness of body weight and the levels of serum lipids and blood pressure.

TABLE 6-2
DIAGNOSTIC TESTS USED IN NUTRITION ASSESSMENT

AREA OF CONCERN	POSSIBLE DEFICIENCY	COMMENTS
SERUM PROTEINS		
Decrease of serum albumin, transferrin (iron transport protein), or thyroxine-binding prealbumin*	Protein	These proteins are produced in the liver, are depressed in hepatic failure, and are falsely low in fluid volume excess and elevated in volume deficit. Albumin has a long half-life (14-20 days) and is slow to change in malnutrition and repletion; transferrin has a half-life of 7-8 days, but levels increase in iron deficiency, and prevalence of iron deficiency limits usefulness in diagnosing protein deficits; prealbumin half-life is 2-3 days.
HEMATOLOGIC VALUES		
Anemia (decreased Hct, Hgb)		Hct and Hgb are falsely low in fluid volume excess and falsely high in fluid volume deficit.
Normocytic (normal MCV, MCHC)	Protein	
Microcytic (decreased MCV, MCH, MCHC)	Iron, copper	
Macrocytic (increased MCV)	Folate, vitamin B_{12}	
Total lymphocyte count (TLC = WBC × % lymphocytes)		
TLC of <1200/mm³	Protein	TLC is decreased in severe debilitating disease.
URINARY CREATININE		
Creatinine excretion of <17 mg/kg/day (women), <23 mg/kg/day (men)	Protein (reflection of lean body mass)	Collecting accurate 24-hr urine is difficult. Creatinine excretion varies widely from day to day; levels decline with age as percentage of lean body mass declines.
NITROGEN BALANCE†		
Negative values	Protein, calories (during calorie deficit, protein metabolized to provide calories)	Negative values occur when more nitrogen is excreted than consumed (reflects inadequate intake or increased needs); positive values occur when more is consumed than lost (e.g., during nutrition repletion, growth, pregnancy); normal healthy adults excrete exactly what they consume. Limitations: collecting accurate 24-hr urine is difficult; retention of nitrogen does not necessarily mean that it is being used for tissue synthesis.

Hct, Hematocrit; *Hgb*, hemoglobin; *MCV*, mean corpuscular volume; *MCHC*, mean corpuscular hemoglobin concentration; *MCH*, mean corpuscular hemoglobin; *TLC*, total lymphocyte count; *WBC*, white blood cell.
*Evaluation of at least one of these is a part of almost every nutritional assessment.
†Protein is 16% nitrogen. Thus nitrogen balance = [24-hr protein intake (g) × 0.16] − [24-hr urine urea nitrogen (g) + 4 g]. The 4 g is an estimate of fecal, skin, and other minor losses.

Nutritional intervention in cardiovascular alterations

MYOCARDIAL INFARCTION. The following guidelines will assist nurses in providing appropriate nutritional care for patients in the immediate post–myocardial infarction (MI) period:

1. Limit meal size for patients with severe myocardial compromise or postprandial angina.
2. Monitor the effect of caffeine on patients if caffeine is included in the diet.
3. Avoid serving foods at temperature extremes.

TABLE 6-3
NUTRITIONAL ASSESSMENT OF CARDIOVASCULAR PATIENTS

	SIGNIFICANT FINDINGS		
AREA OF CONCERN	HISTORY	PHYSICAL ASSESSMENT	LABORATORY DATA
Overweight/obesity	Excessive kcal intake (consult dietitian regarding nutrition history) Sedentary lifestyle	Weight >120% of desirable Triceps skinfold measurement of >90th percentile*	

Protein-calorie malnutrition (cardiac cachexia)	Chronic cardiopulmonary disease causing the following:
	  Decreased food intake related to angina, respiratory embarrassment, or fatigue during eating
	  Malabsorption of nutrients caused by hypoxia of the gut
	  Medications that impair appetite (e.g., digitalis, quinidine)
		Weight <85% of desirable
		Triceps skinfold measurement of <10th percentile†
		Muscle wasting
		Loss of subcutaneous fat
			Serum albumin <3.5 g/dl (or low serum transferrin or prealbumin level)
			Negative nitrogen balance
			Creatinine excretion <17 mg/kg/day (women) or <23 mg/kg/day (men)

Elevated serum lipid levels	Frequent or daily use of foods high in cholesterol and saturated fat, including red meat, cold cuts, bacon or sausage, butter, cream or nondairy creamer, foods containing shortening or lard or fried in those products, eggs, organ meats, cheese, ice cream Sedentary lifestyle Family history of hyperlipidemia Overweight or obesity	Xanthomas, or yellowish plaques deposited in the skin (uncommon)	Serum cholesterol >200 mg/dl Low-density lipoprotein cholesterol >130 mg/dl
Elevated blood pressure	Daily use of high-sodium foods and salt at the table Consumption of >2 oz of alcohol/day		

Modified from Moore MC: *Pocket guide to nutrition and diet therapy*, ed 2, St Louis, 1993, Mosby.
*20 mm for men and 34 mm for women.
†6 mm for men and 14 mm for women.

HYPERTENSION. The primary nutritional intervention for hypertensive patients is to limit sodium intake, usually to no more than 2 g/day. To achieve this level of intake, patients usually require help in avoiding foods high in sodium. The primary sodium source in the American diet is salt (sodium chloride) added during food processing and preparation or at the dinner table. One teaspoon of salt provides about 2.3 g of sodium. Most salt substitutes contain potassium chloride and may be used with the physician's approval by patients who have no renal impairment.

HEART FAILURE. Nutritional intervention in heart failure (HF) is designed to reduce fluid retained within the body and thereby reduce the preload. Because fluid accompanies sodium, limiting sodium is necessary to reduce fluid retention. Specific interventions include (1) limiting sodium intake, usually to 2 g/day or less, and (2) limiting fluid intake as appropriate. The amount ordered is usually 1.5 to 2 L/day, to include both fluids in the diet and those given with medications and for other purposes.

CARDIAC CACHEXIA. Severely malnourished cardiac patients often suffer from congestive heart failure (CHF). Therefore sodium and fluid restriction, as previously described, are appropriate. It is important to concentrate nutrients into as small a volume as possible and to serve small amounts frequently, rather than three large meals daily, which may overwhelm patients. Patients also can be given calorie-dense foods and supplements.

Because patients are likely to tire quickly and suffer from anorexia, tube feeding or total parenteral nutrition (TPN) may be necessary. When tube feeding is needed, formulas with 2 or more calories/ml are preferable. (Most commonly used formulas provide 1 calorie/ml.) Formulas appropriate for fluid-restricted patients include Magnacal (Sherwood), Isocal HCN (Mead Johnson), TwoCal HN (Ross), and Nutrisource (Sandoz). During TPN, 20% lipid emulsions with 2 calories/ml provide a concentrated energy source. (The 10% emulsions, in contrast, contain only 1.1 calorie/ml.)

Nurses must monitor the fluid status of these patients carefully when they are receiving nutritional support.

Body weight must be recorded daily; a consistent gain of more than 0.11 to 0.22 kg ($^1/_4$ to $^1/_2$ lb) a day usually indicates fluid retention rather than gain of fat and muscle mass. Nurses also must check patients frequently for increasing pulmonary and peripheral edema.

Nutrition and Pulmonary Alterations

Malnutrition has extremely adverse effects on respiratory function, decreasing both surfactant production and vital capacity.[7] Moreover, individuals who lose weight lose proportionately more mass from the diaphragm than total body mass, which further impairs ventilation.[7] Early detection and treatment of nutritional deficits seem to be especially important in patients with pulmonary alterations, who often find it difficult to consume adequate oral nutrients and can rapidly become malnourished.

Nutritional assessment in pulmonary alterations
Nutritional assessment is summarized in Table 6-4. Patients with respiratory compromise are especially vulnerable to the effects of fluid volume and carbohydrate excess and must be assessed continually for these complications.

Nutritional intervention in pulmonary alterations
PREVENT OR CORRECT UNDERNUTRITION AND UNDERWEIGHT. Nurses and dietitians can work together to encourage oral intake in undernourished or potentially undernourished patients who are capable of eating. Small, frequent feedings are especially important because a very full stomach can interfere with diaphragmatic movement. Mouth care needs to be provided before meals and snacks to clear the palate of the flavors of sputum and medications. Administering bronchodilators with food can help reduce gastric irritation.

AVOID EXCESS CARBOHYDRATE ADMINISTRATION. The production of carbon dioxide increases when carbohydrate is relied on as the primary energy source, and this raises the respiratory quotient. This development is usually insignificant in patients who are eating foods. Instead, it is an iatrogenic complication of TPN, in which glucose is often the predominant calorie source, or occasionally of tube feeding with a very high carbohydrate formula.[8] Excessive carbohydrate intake can raise the $Paco_2$ level sufficiently to make it difficult to wean patients from the ventilator. Patients who are not dependent on a ventilator may experience tachypnea or shortness of breath on a high carbohydrate regimen.

Nurses who note increasing $Paco_2$ in patients receiving carbohydrate-based TPN should discuss with physicians the possibility of providing daily lipid infusions for these patients. A regimen with both lipids and carbohydrates providing the nonprotein calories is optimal for patients with respiratory compromise.

AVOID EXCESSIVE SERUM LIPID LEVELS. Excessive lipid intake can impair capillary gas exchange in the lungs, although not usually enough to produce an increase in $Paco_2$ or decrease in Pao_2 values. However, patients with severe respiratory alteration may be further compromised by lipid overdose. If lipid intake is maintained at no more than 2 g/kg/day, lipid excess is rarely a problem. Lipids are available as 20 g lipid/100 ml (20% lipid emulsion) and 10 g/100 ml (10% emulsion). Serum triglyceride levels are usually maintained at less than 150 mg/dl. Higher levels may indicate inadequate clearance and the need to decrease the lipid dosage.

PREVENT FLUID VOLUME EXCESS. Pulmonary edema and failure of the right side of the heart, which may result from fluid volume excess, further worsen the status of patients with respiratory compromise. Strict intake records must be maintained to allow accurate totals of fluid intake. Usually patients require no more than 35 to 50 ml/kg/day of fluid. For patients receiving nutritional support, fluid intake can be reduced by using 20% lipid emulsions as a source of calories, using tube feeding formulas providing at least 2 calories/ml (the dietitian can suggest appropriate choices), and choosing oral supplements that are low in fluid. Some examples are cottonseed oil (Lipomul [Upjohn]), an oral lipid supplement providing 6 cal/ml, and powdered glucose polymers, which increase caloric intake without increasing volume.

Nutrition and Neurologic Alterations

Because neurologic disorders tend to be long-term problems, they necessitate good nutritional care to prevent nutritional deficits and promote well-being.

Nutritional assessment in neurologic alterations
Nutrition-related assessment findings vary widely in patients with neurologic alterations depending on the type of disorder present. Some common findings are shown in Table 6-5.

Nutritional intervention in neurologic alterations
PREVENTION OR CORRECTION OF NUTRITIONAL DEFICITS

ORAL FEEDINGS. Patients with dysphagia or weakness often experience the greatest difficulty in swallowing dry foods or thin liquids that are difficult to control such as water. For these patients, nurses and dietitians can work together to plan suitable meals and evaluate patient acceptance and tolerance.

TUBE FEEDINGS OR TPN. Patients who are unconscious or unable to eat because of severe dysphagia, weakness, ileus, or other reasons will need tube feedings or TPN. Prompt initiation of nutritional support must be a priority for patients with neurologic impairments. Infection and fever, as may occur with encephalitis and meningitis, increase the need for protein and calories. Needs for protein, calories, zinc, and vitamin C increase during wound healing, as occurs in trauma patients and patients with decubitus ulcers.

Tube feeding can be successful in some patients with neurologic impairment. Because these patients have an increased risk of certain complications, particularly pulmonary aspiration, they require especially careful nursing care. Patients of most concern are (1) those with an

TABLE 6-4

NUTRITIONAL ASSESSMENT OF PATIENTS WITH PULMONARY CONDITIONS

AREA OF CONCERN	SIGNIFICANT FINDINGS		
	HISTORY	PHYSICAL ASSESSMENT	LABORATORY DATA
Protein-calorie malnutrition	Chronic lung disease: Poor intake of protein and calories because of the following: Breathing difficulty from pressure of a full stomach on the diaphragm Unpleasant taste in the mouth from chronic sputum production Gastric irritation from bronchodilator therapy Increased energy expenditure from increased work of breathing	Muscle wasting Loss of subcutaneous fat Recent weight loss or weight measurement of <90% of desirable Triceps skinfold measurement of <10th percentile*	Serum albumin <3.5 g/dl or low transferrin or prealbumin level Total lymphocyte count <1200/mm³ Creatinine excretion <17 mg/kg (women) or <23 mg/kg (men)
	Acute respiratory alterations: Inadequate intake of protein and calories because of the following: Upper airway intubation Altered state of consciousness Dyspnea Increased protein and calorie requirements caused by increased work of breathing or acute pulmonary infections Catabolism resulting from corticosteroid use	Same as for chronic disease	Same as for chronic disease
Overweight/obesity (in patients with chronic lung disease)	Decreased caloric needs resulting from decreasing metabolic rate with aging (metabolic rate declines by 2% per decade after age 30) or decreased activity to compensate for impaired respiratory function	Weight >120% of desirable Triceps skinfold measurement >90th percentile†	
Elevated respiratory quotient (RQ)‡	Use of glucose or other carbohydrate to provide 70% or more of nonprotein calories Consumption of excess calories	Tachypnea, shortness of breath	RQ ≥1 Elevated V_{O_2} and V_{CO_2} Elevated Pa_{CO_2} (not always present)
Fluid volume excess	Administration of more than 35-50 ml fluid/kg/day Increased antidiuretic hormone (ADH) release resulting from stress and ventilator dependency	Dependent edema Pulmonary rales Bounding pulse Shortness of breath	Serum sodium <135 mEq/L BUN, hematocrit, and serum albumin decreased from previous values
Excess lipid intake	Administration of IV lipids		Serum triglyceride >150 mg/dl Low V_A/Q§

BUN, Blood urea nitrogen.
*6 mm for men and 14 mm for women.
†20 mm for men and 34 mm for women.
‡RQ, or CO₂ produced ÷ O₂ consumed, is measured by indirect calorimetry, which is not available in all institutions. However, pulmonary function tests can provide some indication of RQ, as the "laboratory data" column demonstrates. Carbon dioxide production (and RQ) rises in the patient who is depending primarily on carbohydrate for fuel (e.g., the patient receiving TPN in whom dextrose is supplying almost all calories rather than receiving a balance between dextrose and lipid calories) and especially in the patient who is being overfed so that adipose tissue is being accumulated.
§The defect is not usually sufficient to alter Pa_{O_2} or Pa_{CO_2} except in patients with the most severe lung disease.

NUTRITION ASSESSMENT OF PATIENTS WITH NEUROLOGIC ALTERATIONS

AREA OF CONCERN	SIGNIFICANT FINDINGS		
	HISTORY	PHYSICAL ASSESSMENT	LABORATORY DATA

DISORDERS OF PROTEIN AND CALORIE NUTRITURE

AREA OF CONCERN	HISTORY	PHYSICAL ASSESSMENT	LABORATORY DATA

Protein-calorie malnutrition	Decreased intake because of the following:
	  Coma or confusion
	  Feeding/swallowing difficulties such as dribbling of food and beverages from mouth, dysphagia, weakness of muscles involved in chewing and swallowing
	  Ileus resulting from spinal cord injury or use of pentobarbital
	  Anorexia resulting from depression
	Increased needs because of the following:
	  Hypermetabolism and catabolism after head injury
	  Catabolism resulting from corticosteroid use
	  Trauma and surgical wounds
	Loss of protein from decubitus ulcers
		Muscle wasting
		Loss of subcutaneous fat
		Weight <90% of desirable
		Triceps skinfold measurement <10th percentile*
		Change in hair texture, loss of hair
			Serum albumin <3.5 g/dl (or low transferrin or prealbumin values)
			Negative nitrogen balance
			Total lymphocyte count <1200/mm^3
			Creatinine excretion <17 mg/kg/day (women) or <23 mg/kg/day (men)

Overweight/obesity	Decreased caloric needs resulting from inactivity Reliance on soft or pureed foods, which are often more dense in calories than higher fiber foods Increased food intake resulting from depression/boredom	Weight >120% of desirable Triceps skinfold >90th percentile†	

VITAMIN AND MINERAL DEFICIENCIES

AREA OF CONCERN	HISTORY	PHYSICAL ASSESSMENT	LABORATORY DATA
Iron (Fe)	Poor intake of meats resulting from chewing difficulties (e.g., as occurs with myasthenia gravis) Loss of blood in trauma	Pallor, blue sclerae Koilonychia	Microcytic anemia (low Hct, Hgb, MCV, MCH, MCHC) Serum Fe <50 µg/ml
Zinc (Zn)	Poor intake of meat resulting from chewing problems Increased needs for healing decubitus ulcers, trauma, or surgical wounds	Hypogeusia, dysgeusia Diarrhea Seborrheic dermatitis Alopecia	Serum Zn <60 µg/ml

FLUID ALTERATIONS

AREA OF CONCERN	HISTORY	PHYSICAL ASSESSMENT	LABORATORY DATA
Fluid volume deficit	Poor intake resulting from difficulty swallowing (e.g., as occurs with cerebrovascular accident), inability to express thirst, fluid restriction in an effort to reduce intracranial edema	Poor skin turgor Decreased urinary output Dry, sticky mucous membranes	Serum sodium >145 mEq/L Serum osmolality >300 mOsm/kg Increased BUN and Hct levels Urine specific gravity >1.030

From Moore MC: *Pocket guide to nutrition and diet therapy*, St Louis, 1993, Mosby.
Hct, Hematocrit; *Hgb*, hemoglobin; *MCV*, mean cell volume; *MCH*, mean cell hemoglobin; *MCHC*, mean cell hemoglobin concentration; *BUN*, blood urea nitrogen.
*6 mm for men and 14 mm for women.
†20 mm for men and 34 mm for women.

impaired gag reflex, such as some patients with cerebral vascular accident; (2) those with delayed gastric emptying, such as patients in the early period after spinal cord injury and patients with head injury treated with barbiturate coma; and (3) patients likely to experience seizures. To help prevent pulmonary aspiration, nurses should keep patients' heads elevated at 30 degrees if possible; when elevating the head is not possible, administering feedings with patients in the prone or lateral positions allows free drainage of emesis from the mouth and decreases the risk of aspiration.

Although formulas for enteral feeding can interfere with phenytoin absorption,[9] two investigations failed to find any effect on overall absorption of phenytoin.[10,11] Until this issue has been resolved, phenytoin levels should be monitored carefully in patients receiving enteral feedings.

Hyperglycemia is a common complication in patients receiving corticosteroids. Patients treated with these drugs should have blood glucose levels monitored regularly and may require insulin to prevent substantial loss of glucose in the urine, as well as osmotic diuresis, loss of excessive amounts of potassium, and other fluid and electrolyte disturbances.

Tube feedings may not be possible in some patients with neurologic alterations.[12] Certain patients with head injuries may not tolerate tube feedings for a prolonged period because of vomiting and poor gastrointestinal motility. Patients with frequent or uncontrolled seizures are also poor candidates.

TPN is needed by most patients who fail to tolerate tube feedings or those who cannot be enterally fed for at least 5 to 7 days. Prompt use of TPN is especially important for patients with head injuries because head injury causes marked catabolism,[13] even in patients who receive barbiturates, which should decrease metabolic demands.[13,14] Patients with head injuries rapidly exhaust glycogen stores and begin to utilize body proteins to meet energy needs, a process that can quickly cause PCM. The catabolic response to head injury is partly a result of the corticosteroids often used in treatment. However, the hypermetabolism and hypercatabolism are also caused by dramatic hormonal responses to this type of injury.[13] Levels of cortisol, epinephrine, and norepinephrine increase, with levels of norepinephrine elevating as much as sevenfold. These hormones increase the metabolic rate and caloric demands, causing mobilization of body fat and proteins to meet the increased energy needs. Furthermore, patients with head injuries undergo an inflammatory response and may be febrile, creating increased needs for protein and calories. Improved survival rates have been observed in these patients who receive adequate nutrition support early in the hospital course.[13]

Nutrition and Renal Alterations

Providing adequate nutritional care for patients with renal disease can be extremely challenging. Although renal disturbances and their treatments can markedly increase needs for nutrients, necessary restrictions in intake of fluid, protein, phosphorus, and potassium make delivery of adequate calories, vitamins, and minerals difficult.

Nutritional assessment in renal alterations

Assessment is summarized in Table 6-6.

Nutritional intervention in renal alterations

The goal of nutritional interventions is to administer adequate nutrients, including calories, protein, vitamins, and minerals, while avoiding excesses of fluid, protein, electrolytes, and other potentially toxic nutrients.

PROTEIN. Evidence suggests that a low-protein diet retards the progression of renal damage. It is postulated that a high-protein intake increases glomerular flow and pressures because the kidney attempts to excrete the urea and other nitrogenous products derived from the protein. The increase in glomerular pressures may hasten the death of the glomeruli.[15] Consequently, decreased protein intake (0.6 g/kg/day compared with the 0.8 g/kg/day recommended for the healthy person and the 1.7 g/kg/day actually consumed by the average American) is recommended for patients with renal failure who are undialyzed. Although uremia necessitates control of protein intake, patients with renal failure often have many problems that actually increase protein/amino acid needs: losses in dialysis, wounds, and fistulae; use of corticosteroid drugs that exert a catabolic effect; increased endogenous secretion of catecholamines, corticosteroids, glucagon, and parathyroid hormone, all of which can cause or aggravate catabolism; and catabolic conditions, such as trauma, surgery, and sepsis associated or coincident with the renal disturbances. Therefore protein needs may actually increase. During hemodialysis and arteriovenous hemofiltration, amino acids are freely filtered and lost but proteins such as albumin and immunoglobulin are not. Both proteins and amino acids are removed during peritoneal dialysis, creating a greater nutritional requirement for protein.[16] Protein needs are estimated at approximately 1.0 g/kg/day or more for patients receiving hemodialysis or hemofiltration[17] and 1.2 to 1.5 g/kg/day for those receiving peritoneal dialysis.[16] Although these amounts are greater than the recommended daily level for healthy adults, they are lower than the amount found in the diet of most adults, and thus most patients will perceive them as restrictions.

Controversy exists regarding the type of amino acids to be provided to patients in renal failure. Some authorities advocate using primarily essential amino acids, those the body cannot make, with the idea that patients will form adequate amounts of nonessential amino acids via the process of transamination (transfer of amine groups from one carbon backbone to another). However, it is not clear that outcome is improved in patients receiving essential amino acid preparations. Many physicians now recommend the use of more balanced preparations con-

TABLE 6-6

NUTRITIONAL ASSESSMENT OF PATIENTS WITH RENAL CONDITIONS

AREA OF CONCERN	HISTORY	PHYSICAL ASSESSMENT	LABORATORY DATA
Protein-calorie malnutrition	Poor dietary intake because of the following: 　Dietary restrictions on protein-containing foods 　Anorexia caused by Zn deficiency (lost in dialysis or decreased in diet because of restrictions on meats, whole grains, legumes) 　Increased protein and amino acid losses from the following: 　　Dialysis (hemodialysis losses ≈ 10-13 g/session; CAPD losses ≈ 5-15 g/day)† 　　Tissue catabolism resulting from corticosteroid use 　　Proteinuria (e.g., as occurs with nephrotic syndrome) 　　Increased needs for protein and calories during peritonitis and other infections	Muscle wasting Loss of subcutaneous tissue Weight <90% of desirable Triceps skinfold <10th percentile* (Loss of weight and subcutaneous fat may be masked by edema) Loss of hair, change of hair texture	Serum albumin <3.5 g/dl or low transferrin or prealbumin levels Total lymphocyte count <1200/mm^3 Negative nitrogen balance
Altered lipid metabolism	Nephrotic syndrome, with elevated cholesterol levels Excess carbohydrate (CHO) consumption from the following: 　Emphasis on CHO in the diet to replace some of the calories normally provided by protein 　Use of glucose as an osmotic agent in dialysis		Serum cholesterol >250 mg/dl Serum triglyceride >180 mg/dl
Potential fluid volume excess	Oliguria or anuria Patient knowledge deficit about or noncompliance with fluid restriction	Edema Hypertension Acute weight gain (≥1%-2% of body weight)	Hematocrit decreased from previous levels

DISORDERS OF MINERALS/ELECTROLYTES

AREA OF CONCERN	HISTORY	PHYSICAL ASSESSMENT	LABORATORY DATA
Phosphorus (P) excess	Oliguria or anuria	Tetany	Serum P >4.5 mg/dl Calcium × P product (Ca in mg/dl × P in mg/dl) >70
Zinc (Zn) deficit	Poor intake because of restriction of protein-containing foods Loss in dialysis	Hypogeusia, dysgeusia Alopecia Seborrheic dermatitis Diarrhea	Serum Zn <60 µg/ml
Iron (Fe) deficit	Decreased intake because of restriction of protein-containing foods Loss of blood in dialysis tubing	Fatigue Pallor, blue sclerae Koilonychia	Hematocrit <37% (women) or <42% (men); hemoglobin <12 g/dl (women) or <14 g/dl (men); low MCV, MCH, MCHC levels
Sodium excess	Oliguria or anuria	Edema Hypertension	
Potassium (K$^+$) excess	Oliguria or anuria	Weakness, flaccid muscles	Serum K$^+$ >5 mEq/L Elevated T wave and depressed ST segment on ECG

From Moore MC: *Pocket guide to nutrition and diet therapy*, St Louis, 1993, Mosby.
CAPD, Continuous ambulatory peritoneal dialysis; *MCV*, mean cell volume; *MCH*, mean cell hemoglobin; *MCHC*, mean cell hemoglobin concentration.
*6 mm for men, and 14 mm for women.
†Increased by 50%-100% in peritonitis.

Continued.

TABLE   6 - 6

NUTRITIONAL ASSESSMENT OF PATIENTS WITH RENAL CONDITIONS—CONT'D

AREA OF CONCERN	HISTORY	PHYSICAL ASSESSMENT	LABORATORY DATA
Aluminum (Al) excess	Use of aluminum-containing phosphate binders Al contamination of TPN constituents	Ataxia, seizures Dementia Renal osteodystrophy with bone pain and deformities	Plasma Al >100 µg/L
DISORDERS OF VITAMIN NUTRITURE			
A excess	Oliguria or anuria Daily administration of tube feedings, TPN, or oral supplement with vitamin A	Anorexia Alopecia, dry skin Hepatomegaly Fatigue, irritability	Serum retinol level of >80 µg/dl
C deficit	Loss in dialysis Decreased intake due to restriction of K^+-containing fruits and vegetables	Gingivitis Petechiae, ecchymoses	Serum ascorbate <0.4 mg/dl
B_6	Failure of the diseased kidney to activate vitamin B_6 Loss in dialysis	Dermatitis Ataxia Irritability, seizures	Plasma pyridoxal phosphate <34 nmol (normal levels not well established)
Folic acid	Loss in dialysis Decreased intake resulting from restriction of meats, fruits, and vegetables	Glossitis (inflamed tongue) Pallor	Hematocrit $<37\%$ (women) or $<42\%$ (men), elevated MCV level Serum folate <6 ng/ml

taining both essential and nonessential amino acids because protein synthesis may be improved if both types of amino acids are consumed.[18] For patients with renal disease who are stressed and catabolic, provision of adequate amounts of all types of amino acids required for anabolism appears to be more important than delaying initiation of dialysis.

FLUID. Patients are usually limited to a fluid intake resulting in a gain of no more than 0.45 kg (1 pound) per day on the days between dialysis. This generally means a daily intake of 500 ml plus the volume lost in urine, diarrhea, and vomitus. Continuous peritoneal dialysis, hemofiltration, and arteriovenous hemodialysis can liberalize the fluid intake. A liberal fluid allowance permits more adequate nutrient delivery, whether by oral, tube, or parenteral feedings. Enteral formulas providing 2 cal/ml or more—such as Nutrisource (Sandoz), TwoCal HN (Ross), Isocal HCN (Mead Johnson), and Magnacal (Sherwood)—are useful in providing a concentrated source of calories for patients being tube fed who require fluid restriction. Intravenous lipids, particularly 20% emulsions, can be used to supply concentrated calories for patients receiving TPN.

CALORIES. Patients with renal disease must receive an adequate number of calories to prevent catabolism of body tissues to meet energy needs. Catabolism not only reduces the mass of muscle and other functional body tissues but also releases nitrogen that must be excreted by the kidney. Adults with renal failure need about 30 to 40 calories/kg/day compared with the 25 to 30 calories/kg needed by healthy adults to prevent catabolism and ensure that all protein consumed is used for anabolism rather than to meet energy needs. After renal transplantation, when patients usually receive large doses of corticosteroids, ensuring that adequate caloric intake continues to prevent undue catabolism is especially important.

High-carbohydrate foods such as hard candies, sugar, honey, jelly, jellybeans, and gumdrops are often used as a means of supplying calories to patients with renal failure because these foods are low in sodium and potassium, which are retained in renal failure. However, a substantial number of patients with renal disorders also suffer from hypertriglyceridemia. This condition is worsened by excessive intake of simple refined sugars such as sucrose (table sugar) or glucose. When hypertriglyceridemia is a concern, carbohydrate intake can be reduced, with the emphasis placed on complex carbohydrates (starches and fibers). When glucose is used as the osmotic agent in peritoneal dialysis and arteriovenous hemodialysis, approximately 70% of the glucose in the dialysate may be absorbed and must therefore be considered part of the

T A B L E 6 - 7		
DAILY NUTRITIONAL RECOMMENDATIONS FOR PATIENTS WITH RENAL FAILURE		

NUTRIENT	RECOMMENDED DIETARY ALLOWANCE (RDA) FOR HEALTHY ADULTS	DAILY AMOUNT IN RENAL FAILURE
Protein or amino acids (g/kg)	0.8	0.6 (undialyzed)* 1.0+ (hemodialysis)* 1.2-1.5 (peritoneal dialysis)*
Calories/kg	25-30	30-40
Electrolytes and minerals†		
Sodium	Unspecified	87-109 mEq (2-2.5 g)‡
Potassium	Unspecified	70-80 mEq (2.7-3.1 g)
Calcium (mg)	800	1000-2000
Phosphorus (mg)	800	700-800
Magnesium (mg)	280-350	200-300
Trace minerals		
Iron (mg)	10-15	15 mg +, as needed to prevent deficiency
Zinc (mg)	12-15	15 mg +, as needed to prevent deficiency
Vitamins		
C (mg)	60	70-100
B$_6$ (mg)	1.6-2.0	5-10
Folic acid (µg)	180-200	1000

From Feinstein EI: *Nutr Clin Prac* 3:9, 1988; Kopple JD, Blumenkrantz MJ: *Kidney Int Suppl* 16:S295, 1983; Oldrizzi L and others: *Nutr Clin Prac* 9:3, 1994; and *Recommended dietary allowances,* Washington, DC, 1989, National Academy of Sciences—National Research Council.
*Based on estimated dry weight.
†Dosages given are representative ranges; serum levels and physical findings help to determine actual individual intake. For instance, the presence of edema and hypertension usually necessitates a reduced sodium allowance. These are enteral recommendations, and parenteral levels may be lower.
‡Levels for continuous ambulatory peritoneal dialysis (CAPD) may be higher.

patient's carbohydrate intake.[19] The glucose monohydrate used in intravenous and dialysate solutions supplies 3.4 calories/g. Thus if patients receive 4.25% glucose (4.25 g glucose/100 ml solution) in the dialysate, they receive the following:

42.5 g/L × 70% × 3.4 calories/g = 101 calories/L of dialysate

For patients who are tube fed, enteral formulas that contain some fiber, such as Compleat (Sandoz) and Enrich (Ross), may help to control hypertriglyceridemia.

To help control hypertriglyceridemia and provide concentrated calories in minimum amounts of fluid, fat should supply about half or more of patients' calories. Because hypercholesterolemia is frequently found in patients with renal failure, polyunsaturated fats and oils are preferred over saturated fats, which tend to raise cholesterol levels. The necessary restriction of meat, milk, and other protein foods in the diet help lower cholesterol and saturated fat intake. For patients who need a caloric supplement, Lipomul (Upjohn) is a palatable oral lipid supplement providing 6 calories/ml with minimum amounts of sodium and potassium. Intravenous lipids and the long-chain fats found in most enteral formulas, except those prepared from blended foods, are primarily polyunsaturated. Some formulas are rich in medium-chain triglycerides, or fats. Although these triglycerides are saturated, they do not contribute to hypercholesterolemia and may be used for patients with renal disease.

OTHER NUTRIENTS. Table 6-7 summarizes the recommended nutrient intake for patients with renal disorders, for whom recommendations are different from those for healthy adults. The recommendations for healthy adults are included to provide a basis for comparison.

Nutrition and Gastrointestinal Alterations

Because the gastrointestinal (GI) tract is so inherently related to nutrition, it is not surprising that catastrophic occurrences in the GI tract—hemorrhage, perforation, infarct, and related organ failure—have acute and severe adverse effects on nutritional status.

Nutritional assessment in gastrointestinal alterations

Assessment is summarized in Table 6-8. The area and amount of the GI tract affected largely determine the likelihood and degree of nutritional deficits because each portion of the bowel has a role to play in absorption. The ileum is among the most nutritionally important areas.

T A B L E   6 - 8

NUTRITIONAL ASSESSMENT OF THE PATIENT
WITH A GASTROINTESTINAL DISORDER

AREA OF CONCERN	HISTORY	PHYSICAL ASSESSMENT	LABORATORY DATA

Protein-calorie malnutrition	Decreased oral intake caused by the following:
	  Fear of symptoms—pain, cramping, diarrhea—associated with eating (e.g., as occurs with peptic ulcer, dumping syndrome)
	  Alcohol abuse
	  Nausea, vomiting, anorexia
	Increased losses because of the following:
	  Maldigestion or malabsorption (e.g., as occurs with inadequate bile salt production, increased loss of bile salts in short bowel syndrome, diarrhea, inadequate absorptive area in short bowel syndrome)
	  GI bleeding
	  Fistula drainage
	Increased requirements caused by needs for healing (e.g., surgical wounds, fistulae)
		Muscle wasting
		Loss of subcutaneous fat
		Weight <90% of desirable or recent weight loss
		Triceps skinfold measurement <10th percentile*
		Hair loss or change in hair texture
			Serum albumin <3.5 g/dl or low transferrin level
			Total lymphocyte count <1200/ mm^3
			Creatinine excretion <17 mg/ kg/day (women) or <23 mg/ kg/day (men)
			Negative nitrogen balance
			Fecal fat >5 g/day or >5% of intake

Potential fluid volume deficit	Losses caused by severe vomiting or diarrhea (e.g., as occurs with GI obstruction, short bowel syndrome)	Poor skin turgor Dry, sticky mucous membranes Complaint of thirst Loss of ≥0.23 kg (0.5 lb) in 24 hr	Hct >52% (men) or >47% (women) BUN >20 mg/dl Serum sodium >145 mEq/L Serum osmolality >300 mOsm/kg Urine specific gravity >1.030

DISORDERS OF MINERAL/ELECTROLYTE NUTRITURE

AREA OF CONCERN	HISTORY	PHYSICAL ASSESSMENT	LABORATORY DATA
Calcium (Ca)	Increased loss because of steatorrhea (Ca forms soaps with fat in the stool and thus becomes unabsorbable)	Tingling of fingers Muscular tetany and cramps Carpopedal spasm Convulsions	Serum Ca level of <8.5 mg/dl (severe deficits only)

Magnesium (Mg)	Inadequate intake because of poor diet in alcoholism
	Increased losses because of the following:
	  Diarrhea or steatorrhea
	  Loss of small bowel fluid (e.g., as occurs with short bowel syndrome, fistulae)
		Tremor
		Hyperactive deep reflexes
		Convulsions
			Serum Mg <1.5 mEq/L

Iron (Fe)	Blood loss Impaired absorption because of decreased upper GI acidity with gastrectomy or use of antacids and cimetidine Inadequate intake (e.g., restriction of protein foods in hepatic failure)	Pallor, blue sclerae Fatigue Koilonychia	Hct <42% (men) or <37% (women); Hgb <14 g/dl (men) or <12 g/dl (women); low MCV, MCH, MCHC Serum Fe <60 μg/dl

Modified from Moore MC: *Pocket guide to nutrition and diet therapy,* ed 2, St Louis, 1993, Mosby.
Hct, Hematocrit; *BUN,* blood urea nitrogen; *Hgb,* hemoglobin; *MCV,* mean cell volume; *MCH,* mean cell hemoglobin; *MCHC,* mean cell hemoglobin concentration; *Ca,* calcium.
*6 mm for men and 14 mm for women.

TABLE 6-8

NUTRITIONAL ASSESSMENT OF THE PATIENT WITH A GASTROINTESTINAL DISORDER—CONT'D

AREA OF CONCERN	HISTORY	PHYSICAL ASSESSMENT	LABORATORY DATA
Zinc (Zn)	Increased losses caused by the following: Diarrhea, steatorrhea; Loss of small bowel fluid; Diuretic use (in hepatic failure); Increased urinary losses in alcoholism. Inadequate intake caused by the following: Protein restriction in hepatic failure; Poor diet in alcoholism	Anorexia; Hypogeusia, dysgeusia; Seborrheic dermatitis	Serum Zn <60 µg/dl
Potassium (K$^+$)	Increased loss caused by the following: Diarrhea; Diuretic use; Hyperaldosteronism (in hepatic failure); GI suction	Muscle weakness, ileus; Diminished reflexes	Serum K$^+$ <3.5 mEq/L
DISORDERS OF VITAMIN NUTRITURE			
A	Increased loss in steatorrhea (vitamin A dissolves in fatty stools). Impaired release of vitamin A from storage in the liver because of inadequate production of retinol-binding protein, the transport protein, in malnutrition or liver failure	Drying of skin and cornea; Poor wound healing; Follicular hyperkeratosis (resembles gooseflesh)	Serum retinol <20 µg/dl
K	Impaired absorption in steatorrhea. Decreased production because of destruction of intestinal bacteria by antibiotic usage	Petechiae, ecchymoses; Prolonged bleeding	Prothrombin time >12.5 sec (not accurate in liver failure)

Absorption of fat and bile salt occurs in this area, as does absorption of vitamin B_{12}. Patients with ileal disease or resection are likely to become malnourished as a result of significant loss of calories as well as vitamins and minerals in the feces. The ileocecal valve is especially critical in maintaining adequate nutrition. It not only slows the entry of GI contents into the large bowel, allowing more time for absorption to take place in the small bowel, but also helps prevent migration of the microorganisms from the large bowel into the small bowel. Proliferating microorganisms in the small bowel deconjugate the bile salts, impairing fat absorption. Deconjugated bile salts also irritate the intestinal mucosa and raise the osmolality level within the bowel, promoting diarrhea.[20] The ileum can absorb most of the nutrients normally absorbed in the upper half of the small bowel, but the duodenum and jejunum cannot compensate for the loss of the ileum.

Nutritional intervention in gastrointestinal alterations

The GI tract is the preferred route for delivery of nutrients in GI disease, as it is in all other disease states. However, after damage or resection, enteral nutrition support may be inadequate or impossible at least temporarily. Because bowel resection and hepatic failure are two of the most nutritionally challenging GI alterations, most of this discussion is devoted to them.

SHORT BOWEL SYNDROME (BOWEL RESECTION)

ADMINISTRATION OF FLUIDS AND ELECTROLYTES. Extensive bowel resection is associated with marked gastric hypersecretion. The increase in gastric juices, coupled with the sudden loss of absorptive area, results in the loss of several liters of fluid daily, along with potassium, magnesium, and zinc. The role of nurses in management of these patients includes (1) keeping strict intake and output records, including volume or weight of stools if they are frequent or loose; (2) continually assessing patients' state of hydration; and (3) administering fluids and electrolytes and evaluating patients' responses—including daily weight measurements—to evaluate the adequacy of fluid replacement.

ADMINISTRATION OF NUTRITION SUPPORT. The major nutritional problems associated with bowel resection are loss of absorptive area, with increased fecal losses of fluids, electrolytes, fat, protein, and other nutrients; increased loss of bile salts, especially if the terminal ileum was resected, with further malabsorption of fat; and micronutrient deficiencies resulting from trapping of minerals and fat-soluble vitamins within the excreted fat. After bowel resection the remaining intestine undergoes marked hyperplasia, with increasing length of the remaining villi, which increases the available absorptive area. The result is improved absorption of water, electrolytes, and glucose.[20] Some patients with 70% to 80% resection of the small bowel can eventually be maintained on enteral feedings only, especially if the terminal ileum and ileocecal valve are retained, but patients with resection of more than 90% of the small bowel usually require permanent TPN.[21]

The first priority in nutritional support of patients with short bowel syndrome is stabilization of fluid and electrolyte balance. After that is accomplished, TPN is initiated. Patients begin with small enteral feedings to stimulate adaptation of the remaining bowel. Feedings may consist of an elemental, or predigested, diet given by tube. Because fat is the most difficult nutrient to absorb, the formula will ordinarily be very low in fat or high in medium-chain triglycerides, which are more readily absorbed than the long-chain triglycerides predominating in most foods. Tube feedings should be given continuously to promote optimal absorption. Intragastric rather than transpyloric feedings are preferable to use every available centimeter of intestinal surface area. Alternatively, a low-fat, high-starch diet may be given by mouth.[22] Lactose, or milk sugar, is often tolerated poorly by patients with bowel resection, but low-fat cottage cheese and yogurt, which are relatively low in lactose, may be tolerated.

ADMINISTRATION OF MEDICATIONS. In some patients with short bowel syndrome in whom diarrhea is prolonged or especially severe and causes anal excoriation or copious ostomy output, antidiarrheal agents such as diphenoxylate with atropine or codeine may be beneficial. Anticholinergic drugs such as glycopyrrolate can also be used to counteract the gastric hypersecretion.

HEPATIC FAILURE. Hepatic failure is associated with a wide spectrum of metabolic alterations. The diseased liver's impaired ability to deactivate hormones elevates levels of circulating glucagon, epinephrine, and cortisol. These hormones promote catabolism of body tissues.

Glycogen stores are rapidly exhausted. Although release of lipids from their storage depots accelerates, the liver has decreased ability to metabolize them for energy. Furthermore, as many as half the patients with hepatic failure may have malabsorption of fat because of inadequate production of bile salts by the liver. Therefore body proteins are increasingly used for energy sources, producing rapid tissue wasting.

MONITORING OF FLUID AND ELECTROLYTE STATUS. Ascites and edema result from decreased colloid osmotic pressure in the plasma because the diseased liver produces less albumin and other plasma proteins, increased portal pressure caused by obstruction, and renal sodium retention from secondary hyperaldosteronism. Restriction of sodium (usually 500 to 1500 mg, or 20 to 65 mEq, daily) and fluid (1500 ml or less) is generally necessary in conjunction with administration of diuretics to control fluid retention. Patients must be weighed daily to evaluate the success of treatment. In addition, laboratory and physical status must be closely observed for potassium deficits caused by diuretic therapy and hyperaldosteronism.

PROVISION OF A NUTRITIOUS DIET AND EVALUATION OF RESPONSE TO DIETARY PROTEIN. Nutrition intervention in hepatic failure is based on the metabolic alterations. Initially, protein allowances are increased to 1 to 1.5 g/kg/day in an effort to suppress catabolism and promote liver regeneration. However, if encephalopathy occurs or appears to be impending, protein intake is reduced to 0.5 g/kg/day or less. A high-calorie diet (45 to 50 calories/kg/day, compared with approximately 25 to 30 calories for the healthy adult) is provided to help prevent catabolism and the use of dietary protein for energy needs. Moderate amounts of fat are given unless the patient has steatorrhea, in which case it is necessary to rely heavily on carbohydrates and mean circulation times to meet caloric needs. Soft foods are preferred because patients may have esophageal varices that might be irritated by high-fiber foods. Because alcoholism is often the cause of hepatic failure and the diets of alcoholics have been shown to be low in zinc, vitamin B complex, folate, and magnesium, supplements of these nutrients are usually provided daily.[23] Anorexia, malaise, and confusion may interfere with oral intake, and nurses may need to encourage patients to eat adequately. Small, frequent feedings are usually better accepted by patients with anorexia than are three large meals daily. Nurses must assess patients' neurologic status daily to evaluate tolerance of dietary protein. Increasing lethargy, confusion, or asterixis may signal the need for decreased protein intake. Anorexia—coupled with the unpalatable nature of the very low-sodium, low-protein diet required in impending coma—may result in a need for tube feedings.

Nutrition and Endocrine Alterations

Because of the far-reaching effects on all body systems, endocrine alterations have an impact on nutritional status in a variety of ways.

Nutritional assessment in endocrine alterations

The nutrition assessment process is summarized in Table 6-9. Because of the prevalence of patients with non–insulin-dependent diabetes mellitus (NIDDM) among the hospitalized population, the nutritional problems most commonly noted in patients with endocrine alterations are overweight and obesity.

Nutritional intervention in endocrine alterations

Underweight and malnourished patients. The most severely undernourished patients are usually those with pancreatitis because of loss of pancreatic exocrine function. Pancreatic insufficiency—with inadequate re-

lease of trypsin, chymotrypsin, and pancreatic lipase and amylase—results in impaired digestion and subsequent loss of nutrients in the stool. Fat malabsorption is the most marked effect of pancreatic insufficiency. Fat lost in the stools is accompanied by calcium, zinc, and other minerals, along with the fat-soluble vitamins.

Patients with insulin-dependent diabetes mellitus (IDDM) or endocrine dysfunction caused by pancreatitis often have weight loss and malnutrition as a result of tissue catabolism because they cannot use dietary carbohydrates to meet energy needs. Although patients with NIDDM are more likely to be overweight than underweight, they too may become malnourished as a result

TABLE 6-9

NUTRITIONAL ASSESSMENT OF PATIENTS WITH ENDOCRINE DISORDERS

AREA OF CONCERN	HISTORY	PHYSICAL FINDINGS	LABORATORY DATA
Underweight or protein-calorie malnutrition	Increased losses of calories in urine or feces caused by the following: Impaired glucose metabolism and glucosuria in type I diabetes mellitus; Steatorrhea in pancreatitis. Decreased intake because of the following: Discomfort with eating (in pancreatitis); Alcoholism (often a cause of pancreatitis)	Weight of <90% of desirable; Recent weight loss; Wasting of muscle and subcutaneous tissue; Triceps skinfold measurement of <10th percentile*	Urine glucose >0.5%; Fecal fat >5 g/24 hr or <95% of intake; Serum albumin <3.5 g/dl, or low transferrin or prealbumin levels; Total lymphocyte count (<1200/mm³; Creatinine excretion <17 mg/kg/day (women) or <23 mg/kg/day (men)
Overweight	NIDDM; Sedentary lifestyle	Weight of >120% of desirable; Triceps skinfold measurement of >90th percentile†	
Risk for fluid volume deficit	Diuresis (from diabetes insipidus or osmotic diuresis of HHNK or ketoacidosis)	Poor skin turgor; Dry, sticky mucous membranes; Thirst; Loss of >0.23 kg (0.5 pound) in 24 hr; Increased urine output	Serum glucose >250 mg/dl; Urine glucose >0.5%; Serum sodium >145 mEq/L; Increasing Hct; BUN >20 mg/dl
Risk for fluid volume excess	Fluid retention caused by SIADH	Edema (peripheral and/or pulmonary); Gain of >0.23 kg (0.5 lb) in 24 hr	Serum sodium <135 mEq/L; Decreasing Hct
Potential zinc deficiency	Impaired absorption in steatorrhea associated with pancreatitis; Increased urinary losses in diuresis, diabetes mellitus, and alcoholism; Poor intake in alcoholism	Hypogeusia, dysgeusia; Alopecia; Seborrheic dermatitis; Impaired wound healing	Serum zinc <60 µg/ml

Modified from Moore MC: *Pocket guide to nutrition and diet therapy*, ed 2, St Louis, 1993, Mosby.
Hct, Hematocrit; *BUN,* blood urea nitrogen; *HHNK,* hyperosmolar hyperglycemic nonketotic coma; *SIADH,* syndrome of inappropriate secretion of antidiuretic hormone.
*6 mm for men and 14 mm for women.
†20 mm for men, and 34 mm for women.

of chronic or acute infections, trauma, major surgery, or other illnesses. Delivery of nutritional support in these patients, especially control of blood glucose, can be challenging. Blood glucose should be monitored regularly, usually several times a day until patients are stable.

Adding regular insulin to the solution is the most common method of managing hyperglycemia in patients receiving TPN. The dosage required may be larger than the usual subcutaneous dose because some of the insulin adheres to glass bottles and plastic bags or administration sets. Continuous subcutaneous infusion of insulin also may be used. Hyperglycemia is another common problem in patients who are tube fed, particularly when feedings are given continuously. Twice-daily doses of intermediate-acting insulin or more frequent doses of regular insulin may be inadequate to control hyperglycemia in these patients. One solution is to administer feedings intermittently on a meal-type schedule and to administer oral hypoglycemics, regular insulin, or intermediate-acting insulin based on this schedule.[24] However, some patients with diabetes require continuous feedings. For example, patients with severe gastroparesis may need transpyloric feedings because poor gastric emptying makes intragastric feedings impossible or inadequate. Transpyloric feedings must almost always be given continuously because dumping syndrome and poor absorption often occur if feedings are given rapidly into the small bowel. For patients with diabetes who are continuously tube fed, control of blood glucose may be improved either with continuous insulin infusion or by use of a formula containing fiber such as Compleat (Sandoz) and Enrich (Ross). Fiber slows the absorption of the carbohydrate in the formula, producing a more delayed and sustained glycemic response.

OVERWEIGHT PATIENTS. Aggressive attempts at weight loss are rarely warranted among very ill patients, although weight loss in overweight patients with NIDDM improves glucose tolerance. Instead of suggesting a low-calorie diet, nurses should encourage patients to select foods providing fiber and starches. Diets rich in complex carbohydrates have been shown to lower insulin requirements, increase the sensitivity of the peripheral tissues to insulin, and decrease serum cholesterol levels.[25]

Nutritional support should not be neglected simply because patients are obese because PCM develops even among such patients. When patients are not expected to be able to eat for at least 5 to 7 days or inadequate intake persists for that period, nurses should consult with physicians regarding initiation of tube feedings or TPN if no steps have been taken to do so.

SEVERE VOMITING OR DIARRHEA IN PATIENTS WITH IDDM. When patients with IDDM experience vomiting and diarrhea severe enough to interfere significantly with oral intake or result in excessive fluid and electrolyte losses, adequate carbohydrates and fluids must be supplied. Blood glucose and urine ketone levels should be monitored frequently and physicians notified of increasing hyperglycemia, ketonuria, difficulty retaining fluids, and signs of dehydration.

Administering Nutritional Support
Enteral Nutrition Support

Whenever possible, the enteral route is the preferred method of feeding because it is generally safer, more physiologic, and much less expensive than parenteral feeding. There are a variety of enteral feeding products, some of which are designed to meet the specialized needs of very sick patients. Some products can be consumed orally, but many of the specialized ones are so unpalatable that they are reserved solely for tube feeding. Table 6-10 provides more information about the major categories of products.

Oral supplementation

For patients who can eat and have normal digestion and absorption but simply cannot consume enough regular foods to meet caloric and protein needs, oral supplementation may be necessary. Patients with mild to moderate anorexia, burns, or trauma sometimes fall into this category.

Enteral tube feedings

Tube feedings are used for patients who have at least some digestive and absorptive capability but are unwilling or unable to consume enough by mouth. Patients with profound anorexia and those experiencing severe stress that greatly increases their nutritional needs[26] (e.g., those with major burns, trauma) often benefit from tube feedings. Individuals who require elemental formulas because of impaired digestion or absorption or the specialized formulas for altered metabolic conditions (see Table 6-10) usually require tube feeding because the unpleasant flavors of the free amino acids, peptides, and protein hydrolysates used in these formulas are very difficult to mask.

LOCATION AND TYPE OF FEEDING TUBE. Whether temporary tubes (nasogastric or nasoduodenal/nasojejunal) or more permanent ones (gastrostomy or jejunostomy) are used depends largely on the length of time that feedings are anticipated to be needed. Usually 3 months or longer constitutes long-term feedings. However, patients who are extremely agitated or confused or for some other reason do not tolerate nasal intubation may require a permanent tube earlier. In addition, the advent of the percutaneous gastrostomy tube, which can be inserted without a general anesthetic, has made gastrostomy increasingly popular, even in patients who do not require long-term feeding.

The site for intubation is determined by patient need. Nasoduodenal, nasojejunal, or jejunostomy tubes are most often used when there is a high risk for pulmonary aspiration because the pyloric sphincter is believed to provide a barrier that lessens the risk of regurgitation and

TABLE 6-10
ENTERAL FORMULAS

FORMULA TYPE	EXAMPLES OF FORMULAS	ORAL OR TUBE FEEDING	NUTRITIONAL PROBLEM	CLINICAL EXAMPLES
Complete diet with intact protein and LCT* (some contain blended foods)	Ensure and Osmolite (Ross), Sustacal and Isocal (Mead Johnson Nutritional), Meritene and Compleat (Sandoz); for fluid restriction: Magnacal (Sherwood Medical), Isocal HCN (Mead Johnson Nutritional), TwoCal HN (Ross)	Some suited to both (e.g., Ensure), some primarily to oral (e.g., Sustacal, Meritene), and some primarily to tube feeding (e.g., Compleat, Osmolite, Isocal)	Inability to ingest food Inability to ingest enough food to meet needs	Oral or esophageal cancer Coma Anorexia resulting from chronic illness Burns or trauma
Elemental diets†	Criticare HN (Mead Johnson Nutritional), Vital High Nitrogen (Ross), Reabilan (O'Brien), Vivonex and Vivonex T.E.N. (Norwich Eaton), Petamen (Clintec Nutrition)	Tube feeding	Impaired digestion and/or absorption	Pancreatitis Inflammatory bowel disease Radiation enteritis Short bowel syndrome Malnutrition
SPECIALIZED DIETS FOR METABOLIC ALTERATIONS				
Diets high in branched chain amino acids, low in aromatic amino acids‡	Hepatic-Aid II (Kendal McGaw), Travasorb Hepatic (Clintec Nutrition)	Both (especially tube)	Hepatic failure	Impending hepatic coma
Diets high in branched chain amino acids‡§	Stresstein (Sandoz), TraumaCal (Mead Johnson Nutritional), Traum-Aid HBC (Kendall McGaw)	Both (especially tube)	Stress	Trauma and injury Sepsis

LCT, Long-chain triglycerides or fat (used in formulas for patients with no digestive or absorptive abnormality).
*Some of these formulas contain lactose. If the patient has a lactose intolerance, the dietitian can recommend an appropriate lactose-free formula.
†Contain "predigested" nutrients: protein in the form of amino acids and/or peptides or protein hydrolysates, fat as medium chain triglycerides (which require less emulsification by bile salts and enzymatic digestion than LCT) or minimal fat, and easily digested carbohydrates (no lactose).
‡Not conclusively proven to improve patient outcome.
§Branched-chain amino acids (leucine, isoleucine, and valine) contain a branch in their carbon chain structure. They are required for protein synthesis, but they are especially important because they serve as a valuable energy source after injury.

aspiration.[27,28] However, one small prospective study failed to find any reduction in aspiration with transpyloric tubes in comparison with intragastric ones.[29] Jejunostomy tubes have the added advantage of being able to bypass an upper GI obstruction.

NURSING MANAGEMENT. The role of nurses in delivery of tube feedings usually includes insertion of the tube if a temporary tube is used, maintenance of the tube, administration of the feedings, prevention of complications associated with this form of therapy, and participation in assessment of patients' responses to tube feedings.[30] Tubes with mercury, stainless steel, or tungsten weights on the proximal end are often used when transpyloric tube placement is desired, in the belief that the weight encourages transpyloric passage of the tube or helps the tube maintain its position once it passes into the bowel. However, unweighted tubes are just as likely as weighted ones to migrate through the pylorus.[31-33] Furthermore, weighted tubes appear no more likely to remain in place than unweighted ones.[32] Because the weights sometimes cause discomfort during nostril insertion, unweighted tubes may be preferable. Administering metoclopramide hydrochloride before inserting the tube has been shown to promote transpyloric passage. Administering the drug after the tube's proximal tip is already in the stomach is much less effective.[34,35]

Maintenance of the tube includes regular irrigation of the tube to maintain patency, skin care around the insertion site, and mouth care. The newer, small-bore (usually 8 French) "nonreactive" tubes made of polyurethane, silicone rubber, and similar materials are much more comfortable for patients than are the older polyethylene or polyvinylchloride tubes (usually 12 to 16 French), and patient complaints of discomfort and nasal and skin erosion have decreased with the use of the nonreactive tubes. Unfortunately, these small tubes tend to clog readily. Regular irrigation helps prevent tube occlusion. Generally, 30 to 60 ml of irrigant every 3 to 4 hours or after each feeding is appropriate, but the volume of irrigant may have to be reduced during fluid restriction. The irrigant is usually water, but other fluids, such as cranberry juice and cola beverages, are sometimes used in an effort to reduce the incidence of tube occlusion. Polyurethane tubes clog less readily than those made of silicone rubber, an important consideration for nurses when selecting a feeding tube.[36]

Careful attention to administration of tube feedings can prevent many complications. Hygienic techniques in the handling and administration of the formula can help prevent bacterial contamination and resultant infections.[37] The schedule for delivery of feedings is also important. Tube feedings may be administered intermittently or continuously. Intermittent feedings are best suited to those patients who are disoriented and attempt to remove the feeding tube when they are alone. Bolus feedings, which are intermittent feedings delivered rapidly into the stomach or small bowel, are likely to cause distention, vomiting, and dumping syndrome with diarrhea.[38] Instead of using bolus feedings, nurses should gradually drip intermittent feedings, with each feeding lasting 20 to 30 minutes or longer, to promote optimal assimilation. Regardless of how slowly intermittent feedings are given, however, continuous feedings are usually better absorbed by patients who have compromised digestion or absorption. Even patients who might be expected to have normal GI function such as those with burns or trauma have been shown to absorb the feedings better, tolerate larger volumes of formula, and experience less diarrhea with continuous feedings than with intermittent ones.[39] Therefore continuous feedings are usually preferable for very sick patients.

PREVENTION AND CORRECTION OF COMPLICATIONS. Some of the more common and serious complications of tube feeding are pulmonary aspiration,[40,41] diarrhea, constipation, tube occlusion, and delayed gastric emptying. Delayed gastric emptying limits the amount of feeding that patients can tolerate and thus interferes with ad-

equate nutrition support. Nursing management of these problems is detailed in Table 6-11.

Total Parenteral Nutrition

Total parenteral nutrition (TPN) refers to the delivery of all nutrients by the intravenous route. TPN is generally not worthwhile when enteral intake is expected to be adequate within 5 to 7 days. Likely candidates for TPN include patients who are unable to ingest or absorb nutrients via the GI tract, as in short bowel syndrome; have severe disease of the small bowel (e.g., inflammatory bowel disease, collagen-vascular diseases, intestinal pseudoobstruction, radiation enteritis); or are experiencing intractable vomiting. TPN may be warranted in patients receiving high-dose chemotherapy, radiation, and bone marrow transplantation, after which nutritional intake is likely to be poor for several weeks because of stomatitis, nausea, vomiting, diarrhea, and anorexia. It may also be useful for patients who can benefit from a period of bowel rest, including those with moderate to severe pancreatitis or enterocutaneous fistulae. In both cases, enteral intake (which stimulates secretion of digestive enzymes) is likely to exacerbate the condition, whereas bowel rest may promote healing. In addition, some postoperative, trauma, or burn patients may need temporary TPN.

Routes for TPN

TPN may be delivered through either central or peripheral veins. Because it requires an indwelling catheter, central vein TPN carries an increased risk of sepsis as well as potential insertion-related complications such as pneumothorax and hemothorax. Air embolism is also more likely with central vein TPN. However, central venous catheters provide very secure intravenous access and allow delivery of more hyperosmolar solutions than peripheral TPN. An inexpensive source of calories, TPN solutions containing 25% to 35% dextrose are commonly used via central veins. It is increasingly common for patients requiring multiple IV therapies and frequent blood sampling to have multilumen central venous catheters and for TPN to be infused via these catheters. Infection rates in patients receiving TPN via multilumen catheters have been reported to be as much as three times higher than those in patients with single-lumen catheters.[42] Scrupulous aseptic technique is essential in maintaining multilumen catheters; the manipulation involved in frequent changes of intravenous fluid and obtaining blood specimens through these catheters increases the risk of catheter contamination. Moreover, patients requiring these catheters are likely to be very ill and immunocompromised.

Peripheral TPN is rarely associated with serious infectious or mechanical complications[43] but does necessitate good peripheral venous access. Therefore it may not be appropriate for long-term nutrition support or for patients receiving multiple IV therapies. Furthermore, pe-

NURSING MANAGEMENT OF ENTERAL TUBE FEEDING COMPLICATIONS

COMPLICATION	CONTRIBUTING FACTOR(S)	PREVENTION/CORRECTION
Pulmonary aspiration	Feeding tube positioned in esophagus or respiratory tract	Check tube placement before intermittent feeding and every 4-6 hr during continuous feedings; be aware that an inrush of air can sometimes be auscultated over the right upper quadrant even when the distal tip of the tube is in the esophagus or respiratory tract; if there is a question about the tube position, check the pH level of fluid aspirated from the tube (usually gastric juice pH is 1.0-3.5) or perform an x-ray examination. Some tubes are made with a pH detector implanted in the tube.
	Regurgitation of formula (most common in patients with inadequate gag reflex, artificial airways, or altered state of consciousness and also in those with delayed gastric emptying)	Add food coloring (usually blue, to avoid mistaking it for any body secretion) to all formula to facilitate diagnosis of aspiration.
		Elevate head to 30 degrees during feedings; if it is impossible to raise the head, position patient in lateral or prone position to improve drainage of vomitus from the mouth (the right lateral position is especially advantageous because it facilitates gastric emptying); if head must be in a dependent position (e.g., for postural drainage), discontinue feedings 30-60 min earlier and restart them only when the head can be raised.
		Keep cuff of endotracheal or tracheostomy tube inflated during feedings if possible.
		Measure gastric residual before each intermittent feeding and at least every 4-6 hr during continuous feedings; guidelines vary, but often a volume of >150 ml or 110%-120% of the hourly rate is considered excessive; it is difficult to aspirate GI contents via small-bore nonreactive tubes without collapsing the tube, but use of large syringes (35-60 ml) is least likely to cause tube collapse. If a patient is at risk for pulmonary aspiration and it proves impossible to measure gastric residuals with an 8-French tube, substitute a 10- or 12-French one.
Diarrhea	Medications with GI side effects (antibiotics, which can alter gut flora, are common culprits, but others include digitalis, laxatives, magnesium-containing antacids, and quinidine)	Evaluate the patient's medications to determine their potential for causing diarrhea, consulting the pharmacist if necessary.
	Hypertonic formula or medications (e.g., oral suspensions of antibiotics, potassium, or other electrolytes), which cause fluid to be drawn into the gut to dilute the hypertonic load	Consult the physician about using continuous feedings (if feedings are currently intermittent) or diluting or slowing tube feedings temporarily; dilute enteral medications well.
	Malnutrition (hypoalbuminemia impairs absorption by decreasing plasma oncotic pressure; malnutrition also results in loss of intestinal microvilli, reducing brush border enzymes needed for digestion as well as the absorptive area)	Consult with the physician about using continuous feedings, which may facilitate absorption.
	Bacterial contamination	Use scrupulously clean technique in administering tube feedings; keep opened containers of formula refrigerated and discard them within 24 hr; discard enteral feeding containers and administration sets every 24 hr, hang formula for no more than 4-8 hr unless it comes prepackaged in sterile administration sets; be especially careful with feedings given to patients being fed transpylorically or those receiving cimetidine or antacids because these patients lack the normal antibacterial barrier of the stomach's hydrochloric acid.

TABLE 6-11		
NURSING MANAGEMENT OF ENTERAL TUBE FEEDING COMPLICATIONS—CONT'D		
COMPLICATION	**CONTRIBUTING FACTOR(S)**	**PREVENTION/CORRECTION**
	Fecal impaction with seepage of liquid stool around the impaction	Perform a digital rectal examination to rule out impaction; see guidelines for prevention of constipation (below).
Constipation	Low-residue formula, creating little fecal bulk	Consult with the physician regarding the use of fiber-containing formula (e.g., Enrich [Ross], Compleat [Sandoz]), although this is not possible if the patient requires an elemental diet; consult with the physician about adding bran or bulk-type laxatives to the patient's regimen.
	Inadequate fluid intake	Check patient's fluid intake to see that it totals 50 ml/kg/day unless there is need for fluid restriction.
Tube occlusion	Giving medications via tube (medications may physically plug the tube or may coagulate the formula, causing it to clog the tube)	If medications must be given by tube, avoid use of crushed tablets; consult with the pharmacist to see whether medications can be dispensed as elixirs or suspensions; irrigate tube with water before and after administering any medication; never add any medication to the tube-feeding formula unless the two are known to be compatible.
	Sedimentation of formula	Irrigate tube every 4-8 hr during continuous feedings and after every intermittent feeding.
Gastric retention	Delayed gastric emptying resulting from neural impairment or serious illness (e.g., diabetic gastroparesis, trauma)	Measure gastric residual at least every 4-6 hr or before every feeding; consult with physician about use of transpyloric feedings, temporary reduction of formula volume, or metoclopramide hydrochloride to stimulate gastric emptying; encourage patient to lie in right lateral position frequently unless contraindicated.

ripheral veins tolerate very hyperosmolar solutions poorly, and thus peripheral solutions are limited to about 10% dextrose. Daily use of intravenous lipid emulsions, which are isotonic, is necessary to provide adequate calories during peripheral TPN, unless patients are consuming substantial amounts by mouth and the TPN is being used only as a supplement.

Nursing management

Nursing care of patients receiving TPN includes catheter care, administration of solutions, prevention or correction of complications, and evaluation of patient responses to intravenous feedings (Table 6-12).

The indwelling central venous catheter provides an excellent nidus for infection.[44-46] Nurses have a major role in preventing this complication of TPN therapy. Catheter care includes maintaining an intact dressing at the catheter insertion site and manipulating the catheter and administration tubing with aseptic technique. Dressings for TPN catheters may consist of either gauze and tape or transparent film. Usually gauze dressings are changed three times weekly, and transparent dressings are changed every 5 to 7 days. Both types are also changed whenever they become wet, soiled, or nonadherent. These types of dressings have comparable rates of catheter-related sepsis,[47,48] but the transparent dressings usually decrease nursing time spent on dressing changes and may reduce

irritation of sensitive skin.[47,48] After removal of the old dressing, the skin at the insertion site is commonly cleansed with povidone iodine, which is used because it has both antibacterial and antifungal activity. Chlorhexidine hydrochloride can be substituted for povidone iodine for patients allergic to iodine.

TPN solutions usually consist of amino acids, dextrose, electrolytes, vitamins, minerals, and trace elements. Although dextrose-amino acid solutions are commonly thought of as good growth media for microorganisms, they actually suppress the growth of most organisms usually associated with catheter-related sepsis except yeasts. However, because the many manipulations required to prepare solutions increase the possibility of contamination, TPN solutions are best used with caution. They should be prepared under laminar flow conditions in the pharmacy and protected from additions on the nursing unit. Solution containers should be inspected for cracks or leaks before hanging, and solutions should be discarded within 24 hours of hanging. An in-line 0.22-μm filter, which eliminates all microorganisms but not endotoxins, may be used in administration of solutions. Use of the filter, however, should not be substituted for scrupulous aseptic technique because there is no conclusive evidence that filters decrease sepsis rates.

In contrast to dextrose–amino acid solutions, intravenous lipid emulsions support the proliferation of many

TABLE 6-12

NURSING MANAGEMENT OF TPN COMPLICATIONS

COMPLICATION	CLINICAL MANIFESTATIONS	PREVENTION/CORRECTION
Catheter-related sepsis	Fever, chills, glucose intolerance, positive blood culture	Maintain an intact dressing, change if contaminated by vomitus, sputum, and so on; use aseptic technique when handling catheter, IV tubing, and TPN solutions; hang a bottle of TPN no longer than 24 hr, lipid emulsion no longer than 12-24 hr; use an in-line 0.22-μm filter with TPN to remove microorganisms; avoid drawing blood, infusing blood or blood products, piggybacking other IV solutions into medications into TPN IV tubing, or attaching manometers or transducers via the TPN infusion line if at all possible. If catheter-related sepsis is suspected, remove catheter or assist in changing the catheter over a guidewire and administer antibiotics as ordered.
Air embolism	Dyspnea, cyanosis, apnea, tachycardia, hypotension, "millwheel" heart murmur; mortality rate estimated at 50% (depends on quantity of air entering)	Secure all connections well; use an in-line 0.22-μm air-eliminating filter; have patient perform Valsalva maneuver during tubing changes; if the patient is on a ventilator, change tubing quickly at end expiration; maintain occlusive dressing over catheter site for at least 24 hr after removing catheter to prevent air entry through catheter tract. If air embolism is suspected, place patient in left lateral decubitus and Trendelenburg's position (to trap air in the apex of the right ventricle, away from the outflow tract) and administer oxygen and CPR as needed; immediately notify physician, who may attempt to aspirate air from the heart.
Pneumothorax	Chest pain, dyspnea, hypoxemia, hypotension, radiographic evidence, needle aspiration of air from pleural space	Thoroughly explain catheter insertion procedure to patients because when they move or breathe erratically they are more likely to sustain pleural damage; perform x-ray examination after insertion or insertion attempt. If pneumothorax is suspected, assist with needle aspiration or chest tube insertion if necessary; chest tubes are usually used for pneumothorax of >25%.
Central venous thrombosis	Edema of neck, shoulder, and arm on same side as catheter; development of collateral circulation on chest; pain in insertion site; drainage of TPN from the insertion site; positive findings on venogram	Follow measures to prevent sepsis; repeated or traumatic catheterizations are most likely to result in thrombosis. If thrombosis is suspected, remove catheter and administer anticoagulants and antibiotics as ordered.
Catheter occlusion or semiocclusion	No flow or a sluggish flow through the catheter	If infusion is stopped temporarily, flush catheter with heparinized saline. If catheter appears to be occluded, attempt to aspirate the clot; if this is ineffective, physician may order thrombolytic agent such as streptokinase or urokinase instilled in the catheter.
Hypoglycemia	Diaphoresis, shakiness, confusion, loss of consciousness	Infuse TPN within 10% of ordered rate; observe patients carefully for signs of hypoglycemia after discontinuance of TPN. If hypoglycemia is suspected, administer oral carbohydrate; if patients are unconscious or oral intake is contraindicated, the physician may order a bolus of IV dextrose.
Hyperglycemia	Thirst, headache, lethargy, increased urinary output	Administer TPN within 10% of ordered rate; monitor blood glucose level at least daily until stable; patients may require insulin added to the TPN if hyperglycemia is persistent; sudden appearance of hyperglycemia in patients who were previously tolerating the same glucose load may indicate onset of sepsis.

microorganisms. Furthermore, lipid emulsions cannot be filtered through an in-line 0.22-μm filter because some particles in the emulsions have larger diameters than this. Lipid emulsions should be handled with strict asepsis and discarded within 12 to 24 hours of hanging. There is a trend toward mixing lipid emulsions with dextrose–amino acid TPN solutions. Although this saves nursing time, nurses must be extremely careful in administering these solutions. TPN solutions containing lipids cannot be filtered through an in-line 0.22-μm filter, and they support the growth of most bacteria and *Candida albicans* better than dextrose–amino acid TPN solutions.

Prevention or correction of complications

Some more common and serious complications of TPN include catheter-related sepsis, air embolism, pneumothorax, central venous thrombosis, catheter occlusion, and metabolic imbalances such as hypoglycemia and hyperglycemia. These complications, along with nursing approaches to their management, are described in Table 6-12.

References

1. McClave SA, Snider HL: Understanding the metabolic response to critical illness: factors that cause patients to deviate from the expected pattern of hypermetabolism, *New Horiz* 2(2):139, 1994.
2. Evans NJ, Sorouri BK, Feurer ID: Constraints of nutrient supply in the intensive care unit, *JPEN* 15(1):34S, 1991.
3. Mainous MR, Block EF, Deitch EA: Nutritional support of the gut: how and why, *New Horiz* 2(2):193, 1994.
4. Meyer NA, Muller MJ, Herndon DN: Nutrient support of the healing wound, *New Horiz* 2(2):202, 1994.
5. Long CL, Lowry SF: Hormonal regulation of protein metabolism, *JPEN* 14(6):555, 1990.
6. Messner RL and others: Effect of admission nutritional status on length of hospital stay, *Gastroenterol Nurs* 13:202, 1991.
7. Grant JP: Nutrition care of patients with acute and chronic respiratory failure, *Nutr Clin Pract* 9:11, 1994.
8. Benotti PN, Bistrian B: Metabolic and nutritional aspects of weaning from mechanical ventilation, *Crit Care Med* 17:181, 1989.
9. Olsen KM and others: Effect of enteral feedings on oral phenytoin absorption, *Nutr Clin Pract* 4:176, 1989.
10. Nishimura LY and others: Influence of enteral feedings on phenytoin sodium absorption from capsules, *DICP* 22:130, 1988.
11. Marvel ME, Bertino JS Jr: Comparative effects of an elemental and a complex enteral feeding formulation on the absorption of phenytoin suspension, *JPEN* 15:316, 1991.
12. Chin DE, Kearns P: Nutrition in the spinal-injured patient, *Nutr Clin Pract* 6:213, 1991.
13. Ott L, Young B: Nutrition in the neurologically injured patient, *Nutr Clin Pract* 6:223, 1991.
14. Lander V and others: Enteral feeding during barbiturate coma, *Nutr Clin Pract* 2:56, 1987.
15. Rodriguez DJ and others: Obligatory negative nitrogen balance following spinal cord injury, *JPEN* 15:319, 1991.
16. Shizgal HM and others: Body composition in quadriplegic patients, *JPEN* 10:364, 1986.
17. Cox SAR and others: Energy expenditure after spinal cord injury: an evaluation of stable rehabilitating patients, *J Trauma* 25:419, 1985.
18. Ihle BU and others: The effect of protein restriction on the progression of renal insufficiency, *N Engl J Med* 321:1773, 1989.
19. Gahl GM, Hain H: Nutrition and metabolism in continuous ambulatory peritoneal dialysis, *Contrib Nephrol* 84:36, 1990.
20. Purdum PP III, Kirby DF: Short-bowel syndrome: a review of the role of nutrition support, *JPEN* 15:93, 1991.
21. American Society for Parenteral and Enteral Nutrition Board of Directors: Guidelines for the use of enteral nutrition in the adult patient, *JPEN* 11:435, 1987.
22. Beyer PL, Frankenfield DC: Enteral nutrition in extreme short bowel, *Nutr Clin Pract* 2:60, 1987.
23. Hiyama DT, Fischer JE: Nutritional support in hepatic failure: current thought in practice, *Nutr Clin Pract* 3:96, 1988.
24. Phillips ML: Enteral nutrition support in diabetes mellitus, *Nutr Clin Pract* 2:152, 1987.
25. Anderson JW and others: Dietary fiber and diabetes: a comprehensive review and practical application, *J Am Diet Assoc* 87:1189, 1987.
26. Moore F and others: Enteral feeding reduces postoperative septic complications, *JPEN* 15(1):22S, 1991.
27. Treloar DM, Stechmiller J: Pulmonary aspiration in tube-fed patients with artificial airways, *Heart Lung* 13:667, 1984.
28. Minard G, Kudsk KA: Is early feeding beneficial? How early is early? *New Horiz* 2(2):156, 1994.
29. Strong RM and others: Equal aspiration rates from postpylorus and intragastric-placed small-bore nasoenteric feeding tubes: a randomized, prospective study, *JPEN* 16:59, 1992.
30. Estoup M: Approaches and limitations of medication delivery in patients with enteral feeding tubes, *Crit Care Nurs* Feb 1994, p 68.
31. Levenson R and others: Do weighted nasoenteric feeding tubes facilitate duodenal intubations? *JPEN* 12:135, 1988.
32. Rees RGP and others: Spontaneous transpyloric passage and performance of fine-bore polyurethane feeding tubes: a controlled clinical trial, *JPEN* 12:469, 1988.
33. Rakel and others: Nasogastric and nasointestinal feeding tube placement: an integrative review of research, *AACN Clin Issues* 5(2):194, 1994.
34. Kittinger JW, Sandler RS, Heizer WD: Efficacy of metoclopramide as an adjunct to duodenal placement of small-bore feeding tubes: a randomized, placebo-controlled, double-blind study, *JPEN* 11:33, 1987.
35. Whatley K and others: When does metoclopramide facilitate transpyloric intubation? *JPEN* 8:679, 1984.
36. Metheny N, Eisenberg P, McSweeney M: Effect of feeding tube properties and three irrigants on clogging rates, *Nurs Res* 37:165, 1988.
37. Kohn CL: The relationship between enteral formula contamination and length of enteral delivery set usage, *JPEN* 15:567, 1991.
38. Guenter PA and others: Tube feeding–related diarrhea in acutely ill patients, *JPEN* 15:277, 1991.
39. Hiebert JM and others: Comparison of continuous vs intermittent tube feedings in adult burn patients, *JPEN* 5:73, 1981.
40. Sands JA: Incidence of pulmonary aspiration in intubated patients receiving enteral nutrition through wide- and narrow-bore nasogastric feeding tubes, *Heart Lung* 20(1):75, 1991.
41. Mullan H, Roubenoff RA, Roubenoff R: Risk of pulmonary aspiration among patients receiving enteral nutrition support, *JPEN* 16:160, 1992.
42. Clark-Christoff N and others: Use of triple lumen subclavian catheters for administration of TPN, *JPEN* 17:297, 1993.

43. Payne-James JJ, Khawaja HT: First choice for total parenteral nutrition: the peripheral route, *JPEN* 17:468, 1993.

44. Corona ML and others: Infections related to central venous catheters, *Mayo Clin Proc* 65:979, 1990.

45. Armstrong CW and others: Clinical predictors of infection of central venous catheters used for total parenteral nutrition, *Infect Control Hosp Epidemiol* 11(2):71, 1990.

46. Horowitz HW and others: Central catheter-related infections: comparison of pulmonary artery catheters and triple lumen catheters for the delivery of hyperalimentation in a critical care setting, *JPEN* 14(6):588, 1990.

47. Kellam B, Fraze DE, Kanarek KS: Central line dressing material and neonatal skin integrity, *Nutr Clin Pract* 3:65, 1988.

48. Young GP and others: Catheter sepsis during parenteral nutrition: the safety of long-term OpSite dressings, *JPEN* 12:365, 1988.

7

Gerontologic Alterations

MARIANN REBENSON-PIANO

CHAPTER OBJECTIVES

- Describe the age-associated physiologic changes that occur in the cardiovascular, respiratory, renal, gastrointestinal, hepatic, integumentary, and central nervous systems.
- State the clinical significance of age-related physiologic changes and the expected nursing considerations or interventions used in caring for older critical care patients.

- Relate the age-related changes in hepatic function and accompanying pharmacokinetic changes to the administration of various cardiovascular medications.

KEY TERMS

arteriosclerosis, p. 73.

baroreceptor function, p. 72.

intrinsic heart rate, p. 71.

osteoporosis, p. 81.

presbyesophagus, p. 76.

More than 50% of critical care patients are older than 65 years of age.[1] Patients who are 65 years or older are hospitalized for longer periods in the critical care unit.[1,2] Henning and others[2] found the average length of stay in the critical care unit for an older person (i.e., >59.5 years of age) was 3.7 days, compared with 2.1 days for younger adults (i.e., <56.5 years of age). The survival rate for the former group was 81%, compared with 98% for the latter group.[1] In critical care patients, sepsis

is a leading cause of mortality. Sepsis is the third overall leading cause of death in older people.[3]

Advancing age is accompanied by physiologic changes in the cardiovascular, respiratory, renal, gastrointestinal, hepatic, integumentary, and central nervous systems. With advancing age the incidence of disease increases, with cardiovascular and neoplastic diseases being the most common causes of death.[4,5] However, although physiologic decline and disease processes influence each other, physiologic decline occurs independently of disease. Therefore critical care nurses should consider changes in physiologic function when caring for older patients.[4] The purpose of this chapter is to acquaint critical care nurses with literature and research on the age-associated changes in physiologic function in healthy older adults and to describe implications for this population in critical care.

Cardiovascular System

Advancing age has many effects on the cardiovascular system. With advancing age both the myocardium and vascular system undergo a multitude of anatomic and cellular changes that alter the function of the myocardium and peripheral vascular system.[6]

Age-Related Morphologic Changes in the Myocardium

Myocardial collagen content increases with age.[7,8] Collagen is the principal noncontractile protein occupying the cardiac interstitium.[9] Increased myocardial collagen content renders the myocardium less compliant.

The decrease in myocardial compliance can adversely affect diastolic filling (through decreased distensibility and dilation) and myocardial relaxation. Consequently the left ventricle must develop a higher filling pressure for a given increase in ventricular volume. The functional consequence could be an increase in myocardial oxygen consumption.

Under normal physiologic conditions an increase in myocardial oxygen demand is met with a corresponding increase in coronary artery blood flow. However, in the presence of coronary artery disease, coronary artery blood flow can be limited because of atherosclerotic-mediated narrowing of the coronary arteries. Hence the patient is at risk for developing myocardial ischemia and/or infarction. Clinical manifestations of myocardial ischemia include electrocardiographic changes and chest pain. However, Muller and others[10] found that complaints of chest pain were absent in 75% of older patients (over the age of 85 years) who sustained a myocardial infarction. Others[11] have also reported that chest pain is less intense and of shorter duration and originates in other areas of the chest besides the substernal region.

The aging heart undergoes a modest degree of hypertrophy similar to pressure-overload–induced hypertrophy. Such hypertrophy entails a thickening of the left ventricular wall without appreciable changes in the size of the left ventricular chamber (dilatation).[12]

Functional Changes: Myocardial Contraction and Relaxation

In the aging human myocardium, several indexes of relaxation—such as the isovolumic phase of diastole and early diastolic filling—are prolonged.[13,14] The duration of the QT interval on the electrocardiogram (ECG) also increases.[15] Theoretically, impaired relaxation can affect ventricular filling and myocardial perfusion because most of the myocardial layers are perfused during diastole. In healthy older people, impaired relaxation may not cause any appreciable change in ventricular filling and therefore cardiac output (CO) or myocardial perfusion. However, in older people with ischemic heart disease the delay in the rate of relaxation could compromise perfusion of the myocardium, especially the subendocardial layer.[16]

Hemodynamics and the Electrocardiogram

Resting (supine) heart rate decreases with age. By age 70 there is approximately a 16 beat/min decrease in the resting heart rate, as compared with the heart rate values of younger adults.[17,18] Heart rate is an important determinant of CO, and the normal resting heart beats approximately 70 times a minute. At rest or with minimal activity, older people probably will not experience any untoward cardiovascular effect (i.e., a decrease in CO) with a lower heart rate. However, if heart rate response is attenuated during exercise, older people may experience a limited capacity for exercise.

Intrinsic heart rate also decreases with aging.[19] Both divisions of the autonomic nervous system modulate resting heart rate. In healthy resting individuals, parasympathetic (cholinergic) influences predominate, which causes a heart rate of approximately 70 beats/min.[16] Without parasympathetic and sympathetic influences the heart rate of young adults averages about 100 beats/min and is referred to as the ***intrinsic heart rate.*** Jose[19] found that the intrinsic heart rate (in the presence of sympathetic and parasympathetic blockers) in a 20-year-old person was 100 beats/min, as compared with a heart rate of 74 beats/min in an 80-year-old man. This decrease in intrinsic heart rate may in part explain the decrease in the resting (supine) heart rate that occurs with aging.

Early reports indicate that resting CO and stroke volume decrease with advancing age.[20] At rest, left ventricular end-diastolic volume (preload), end-systolic volume (the volume of blood remaining in the ventricle after systole), and the ejection fraction are not affected by age.[20] In addition, Kennedy and Caird[21] reported that pulmonary artery pressures are similar between young and older subjects.

Advancing age produces changes in the ECG. The incidence of asymptomatic cardiac dysrhythmias also increases in older patients.[22] R-wave and S-wave amplitude significantly decrease in persons over 49 years of age, whereas Q-T duration increases (Table 7-1).[15] The increase in the duration of the Q-T interval reflects the prolonged rate of relaxation.[15] There is also a downward shift in the frontal plane axis from 48.93 to 38.83 degrees between the ages of 30 and 49, which suggests a modest degree of cardiac enlargement or hypertrophy.[15]

The types of dysrhythmias occurring most frequently in older individuals are premature ventricular contrac-

| TABLE 7-1 |
| AGE-RELATED CHANGES IN ELECTROCARDIOGRAPHIC VARIABLES |

ECG VARIABLE	<30 YEARS	30-39 YEARS	40-49 YEARS	>49 YEARS
R-wave amplitude (mm)	10.43	10.53	9.01	9.25
S-wave amplitude (mm)	15.21	14.21	12.22	12.42
Frontal plane axis (degrees)	48.93	48.13	36.50	38.83
P-R duration (ms)	15.89	16.23	16.04	16.25
QRS duration (ms)	7.64	7.51	7.36	8.00
Q-T duration (ms)	37.83	37.50	37.99	39.58
T-wave amplitude (ms)	5.21	4.57	4.31	4.42

Modified from Bachman S, Sparrow D, Smith LK: *Am J Cardiol* 48:513, 1981.

tions (PVCs). Camm and others[23] and Fleg and Kennedy[24] report that 70% to 80% of all patients over 60 years of age experience PVCs. In a healthy geriatric population (60 to 85 years of age), 24-hour ambulatory electrocardiographic recordings revealed that 80% of the 98 subjects studied experienced asymptomatic ventricular ectopic beats. The findings of this study suggest that aging itself is associated with an increase in the occurrence of PVCs.

Other common types of dysrhythmias include atrial fibrillation, atrial flutter, paroxysmal supraventricular tachycardia, and atrioventricular conduction disturbances.[22-24] Because the majority of patients are asymptomatic, the use of antidysrhythmics is generally not recommended. The side effects and toxic effects of antidysrhythmics impose more risks than those associated with dysrhythmia.[22] However, in patients who are symptomatic and have malignant ventricular dysrhythmias (sustained ventricular tachycardia and/or fibrillation), pharmacologic therapy is warranted.[22]

Age-Related Changes in Baroreceptor Function

Aging alters baroreceptor-reflex function.[25] The change in **baroreceptor function** may explain in part the occurrence of postural or orthostatic hypotension in older people. When position changes from supine to standing, the distribution of blood volume also changes, which can result in a reduction in CO and hence blood pressure.[16] However, with these changes in position, there are simultaneous baroreceptor-mediated increases in the heart rate that serve to maintain the blood pressure by increasing the CO. The baroreceptor reflex response also mediates changes in the peripheral resistance and force of myocardial contraction, which likewise serve to offset the drop in blood pressure. Postural hypotension was once believed to occur more frequently in older subjects. However, recent studies have shown that the prevalence of postural hypotension is quite low among older people.[26,27] The prevalence of orthostatic hypotension is greater in institutionalized older patients who receive antihypertensive medications.[28]

Left Ventricular Function in Older Persons at Rest and During Exercise

The decreased ability of older people to exercise is well established.[15] During exercise, CO is increased by four mechanisms: an increased heart rate, increased inotropic state of the myocardium, decreased aortic impedance or afterload, and increased dependence on Starling's law of the heart.[29] With advancing age, exercise causes decreases in the first three mechanisms; however, there is a striking increase in the left ventricular end-diastolic volume, which suggests an increased dependence on Starling's law of the heart. This means that at the same end-diastolic volume the older myocardium develops more force as compared with a younger myocardium. Because the former contracts more forcefully, it achieves a greater stroke volume and CO but at the same end-diastolic volume. In older subjects during exercise, CO is augmented through Starling's law of the heart, thereby compensating for the attenuated heart rate response, inotropic response, and reduced afterload response.[29]

The Peripheral Vascular System

Blood pressure changes

The gradual but linear rise in systolic blood pressure reflects the effects of aging on the peripheral vascular system.[30,31] Diastolic blood pressure is less affected by age and generally remains the same or decreases.[31] Important determinants of systolic blood pressure include the compliance of the vasculature and the blood volume within the vascular system. As with the heart, the compliance of the vasculature is determined by its composition. With advancing age the intimal layer thickens, principally because of an increase in smooth muscle cells (which have migrated from the medial layer), and the amount of connective tissue (collagen and elastic tissue) increases.[30] These changes occur in the intima of the large and distal arteries. This gradual decrease in arterial compliance or "stiffening of the arteries" is sometimes referred to as ***arteriosclerosis.***

Arteriosclerotic changes are also accompanied by changes caused by atherosclerosis. Because of arteriosclerotic and atherosclerotic processes, the arteries become progressively less distensible and the vascular pressure-volume relationship is altered. These changes are clinically significant because small changes in intravascular volume are accompanied by disproportionate increases in systolic blood pressure.[32] The decrease in arterial compliance and disproportionate increase in systolic blood pressure may lead to an increase in afterload and the development of concentric (pressure-induced) ventricular hypertrophy in older patients.[32]

Lipoprotein changes

Lipoprotein levels increase with advancing age. However, innumerable factors can influence the serum lipoprotein level, making determining whether such changes contribute to the aging of the peripheral vascular system very difficult.[33,34]

In men the serum total cholesterol level (all of the lipoproteins combined) increases progressively from 150 to 200 mg/dl between the ages of 20 and 50 years and remains relatively unchanged until the age of 70 years.[34] As predicted, the age-related changes in serum low-density lipoprotein (LDL) levels parallel the changes in the total serum cholesterol level. All lipoprotein fractions transport cholesterol; however, in healthy people, three fourths of the total cholesterol is transported within the LDL. There are relatively few age-related changes in very low-density lipoprotein (VLDL) and high-density lipoprotein (HDL) levels in men. In men, serum triglyceride levels peak at approximately age 40 and then decrease.[33,34]

In women, serum total cholesterol levels are low between the ages of 20 and 50 years.[33,34] However, between the ages of 55 to 60 years, serum total cholesterol levels progressively increase, usually with simultaneous changes in the hormonal production of estrogen.[34] The increase in total serum cholesterol level is primarily the result of an increase in the LDL fraction and, to a lesser extent, the VLDL and HDL fractions, which do not change appreciably with age in women. In women, serum triglyceride levels progressively increase with age.[34]

Arterial pressure changes

Arterial pressure is also governed by the amount of blood volume, which in turn is regulated by plasma levels of sodium and water and the activity of the renin-angiotensin system (RAS).[35] Plasma renin activity declines with age, and aging itself has no appreciable effect on sodium and water homeostasis.[36,37] However, as noted earlier, there are age-related changes in tubular

function as well as a decrease in the glomerular filtration rate (GFR), both of which can affect overall sodium and water homeostasis. Circulating levels of sodium-regulating hormones—such as natriuretic hormone, aldosterone, and antidiuretic hormone (ADH)—are not appreciably altered by advancing age.[37,38] However, a delayed natriuretic response after sodium loading and plasma volume expansion and diminished renal response to ADH secretion have been reported in older people.[38]

Respiratory System

Many of the changes in the pulmonary system that occur with aging are reflected in tests of pulmonary function and include changes in thoracic wall expansion, respiratory muscle strength, and morphology of alveolar parenchyma and decreases in arterial oxygen tension (Pao_2).[39] These changes occur progressively as age advances and should not alter the ability of older people to breathe effortlessly.

Thoracic Wall and Respiratory Muscles

The chest wall (thoracic skeleton) and vertebrae undergo a small degree of osteoporosis, and at the same time the costal cartilages connecting the rib cage become calcified and stiff. These changes may produce kyphosis and reduce chest wall compliance, respectively (Fig. 7-1).[39-41] The functional effect is a decrease in thoracic wall excursion. Factors such as an increase in abdominal girth and change in posture also decrease thoracic excursion. These anatomic structural changes are reflected by an increase in residual volume and decrease in vital capacity.

There is a gradual decrease in the strength of the respiratory muscles: the diaphragm and both the external and internal intercostal muscles. During aging, skeletal muscle progressively atrophies and its energy metabolism decreases, which may partially explain the declining strength of the respiratory muscles.[42,43] In addition, there is an age-associated decrease in the effectiveness of the cough reflex, possibly caused by a decrease in ciliary responsiveness and motion.[44] These changes underscore the importance of deep breathing and coughing for bedridden older patients in the critical care unit.

As noted previously, age-associated changes in pulmonary function do not alter the ability of older people to breathe effortlessly. However, the decrease in respiratory muscle strength may limit exercise because the respiratory muscles—specifically the accessory inspiratory muscles (sternocleidomastoid, scalene, and trapezius)—facilitate inspiration during exercise.

Alveolar Parenchyma

With advancing age a diminished recoil (or increased compliance) of the lung occurs, as exemplified by a leftward shift in the pressure-volume curve.[45] The reduced recoil results from the increase in the ratio of elastin to collagen content that occurs with aging.[46] Whereas total lung collagen remains unaltered, the amount of elastin increases with age in the interlobular septa and pleura and possibly within the bronchi and their vessels.[47,48] An increase in residual volume and a decrease in forced expiratory volume reflect these anatomic structural changes.

An additional anatomic structural change is the increase in the size of the alveolar ducts, which occurs after 40 years of age.[39] The bronchial enlargement displaces inhaled air volume away from the alveoli that line the alveolar ducts (Fig. 7-1).[39] Ventilation and the process of oxygen and carbon dioxide exchange (diffusion) depend on numerous factors, one of which is the surface area available for diffusion. A displacement of inhaled air volume away from the alveoli limits the surface area available for gas exchange. This may partly explain the progressive and linear decrease in the pulmonary diffusion capacity, which depends on both the surface area and capillary blood volume. Capillary blood volume decreases with advancing age according to some reports.[49]

Pulmonary Gas Exchange

PaO_2 decreases with age, such that the median PaO_2 for healthy persons over 60 years of age is 74.3 mm Hg compared with 94 mm Hg for younger adults.[50] In contrast, arterial carbon dioxide ($PaCO_2$) does not change with advancing age (Table 7-2).[50]

The decrease in PaO_2 may be the result of an increase in the closing volume in the dependent lung zones during resting tidal breathing in older subjects.[51,52] Consequently, dependent lung zones may be ventilated intermittently, leading to regional differences in ventilation. Alterations in blood volume and vascular resistance within the pulmonary circulation possibly contribute to ventilation/perfusion (V/Q) mismatching. Factors such

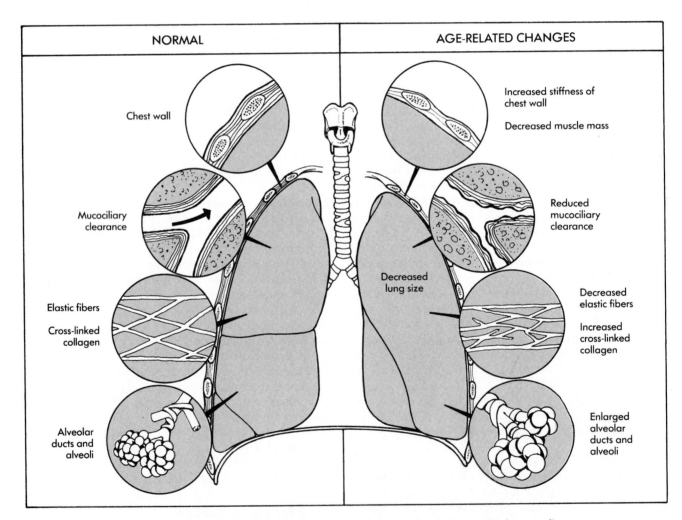

| NORMAL | AGE-RELATED CHANGES |

Chest wall — Increased stiffness of chest wall / Decreased muscle mass

Mucociliary clearance — Reduced mucociliary clearance

Decreased lung size

Elastic fibers / Cross-linked collagen — Decreased elastic fibers / Increased cross-linked collagen

Alveolar ducts and alveoli — Enlarged alveolar ducts and alveoli

FIG. 7-1 Age-related changes in the respiratory system. With advancing age the compliance of the chest wall and lung tissue change. There is also a reduced clearance of mucus by the cilia that line the pulmonary tree and an enlargement of the alveolar ducts and alveoli. More age-related changes in respiratory function are described in the text. (From Webster JR, Kadah H: *Geriatrics* 46:31, 1991.)

as smoking and pulmonary disease also have an impact on the level of arterial oxygenation.

Lung Volumes and Capacities

With advancing age, total lung capacity and tidal volume do not change.[40] Residual volume (RV) increases with age, paralleling the decrease in chest wall compliance and reduced strength of the respiratory muscles.[39] The increase in RV may also add to the diminished strength of the inspiratory muscles by stretching the diaphragm and altering the tension-length relationship. (Age-related changes in various pulmonary function tests are summarized in Table 7-3.)

Renal System

Aging produces changes in renal structure and function, many of which begin at approximately 30 to 40 years of age.[53] One prominent change is a decrease in the number and size of the nephrons, which begins in the cortical regions and progresses toward the medullary portions of the kidney.[54] The decrease in the number of nephrons corresponds to a 20% decrease in the weight of the kidney between 40 and 80 years of age.[54] Initially, this loss of nephrons does not appreciably alter renal function because of the large renal reserve: the kidney contains approximately 2 to 3 million nephrons, all of which are not required to maintain adequate fluid and acid-base homeostasis. However, with time, geriatric patients also lose this "renal reserve."[54]

Nephron loss is caused by a gradual reduction in blood flow to the glomerular capillary tuft.[55] Total renal blood flow declines after the fourth decade of life[53] because of hyaline arteriolosclerosis.[55,56] The etiology of this vascular lesion within the glomerular tuft is unknown. By the eighth decade of life, 50% of the glomeruli are lost as a result of this arteriolar hyalinization.[54]

The GFR decreases with advancing age.[53,54] The GFR is the volume of fluid traversing the glomerular membrane in a given period and is an important regulator of water and solute excretion. GFR depends on the permeability of the glomerular capillary and the surface area available for filtration as well as the balance of pres-

TABLE 7-2
PROGRESSIVE CHANGES IN ARTERIAL OXYGEN TENSION (Pa_{O_2}) AND CARBON DIOXIDE TENSION (Pa_{CO_2})

AGE-GROUPS	Pa_{O_2} (mm Hg)	Pa_{CO_2} (mm Hg)
<30 years	94	39
31-40	87	38
41-50	84	40
51-60	81	39
>60	74	40

Adapted from Sorbini CA and others: *Respiration* 25:3, 1968.

TABLE 7-3
AGE-RELATED CHANGES IN FREQUENTLY PERFORMED PULMONARY FUNCTION TESTS

PULMONARY FUNCTION TESTS	DESCRIPTIONS	STANDARD LUNG VOLUMES AND CAPACITIES (ML)	AGE-RELATED CHANGES (ML)
Total lung capacity	Vital capacity plus residual volume	6000	6000
Vital capacity	Amount of air exhaled after a maximal inspiration	5000	↓ 3750
Tidal volume (V_T) (ml)	Amount of air inhaled or exhaled with each breath	500	500
Residual volume (RV) (ml)	Amount of air left in lungs after forced exhalation	1200	↑ 1800
Inspiratory reserve volume (IRV)	Amount of air that can be forcefully inhaled after inspiring a normal V_T	3100	↓ 2800
Expiratory reserve volume (ERV)	Amount of air that can be forcefully exhaled after expiring a normal V_T	1200	↓ 1000
Forced expiratory volume in 1 sec (FEV_1)	Volume exhaled in the first second of a single forced expiratory volume; expressed as a percent of the forced vital capacity	80%	↓ 75%

sure gradients between the glomerular capillary and Bowman's space.[35] In older people the decrease in GFR is most likely caused by the decrease in nephrons as well as the decrease in renal blood flow.[53] Even though the remaining nephrons adapt to the loss of nephrons by glomerular hyperfiltration and increased solute load per nephron, the reduced GFR predisposes older patients to adverse drug reactions and drug-induced renal failure. Some drugs are excreted unchanged in the urine, whereas others have active or nephrotoxic metabolites that are excreted in the urine. The senescent kidney is also more susceptible to injury by hypotensive episodes because of the age-related decrease in renal blood flow and reduced pressure gradient across the afferent arteriole.[57]

Aging also produces changes in tubular function. The primary functions of the renal tubules are sodium and water concentration and conservation and acidification of the urine.[35] These functions are governed by the amount of sodium and water delivered to the tubules and overall acid-base balance. Age-related changes in tubular function become apparent when there are extreme changes in the body fluid composition or acid-base balance. For example, with systemic acidosis the rate and amount of total acid excretion (bicarbonate, titratable acid, and ammonium) are reduced.[53,57] This predisposes older patients to metabolic acidosis, volume depletion, and hyperchloremia. However, at a normal pH level the senescent kidney is able to maintain acid-base homeostasis.

The ability of the senescent kidney to excrete a free water load, conserve water during periods of dehydration, and conserve sodium during periods of low salt intake diminishes.[53] There are also age-related changes in extrarenal mechanisms, such as the decreased activity and responsiveness of the senescent kidney to the sympathetic nervous system and RAS, which are important in integrating overall fluid homeostasis and maintaining blood pressure in response to changes in body position.[36]

Gastrointestinal System

Age-related gastrointestinal changes occur in the processes of swallowing, motility, and absorption.[58,59] Swallowing may be difficult for older people because of incomplete mastication of food.[59] Deteriorating dentition, diminished lubrication, and ill-fitting dentures result in insufficient mastication of food within the oral cavity, thereby predisposing older patients to aspiration.[58] In addition, the number and velocity of the peristaltic contractions of the senescent esophagus decrease, and the number of nonperistaltic contractions increases.[59] These changes in esophageal motility are referred to as *presbyesophagus*. These changes may predispose patients to erosion of the esophageal wall (recurrent esophagitis) because food will remain in the esophagus longer. In addition, bed rest and reclining in a supine position for a prolonged period can cause esophageal reflux, which also can lead to esophagitis.

The aging process produces thinning of the smooth muscle within the gastric mucosa.[60] The epithelial layer of the gastric mucosa, which contains the chief and parietal cells, undergoes a modest degree of atrophy, resulting in the hyposecretion of pepsin and acid, respectively.[61] Furthermore, mucin secretion from the mucus cells decreases, thereby altering the protective function of the gastric mucosal (bicarbonate) barrier. Because of this, the stomach wall is more susceptible to acid injury, thus increasing the incidence of gastric ulcerations.[62] Aging does not appreciably alter gastric emptying of solid foods. However, Moore and others[63] found a delay in the emptying of liquids from the stomach in older subjects.

Alterations within the small intestine include a decrease in intestinal weight after the age of 50 and a flattening of jejunal villi.[64] Age produces no change in the small intestine's absorption of fats and proteins; however, decreased carbohydrate absorption has been reported.[65,66] There is essentially no change in vitamin or mineral absorption, except for a decrease in calcium absorption from the aged duodenum.[59]

The Liver

With advancing age, hepatocyte number and liver weight decrease.[67] There is also a significant decrease in total liver blood flow, such that between 25 and 65 years of age, there is a 50% decrease in total liver blood flow.[67-69] The liver has many complex functions, including carbohydrate storage, ketone body formation, reduction and conjugation of adrenal and gonadal steroid hormones, synthesis of plasma proteins, deamination of amino acids, storage of cholesterol, urea formation, and detoxification of toxins and drugs. However, despite changes in hepatocyte number and blood flow, liver function is not appreciably altered.[69] Several tests of liver function—such as serum bilirubin, alkaline phosphatase, and glutamic oxaloacetic transaminase levels—are not altered with advancing age.

The most important age-related change in liver function is the decrease in the liver's capacity to metabolize drugs.[70,71] Although clinical tests of liver function do not reflect this change in metabolism, it is widely recognized that drug side effects and toxic effects occur more frequently in older adults than young adults.[71] This reduced drug-metabolizing capacity is caused by a reduction in the activity of the drug-metabolizing enzyme system (MEOS) and decrease in total liver blood flow.[68,72]

Changes in Pharmacokinetics and Pharmacodynamics

There are many age-related changes in drug pharmacokinetics, which is the manner in which the body absorbs, distributes, metabolizes, and excretes a drug.[72,73] The aging process alters various gastrointestinal properties, such as the gastric pH level, which can alter the ionization or solubility of a drug and hence its absorption (Table 7-4).[71,72]

TABLE 7 - 4
AGE-RELATED CHANGES IN PHARMACOKINETICS

PHARMACOKINETIC PARAMETERS	DEFINITIONS	AGE-RELATED CHANGES
Absorption	Receptor-coupled or diffusional uptake of drug into tissue	Decreased absorptive surface area of small intestine Decrease in splanchnic blood flow Increase in gastric acid pH Decrease in gastrointestinal motility
Distribution	Theoretic space (tissue) or body compartment into which free form of drug distributes	Decreased lean body mass and total body water Increased total body fat Decreased serum albumin level Increased alpha-acid glycoprotein
Metabolism	Chemical change in drug that renders it active or inactive	Decreased liver mass Decrease in activity of microsomal drug-metabolizing enzyme system Decrease in total liver blood flow
Excretion	Removal of drug through an eliminating organ, which is often the kidney; some drugs are excreted in the bile or feces, in the saliva, or via the lungs	Decreased renal blood flow and GFR Decrease in distal renal tubular secretory function

From Gilman and others, editors: *Goodman and Gilman's the pharmacological basis of therapeutics,* London, 1990, Pergamon Press, and Vestal RE, Cusack BJ: *Pharmacology and aging.* In Schneider EL, Rowe JW, editors: *Handbook of the biology of aging,* San Diego, 1990, Academic Press.

Drug distribution depends on body composition as well as the physiochemical properties of the drug. With advancing age, fat content increases and intracellular water concentration decreases, which can alter the drug disposition.[72] For example, because of the increase in the ratio of body fat content to body weight, lipophilic drugs have a greater volume of distribution per body weight in older persons. Other age-related factors affecting drug disposition are listed in Table 7-4.

As noted previously the senescent liver has a decreased ability to metabolize drugs, which also affects the clearance of some drugs. For example, there is altered metabolism of loop diuretics in older patients, which reduces the peak plasma concentration of the diuretic and decreases the magnitude of the diuretic response.[74] Other drugs—such as angiotensin II–converting enzyme (ACE) inhibitors—have delayed excretion, increased serum concentration, and more prolonged duration of action.[75] GFR progressively decreases with aging. Table 7-4 summarizes age-related changes in drug pharmacokinetics, and Table 7-5 outlines the potential side effects, nursing interventions, and/or special considerations for frequently-used pharmacologic agents used with older patients in the critical care unit.

Age-related changes in pharmacodynamics reportedly exist. *Pharmacodynamics* refers to the pharmacologic or physiologic response to a drug that occurs after the drug interacts with its receptor on the plasma membrane. The chronotropic and inotropic effects of beta-adrenergic agonists reportedly decrease in older patients.[76,77] There also are reports that age produces no change in heparin-stimulated increases in partial thromboplastin time, whereas there is a diminished effect of coumadin (less of an increase in the prothrombin time). Schwertz and Bushmann[73] provide an extensive review of the pharmacologic considerations for older patients in the critical care unit.

Central Nervous System

In some individuals, changes in cognitive function such as impairments in short-term memory, speed of cognitive processing, and verbal intelligence occur with age. Some older people also experience changes in sensorimotor function; for example, vision and hearing are less acute, and gait may become slightly unsteady. Some of these changes are thought to be related to the numerous structural and morphologic changes that occur in the aging brain.[78]

Changes in neurologic function generally do not interfere with the ability of older people to carry out activities of daily living. However, neurologic disorders—such as Alzheimer's disease, stroke, and Parkinson's disease—account for almost 50% of the functional incapac-

TABLE 7-5

PHARMACOLOGIC AGENTS USED IN THE CRITICAL CARE UNIT AND FREQUENT SIDE EFFECTS EXPERIENCED BY THE GERONTOLOGIC PATIENT

PHARMACOLOGIC AGENT	DRUG ACTIONS	ADVERSE DRUG EFFECTS*	NURSING INTERVENTIONS AND/OR SPECIAL CONSIDERATIONS
ACE INHIBITORS			
Enalapril	Inhibits the conversion of angiotensin I to angiotensin II	Hypotension, especially in patients taking diuretics	Monitor HR and BP.
			Monitor serum creatinine level.
		Hypokalemia	Monitor serum K^+ level.
			Excreted by the kidney so the dosage should be reduced if the GFR is reduced.
DIURETICS			
Lasix	Inhibits Na^+ and Cl^- absorption from the proximal tubule and loop of Henle	Hypokalemia Volume depletion	Reduced rate of clearance and magnitude of the diuretic response.
CARDIAC GLYCOSIDES			
Digoxin	Inhibits the sarcolemmal Na^+K^+-ATPase	Digitalis toxicity	Monitor HR and serum K^+ and serum digoxin levels.
			Verapamil, quinidine, and amidarone increase serum digoxin levels.
ANTIDYSRHYTHMICS			
Procainamide	Decreases myocardial conduction velocity and excitability and prolongs myocardial refractoriness	Procainamide toxicity	Procainamide is converted to its active metabolite N-acetyl-procainamide (NAPA) in the liver. NAPA may accumulate and cause side effects, even though the procainamide plasma level is within therapeutic range.
Lidocaine	Decreases automaticity (especially in Purkinje fibers) and prolongs conduction and refractoriness	Dizziness, paresthesia, and drowsiness at lower plasma concentrations	Can be administered only parenterally.
CALCIUM CHANNEL BLOCKERS			
Verapamil	Blocks the entry of Ca^{2+} through voltage-dependent Ca^{2+} channels and decreases SA automaticity and AV conduction	Constipation May alter liver function	Monitor liver function tests. Contraindicated in heart failure, sick sinus syndrome, or first-degree AV block.
Nifedipine	Same as verapamil	Headaches, tachycardia, palpitations, flushing, and ankle edema	Calcium channel blockers have a negative inotropic effect, but nifedipine produces less of a negative inotropic effect as compared with verapamil.
Diltiazem	Same as verapamil	Constipation	Monitor liver function tests. Contraindicated in heart failure, sick sinus syndrome, or first-degree AV block.

From Creasy WA and others: *J Clin pharmacol* 26:264, 1986; Gilman AG and others, editors: *Goodman and Gilman's the pharmacological basis of therapeutics,* London, 1990, Pergamon Press; Hockings N, Ajayi AA, Reid JL: *Br J Pharmacol* 21:341, 1986; Lynch RA, Horowitz LN: *Geriatrics* 46:41, 1991; Pederson KE: *Acta Med Scand* 697(suppl 1):1, 1985; Vidt GD, Borazanian RA: *Geriatrics* 46:28, 1991; Wall RT: *Clin Geriatr Med* 6:345, 1990; and Watters JM, McClaran JC: *The elderly surgical patient.* In Wilmore DW and others, editors: *In care of the surgical patient,* vol III, Special problems, New York, 1990, Scientific American.

*Not all side effects are listed for each drug.

BP, blood pressure; *SA,* sinus node; *AV,* atrioventricular node; *CNS,* central nervous system; *HR,* heart rate.

PHARMACOLOGIC AGENT	DRUG ACTIONS	ADVERSE DRUG EFFECTS*	NURSING INTERVENTIONS AND/OR SPECIAL CONSIDERATIONS
NARCOTIC ANALGESICS			
Demerol	Blocks the transmission of pain and inhibits the release of substance P; site of action is within the CNS	Respiratory depression and oversedation Tremors and muscle twitches related to effects of the metabolite normeperidine	Accumulation of normeperidine can produce CNS hyperexcitability.
Morphine	Synthetic analgesic; mechanism similar to demerol	Respiratory depression and oversedation	The volume of distribution for morphine is small; hence plasma and tissue levels are greater at a specific plasma concentration.

ity experienced by older people.[78,79] As with other aging processes, age-associated changes in neurologic function occur at different rates and may be exaggerated by the coexistence of other neurologic disorders or nutritional alterations. In contrast, some older adults may experience little or no neurologic deficit or decline in cognitive or memory function. Finally, it also becomes difficult to distinguish between normal and disease-associated changes in neurologic functioning when patients are over 85 years of age.[79]

Changes in Structure and Morphology

The brain decreases approximately 20% in size between 25 and 95 years of age (Fig. 7-2).[78] The reduced brain weight may be related in part to the overall decrease in the number of neurons that occurs with advancing age. The cerebral ventricles enlarge and develop an asymmetric appearance.[80] Cerebrospinal fluid (CSF) also accumulates in the ventricles; however, total brain CSF is not increased.[80]

Accompanying the loss of neurons are changes in the ultrastructure and intracellular structures of the neuron.[81] These changes may affect the transmitting and processing of sensory and motor information, thereby affecting learning, memory, and other complex, integrative intellectual functions.[78]

In the senescent brain, synaptogenesis (synaptic regeneration) still occurs after partial nerve degeneration.[81] After a nerve fiber is damaged, neighboring undamaged neurons often sprout new fibers and form new connec-tions. However, synaptogenesis occurs at a slower rate in the older brain.[81]

Neurotransmitter Synthesis

Advancing age is associated with changes in neurotransmitter function. Altered neurotransmitter function can result from changes in the available precursors for neurotransmitter synthesis, changes in the neurotransmitter receptor, and changes in the activity of the enzymes that synthesize and degrade the neurotransmitter. These neurotransmitters have many functions within the central nervous system and are localized in different areas of the brain. Gottstein and Held[82] suggested that age-related changes in neurotransmitter levels may cause a "desynchronization" in neurotransmission, thereby affecting many neurologic functions.

Cerebral Metabolism and Blood Flow

Cerebral blood flow (CBF) decreases with advancing age. This decrease parallels the decrease in brain weight and is most likely caused by the reduction in neurons and metabolic needs of the cerebral tissue.[83]

Integumentary and Musculoskeletal Systems

As noted previously, the loss of elastic and connective tissue causes the skin to wrinkle and sag over many

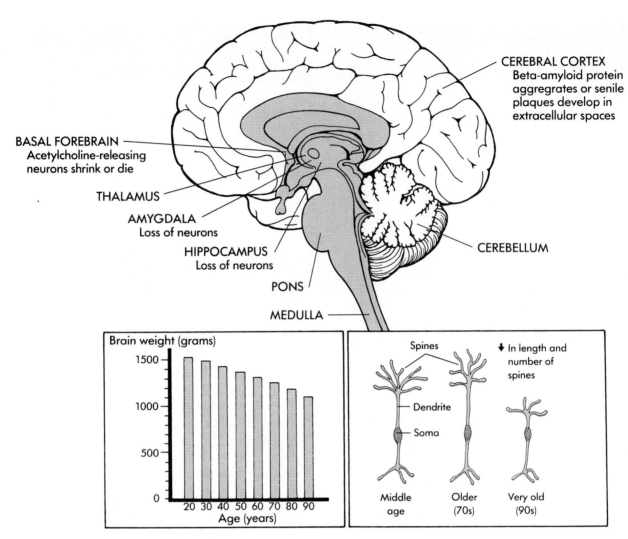

FIG. 7-2 Summary of age-related changes in the brain. (From Selkoe DJ: *Sci Am* 267:135, 1992.)

areas of the body. The appearance and number of skin wrinkles depend greatly on environmental agents and the degree of exposure to ultraviolet rays.[84] Underlying structures such as the veins and muscles are more visible because of the skin's transparency. Because of the loss of skin turgor, especially in the hands, nurses should assess for dehydration by pinching the skin over the sternum or forehead. Table 7-6 summarizes age-related changes in the skin and underlying mechanisms.

Nurses may also find multiple ecchymotic areas caused by decreased protective subcutaneous tissue layers, increased capillary fragility, and flattening of the capillary bed.[85-87] In conjunction with frequent aspirin use, these physiologic factors result in increased bleeding and the appearance of ecchymotic areas. However, areas of ecchymosis may also indicate abuse. Nurses should be alert to discrepancies between patients' histories and physical findings. Patients at risk for abuse are those who require

maximal physical assistance in the home setting.[88] Caregivers may express frustration by physical assault.

Changes that occur in the musculoskeletal system are a decrease in lean body mass; a compression of the spinal column, which results from the thinning of cartilage between vertebra; and a decrease in the mobility of skeletal joints.[88] Despite the ubiquitous finding of reduced joint mobility, no exact physiologic process is known to cause altered mobility. The reduced synovial fluid production that occurs with aging possibly causes changes in function. Muscle rigidity also increases, especially in the neck, shoulders, hips, and knees.[88] These changes may affect range of motion.

Bone demineralization afflicts both men and women as they age but occurs four times more frequently in women. *Bone demineralization* refers to an increase in osteoclast activity, which decreases calcium absorption into the bone.[89] Mineral loss (calcium and phosphorous),

TABLE 7-6

AGE-RELATED CHANGES IN THE INTEGUMENTARY SYSTEM

SKIN PROBLEMS	NURSING INTERVENTIONS	RATIONALE
Delayed wound healing	Use nonrestrictive dressings. Weigh patient daily. Support nutritional needs.	↓ Vascular supply to dermis ↓ Connective tissue layer ↓ SQ tissue layer Impaired inflammatory response ↓ New connective tissue proliferation
Thermoregulation	Monitor room temperature.	↓ SQ tissue layer ↓ Number of capillary arterioles supplying skin ↓ Number of eccrine (sweat) glands
Pressure ulcers	Reposition patient every 2 hours. Use pressure-relieving devices.	↓ Flattening of capillary bed ↓ Thinning of epidermis
IV infiltrations	Monitor peripheral IV site hourly. Discontinue IV at first sign of infiltration.	↓ Connective tissue layer Vascular fragility
Diminished skin turgor	Bathe with tepid water. Avoid use of deodorant soap.	↓ Connective tissue layer ↓ Eccrine and sebaceous gland activity

CBC, complete blood cell count; *IV*, intravenous; *SQ*, subcutaneous.

along with a decrease in bone mass, is referred to as ***osteoporosis***.[89] Osteoporosis produces bones that are more "porous" or fragile. With extensive bone demineralization, older patients may sustain multiple fractures. An accelerated incidence of osteoporosis occurs in women who have experienced menopause. A decrease in estrogen is implicated in this process because estrogen replacement may arrest, although it will not reverse, osteoporosis.

Summary

Older patients require more intense observation and consideration in the critical care unit because their systems have become less adaptable to stress and illness. Box 7-1 lists the effects of aging on various laboratory values commonly used in diagnostic testing.

Table 7-7 summarizes the major changes in the various systems, along with clinical considerations.[90] As shown in Fig. 7-3, many physiologic changes occur with advancing age, and each change may render a particular system less adaptable to stress. Moreover, the change in one system may affect another system in the presence of disease.

Critical care nurses must also be aware of socioeconomic factors that affect older patients, as well as lifestyle adjustments such as the death of a spouse or friend. Changes in the Medicare system have also placed a financial burden on many patients. To provide the best care and prevent iatrogenic complications, critical care nurses must consider all physiologic and psychologic factors affecting older patients.

BOX 7-1

EFFECTS OF AGING ON VARIOUS LABORATORY VALUES

VALUES THAT DO NOT CHANGE WITH AGE

Hemoglobin/hematocrit
Platelet count
White blood cell count with differential
Serum electrolytes
Coagulation profile
Liver function tests
Thyroid function tests
↔ or ↓ Blood urea nitrogen
↔ or ↓ Creatinine

VALUES THAT CHANGE WITH AGE BUT HAVE LITTLE CLINICAL SIGNIFICANCE

↓ Calcium
↑ Uric acid

VALUES THAT CHANGE WITH AGE AND HAVE CLINICAL SIGNIFICANCE

↓ Erythrocyte sedimentation rate
↓ Arterial oxygen pressure
↑ Blood glucose
↓ or ↑ Serum lipid profile
↓ Albumin

From Duthie EH, Abbasi AA: *Geriatrics* 46:41, 1991.
↓, decrease; ↑, increase; ↔ no change.

TABLE 7-7

SUMMARY OF AGE-RELATED PHYSIOLOGIC CHANGES AND RELATED CLINICAL CONSIDERATIONS

AGE-RELATED EFFECTS	CLINICAL CONSIDERATIONS
CARDIOVASCULAR SYSTEM	
↓ Inotropic and chronotropic response of myocardium to catecholamine stimulation	The increase in CO achieved during stress or exercise is achieved by an increase in diastolic filling (increased dependence on Starling's law of the heart)
↑ Myocardial collagen content	Leads to a decrease in the compliance of the ventricle (higher filling pressures are needed to maintain stroke volume)
↓ Baroreceptor sensitivity	↑ Tendency for orthostatic hypotension after prolonged bed rest, or if patient is taking antihypertensive medication or has systolic hypertension
Prolonged rate of relaxation	May predispose the elderly patient to hemodynamic derangements in the presence of tachydysrhythmias, hypertension, or ischemic heart disease
↓ Compliance of blood vessels	↑ Peripheral vascular resistance and blood pressure
RESPIRATORY SYSTEM	
↓ Strength of the respiratory muscles, recoil of lungs, chest wall compliance, and efficiency and number of cilia in airways	↑ Susceptibility to aspiration, atelectasis, and pulmonary infection
	Patient may require more frequent deep breathing, coughing, and position change
↓ Pa_{O_2} level	↓ Ventilatory response to hypoxia and hypercapnia
	↑ Sensitivity to narcotics
RENAL SYSTEM	
↓ GFR	Careful observation of patient when administering aminoglycosides, antibiotics, and contrast dyes
↓ Ability to concentrate and conserve water	May predispose patient to development of dehydration and hypernatremia, especially if patient is fluid restricted and insensible losses are high (e.g., during mechanical ventilation or fever)
↓ Ability to excrete salt and water loads, as well as urea, ammonia, and drugs	Observe for clinical manifestations of fluid overload and drug reactions
↓ Response to an acid load	After an acid load (i.e., metabolic acidosis) the older patients may be in a state of uncompensated metabolic acidosis for a longer period
LIVER	
↓ Total liver blood flow	Adverse drug reactions, especially with polypharmacy
GASTROINTESTINAL SYSTEM	
Diminished ability to swallow	May predispose older patients to aspiration pneumonia
	Assess for proper fit of dentures and ability to chew
	Flex head forward 45 degrees
Impaired esophageal motility	Develop awareness for complaints of food or medications "sticking in throat"
	Assess for complaints of heartburn or epigastric discomfort
	Avoid prolonged supine position
Delayed emptying of liquids	Examine abdomen for distention
	Investigate complaints of anorexia
↓ Stool weight and transit time	Obtain thorough bowel history, and note routine use of laxatives
	Increase intake of dietary fiber, and assess for fecal incontinence and impaction
NEUROLOGIC SYSTEM	
↑ In cranial dead space	Older persons may sustain a significant amount of hemorrhage before symptoms are apparent
↓ In number of neurons and dendrites and length of dendrite spines	Delayed or impaired processing of sensory and motor information
Delay in the rate of synaptogenesis	
Changes in neurotransmitter turnover	May cause desynchronization of neurotransmission

Modified from Rebenson-Piano M: *Crit Care Q* 12:1, 1989.

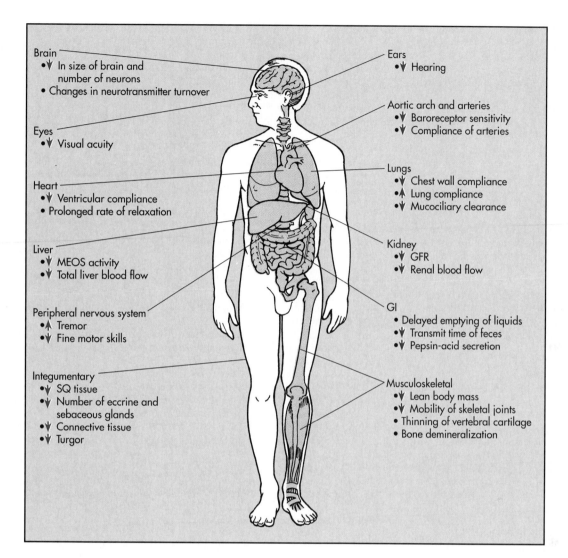

Brain
- •↓ In size of brain and number of neurons
- • Changes in neurotransmitter turnover

Eyes
- •↓ Visual acuity

Heart
- •↓ Ventricular compliance
- • Prolonged rate of relaxation

Liver
- •↓ MEOS activity
- •↓ Total liver blood flow

Peripheral nervous system
- •↑ Tremor
- •↓ Fine motor skills

Integumentary
- •↓ SQ tissue
- •↓ Number of eccrine and sebaceous glands
- •↓ Connective tissue
- •↓ Turgor

Ears
- •↓ Hearing

Aortic arch and arteries
- •↓ Baroreceptor sensitivity
- •↓ Compliance of arteries

Lungs
- •↓ Chest wall compliance
- •↑ Lung compliance
- •↓ Mucociliary clearance

Kidney
- •↓ GFR
- •↓ Renal blood flow

GI
- • Delayed emptying of liquids
- •↓ Transmit time of feces
- •↓ Pepsin-acid secretion

Musculoskeletal
- •↓ Lean body mass
- •↓ Mobility of skeletal joints
- • Thinning of vertebral cartilage
- • Bone demineralization

FIG. 7-3 Summary of physiologic changes that occur in all systems and that critical care nurses should consider in caring for older patients in the critical care unit. NOTE: *MEOS,* microsomal enzyme oxidative system; *GFR,* glomerular filtration rate; *GI,* gastrointestinal.

References

1. Munoz E and others: Diagnosis-related groups, costs, and outcome for patients in the intensive care unit, *Heart Lung* 18(6):627, 1989.
2. Henning RJ and others: Clinical characteristics and resource utilization of ICU patients: implications for organization of intensive care, *Crit Care Med* 15(3):264, 1987.
3. Stengle J, Dries D: Sepsis in the elderly, *Crit Care Nurs Q* 6(2):421, 1994.
4. Abrass IB: *Biology of aging.* In Wilson JD and others, editors: *Harrison's principles of internal medicine,* New York, 1991, McGraw-Hill.
5. Abrams WB: Cardiovascular drugs in the elderly, *Chest* 98:980, 1990.
6. Weisfeldt ML, Lakatta EG, Gerstenblith G: *Aging and the heart.* In Braunwald E, editor: *Heart disease,* Philadelphia, 1992, WB Saunders.
7. Eghbali M and others: Collagen accumulation in heart ventricles as a function of growth and aging, *Cardiovasc Res* 23:723, 1989.

8. Wegelius O, von Knorring J: The hydroxyproline and hexosamine content in human myocardium at different ages, *Acta Med Scand Suppl* 412:233, 1964.
9. Katz AM: *Heart failure.* In Fozzard HA and others, editors: *The heart and cardiovascular system,* New York, 1991, Raven Press.
10. Muller RT and others: Painless myocardial infarction in the elderly, *Am Heart J* 119:202, 1990.
11. Mukerji V, Holman AJ, Alpert MA: The clinical description of angina pectoris in the elderly, *Am Heart J* 117:705, 1989.
12. Gerstenblith G and others: Echocardiographic assessment of normal adult aging population, *Circulation* 56:273, 1977.
13. Bonow RO and others: Effects of aging on asynchronous left ventricular regional function and global ventricular filling in normal human subjects, *J Am Coll Cardiol* 11:50, 1988.
14. Miller TR and others: Left ventricular diastolic filling and its association with age, *Am J Cardiol* 58:531, 1986.
15. Bachman S, Sparrow D, Smith LK: Effect of aging on the electrocardiogram, *Am J Cardiol* 48:513, 1981.
16. Opie LH: *The physiology of the heart and metabolism,* New York, 1991, Raven Press.

17. Cinelli P and others: Effects of age on mean heart rate variability, *Age* 10:146, 1987.

18. Ribera JM and others: Cardiac rate and hyperkinetic rhythm disorders in healthy elderly subjects: evaluation by ambulatory electrocardiographic monitoring, *Gerontology* 35:158, 1989.

19. Jose AD: Effect of combined sympathetic and parasympathetic blockage on heart rate and cardiac function in man, *Am J Cardiol* 18:476, 1966.

20. Lakatta EG: *Heart and circulation*. In Schneider EL, Rowe JW, editors: *Handbook of the biology of aging*, San Diego, 1990, Academic Press.

21. Kennedy RD, Caird FI: *Physiology of heart*. In Noble RJ, Rothbaum RA, editors: *Geriatric cardiology*, Philadelphia, 1981, FA Davis.

22. Horwitz LN, Lynch RA: Managing geriatric arrhythmias. I. General considerations, *Geriatrics* 46:31, 1991.

23. Camm AJ and others: The rhythm of the heart in active elderly subjects, *Am Heart J* 99:598, 1980.

24. Fleg JL, Kennedy HL: Cardiac arrhythmias in a healthy elderly population detection by a 24-hour ambulatory electrocardiography, *Chest* 81:302, 1982.

25. Docherty JR: Cardiovascular responses in aging: a review, *Pharmacol Rev* 42:103, 1990.

26. Smith JJ and others: The effect of age on hemodynamic response to graded postural stress in normal men, *J Gerontol* 42:406, 1987.

27. Dambrink JHA, Wieling W: Circulatory response to postural change in healthy male subjects in relation to age, *Clin Sci* 72:335, 1987.

28. Applegate WB and others: Prevalence of postural hypotension at baseline in the systolic hypertension in the elderly program (SHEP) cohort, *J Am Geriatr Soc* 39:1057, 1991.

29. Rodeheffer RJ and others: Exercise cardiac output is maintained with advancing age in human subjects: cardiac dilation and increased stroke volume compensate for a diminished heart rate, *Circulation* 69:203, 1984.

30. Bierman EL: *Arteriosclerosis and aging*. In Finch CE, Schneider EL, editors: *Handbook of the biology of aging*, New York, 1985, Van Nostrand Reinhold.

31. Schoenberger JA: Epidemiology of systolic and diastolic systemic blood pressure elevation in the elderly, *Am J Cardiol* 57:45c, 1986.

32. Rowe JW: Clinical consequences of age-related impairments in vascular compliance, *Am J Cardiol* 60:68G, 1987.

33. Kreisberg RA, Kasim S: Cholesterol metabolism and aging, *Am J Med* 82:54, 1987.

34. Davis CE and others: Lipoprotein-cholesterol distributions in selected North American populations: the Lipid Research Clinics Program Prevalence Study, *Circulation* 2:302, 1980.

35. Rose BD: *Clinical physiology of acid-base and electrolyte disorders*, New York, 1989, McGraw-Hill.

36. Hall JE, Coleman TG, Guyton AC: The renin-angiotensin system: normal physiology and changes in older hypertensives, *J Am Geriatr Soc* 37:801, 1989.

37. Crane MG, Harris JJ: Effect of aging on renin activity and aldosterone excretion, *J Lab Clin Med* 87:947, 1976.

38. Sica DA, Harford A: *Sodium and water disorders in the elderly*. In Zawada ET, Sica DA, editors: *Geriatric nephrology and urology*, Littleton, Mass, 1985, PSG Publishing.

39. Webster JR, Kadah H: Unique aspects of respiratory disease in the aged, *Geriatrics* 46:31, 1991.

40. Levitzky MG: Effects of aging on the respiratory system, *Physiologist* 27:102, 1984.

41. Mittman C and others: Relationship between chest wall and pulmonary compliance and age, *J Appl Physiol* 20:1211, 1965.

42. Rizzato G, Marazzine L: Thoracoabdominal mechanisms in elderly men, *J Appl Physiol* 28:457, 1970.

43. Gutmann E, Hanzlikova V: Fast and slow motor units in aging, *Gerontology* 22:280, 1976.

44. Pontoppidan HH, Beecher HK: Progressive loss of protective reflexes in the airway with advance of age, *JAMA* 1974:2209, 1960.

45. Knudson RJ and others: Changes in the normal maximal expiratory flow-volume curve with growth and aging, *Am Rev Respir Dis* 127:725, 1983.

46. Turner JM, Mead J, Wohl ME: Elasticity of human lungs in relation to age, *J Appl Physiol* 25:664, 1968.

47. Pierce JA, Hocott JB: Studies on the collagen and elastin content of the human lung, *J Clin Invest* 39:8, 1960.

48. Pierce JA, Ebert RV: Fibrous network of the lung and its change with age, *Thorax* 20:469, 1965.

49. Semmens M: The pulmonary artery in the normal aged lung, *Br J Dis Chest* 64:65, 1970.

50. Sorbini CA and others: Arterial oxygen tension in relation to age in healthy subjects, *Respiration* 25:3, 1968.

51. LeBlanc P, Ruff F, Milic-Emili J: Effects of age and body position on "airway closure" in man, *J Appl Physiol* 28:448, 1970.

52. Holland J and others: Regional distribution of pulmonary ventilation and perfusion in elderly subjects, *J Clin Invest* 47:81, 1968.

53. Weder AB: The renally compromised older hypertensive: therapeutic considerations, *Geriatrics* 46:36, 1991.

54. Gilbert BR, Vaughan ED: Pathophysiology of the aging kidney, *Clinics Geriatr Med* 6(1):12, 1990.

55. Kasiske BL: Relationship between vascular disease and age-associated changes in the human kidney, *Kidney Int* 31:1153, 1987.

56. Anderson S, Brenner BM: Effects of aging on the renal glomerulus, *Am J Med* 80:435, 1986.

57. Watters JM, McClaran JC: *The elderly surgical patient*. In Wilmore DW and others, editors: *In care of the surgical patient*, vol VII, Special problems, New York, 1990, Scientific American.

58. Brandt LJ: *Gastrointestinal disorders in the elderly*. In Rossman I, editor: *Clinical geriatrics*, ed 3, Philadelphia, 1986, JB Lippincott.

59. Williams SA, Fogel RP: Common gastrointestinal problems in the elderly, *JAMA* 87:29, 1989.

60. Altman DF: Changes in gastrointestinal, pancreatic, biliary and hepatic function in aging, *Gastroenterol Clin North Am* 19(2):227, 1990.

61. Thomson AB, Keelan M: The aging gut, *Can J Physiol Pharmacol* 64:30, 1986.

62. Bansal SK and others: Upper gastrointestinal haemorrhage in the elderly: a record of 92 patients in a joint geriatric/surgical unit, *Age Ageing* 16:279, 1987.

63. Moore JG and others: Effect of age on gastric emptying of liquid-solid meals in man, *Dig Dis Sci* 28(4):340, 1983.

64. Schuster MM: Disorders of the aging GI system, *Hosp Prac* 11:95, 1976.

65. Curran J: Overview of geriatric nutrition, *Dysphagia* 5:72, 1990.

66. Ausman LM, Russel RM: *Nutrition and aging*. In Schneider EL, Rowe JW, editors: *Handbook of the biology of aging*, San Diego, 1990, Academic Press.

67. Sato TG, Miwa T, Tauchi H: Age changes in the human liver of the different races, *Gerontologia* 16:368, 1970.

68. Bach B and others: Disposition of antipyrine and phenytoin correlated with age and liver volume in man, *Clin Pharmacokinet* 6:389, 1981.

69. Kampmann JP, Sinding J, Moller-Jorgensen I: Effect of age on liver function, *Geriatrics* 30:91, 1975.
70. Schmucker DL, Wang RK: Age-related changes in liver drug metabolism: structure versus function, *Proc Soc Exp Biol Med* 165:178, 1980.
71. Vestal RE, Cusack BJ: *Pharmacology and aging.* In Schneider EL, Rowe JW, editors: *Handbook of the biology of aging,* San Diego, 1990, Academic Press.
72. Yuen GJ: Altered pharmacokinetics in the elderly, *Clin Geriatr Med* 6:257, 1990.
73. Schwertz DW, Buschmann MT: Pharmacogeriatrics, *Crit Care Q* 12:26, 1989.
74. Mooradian AD: An update of the clinical pharmacokinetics, therapeutic monitoring techniques and treatment recommendations, *Clin Pharmacokinet* 18:165, 1988.
75. Creasy WA and others: Pharmacokinetics of captopril in elderly healthy male volunteers, *J Clin Pharmacol* 26:264, 1986.
76. Bertel O and others: Decreased beta-adrenoreceptor responsiveness as related to age, blood pressure and plasma catecholmines in patients with essential hypertension, *Hypertension* 2:130, 1980.
77. Kendall MJ and others: Responsiveness to beta-adrenergic receptor stimulation: the effects of age are cardioselective, *Br J Clin Pharmacol* 14:821, 1982.
78. Selkoe DJ: Aging brain, aging mind, *Sci Amer* 267:134, 1992.
79. Morris JC, McManus DQ: The neurology of aging: normal versus pathologic change, *Geriatrics* 46:47, 1991.
80. Coleman PD, Flood DG: Neuron numbers and dendritic extent in normal aging and Alzheimer's disease, *Neurobiol Aging* 8:521, 1987.
81. Cotman CW: *Synaptic plasticity, neurotropic factors and transplantation in the aged brain.* In Schneider EL, Rowe JW, editors: *Handbook of the biology of aging,* San Diego, 1990, Academic Press.
82. Gottstein U, Held K: Effects of aging on cerebral circulation and metabolism in man, *Acta Neurol Scand Suppl* 72:54, 1979.
83. Fields SD: History-taking in the elderly: obtaining useful information, *Geriatrics* 46(8):26, 1991.
84. Lapiere CM: The ageing dermis: the main cause for the appearance of "old skin," *Br J Dermatol* 122(suppl 35):5, 1990.
85. Jones PL, Millman A: Wound healing and the aged patient, *Nurs Clin North Am* 25(1):263, 1990.
86. Kelly L, Mobily PR: Iatrogenesis in the elderly, *J Gerontol Nurs* 17(9):24, 1991.
87. Shenefelt PD, Fenske NA: Aging and the skin: recognizing and managing common disorders, *Geriatrics* 45(10):57, 1990.
88. Exton-Smith AN: *Mineral metabolism.* In Finch CE, Schneider EL, editors: *Handbook of the biology of aging,* New York, 1985, Van Nostrand Reinhold.
89. Ganong WF: *Review of medical physiology,* Norwalk, Conn, 1991, Appleton & Lange.
90. Piano MR: The physiologic changes that occur with aging, *Crit Care Q* 12:1, 1989.

UNIT THREE

Cardiovascular Alterations

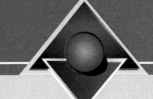

8

Cardiovascular Assessment and Diagnosis

MARY LOUGH

MARTHA LOVE

JENNIFER BLOOMQUIST

CHAPTER OBJECTIVES

- Explain jugular venous distention and its importance as an assessment of central venous pressure.
- Describe the normal heart sounds S_1 and S_2 and the abnormal heart sounds S_3 and S_4.
- Identify correct placement of the electrodes for cardiac monitor leads II, MCL_1, and MCL_6.

- State important ECG findings for each of the cardiac dysrhythmias.
- Discuss nursing management priorities for care of patients with central venous pressure, pulmonary artery (PA) pressure, and cardiac output monitoring.

KEY TERMS

BOX   8 - 1

DATA COLLECTION FOR CARDIOVASCULAR HISTORY

COMMON CARDIOVASCULAR SYMPTOMS

Chest pain
Palpitations
Dyspnea
Cough
Nocturia
Edema
Dizziness/syncope
Claudication

PATIENT PROFILE

Personal habits
    Use of tea, coffee, alcohol, recreational drugs, over-the-counter drug use, smoking, exercise, and dietary habits
Lifestyle pattern
    Working, relaxing, coping
Recent life changes
    Within the past 6 months
Emotional state
    Evidence of psychologic stress, worry, anxiety
Perception of illness and its meaning for the future

RISK FACTORS

Gender/age (≥45 years in men, ≥55 years in women)
Family history (MI or sudden death in a parent or first-degree relative before age 55)
Hypertension
Diabetes mellitus
Obesity (more than 30% over ideal body weight)
Smoking history
High serum cholesterol (HDL <35 mg/dl)
Sedentary lifestyle
Menopause

FAMILY HISTORY

Coronary artery disease
Myocardial infarction
Hypertension
Stroke
Diabetes mellitus
Lipid disorders

CARDIAC DIAGNOSTIC STUDIES IN PAST

Cardiac catheterization
Cardiac ultrasound
ECG
Exercise tolerance test
Myocardial imaging with radiographic isotopes
Percutaneous transluminal coronary angioplasty
Atherectomy
Valvuloplasty

MEDICAL HISTORY

Childhood
    Murmurs, cyanosis, streptococcal infections, rheumatic fever
Adult
    Heart failure, coronary artery disease, heart valve disease, mitral valve prolapse, myocardial infarction, peripheral vascular disease, diabetes mellitus, hypertension, hyperlipidemia, dysrhythmias, murmurs, endocarditis, psychiatric illnesses
Allergies
    Especially to radiographic contrast agents or iodine
Surgical history
    Coronary artery bypass grafting, valve replacement, peripheral vascular bypasses or repairs

CURRENT MEDICATION USAGE

Digitalis
Diuretics
Potassium
Antidysrhythmics
Beta blockers
Calcium channel blockers
Nitrates
Antihypertensives
Anticoagulants

Clinical Assessment

History

The patient history (Box 8-1) is an important source of data contributing to the cardiovascular diagnosis and treatment plan. Patients set the priorities according to their presenting symptoms, which should take priority and direct the history-taking part of the assessment. Each symptom is further explored with the questions detailed in Table 8-1. Obtaining information about the medical history, current medication usage, and diagnostic studies that may have been performed in the past will assist in treatment of the cardiovascular condition. Taking the time to obtain this information can prevent repetitive tests or ineffective therapy.

Physical Examination

Inspection. The priorities for inspection of patients with cardiovascular disease include (1) assessing general appearance, (2) observing the skin and nailbeds, (3) examining the extremities, (4) estimating jugular venous distention (JVD), (5) measuring CVP using

T A B L E 8 - 1	
CLARIFICATION OF SYMPTOMS BY ASKING SPECIFIC QUESTIONS: EXAMPLE: CHEST PAIN	
DETERMINE	**TYPICAL QUESTION**
Location, radiation	Where is it? Does it move or stay in one place?
Quality	What's it like?
Quantity	How severe is it? How frequent? How long does it last?
Chronology	When did it begin? How has it progressed?
Aggravating and alleviating factors	What are you doing when it occurs? What do you do to get rid of it?
Associated findings	Are there any other symptoms you feel at the same time?
Treatment sought and effect	Have you seen a doctor in the past for this same problem? What was the treatment?

the internal jugular vein, and (6) observing the apical impulse.

Assessing general appearance

To determine whether patients are obese (a cardiac risk factor) or cachectic (underweight), nurses should assess patients' weight in proportion to height and their overall nutritional status. Nurses should observe the color of the skin to determine whether it is cyanotic, pale, or jaundiced, also noting facial expressions of apprehension or pain. Body posture sometimes indicates the amount of effort required to breathe or what positions patients find comfortable. Patients in heart failure need to sit upright, and patients with pericarditis may find that leaning forward is the least painful position.[1] Nurses should observe patients for signs of diaphoresis, confusion, or lethargy, each of which could indicate hypotension or low cardiac output. Respiratory rate, pattern, and effort should also be noted. Nurses should inspect the skin on the chest wall and the abdomen for scars, bruises, wounds, or the bulge of a pacemaker or defibrillator implant.

Observing the skin and nailbeds

Cyanosis, a bluish discoloration of the skin, may be central or peripheral. Central cyanosis is a bluish discoloration of the lips, circumoral area, mucous membranes, and nailbeds that indicates decreased oxygen saturation of the circulating hemoglobin molecule and may occur as a result of right-to-left intracardiac shunts, impaired pulmonary function, or hypoxia.[1] Peripheral cyanosis indicates reduction of peripheral blood flow as a result of vascular disease, decreased cardiac output, or cold.[1] Nurses should examine the nailbeds for signs of clubbing, which may indicate chronic oxygen deficiency. Clubbing is evaluated by assessing the angle between the nail and the nail base, which is normally less than 180 degrees. A flattened angle (180 degrees) with a springy or spongy nail base is "early" clubbing, and an angle greater than 180 degrees with a swollen nail base is "late" clubbing.

B O X   8 - 2
Inspection of the Cardiovascular System: *Extremities*
Nail bed color Nail bed clubbing Skin color Skin condition Hair distribution Presence of edema Presence of varicosities Comparison of circumferences

Examining the extremities

The extremities are examined for signs of vascular disease. If peripheral arterial disease is present, leg hair is sparse or lacking; the skin is dry, scaly, cracked, or shiny; and limb temperature is cool, with a pale or dusky color. If arterial insufficiency is present, pallor appears when the legs are elevated and rubor when the legs are dependent. If venous thrombosis exists, the color of the extremity may be dusky and the circumference of the affected calf or thigh slightly larger compared with that of the other extremity. The lower extremities are inspected for varicosities that may predispose patients to develop thrombophlebitis. Box 8-2 lists the specific information to be obtained by inspecting the extremities.

Estimating JVD

When patients are sitting upright, the jugular veins are normally flat. **Jugular venous distention** (JVD) occurs when central venous pressure is elevated, as in failure of the right side of the heart.[2] The procedure for assessing JVD is described in Box 8-3. JVD is present if distention is greater than 3 cm above the sternal angle (Fig. 8-1). JVD may appear before other changes in clinical status. Prompt treatment may prevent sudden deterioration into acute heart failure.

BOX 8-3

PROCEDURE FOR ASSESSING JVD USING THE EXTERNAL JUGULAR VEIN

1. Patient reclines at a 30- to 45-degree angle.
2. The examiner stands on the patient's right side and turns the patient's head slightly toward the left.
3. If the jugular vein is not visible, light finger pressure is applied across the sternocleidomastoid muscle just above and parallel to the clavicle. This pressure will fill the external jugular vein by obstructing flow (Fig. 8-1).
4. Once the location of the vein has been identified, the pressure is released and the presence of JVD is assessed.
5. Because inhalation decreases venous pressure, JVD should be assessed at the end of exhalation.
6. Any fullness in the vein extending more than 3 cm above the sternal angle is evidence of increased venous pressure. Generally the higher the sitting angle of the patient when JVD is discovered, the higher the central venous pressure.
7. *Documentation:* JVD is reported by including the angle of the head of the bed at the time JVD was evaluated (e.g., "presence of JVD with head of bed elevated to 45 degrees").

BOX 8-4

PROCEDURE FOR ASSESSING NON-INVASIVE CENTRAL VENOUS PRESSURE USING THE INTERNAL JUGULAR VEIN

1. The patient reclines in bed. The highest point of pulsation in the internal jugular vein is observed during exhalation.
2. The vertical distance between this pulsation, which is at the top of the fluid level, and the sternal angle is estimated or measured in centimeters (cm).
3. This number is then added to 5 cm for an estimation of central venous pressure. The 5 cm is the approximate distance of the sternal angle above the level of the right atrium (Fig. 8-2).
4. *Documentation:* The degree of elevation of the patient is included in reporting this finding (e.g. "central venous pressure estimated at 13 cm, using the internal jugular vein pulsation, with the head of the bed elevated 45 degrees").

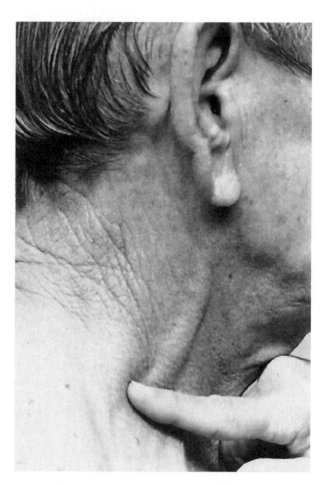

FIG. 8-1 Assessment of jugular vein distention (JVD). Applying light finger pressure over the sternocleidomastoid muscle, parallel to the clavicle, helps identify the external jugular vein by occluding flow and distending it. Release the finger pressure and observe for distention >3 cm above the sternal angle, indicating JVD.

Measuring the CVP using the internal jugular vein

The fluid column of the internal jugular vein is also used to estimate the amount of CVP (in centimeters). This vein lies anterior to the external jugular at the level of the clavicle and follows a parallel path with the carotid artery and the trachea. Central venous pressure elevated greater than 7 cm indicates elevated right atrial pressure.[3] The procedure for CVP measurement is described in Box 8-4.

Observing the apical impulse

The anterior thorax is inspected for the apical impulse, sometimes referred to as the *point of maximal impulse.* The apical impulse occurs as the left ventricle contracts during systole, causing the left ventricular apex to hit the chest wall. The impulse is located just lateral to the left midclavicular line at the fifth intercostal space (Fig. 8-3). The apical impulse is the only normal pulsation visible on the chest wall, and its location, size, and character should be noted if it appears.

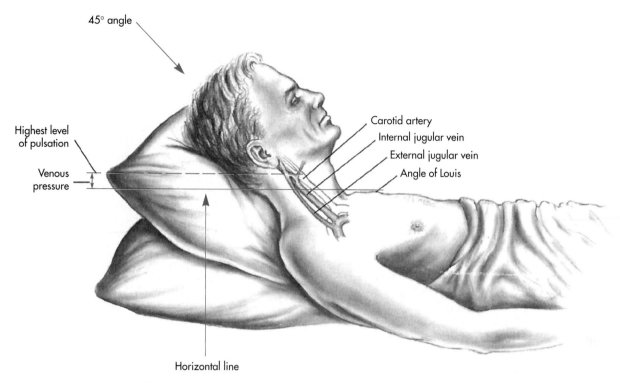

FIG. 8-2 Position of internal and external jugular veins. Pulsation in the internal jugular vein can be used to estimate central venous pressure. (Modified from Thompson JM and others: *Mosby's clinical nursing,* ed 3, St Louis, 1993, Mosby.)

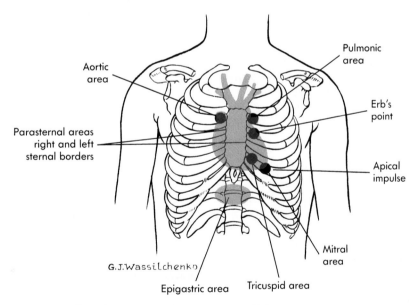

FIG. 8-3 Auscultatory areas for assessment of heart sounds and pulsations.

Palpation

Palpation is a technique that uses the sense of touch. Palpation of the patient includes the following priorities: (1) evaluating arterial pulses, (2) performing the Allen test, (3) confirming capillary refill, (4) quantifying edema, and (5) assessing for signs of thrombophlebitis. The information obtained by palpation reinforces data collected with inspection and is especially important for assessment of the vascular system.

Evaluating arterial pulses

Eight major arterial areas are assessed for pulse palpation. The examination must include bilateral assessment of the carotid, brachial, radial, ulnar, femoral, popliteal, dorsalis pedis, and posterior tibial arterial pulses. The extremity pulses are assessed separately and compared bilaterally to check consistency. Pulse volume is graded on a scale of 0 to 3+ (Box 8-5). Peripheral pulses should be assessed by Doppler ultrasound if they cannot be palpated.

Performing the Allen test

Before a radial artery is punctured or cannulated, the Allen test should be done to assess adequate blood flow to the hand through the ulnar artery. The Allen test is performed as follows:

1. The examiner requests that the patient make a tight fist to squeeze blood from the hand.
2. The examiner uses firm thumb pressure to compress the radial and ulnar arteries.
3. The examiner asks the patient to open the hand, palm side up, and releases the ulnar artery while the radial artery is still occluded.
4. The examiner notes the time it takes for color to return to the hand. If the ulnar artery is patent, the color will return within 3 seconds. Delayed color return (a "failed" Allen test) implies that the ulnar artery is occluded; therefore the radial artery is the only source of blood flow to the hand and should not be punctured or cannulated.

Confirming capillary refill

Capillary refill assessment is performed on the nailbeds to evaluate arterial circulation to the extremity. The nailbed should be compressed to produce blanching, and release of the pressure should result in a return of blood flow and nail color in less than 3 seconds. The more severe the arterial insufficiency, the longer it takes for flow and color to return.

Quantifying edema

Edema is fluid accumulated in the extravascular spaces of the body, such as the abdomen and the dependent tissues of the legs and sacrum. Examiners quantify edema in the extremities by identifying the location and pressing their thumb to the skin of the feet, ankles, or shins against the underlying bone. If the thumb leaves an impression in the tissue, patients have a condition known as *pitting edema*.[4] The extent of the edema may be quantified as shown in Box 8-6.

Assessing for signs of thrombophlebitis

Palpation is used to assess the veins of the lower extremities for thrombophlebitis, an inflammation of the vein with thrombus formation. Venous thrombosis, or deep vein thrombosis, predisposes a patient to pulmonary emboli.[5] In assessment, gentle pressing of the calves against the tibia may elicit pain, tenderness, or tension in the muscle. These signs suggest phlebitis and should alert examiners to check other parameters that may aid in diagnosis, such as comparing leg circumferences and checking for increased heat in the extremity or unexplained fever. Homan's sign, in the presence of the other signs, can assist in the diagnosis of phlebitis.[4] To elicit Homan's sign, examiners should flex patients' knee and forcefully and abruptly dorsiflex patients' foot. If patients report pain in the popliteal region and the calf, the sign is positive.

Percussion

Percussion is rarely used today in the physical examination of the heart. Before the advent of the chest x-ray, percussion was used to outline the left cardiac border.

Auscultation

Auscultation of patients includes the following priorities: (1) measurement of blood pressure, (2) detection of bruits, (3) assessment of normal and abnormal heart sounds, (4) identification of heart murmurs, and (5) recognition of a pericardial friction rub.

Measurement of blood pressure

A thorough cardiovascular assessment includes blood pressure measurements in both arms to rule out aortic or subclavian stenosis.

Detection of bruits

The carotid and femoral arteries are auscultated for bruits. A bruit is a high-pitched "sh-sh," extracardiac vascular sound that vacillates in volume with systole and diastole and results from either normal blood flow through

---

B O X   8 - 5

PULSE PALPATION SCALE

SCALE	DESCRIPTION
0	Not palpable
1+	Faintly palpable (weak and thready)
2+	Palpable (normal pulse)
3+	Bounding (hyperdynamic pulse)

B O X   8 - 6

PITTING EDEMA SCALE

SCALE	DESCRIPTION	DEPTH OF INDENTATION	TIME TO RETURN TO BASELINE
0	None present	0	—
1+	Trace	$0-1/4''$	Rapid
2+	Mild	$1/4-1/2''$	10-15 sec
3+	Moderate	$1/2-1''$	1-2 min
4+	Severe	$>1''$	2-5 min

a tortuous or a partially occluded vessel or increased blood flow through a normal vessel.

Assessment of normal heart sounds (S_1 and S_2)

Normal heart sounds are referred to as *sound one* (S_1) and *sound two* (S_2). S_1 is produced by the rapid deceleration of blood flow when the atrioventricular (mitral and tricuspid) valves close at the beginning of systole. S_2 is heard at the end of systole when the semilunar (aortic and pulmonic) valves reach closure.[1,2] Both sounds are high pitched and best heard with the diaphragm of the stethoscope. Each sound is loudest in an auscultation area located "downstream" from the actual valve because the sound is carried in the direction of blood flow. For example, S_2—which is associated with aortic and pulmo-

nary valve closure—can be best heard at the base of the heart, at the second intercostal space to the right and left of the sternum, and in the areas labeled aortic and pulmonic (Fig. 8-3). Associated with closure of the mitral and tricuspid valves, S_1 is best heard in the mitral and tricuspid areas. Technically both S_1 and S_2 are split sounds (Fig. 8-4) because the left side of the heart contracts milliseconds before the right. However, in the healthy heart the left-sided heart valves, mitral and aortic, are usually the loudest and S_1 and S_2 are heard as a single sound in their respective areas.

Assessment of abnormal heart sounds (S_3 and S_4)

The abnormal heart sounds are identified as *sound three* (S_3) and *sound four* (S_4) and referred to as *gallops* when

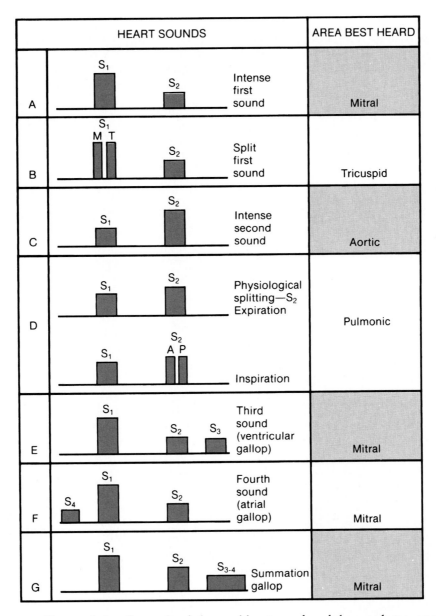

FIG. 8-4 Characteristics of normal and abnormal heart sounds and the auscultatory area where each is best heard.

auscultated during tachycardia. Low pitched, they occur during diastole and are best heard with the bell of the stethoscope positioned lightly over the apical impulse when patients are in the left lateral decubitus position. An S_3 is sometimes referred to as a *ventricular gallop.* Clinically an S_3 can be anticipated in the presence of heart failure. An S_3 occurs when the mitral and tricuspid valves open and blood from the atrium flows into a ventricle that has a greater-than-normal blood volume remaining after systole. The sound occurs after S_2 and resembles a dull thud. An S_3 is considered normal in a young person because of the rapid filling of the healthy ventricle.[6] The S_4 sound is sometimes described as an *atrial gallop* and is produced by atrial contraction just before S_1.

Identification of physiologic murmurs

In children and adolescents, systolic "high flow" murmurs are common, resulting from vigorous ventricular contraction. These murmurs are a normal variant. They have a low-to-medium pitch (best heard with the bell of the stethoscope), grade I to II intensity, and a blowing quality.

Identification of abnormal heart murmurs

Heart murmurs are prolonged extra sounds that occur during systole or diastole. These sounds are vibrations caused by turbulent blood flow through the cardiac chambers. Murmurs are characterized by several characteristics described on page 97 and in Table 8-2:

TABLE 8-2
CHARACTERISTICS OF SOME MURMURS

DEFECT	TIMING IN THE CARDIAC CYCLE	PITCH, INTENSITY, QUALITY	LOCATION, RADIATION
SYSTOLIC MURMURS			
Mitral regurgitation		High / Harsh / Blowing	Mitral area / May radiate to axilla
Tricuspid regurgitation		High / Often faint, but varies / Blowing	Tricuspid RLSB, apex, LLSB, epigastric areas / Little radiation
Ventricular septal defect		High / Loud / Blowing	Left sternal border
Aortic stenosis		Chhhh hh / Medium / Rough, harsh	Aortic area to suprasternal notch, right side of neck, apex
Pulmonary stenosis		Low to medium / Loud / Harsh, grinding	Pulmonic area / No radiation
DIASTOLIC MURMURS			
Mitral stenosis	Atrial kick	Low / Quiet to loud with thrill / Rough rumble	Mitral area / Usually no radiation
Tricuspid stenosis	Atrial kick	Medium / Quiet; louder with inspiration / Rumble	Tricuspid area or epigastrim / Little radiation
Aortic regurgitation		High / Faint to medium / Blowing	Aortic area to LLSB and aorta / Erb's point
Pulmonic regurgitation		Medium / Faint / Blowing	Pulmonic area / No radiation

RLSB, right lower sternal border; *LLSB,* left lower sternal border.

- Timing: systolic or diastolic
- Location and radiation
- Quality: blowing, grating, or harsh
- Pitch: high or low
- Intensity: loudness graded on a scale of I to VI, the higher the number, the louder the murmur, as shown in Box 8-7.

Heart murmur location

When auscultating murmurs, examiners should visualize the cardiac anatomy, specifically the location of the heart valves and the direction of sound transmission with valve closure and murmur. Systolic valvular murmurs generally radiate the sound downstream from the valve that is narrowed. Diastolic valvular murmurs, which indicate a backflow of blood through an incompetent valve, are best auscultated directly over the area of the valve.

Recognition of a pericardial friction rub

A pericardial friction rub is a sound that can occur within the first week after a myocardial infarction or after cardiac surgery and is secondary to pericardial inflammation. A possible indication of a pericardial effusion, it is a high-pitched, grating sound heard during all phases of cardiac motion and best auscultated between the left sternal border and the apex. Because pericardial friction rub may be associated with chest pain, differentiating the pain of pericarditis from that of myocardial ischemia is important.[7]

Laboratory Studies

Potassium

During depolarization and repolarization of nerve and muscle fibers, potassium and sodium exchange occurs intracellularly and extracellularly. Thus either an excess or deficiency of potassium can alter cardiac muscle function. The normal serum level is 3.5 to 5.5 mEq/L (Box 8-8).

Hyperkalemia

High serum potassium, or hyperkalemia, decreases the rate of ventricular depolarization, shortens repolarization, and depresses atrioventricular (AV) conduction. As serum potassium rises above the normal range, changes are seen on the electrocardiograph (ECG) (Fig. 8-5). Tall, peaked T waves are usually, although not uniquely, associated with early hyperkalemia and are followed by widening of the QRS complex and prolongation of the P wave and PR interval. If serum potassium levels rise above 10 to 14 mEq/L, depressed AV conduction leads to cardiac standstill or ventricular fibrillation (VF). Coexisting hyponatremia, hypocalcemia, or acidosis exacerbate the cardiac effects of hyperkalemia.

Hypokalemia

Low serum potassium, or hypokalemia, is commonly caused by gastrointestinal losses, diuretic therapy with insufficient replacement, and chronic steroid therapy. Hy-

---

BOX 8-8

CHEMISTRY VALUES THAT IMPACT CARDIAC CONTRACTILITY

	NORMAL RANGE
Potassium (K^+)	3.5-5.5 mEq/L
Calcium (Ca^{++})	9-11 mg/dl
Magnesium (Mg^{++})	1.5-2.5 mEq/L

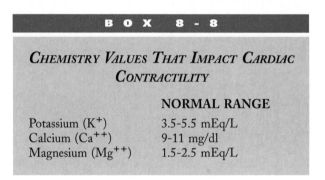
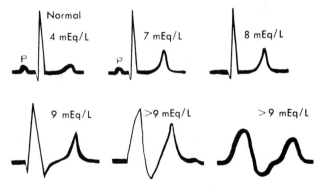

FIG. 8-5 Effects of hyperkalemia: The earliest electrocardiogram (ECG) change with hyperkalemia is peaking (tenting) of the T wave. With progressive increases in the serum potassium level the QRS complexes widen, P waves disappear, and finally ventricular fibrillation develops. These changes do not necessarily occur with a specific serum potassium level. For example, some patients can have a normal ECG with a potassium level of 7 mEq/L, (patients with chronic renal failure), whereas other patients with an *acute* rise in serum potassium to a similar level have ventricular fibrillation. (From Goldberger AL, Goldberger E: *Clinical electrocardiography: a simplified approach,* ed 5, St Louis, 1994, Mosby.)

BOX 8-7

GRADING OF CARDIAC MURMURS

GRADE DESCRIPTION

I/VI	Very faint, may be heard only in a quiet environment
II/VI	Quiet, but clearly audible
III/VI	Moderately loud
IV/VI	Loud; may be associated with a thrill
V/VI	Very loud; thrill easily palpable
VI/VI	Very loud; may be heard with stethoscope off the chest. Thrill palpable and visible

pokalemia is also reflected by the ECG (Fig. 8-6). Myocardial conduction is impaired, and ventricular repolarization is prolonged, as evidenced by a prominent U wave. The U wave is not unique to hypokalemia, but its presence should alert nurses to check the serum potassium level. Another ECG indicator of hypokalemia is the sudden occurrence of supraventricular and ventricular dysrhythmias, which result from the prolonged repolarization phase and exist in most patients with serum potassium levels below 2.6 mEq/L.[8] These rhythm disturbances are reversible with potassium replacement.

Calcium

Maintaining a normal serum calcium (Ca^{++}) level is important because of its effect on myocardial contractility and cardiac excitability. The normal serum level ranges from 9 to 11 mg/dl (see Box 8-8).

Hypercalcemia

High serum calcium, or hypercalcemia, strengthens contractility and shortens ventricular repolarization. The ECG demonstrates this shortened repolarization by a shortened QT interval.

Hypocalcemia

Low serum calcium, or hypercalcemia, has the opposite effect on the myocardium. The ECG shows a prolonged QT interval. Below a level of 6 mg/dl QT prolongation is common, proportional to the amount of hypocalcemia,

and can be reversed with infusion of calcium.[8] Calcium levels are disrupted by tumors of the bone and lung, endocrine disorders, excessive or deficient amounts of vitamin D, intestinal malabsorption of calcium, kidney failure, and pancreatitis.

Magnesium

Magnesium (Mg^{++}) is essential for many enzyme, protein, lipid, and carbohydrate functions in the body. In the bloodstream it is found predominantly within the cells, although an adequate serum level (extracellular) is essential to normal cardiac and skeletal muscle function. The normal serum range is from 1.5 to 2.5 mEq/L (see Box 8-8).

Hypomagnesemia

In the critical care unit low serum magnesium, or hypomagnesemia, is more common than high serum magnesium. Hypomagnesemia can be caused by insufficient intake in the diet or total parental nutrition (TPN), by chronic alcohol abuse, or by diuresis. The use of diuretics to treat heart failure or fluid overload after cardiac surgery often contributes to low serum Mg^{++} levels. Cardiac consequences of hypomagnesemia are demonstrated on the ECG by tall T waves, inverted T waves, and depressed ST segments. In patients with acute cardiac conditions, ventricular dysrhythmias range from premature ventricular contractions (PVCs) to ventricular tachycardia (VT) and VF. In the critical care setting hy-

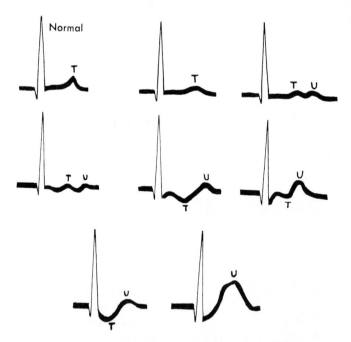

FIG. 8-6   Effects of hypokalemia: Variable ECG patterns—ranging from slight T-wave flattening to the appearance of prominent U waves, sometimes with ST-segment depressions or T-wave inversions—may be seen with hypokalemia. These patterns are not directly related to a specific level of serum potassium. (From Goldberger AL, Goldberger E: *Clinical electrocardiography: a simplified approach,* ed 5, St Louis, 1994, Mosby.)

pomagnesemia and hypokalemia often coexist in the same patient. Because low electrolyte values are caused by diuresis, low Mg^{++} may be overlooked as a potential cause of ventricular dysrhythmias. Administering intravenous magnesium sulphate raises the magnesium level.[9,10]

Cardiac Enzymes

Cardiac enzymes are proteins that are released from irreversibly damaged myocardial tissue cells. The enzymes released by the damaged myocardium include creatine kinase (CK) and lactate dehydrogenase (LDH). When damaged or necrotic, other organs will emit these same enzymes; therefore the enzymes are not cardiac specific when measured as a whole. Each enzyme, however, can be broken into component parts called isoenzymes, the serum level of which yields information of diagnostic value for cardiac disease. Normal values of the cardiac-specific enzymes are shown in Box 8-7. The typical sequence of the appearance of each of the enzymes and isoenzymes is described in Table 8-3.

CK isoenzymes

Creatine kinase (CK) has three isoenzymes composed of varying amounts of muscle, brain, and heart subunits. The brain contains high concentrations of CK-BB, and skeletal muscle contains CK-MM. Myocardial cells contain the CK-MB isoenzyme, which appears in the serum only after myocardial cell death. CK-MB is at present the most specific and sensitive serum index for diagnosing myocardial infarction in patients evaluated within 24 hours of the onset of chest pain.[4,11] Serial samples should be drawn at admission and 12 and 24 hours thereafter to help establish or rule out the diagnosis of myocardial infarction. The serum specimens must be kept on ice if more than 2 hours elapses between the draw and assay time because time and heat will reduce the MB fraction.

LDH isoenzymes

Lactate dehydrogenase (LDH) is composed of five isoenzymes: LDH_1, LDH_2, LDH_3, LDH_4, and LDH_5. Normally LDH_2 is the dominant fraction, followed by LDH_1. Myocardial cells contain a large amount of both LDH_1 and LDH_2. When myocardial infarction occurs, both the LDH_1 and the LDH_2 levels rise and the $LDH_1:LDH_2$ ratio becomes greater than 1 (normally less than 1); in other words the normal situation wherein LDH_2 levels are greater than LDH_1 levels is reversed. An LDH_1 level greater than the LDH_2 level can be used in diagnosis, especially if patients seek medical assistance more than 24 hours after the onset of symptoms and the CK-MB isoenzyme peak is missed.

Hematologic Studies

Hematologic laboratory studies that are routinely ordered for the management of patients with altered cardiovascular status are the red blood cell (RBC or erythrocyte) level, hemoglobin (Hgb) level, hematocrit (Hct) level, erythrocyte sedimentation rate (ESR), and white blood cell (WBC, or leukocyte) count.

Coagulation Studies

Coagulation studies are ordered to determine the effectiveness of serum clotting. For example, patients who have stasis of blood, atrial fibrillation, or a history of thrombosis are at risk for developing a thrombus and may require anticoagulation. Heparin or oral anticoagulating drugs may be administered to prevent the formation or extension of a clot, and coagulation studies are ordered to guide dosage of these drugs. Most coagulation study results record the length of time in seconds it takes for blood to form a clot in the laboratory test tube. Box 8-9 lists normal coagulation values.

Prothrombin time

The prothrombin time (PT) is used to determine the therapeutic dosage of warfarin sodium (Coumadin) necessary to achieve anticoagulation. The PT may be reported in seconds, percents, or as a ratio.

International normalized ratio

Coumadin-type drugs are monitored by the International Normalized Ratio (INR). The INR was developed by the World Health Organization to standardize PT results

---

TABLE 8-3
CARDIAC ENZYME SERUM LEVELS ASSOCIATED WITH MYOCARDIAL INFARCTION

CARDIAC ENZYMES	ELEVATION (HOURS)	PEAK (HOURS)	DURATION (DAYS)
Creatine kinase (CK)	4-8	12-24	3-4
Creatine kinase-MB (CK-MB)	4-8	12-20	2-3
Lactate dehydrogenase (LDH)	12-48	72-144	8-14
$LDH_1:LDH_2$ (normally <1)	($LDH_1:LDH_2$ >1)	72-144	14

NORMAL AND THERAPEUTIC ADULT COAGULATION VALUES

TEST	NORMAL VALUE	THERAPEUTIC VALUE	
PT	11-16 sec*	1.5 to 2.5 times normal	
INR	<2.0	Chronic atrial fibrillation	2.0 to 3.0
		Treatment of DVT/PE	2.0 to 3.0
		Mechanical heart valve	3.0 to 4.5
aPTT	28-38 sec	1.5 to 2.5 times normal	
PTT	60-90 sec	1.5 to 2.5 times normal	
ACT	70-120 sec†	150-190 sec	

*PT normal value may vary by ± 2 sec between different laboratories.
†ACT normal value may vary with type of activator used.
PT = Prothrombin time; INR = international normalized ratio; aPTT = activated partial thromboplastin time; PTT = partial thromboplastin time; ACT = activated coagulation time; DVT = deep vein thrombosis; PE = pulmonary embolism.

TOTAL CHOLESTEROL AND HDL CHOLESTEROL CLASSIFICATIONS

CLASSIFICATION	CHOLESTEROL MEASUREMENT
	TOTAL CHOLESTEROL
Normal*	<200 mg/dL
Borderline-High	200-239 mg/dL
High	≥240 mg/dL
	HDL CHOLESTEROL
Normal*	>35 mg/dL
Low	<35 mg/dL

*Normal in this context describes the more desirable values to prevent CAD.

between clinical laboratories worldwide. Box 8-9 illustrates target INR ranges for different cardiovascular conditions that require anticoagulation.

Partial thromboplastin time

The partial thromboplastin time (PTT) is used to measure the effectiveness of intravenous or subcutaneous heparin administration. Most hospitals use the activated PTT to shorten the length of time necessary to perform the test.

Activated coagulation time

An additional test of heparin effect is the activated coagulation time (ACT). The ACT can be performed outside of the laboratory setting in areas such as the cardiac catheterization laboratory, operating room, and specialized critical care units. Normal and therapeutic values for all of these coagulation studies are shown in Box 8-9.

Lipid Studies

Elevated plasma lipoprotein levels are associated with the development of coronary artery disease (CAD).[12] The term lipoprotein refers to lipids, phospholipids, cholesterol, and triglycerides bound to carrier proteins. Five serum lipoprotein levels are important to measure when evaluating patients' risk of developing or progressing with coronary artery disease:

1. Total cholesterol
2. High density lipoprotein-cholesterol (HDL-C)
3. Low density lipoprotein-cholesterol (LDL-C)
4. Very low density lipoprotein (VLDL-C)
5. Triglycerides

Total cholesterol

The liver produces cholesterol and the lipoproteins that carry it. Excessive cholesterol (greater than 200 mg/dl) in the serum forces the progression of atherosclerosis, a precursor of CAD. Table 8-4 lists normal lipid levels.

LDL-C

Low density lipoproteins are a combination of cholesterol and protein. About 70% of the total cholesterol is contained in the form of LDL-C. High LDL-C levels cause deposition of cholesterol on artery walls (atherosclerosis) and development of CAD.

VLDL-C

Very low density lipoproteins are a combination of triglycerides and protein. High VLDL-C levels also contribute to CAD development.

HDL-C

High density lipoproteins are composed of phospholipids and protein. Approximately 20% to 25% of the serum cholesterol is carried in the form of HDL-C. Normal HDL-C levels protect against CAD, possibly as a result of the role of HDL-C in carrying lipids away from body tissues and to the liver for degradation. In contrast, low HDL-C levels (less than 35 mg/dl) are associated with a higher incidence of CAD. Children and premenopausal women often have an elevated HDL-C concentration, and both groups are considered at low risk for coronary artery disease. HDL-C levels increase in response to exercise, weight loss, and cessation of cigarette smoking.[13]

Triglycerides

Triglycerides are carried in the blood stream by very low-density lipoproteins (VLDL-C).

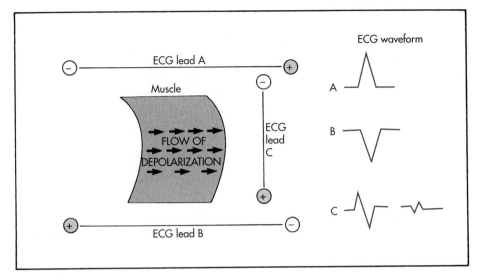

FIG. 8-7 Effect of lead position on the ECG tracing. **A,** Flow of depolarization toward the positive electrode will result in a positive deflection on the ECG. **B,** Flow of depolarization away from the positive electrode will result in a negative deflection on the ECG. **C,** Flow of depolarization perpendicular to the positive electrode will result in a biphasic or nearly isoelectric deflection on the ECG. This basic principle applies to both the P wave and the QRS complex.

Diagnostic Procedures

Electrocardiography

This section on **electrocardiography** provides a general understanding of the dysrhythmias commonly encountered in clinical practice and a basis for understanding the value of the many clinical applications of electrocardiography. The ECG records electrical changes in heart muscle. It does not record mechanical contraction, which usually immediately follows electrical depolarization.

ECG leads

All ECGs use a system of one or more leads designed to record electrical activity. A lead consists of three electrodes: a positive electrode, a negative electrode, and a ground electrode that prevents the display of background electrical interference on the ECG tracing. Leads do not transmit any electricity to patients; they merely sense and record it.

ECG waves

The positive electrode on the skin functions like the lens of a camera. If the wave of depolarization travels toward the positive electrode, an upward wave (or positive deflection) is written on the ECG paper (Fig. 8-7, *A*). If the wave of depolarization travels away from the positive electrode, a downward line (or negative deflection) will be recorded on the ECG (Fig. 8-7, *B*). When depolarization moves perpendicularly to the positive electrode, a biphasic complex will occur. Sometimes the complex appears almost flat (isoelectric) if the electrical forces traveling in opposite directions are equal and, in effect,

cancel each other out (Fig. 8-7, *C*). The size of the muscle mass being depolarized also has an effect, with the larger muscle mass displaying the largest deflection.

Baseline distortion

The portion of the tracing between the various waveforms, referred to as the *baseline,* must be flat. Two forms of artifact can distort the baseline: 60-cycle interference and muscular movement. Figure 8-8, *A* depicts 60-cycle interference, which results from leakage of electrical current somewhere within the system and appears as a generalized thickening of the baseline. It can usually be resolved by ensuring that all electrical equipment at the bedside is well grounded. Unplugging one piece of equipment at a time until the offending device is found is sometimes necessary. Muscular movement (Fig. 8-8, *B*) is displayed as a coarse, erratic disturbance of the baseline.

ECG paper

Specialized ECG paper records the speed and magnitude of electrical impulses on a grid composed of small and large boxes (Fig. 8-9). There are five small boxes in every large box.

ECG speed

Distances along the horizontal axis represent speed and are stated in seconds rather than in millimeters or number of boxes. At a standard paper speed of 25 mm/second, one small box (1 mm) is equivalent to 0.04 of a second, and one large box (5 mm) represents 0.20 of a second.

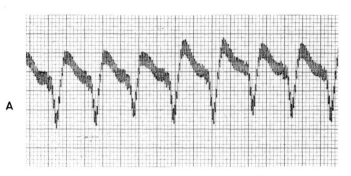

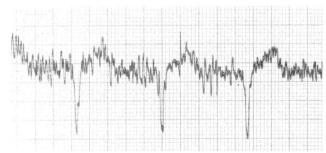

FIG. 8-8   A, Artifact—60-cycle interference. **B,** Artifact—muscular movement.

ECG amplitude

The vertical axis represents magnitude or strength of force. At standard calibration one small box equals 0.1 mV, and one large box equals 0.5 mV. Checking the standardization mark, usually located at the beginning of the tracing, is important. The mark indicates 1 mV and at standard calibration should go up two large boxes (Fig. 8-10).

ECG Waveforms and Intervals

P wave

The P wave represents atrial depolarization (Fig. 8-11).

QRS complex

The letter *Q* is used to describe an initial negative deflection; in other words, only if the first deflection from the baseline is negative will it be labeled a Q wave. The letter *R* applies to any positive deflection. If there are two positive deflections in one QRS complex, the second is labeled *R* (read "R prime"). The letter *S* refers to any subsequent negative deflections. Any combination of these deflections can occur and is collectively called the QRS complex (Fig. 8-12). The QRS duration is normally 0.10 second (2.5 small boxes) or less.

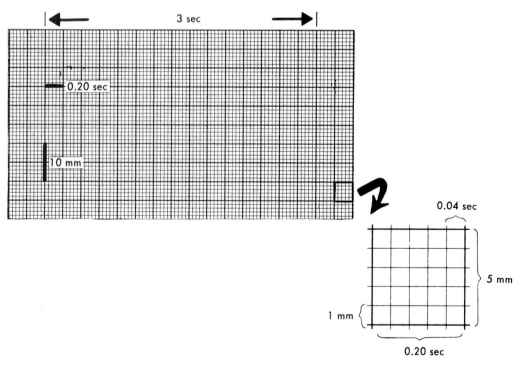

FIG. 8-9   ECG graph paper. The horizontal axis represents time, and the vertical axis represents magnitude of voltage. Horizontally, each small box is 0.04 seconds and each large box is 0.20 seconds. Vertically, each small box is 1 mm and each large box is 5 mm. Markings are present every 3 seconds at the top of the paper for ease in calculating heart rate. (From Goldberger AL, Goldberger E: *Clinical electrocardiography: a simplified approach,* ed 5, St Louis, 1994, Mosby.)

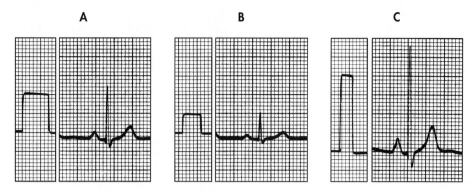

FIG. 8-10 A, Normal standardization mark. The machine is calibrated so that the standardization mark is 10 mm tall. **B,** Half standardization, used whenever QRS complexes are too tall to fit on the paper. **C,** Twice normal standardization, used whenever QRS complexes are too small to be adequately analyzed. (From Goldberger AL, Goldberger E: *Clinical electrocardiography: a simplified approach,* ed 5, St Louis, 1994, Mosby.)

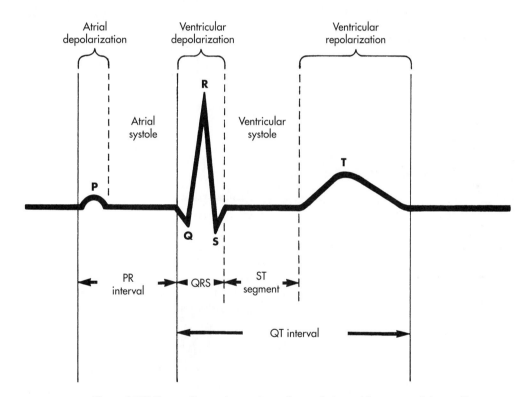

FIG. 8-11 Normal ECG waveforms, intervals, and correlation with events of the cardiac cycle. The **P wave** represents atrial depolarization, followed immediately by atrial systole. The **QRS** represents ventricular depolarization, followed immediately by ventricular systole. The **ST segment** corresponds to phase 2 of the action potential, during which time the heart muscle is completely depolarized and contraction normally occurs. The **T wave** represents ventricular repolarization. The **PR interval** measured from the beginning of the P wave to the beginning of the QRS corresponds to atrial depolarization and impulse delay in the AV node. The **QT interval** measured from the beginning of the QRS complex to the end of the T wave, represents the time from initial depolarization of the ventricles to the end of ventricular repolarization.

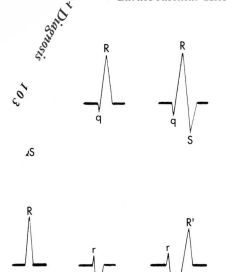

FIG. 8-12 Examples of QRS complexes. Small deflections are labeled with lowercase letters, whereas uppercase letters are used for larger deflections. A second upward deflection is labeled *R'* (read "R prime"). (Modified from Goldberger AL, Goldberger E: *Clinical electrocardiography: a simplified approach,* ed 5, St Louis, 1994, Mosby.)

TABLE 8 - 5	
APPROXIMATE NORMAL LIMITS FOR ADULT QT INTERVALS IN SECONDS*	
HEART RATE PER MINUTE	**QT INTERVAL IN SECONDS**
40	0.45-0.50
46	0.43-0.48
50	0.41-0.46
55	0.40-0.45
60	0.39-0.43
67	0.37-0.41
71	0.36-0.41
75	0.35-0.39
80	0.34-0.38
86	0.33-0.37
93	0.32-0.36
100	0.31-0.35
109	0.30-0.33
120	0.28-0.32
133	0.27-0.30
150	0.25-0.28
172	0.23-0.26

*Adapted from Frye SJ, Lounsbury P: *Cardiac rhythm disorders: an introduction using the nursing process,* Baltimore, 1988, Williams & Wilkins.

T wave

The T wave represents ventricular repolarization (Fig. 8-11).

PR interval

The PR interval is measured from the beginning of the P wave to the beginning of the QRS complex. Normally the PR interval is 0.12 to 0.20 of a second in length. Because most of this time period results from delay of the impulse in the AV node, the PR interval is an indicator of AV nodal function (Fig. 8-11).

ST segment

The portion of the wave that extends from the end of the QRS to the beginning of the T wave is labeled the *ST segment.* The duration is not measured; instead, its shape and location are evaluated. The ST segment should be flat and at the same level as the isoelectric baseline. Many bedside monitor systems are able to monitor the ST segment to detect elevation or depression that may indicate ischemia (Fig. 8-11).

QT interval

The QT interval is measured from the beginning of the QRS complex to the end of the T wave. The length of the QT interval is highly dependent on heart rate. The most accurate method for evaluating a QT interval is to refer to a chart for its normal value at the specific heart rate (Table 8-5).

Cardiac cycle

Although the ECG records only electrical events, understanding the correlation of these intervals to the physiologic events of the cardiac cycle is helpful. Immediately after the P wave and during the PR interval, atrial systole occurs. Similarly, ventricular systole begins immediately after the QRS complex and continues until approximately the midpoint of the T wave (Fig. 8-11).

Bedside Cardiac Monitor Leads

During continuous cardiac monitoring, adhesive, pregelled electrodes are used to obtain an ECG tracing that is similar to one lead of a 12-lead ECG. This technique requires a minimum of three electrodes: one positive, one negative, and one ground (Fig. 8-13, *A*). In many critical care units five electrode systems are used, either to monitor two leads simultaneously or allow selection of several different leads at any time through a lead selector switch on the monitor. Typical placement of the five electrodes in a multi-lead system is shown in Figure 8-13, *B*. The most frequently used leads are II, V_1, MCL_1, and MCL_6. A choice of monitoring leads permits critical care nurses to select the lead that is most appropriate for monitoring dysrhythmias associated with a specific clinical condition.[14,15]

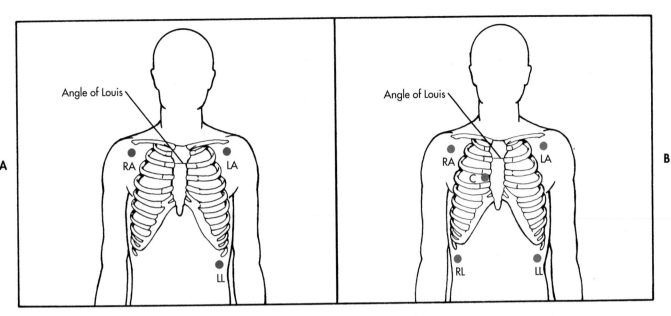

FIG. 8-13 **A,** Three electrodes and lead-wire cables allow monitoring of three of the limb leads (I, II, and III) and can also be rearranged to monitor MCL$_1$ and MCL$_6$. **B,** Five electrodes and lead-wire cables allow monitoring of any of the six standard limb leads (I, II, III, aV$_R$, aV$_L$, or aV$_F$) and any one precordial lead, usually V$_1$ or MCL$_1$. The cable attachments are color coded for quick identification and placement. Accurate electrode placement is essential.

Lead II

Lead II is formed by placing the positive electrode on the lower left side of the torso, below the rib cage. The negative electrode is placed on the right shoulder, and the ground electrode is usually placed on the left shoulder (Fig. 8-14, *A*). Lead II is a popular monitoring lead because the P wave and QRS complex are usually upright and easy to identify with normal conduction (Fig. 8-14, *B*). The waveforms are upright because depolarization normally travels toward the positive electrode.

Leads MCL$_1$ and V$_1$

MCL$_1$ stands for *modified chest lead one* and is equivalent to a V$_1$ lead on a 12-lead ECG. In MCL$_1$ the positive electrode is at the fourth intercostal space just to the right of the sternum, and the negative electrode is placed at the left shoulder (Fig. 8-15, *A*). Many five-lead monitoring systems have a choice of both MCL$_1$ and V$_1$ for bedside monitoring. In V$_1$ the positive electrode is also placed at the right fourth intercostal space, and the negative electrode is calculated by the monitor. In MCL$_1$ and V$_1$ the normal QRS deflection is mostly negative (Fig. 8-15, *B*) because the normal path of left ventricular depolarization is away from the positive electrode.

Dysrhythmia Interpretation

In clinical practice the terms *dysrhythmia* and *arrhythmia* provoke discussion and are often used interchangeably. Both words are correct, and either may be used in practice. This textbook uses *dysrhythmia* as the preferred term

---

B O X   8 - 1 0

EVALUATION OF RHYTHM STRIPS

1. Calculate the ventricular and atrial rates.
2. Determine the rhythm.
3. Analyze the P wave.
4. Measure the PR interval.
5. Determine the QRS duration.
6. Measure the QT interval.
7. Analyze the ST segment.
8. Analyze the T wave.

and defines it as any disturbance in the normal cardiac conduction pathway. Dysrhythmias often occur sporadically; for this reason patients in a critical care unit are monitored continuously, using a single or dual lead system, and ECG strips are recorded routinely as well as any time there is a change in patients' rhythm. A systematic approach to evaluation of a rhythm strip is described, followed by specific criteria for common dysrhythmias encountered in clinical practice. A summary of the key points for evaluation of rhythm strips is found in Box 8-10.

Ventricular heart rate

The first element to assess when evaluating the heart rate from a rhythm strip is the ventricular rate. Regardless of the type of dysrhythmia the ventricular rate indicates

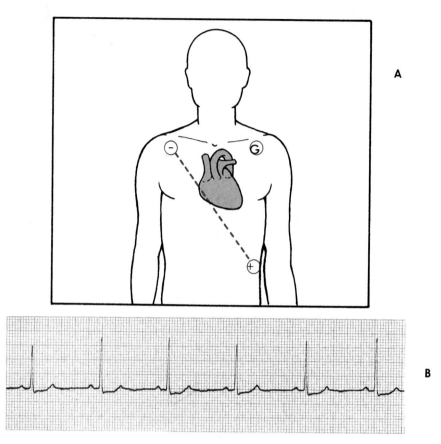

FIG. 8-14 Monitoring lead II: **A,** Electrode placement. The negative electrode is placed below the right shoulder; the positive electrode is placed on the lower left torso (preferably below the rib cage, but at least below the sixth rib); and the ground is usually placed below the left shoulder. **B,** Typical ECG tracing in lead II.

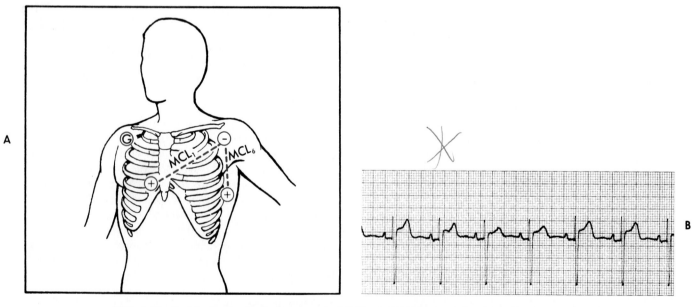

FIG. 8-15 **A,** Monitoring lead placement in MCL$_1$ and MCL$_6$. **B,** Typical ECG tracing in MCL$_1$.

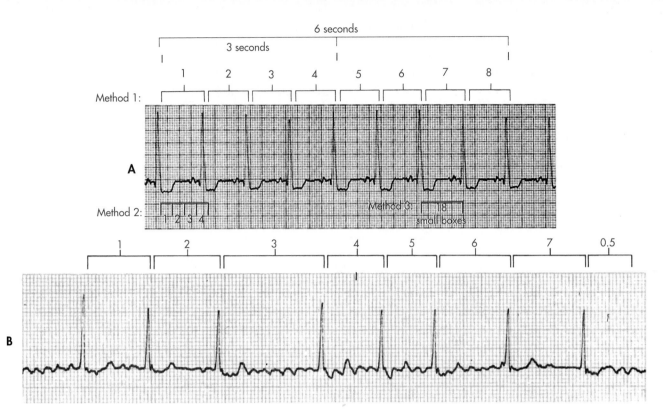

FIG. 8-16 **A,** Calculation of heart rate. *Method 1:* Number of RR intervals in 6 seconds multiplied by 10 (e.g., 8 × 10 = 80/min). *Method 2:* Number of large boxes between QRS complexes divided into 300 (e.g., 300 ÷ 4 = 75/min). *Method 3:* Number of small boxes between QRS complexes divided into 1500 (e.g., 1500 ÷ 18 = 84/min). **B,** Rate calculation if the rhythm is irregular. Only *Method 1* can be used (e.g., 7.5 intervals × 10 = 75/min).

whether patients will be able to tolerate the dysrhythmia—that is, maintain adequate blood pressure, cardiac output, and mentation. If the ventricular rate is consistently greater than 200 or less than 30, emergency measures must be taken to correct the rate; a detailed analysis of the underlying rhythm disturbance can proceed later when the immediate crisis is over. Heart rates may be obtained in several ways. The cardiac monitor gives a ventricular rate, or rate measurement rulers can be purchased to calculate the rate on paper. Three methods for calculating heart rate on paper are described below and illustrated in Figure 8-16.

1. Number of RR intervals in 6 seconds multiplied by 10 (NOTE: ECG paper is marked at the top in 3-second increments, making the 6-second interval easy to identify.)
2. Number of large boxes between QRS complexes divided into 300
3. Number of small boxes between QRS complexes divided into 1500

Atrial heart rate

In the healthy heart the atrial and ventricular rates are the same. However, many dysrhythmias cause the atrial and ventricular rates to differ; thus both must be calculated. The atrial rate can be determined by measuring the P wave to P wave interval, using one of the previously mentioned methods.

Heart rhythm determination

The term *heart rhythm* refers to the regularity with which the P waves or R waves occur. Calipers assist in determining rhythm. One point of the calipers is placed on the beginning of one R wave, and the other point is placed on the very next R wave. Leaving the calipers "set" at this interval, examiners check each succeeding R to R interval to ensure equal width. Regularity is evaluated by the following criteria:

1. Regular rhythms: If the rhythm is regular, the RR intervals are the same within a 10% range.
2. Regular irregular rhythms: If the rhythm is regularly irregular, the RR intervals are not the same but some sort of pattern is involved.
3. Irregular rhythms: If the rhythm is irregular, the RR intervals are not the same and no pattern can be found.

P wave evaluation

The P wave is analyzed by answering the following:

1. Is the P wave present or absent?
2. Is the P wave related to the QRS?
3. Is there only one P wave in front of every QRS?

PR interval evaluation

The duration of the PR interval, which is normally 0.12 to 0.20 second, is measured and all PR intervals on the strip are checked to be sure they are the same duration as the original interval.

QRS evaluation

The entire ECG strip must be evaluated to ensure that the QRS complexes are consistent in shape and width. The normal QRS duration is 0.06 to 0.10 of a second. If more than one QRS shape is on the strip, each QRS must be measured. The QRS is measured from the point at which it leaves the baseline to the point at which it returns to the baseline (Fig. 8-12).

QT interval evaluation

The QT interval is measured as part of the routine analysis and varies with heart rate (Table 8-5).

Text continued on p. 123.

Sinus Rhythms

Normal sinus rhythm (NSR)

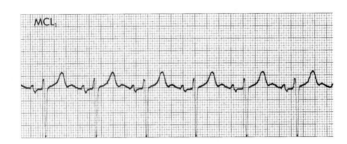

FIG. 8-17

RATE: 60 to 100 beats per minute.
RHYTHM: Regular, plus or minus 10%.

P WAVE: Present, all the same shape, with only one preceding each QRS complex.
PR INTERVAL: 0.12 to 0.20 of a second.
QRS DURATION: 0.06 to 0.10 of a second.

QRS COMPLEX: The shape and whether the deflection is positive or negative will vary depending on lead placement. For example, in lead II the normal complex is positive (Fig. 8-14) and in MCL$_1$ or V$_1$, the normal complex is negative (Fig. 8-15).
ETIOLOGY: Normal conduction.
TREATMENT: None required.

Sinus bradycardia (SB)

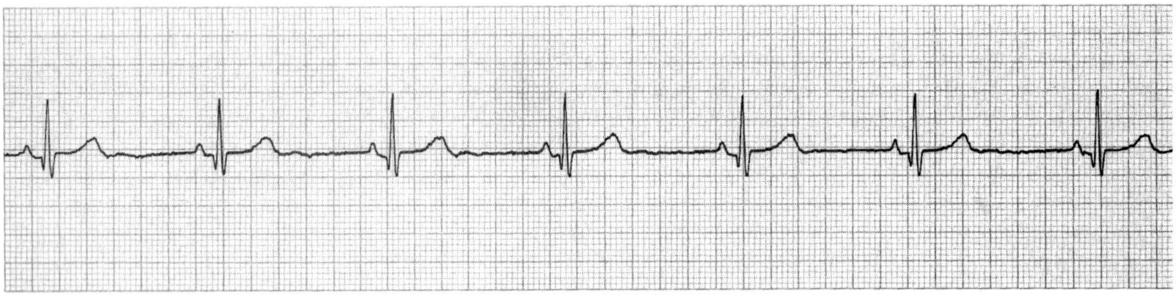

FIG. 8-18

RATE: Less than 60 beats per minute.
RHYTHM: Regular.

P WAVE: Present, all the same shape, with only one preceding each QRS complex.
PR INTERVAL: 0.12 to 0.20 of a second.
QRS DURATION: 0.06 to 0.10 of a second.

QRS COMPLEX: Same as NSR. Narrow complex QRS.
ETIOLOGY: Vagal stimulation, increased intracranial pressure, ischemia of the sinus node caused by an acute inferior wall myocardial infarction or as a side effect of cardiac drugs such as beta blockers or digoxin. SB is also normal in well-conditioned, healthy athletes at rest.
TREATMENT: Only treated if it is accompanied by symptoms of hypoperfusion such as dizziness, chest pain, or changes in level of consciousness.

Sinus tachycardia (ST)

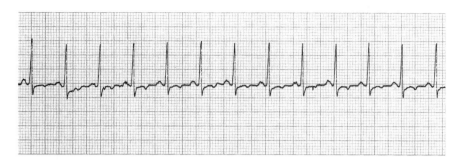

FIG. 8-19

RATE: Greater than 100 beats per minute. Rates may be as high as 180 bpm in young healthy adults during strenuous exercise. However, in the critically ill patient a heart rate above 150 is usually caused by other dysrhythmias.
RHYTHM: Regular.
QRS COMPLEX: Same as NSR. Narrow complex QRS.

P WAVE: Present, all the same shape, with only one preceding each QRS complex.
PR INTERVAL: 0.12 to 0.20 of a second.
QRS DURATION: 0.06 to 0.10 of a second.

ETIOLOGY: Pain, fever, hemorrhage, shock, and acute heart failure. Many medications used in the critical care unit cause sinus tachycardia. A few of these include aminophylline, dopamine, hydralazine, nitroglycerin, epinephrine, and atropine.
PHYSIOLOGY: Tachycardia is detrimental to anyone with ischemic heart disease. The rapid heart rate shortens the time for ventricular filling, decreasing both stroke volume and cardiac output. This occurrence increases myocardial oxygen demand while decreasing oxygen supply because of decreased coronary artery filling time.
TREATMENT: Treatment varies according to the cause. If the cause of the tachycardia is evident (fever or pain), the cause should be treated rather than treating the heart rate directly. If the problem is cardiac-related, both calcium channel blockers and beta blockers are widely used to decrease rapid heart rates. However, clinical assessment is required before these drugs are administered. Cardiac output (CO) is determined by heart rate and stroke volume. If an injured heart can no longer maintain an adequate stroke volume, the body increases heart rate to maintain CO and supply an adequate blood flow to vital body tissues. If a drug is administered to force the sinus node to slow down and the heart cannot increase stroke volume, severe sudden heart failure can result.

Sinus dysrhythmia

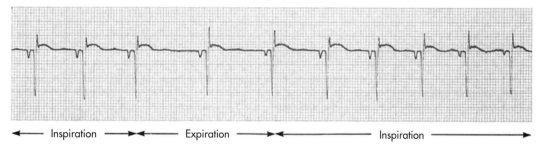

◄——— Inspiration ———►◄——— Expiration ———►◄——— Inspiration ———►

FIG. 8-20 Note the increase in heart rate during inspiration and decrease in heart rate during expiration.

RATE: 60 to 100 beats per minute.
RHYTHM: Irregular, rate varying with the respiratory cycle. It increases with inhalation and decreases with exhalation.
QRS COMPLEX: Same as with NSR. Narrow complex QRS.
ETIOLOGY: Normal variant. Also frequently called sinus arrhythmia.
TREATMENT: None required.

P WAVE: Present, all the same shape, with only one preceding each QRS complex.
PR INTERVAL: 0.12 to 0.20 of a second.
QRS DURATION: 0.06 to 0.10 of a second.

Atrial Dysrhythmias

Premature atrial contraction (PAC)

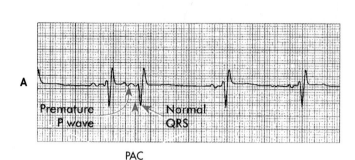

A   Premature P wave   Normal QRS

PAC

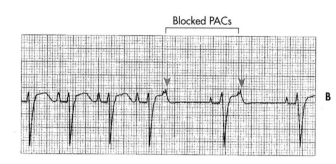

Blocked PACs

B

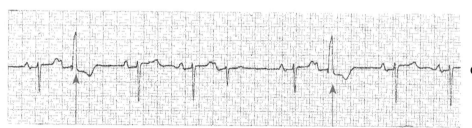

PAC with aberrant conduction

C

FIG. 8-21 **A,** Normally conducted PAC. The early P wave is indicated by the arrow, and the QRS that follows is of normal shape and duration. **B,** Nonconducted (blocked) PACs. The early P waves are indicated by arrows. Note how they distort the T waves, making them appear peaked, compared with the normal T waves seen after the third and fourth QRS complexes. **C,** Right bundle branch block aberration following a PAC.

RATE: Determined by underlying rhythm, which is usually sinus-related.

RHYTHM: Variable. Underlying rhythm may be regular, but PACs create irregularity.

P WAVE: Present, different shape from other P waves, may be inverted. The early P wave may be buried in the preceding T wave.

PR INTERVAL: 0.12 to 0.20 of a second. The PR interval may be longer, shorter, or the same as the PR interval of a sinus beat.

QRS DURATION: 0.06 to 0.10 of a second.

QRS COMPLEX: The QRS usually has a normal appearance because conduction through the AV node and ventricular conduction system is normal (Fig. 8-21, *A*). However, there are exceptions, as shown in Fig. 8-21, *C*.

ETIOLOGY: Can occur normally. Often accentuated by emotional disturbances, caffeine, nicotine, digitalis, mitral valve prolapse, and heart failure.

PHYSIOLOGY: The PAC originates from an ectopic focus in the atria, somewhere other than the sinus node. The ectopic impulse occurs prematurely before the normal sinus impulse is due to occur.

   a. Usually the premature P wave initiates a normal QRS complex (Fig. 8-21, *A*).

   b. If the beat is so early that the AV node remains refractory to stimuli, a pause as a result of a nonconducted PAC is seen (Fig. 8-21, *B*).

   c. Occasionally the early ectopic P wave can be conducted through the AV node, but part of this conduction pathway through the ventricles is blocked. On the ECG, this will appear as an early, abnormal P wave, followed by an abnormally wide QRS (Fig. 8-21, *C*). This is termed *aberrant conduction*.

TREATMENT: None if infrequent. If frequent and the patient is symptomatic, treat the cause. For example, reduce stress, eliminate caffeine and nicotine, modify digitalis dosage, and treat symptoms of heart failure.

Paroxysmal supraventricular tachycardia (PSVT)

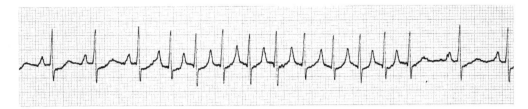

FIG. 8-22 Note that the atrial rate during the tachycardia is 158 beats per minute. The run starts and stops abruptly.

RATE: Greater than 150 to 250 beats per minute (bpm).
RHYTHM: Regular.

P WAVE: Present, may have an abnormal shape. Not all P waves may be conducted to the ventricle.
PR INTERVAL: 0.12 to 0.20 of a second.
QRS DURATION: 0.06 to 0.10 of a second.

QRS COMPLEX: The QRS is usually narrow and normal in appearance.
ETIOLOGY: PSVT has causal factors similar to those of PACs, but it has greater clinical significance. *PSVT* refers to the sudden interruption of sinus rhythm by an atrial ectopic focus that fires repetitively and rapidly and is sustained by a reentry or circular movement. It eventually stops as suddenly as it began. *Paroxysmal* means starting and stopping abruptly.
TREATMENT: PSVT usually responds rapidly to medical treatment. IV adenosine is the drug of choice to slow conduction through the AV node and unmask the ectopic P waves; often it will also restore normal sinus rhythm.[16] Other options include vagal maneuvers, calcium channel blockers, digitalis, or cardioversion.

Atrial flutter (AF)

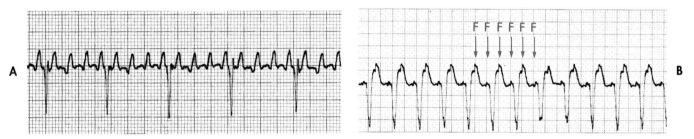

FIG. 8-23 **A,** Atrial flutter with 2:1 conduction through the AV node in a clear saw-toothed pattern. **B,** Atrial flutter with flutter waves hidden in the QRS complexes.

RATE: An atrial rate of 250 to 350 beats per minute. When evaluating the rate of atrial flutter, both the atrial and ventricular rates must be calculated. Usually the atrial rate is faster.
RHYTHM: Regular flutter waves. The ventricular response (QRS complexes) may be regular or irregular.

P WAVE: Flutter (F) waves. When describing atrial flutter, "PR interval" no longer applies; instead, a conduction ratio such as 2:1, 3:1, or 4:1 is used.

The conduction ratio is clearly visible in Fig. 8-23, *A.* However, sometimes the flutter waves are "hidden" by the QRS complex or T wave, as shown in Fig. 8-23, *B.*
PR INTERVAL: 0.12 to 0.20 of a second.
QRS DURATION: 0.06 to 0.10 of a second.

QRS COMPLEX: QRS shape is usually narrow and normal.
PHYSIOLOGY: Atrial flutter (AF) is believed to be caused by a circular reentry pathway through which the wave of depolarization is continually moving. At this rapid rate, individual P waves form the classic saw-tooth pattern shown in Fig. 8-23, *A.*
TREATMENT: The goal of treatment is to decrease the ventricular rate to between 60-100 bpm and eventually to convert patients back to NSR. Medications that slow conduction through the AV node, such as digoxin and calcium channel blockers, are used. Cardioversion is an option for hemodynamically unstable patients or for patients who are unresponsive to drug therapy.

Atrial fibrillation (Af)

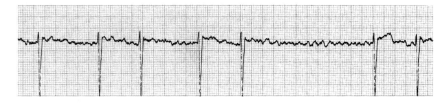

FIG. 8-24   Note the irregularly irregular ventricular rhythm.

RATE: Atrial: 350-600 fibrillatory waves per minute. Ventricular: 60-100 (controlled by medication). Greater than 100 (uncontrolled by medication).

RHYTHM: Irregularly irregular ventricular rhythm.

P WAVE: Replaced by fibrillating baseline or waves.

PR INTERVAL: Absent. Replaced by fibrillating baseline.

QRS DURATION: 0.06 to 0.10 of a second.

QRS COMPLEX: The QRS complex is usually normal because the pathway through the ventricles is unchanged once the impulse leaves the AV node.

ETIOLOGY: Small sections of atrial muscle are activated individually, resulting in quivering of the atrial muscle without effective contraction.

PHYSIOLOGY: When numerous sites in the atria fire spontaneously and rapidly, an organized spread of depolarization can no longer take place and atrial fibrillation results. Atrial fibrillation can be either acute or chronic.

TREATMENT: *Acute atrial fibrillation:* Pharmacologic agents such as digoxin, calcium channel blockers, and beta blockers are used to convert acute atrial fibrillation back to NSR. If medications are not successful, electrical cardioversion is used. However, successful cardioversion that restores NSR may precipitate emboli to the systemic or pulmonary circulations. During atrial fibrillation the atria do not contract; hence blood may pool and clot within the atria. To prevent this, some patients may have a diagnostic echocardiogram to rule out atrial thrombi if the atrial fibrillation has persisted for more than a few days. If clots are present in the atria, anticoagulation therapy is given for several days before the cardioversion.

Chronic atrial fibrillation: digoxin, calcium channel blockers, and beta blockers are used to maintain the ventricular response rate between 60 and 100 beats per minute. Electrical cardioversion does not work if the atrial fibrillation has existed for a long time.

Junctional Dysrhythmias

Premature junctional contraction (PJC)

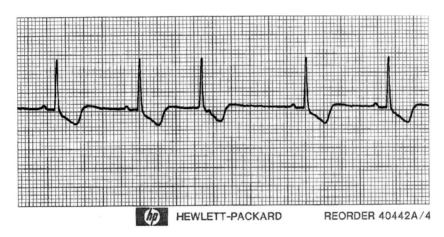

FIG. 8-25 SR with PJC.

RATE: Rate depends on the underlying rhythm, usually a NSR.

RHYTHM: On the ECG, the rhythm is regular from the sinus node except for the early QRS complex (PJC) of normal shape and duration.

P WAVE: **a.** P wave may be entirely absent.
b. P wave may be seen in the T wave.
c. P wave may be inverted with PR interval <0.12 sec.

PR INTERVAL: Usually absent. The lack of a normal PR interval is a defining characteristic of junctional rhythms.

QRS DURATION: 0.06 to 0.10 of a second.

QRS COMPLEX: The QRS complex is usually narrow and normal.

ETIOLOGY: A PJC is a single ectopic impulse that originates in the AV junctional area.

PHYSIOLOGY: Only certain areas of the AV node have the property of automaticity. The entire area around the AV node is collectively called the *junction;* hence impulses generated there are called *junctional.* After an ectopic impulse arises in the junction, it spreads in two directions at once. One wave of depolarization spreads upward into the atria, depolarizes the atria, and causes a P wave that is usually seen following the QRS. At the same time another wave of depolarization spreads downward into the ventricles through the normal conduction pathway and results in a normal QRS complex.

TREATMENT: Usually none required. PJCs have virtually the same clinical significance as do PACs. However, if the patient is receiving digoxin, digitalis toxicity should at least be suspected. Although digoxin slows conduction through the AV node, it also increases automaticity in the junction.

Junctional escape rhythm

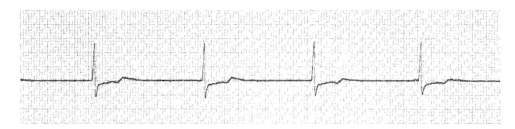

FIG. 8-26 The ventricular rate is 38 beats per minute. P waves are absent, and the QRS is normal width.

RATE: Sometimes the junction becomes the dominant pacemaker of the heart. The intrinsic rate of the junction is 40 to 60 beats per minute.
RHYTHM: Regular.

P WAVE: Same as for PJC.
PR INTERVAL: Usually absent.
QRS DURATION: 0.06 to 0.10 of a second.

QRS COMPLEX: QRS complex is usually narrow and normal because the impulse originates above the ventricles.
ETIOLOGY: A junctional escape rhythm originates in the junction following failure of the sinus node.
PHYSIOLOGY: Under normal conditions the junction never has a chance to "escape" and depolarize the heart because it is overridden by the faster sinus node. However, if the sinus node fails, the junctional impulses can depolarize completely and pace the heart. This junctional escape rhythm is a protective mechanism to prevent asystole in the event of sinus node failure.
TREATMENT: Generally a junctional escape rhythm is well tolerated hemodynamically, although efforts should be directed toward restoring sinus rhythm. Sometimes a pacemaker is inserted as a protective measure because of concern that the junction may fail.

Junctional tachycardia and accelerated junctional rhythm

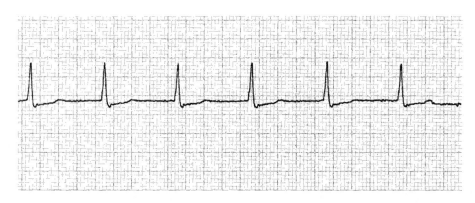

FIG. 8-27 Accelerated junctional rhythm

RATE: Accelerated junctional rhythm: rate 60 to 100 bpm.
    Junctional tachycardia: rate greater than 100 bpm.
RHYTHM: Regular.

P WAVE: Same as PJC.
PR INTERVAL: Usually absent.
QRS DURATION: 0.06 to 0.10 of a second.

QRS COMPLEX: The QRS is usually narrow and normal.
ETIOLOGY: Rapid junctional rhythms originate in the junction. This may indicate irritability in the junctional area caused by AV node ischemia or digitalis toxicity.
PHYSIOLOGY: Accelerated junctional rhythms are usually well tolerated hemodynamically by patients, mainly because the heart rate is within the normal range.
    Junctional tachycardia may not be so well tolerated, depending on patients' tolerance of the rapid rate.
TREATMENT: No treatment if patients have a good blood pressure and no unusual symptoms.
    Drug Toxicity: If this is a recent rhythm change and patients are on digoxin, digitalis toxicity should be suspected. This is because digoxin enhances automaticity of the AV node. If digitalis toxicity is present, the only treatment is to withhold digoxin until the dysrhythmia resolves.

Ventricular Dysrhythmias

Premature ventricular contractions (PVC)

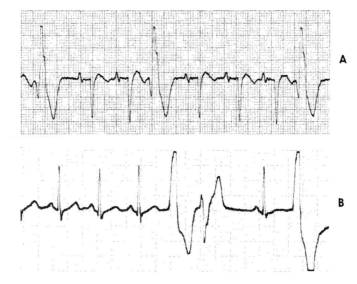

FIG. 8-28 **A,** Unifocal PVCs. **B,** Multifocal PVCs.

RATE: Rate is dependent upon the underlying heart rate, usually NSR.

RHYTHM: Early QRS complexes interrupt the underlying rhythm.

QRS COMPLEX: The QRS complex is wide, with a bizarre shape.

P WAVE: Absent or following the early QRS complex.

PR INTERVAL: Absent.

QRS DURATION: >0.12 of a second. The prolonged width of the QRS is diagnostic for ventricular ectopy.

UNIFOCAL PVCs: If all of the ventricular ectopic beats look the same in a particular lead, they are called *unifocal PVCs,* which means that they probably all result from the same irritable focus (Fig. 8-28, *A*).

MULTIFOCAL PVCs: If the ventricular ectopics are of various shapes in the same lead, they are called *multifocal PVCs* (Fig. 8-28, *B*). Multifocal PVCs are more serious than unifocal ventricular ectopics because they indicate that a greater area of irritable myocardium is involved and they are more likely to deteriorate into ventricular tachycardia or fibrillation.

FUSION BEATS: If a ventricular ectopic impulse and the sinus beat meet in the middle of the ventricles, a fusion beat results. Fusion beats are narrower than are the ventricular beats and look like a cross between patients' sinus QRS and the ventricular ectopic QRS.

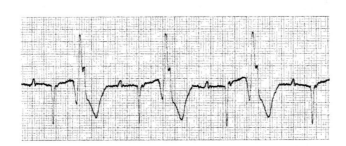

FIG. 8-29 Ventricular bigemeny.

VENTRICULAR BIGEMENY: When a PVC follows each normal beat, it is called *ventricular bigemeny* (Fig. 8-29).

COUPLET: Two consecutive PVCs.

TRIPLET: Three consecutive PVCs.

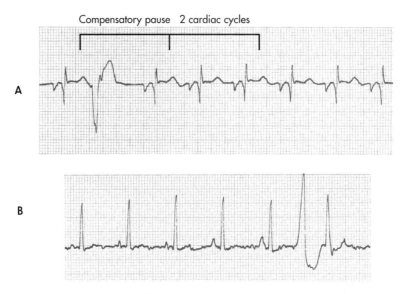

FIG. 8-30 A, PVC with a full compensatory pause. The interval between the two sinus beats that surround the PVC (R_1 and R_2) is exactly 2 times the normal interval between sinus beats (R_3 and R_4). The fully compensatory pause occurs because the sinus node continues to pace despite the PVC. **B,** Interpolated PVC. The PVC falls between two normal QRS complexes without disturbing the rhythm. Note that the RR interval between sinus beats remains the same.

COMPENSATORY PAUSE: If the interval from the last normal QRS preceding the PVC to the one following the PVC is exactly equal to two complete cardiac cycles, it is called a *compensatory pause* (Fig. 8-30, *A*).

INTERPOLATED PVC: (Fig. 8-30, *B*).

R ON T: If a PVC occurs on the T wave during the relative refractory period (latter half of T wave) when only a part of the muscle is repolarized, individual segments of muscle can depolarize separately from each other, resulting in ventricular fibrillation.

ETIOLOGY: The many causes of PVCs include myocardial ischemia; electrolyte imbalances; hypoxia; acidosis; heart diseases such as cardiomyopathy, ventricular aneurysm, and previous MI; and medications that are pro-dysrhythmic.

PHYSIOLOGY: Ventricular dysrhythmias result from an ectopic focus in any portion of the ventricular myocardium. The usual conduction pathway through the ventricles is not used, and the wave of depolarization spreads from cell to cell.

DOCUMENTATION: The underlying rhythm must always be described first: for example, "sinus bradycardia with frequent unifocal PVCs" or "atrial fibrillation with occasional multifocal PVCs."

TREATMENT: Not all ventricular ectopy requires treatment. In individuals without significant underlying heart disease, PVCs do not represent an increased risk for sudden death and are considered benign. Approximately 30% of all patients with ventricular ectopic activity fall into this category.[17]

If possible, the cause of the PVCs should be treated: for example, PVCs caused by hypokalemia and hypomagnesemia are treated by administration of potassium and magnesium. Hypoxia is treated by administration of oxygen, ventilation if required, and correction of acidosis.

Ventricular tachycardia (VT)

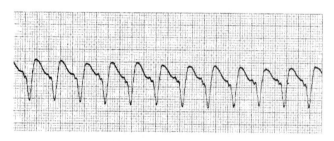

FIG. 8-31

RATE: Greater than 100 beats per minute.
RHYTHM: Mostly regular. May have some irregularities.

P WAVE: P wave is not related to the QRS. In most cases the sinus node is unaffected and will continue to depolarize the atria on schedule. Therefore P waves can sometimes be seen on the ECG tracing. They are not related to the QRS and may even conduct a normal impulse to the ventricles if the timing is just right.
PR INTERVAL: Absent.
QRS DURATION: Greater than 0.12 of a second.
QRS COMPLEX: Wide, with a bizarre shape compared to the sinus QRS.
NONSUSTAINED VT: Three or more consecutive PVCs, rate greater than 110 beats per minute, lasts less than 30 seconds without hemodynamic collapse, and self-terminates.[11] Approximately 65% of all patients with ventricular ectopic activity fall into this category.[18]
SUSTAINED VT: If the VT does not self-terminate, it is described as *sustained*. If there is hemodynamic collapse, CPR* and ACLS† measures will be required. ACLS protocols are described in Appendix A.

---

*CPR = Cardiopulmonary Resuscitation
†ACLS = Advanced Cardiac Life Support

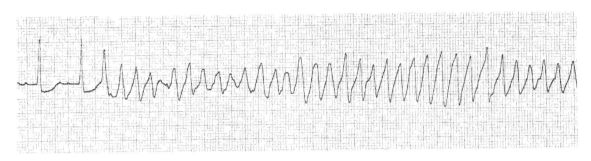

FIG. 8-32 Torsades de pointes.

TORSADES DE POINTES (twisting of the points): This is a specific form of ventricular tachycardia. Its name refers to the twisting appearance of the VT on the ECG strip. It may be precipitated by antidysrhythmic drugs that prolong the QT interval and ventricular refractory period. Quinidine is an example of a drug that prolongs the QT interval.

ETIOLOGY: VT may be caused by all of the same factors that cause PVCs, as described in that section: myocardial ischemia, digitalis toxicity, electrolyte disturbances, and as an adverse side effect of certain antidysrhythmic drugs. Some antidysrhythmic drugs can actually cause more serious dysrhythmias than those they were intended to treat.[17,18]

PHYSIOLOGY: VT results from a repeating ectopic focus in the ventricular myocardium. The usual conduction pathway through the ventricles is bypassed, and the wave of depolarization spreads from cell to cell.

SUDDEN DEATH: In patients with only moderate left ventricular dysfunction, (EF* >30%), the risk of sudden death from VT is only modest, but in patients with severe left ventricular dysfunction (EF <30%), the risk is high. Sudden cardiac death occurs if the VT degenerates into ventricular fibrillation.

TREATMENT: VT may be treated pharmacologically or with electrical cardioversion or defibrillation.

Acute VT: VT that occurs in critically ill patients because of myocardial ischemia or following cardiac surgery is treated emergently by lidocaine, procainamide, and emergency cardioversion or defibrillation. If hypoxia, acidosis, electrolyte imbalances, or drug toxicity is the cause, these must also be corrected to prevent the recurrence of the VT.

Chronic VT: Many patients with underlying heart disease from cardiomyopathy or an old myocardial infarction (MI) have frequent PVCs and episodes of VT. Traditionally these dysrhythmias have been treated aggressively with oral antidysrhythmic drugs. However, a landmark clinical study known as the *Cardiac Arrhythmia Suppression Trial* (CAST) suggests that treatment of this ventricular ectopic activity may increase the risk of sudden cardiac death.[17] For more information on cardiac drugs, see pages 203-205. Another option for treatment of chronic VT is an implantable cardioverter defibrillator (ICD), described in more detail on pages 190-192.

VT versus SVT: Sometimes a supraventricular tachycardia (SVT) takes an unusual path through the ventricles, causing a wide-complex tachycardia that mimics VT. This causes considerable diagnostic difficulty.

Unstable VT/SVT: If patients are hemodynamically unstable, emergency defibrillation is used. (See ACLS guidelines in Appendix A).

Stable VT/SVT: However, if patients are hemodynamically stable, conscious, and with an adequate blood pressure the situation is more complex. Standard treatment for VT includes administration of intravenous (IV) lidocaine, whereas SVT is often managed with IV verapamil. If the diagnosis is incorrect and a SVT is treated with lidocaine, the treatment is ineffective but there is no danger to patients. If a VT is mistakenly diagnosed as SVT and verapamil is given, the AV node may be blocked and patients may develop hypotension or loss of consciousness requiring immediate cardioversion.

VT/SVT Diagnosis: In hemodynamically stable patients, it is important to determine the mechanism of the wide-complex tachycardia before treatment is initiated. A 12-lead ECG will give more clues about the P wave-QRS relationship than a bedside ECG strip, but if this is not diagnostic, IV adenosine will temporarily block the AV node so atrial activity can be visualized if present.[16]

---

*Ejection Fraction

Ventricular fibrillation (VF)

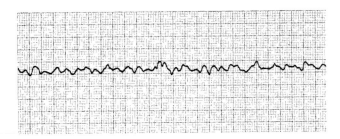

FIG. 8-33

RATE: Indeterminable.

RHYTHM: Irregular, wavy baseline without recognizable QRS complexes.

P WAVE: Absent. Cannot be distinguished from the fibrillating ventricular baseline.

PR INTERVAL: Absent.

QRS DURATION: Absent. No QRS complexes are present.

QRS COMPLEX: The normal QRS is missing. In VF the ECG appears as a wavy baseline. Sometimes VF is described as "coarse" or "fine." Coarse VF is seen on the ECG as large, erratic undulations of the baseline, whereas in fine VF the ECG baseline exhibits only a mild tremor. In either case, patients have no pulse, no blood pressure, and are unconscious.

ETIOLOGY: VT is the most common precursor of VF. Therefore all of the factors that predispose patients to VT apply.

PHYSIOLOGY: Ventricular fibrillation is the result of electrical impulses from single or multiple foci in the ventricles that prevent the ventricles from contracting. The ventricles merely quiver, and there is no forward flow of blood.

TREATMENT: Defibrillation is the emergency treatment of choice. (See Appendix A for Advanced Cardiac Life Support (ACLS) guidelines.) Epinephrine may be used to try to change fine VF to coarse VF and facilitate defibrillation attempts. Antidysrhythmic drugs such as intravenous lidocaine and bretylium are also given if initial attempts at defibrillation fail. As with any cardiac arrest situation, supportive measures such as CPR, intubation, and correction of metabolic abnormalities are performed concurrently with definitive therapy.

Idioventricular rhythm

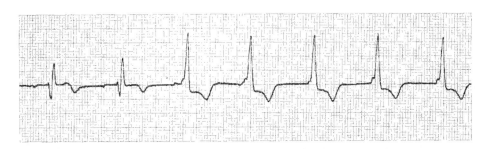

FIG. 8-34   Accelerated idioventricular rhythm (AIVR). The QRS duration is 0.14 second, and the ventricular rate is 65.

RATE: 20-40 beats per minute
RHYTHM: Regular.

P WAVE: Present, but not associated with the QRS complex.
PR INTERVAL: Absent.
QRS DURATION: Greater than 0.12 of a second.

QRS COMPLEX: Wide and bizarre because the complexes originate in the ventricles.

ACCELERATED IDIOVENTRICULAR RHYTHM (AIVR): This occurs when a ventricular focus assumes control of the heart at a rate greater than its intrinsic rate of 40 per minute but less than 100 per minute (Fig. 8-34). If patients have a good blood pressure, this rhythm is not treated pharmacologically, although patients are monitored carefully. A transvenous temporary pacemaker should be inserted electively as a precaution against sudden hemodynamic deterioration.

ETIOLOGY: The SA and AV nodes may be damaged by degenerative heart disease or an acute MI or depressed by drug toxicity.

PHYSIOLOGY: At times an ectopic focus in the ventricle can become the dominant pacemaker of the heart. If both the SA node and the AV junction fail, the ventricles will depolarize at their own intrinsic rate of 20 to 40 times per minute.

TREATMENT: Rather than trying to abolish the ventricular beats, the aim of treatment is to increase the effective heart rate and to reestablish a higher pacing site, such as the SA node or AV junction. The heart rate may be increased pharmacologically with an infusion of isoproteronal (Isuprel). More commonly a transvenous temporary pacemaker is inserted and the heart is paced at a faster rate until the underlying problems that caused failure of faster pacing sites can be resolved.

Precautions: Drugs such as lidocaine are contraindicated in treatment of idioventricular rhythms because if the ventricular ectopic focus is abolished, patients could become asystolic.

Atrioventricular Conduction Disturbance and Heart Blocks

First degree AV block (1° AV block)

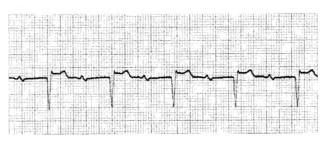

FIG. 8-35 The PR interval is prolonged to 0.44 second.

RATE: Depends on the underlying rhythm, usually normal sinus rhythm.

RHYTHM: Regular if NSR.

QRS COMPLEX: Unaffected by 1° AV block.

P WAVE: Present, normal shape.

PR INTERVAL: Greater than 0.20 of a second.

QRS DURATION: 0.06 to 0.10 of a second.

ETIOLOGY: All atrial impulses that should be conducted to the ventricles are conducted, but the PR interval is prolonged.

TREATMENT: None required. Many older patients have 1° AV block as a chronic condition associated with aging of the AV junction.

Acute MI: Patients with an acute MI should be monitored for degeneration into more serious forms of AV block.

Drug side effect: If the development of 1° AV block is new and related to recent antidysrhythmic drug administration, the medication regimen must be evaluated.

Second degree AV block—Mobitz type I or Wenckebach

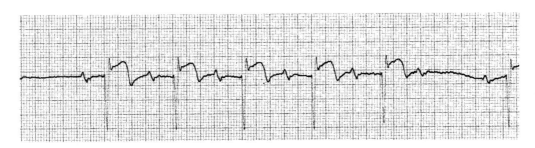

FIG. 8-36 Note that the PR intervals gradually increase from 0.36 to 0.46 second until finally a P wave is not conducted to the ventricles.

RATE: *Atrial:* Depends on the underlying sinus rate.

Ventricular: Depends on the P wave to QRS ratio.

RHYTHM: Regular, irregular pattern. P waves will be regular. As part of the Mobitz 1 pattern the R to R intervals become progressively shorter until the sinus P wave is not conducted. This causes a pause. After the pause the cycle repeats itself.

QRS COMPLEX: The conducted QRS complexes are normal.

P WAVE: Normal shape.

PR INTERVAL: The PR intervals progressively lengthen until a P wave is not conducted to the ventricles and is therefore not followed by a QRS.

QRS DURATION: 0.06 to 0.10 of a second.

ETIOLOGY: In Mobitz type I block the anatomic site of the block is at the level of the AV node. If it is associated with an acute inferior wall MI, the block is caused by ischemia and is usually transient.

PHYSIOLOGY: In Mobitz type I block the AV conduction time progressively lengthens until a P wave is not conducted to the ventricles.

DOCUMENTATION: The P wave to QRS complex ratio is documented. For example, if four P waves are conducted to the ventricles and the fifth one is not, a 5:4 conduction ratio is present (five P waves to four QRS complexes).

TREATMENT: No treatment is required if the ventricular rate is sufficient to sustain hemodynamic stability. In certain clinical conditions, such as an acute MI, the possibility of progression to a more serious conduction disturbance exists, and patients are closely monitored. If hemodynamic compromise is present or deemed likely, a temporary transvenous pacemaker may be inserted.

Second degree AV block (Mobitz type II)

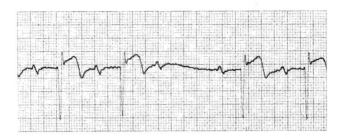

FIG. 8-37 The PR intervals of the conducted beats remain constant.

RATE: *Atrial:* Usually 60-100 range.

    Ventricular: The ventricular rate is slower and depends upon the number of conducted P waves.

RHYTHM: *Regular:* If the AV node conducts every second or third P wave in a consistent pattern.

    Irregular: If the P waves are conducted irregularly.

P WAVE: Normal in shape. There are more P waves than QRS complexes.

PR INTERVAL: 0.12 to 0.20 of a second. The PR interval is constant for the P waves that conduct to the ventricles.

QRS DURATION: 0.06 to 0.10 of a second. Will be wider if a bundle branch block (BBB) is present.

QRS COMPLEX: May be narrow and normal or widened due to a coexisting BBB.

ETIOLOGY: Usually Mobitz II indicates block below the AV node, either in the His bundle or in both bundle branches. It most frequently occurs when one bundle branch is blocked and the other is ischemic. Mobitz II block is more ominous clinically than Mobitz I and often progresses to complete AV block.

PHYSIOLOGY: Mobitz type II block occurs in the presence of a long absolute refractory period with virtually no relative refractory period. This results in an "all or nothing" situation. Sinus P waves may be conducted. When conduction does occur, all PR intervals are the same.

TREATMENT: Mobitz II can be serious and often precedes complete AV block. Use of a temporary transvenous pacemaker is usually necessary, but its insertion can be elective if patients remain hemodynamically stable.

Third-degree AV block (3° AV block)

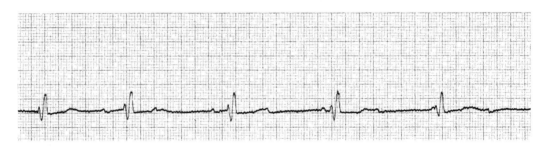

FIG. 8-38

RATE: Depends on underlying rhythm.

RHYTHM: Usually regular.

P WAVE: Normal shape.

PR INTERVAL: P waves are not related to the QRS complexes, so the PR intervals will vary widely.

QRS DURATION: Greater than 0.10 of a second.

QRS COMPLEX: *Junctional focus:* If a junctional focus is pacing the heart, the QRS complex looks normal but is not related to the P waves.

    Ventricular focus: If a ventricular focus is pacing the heart, the QRS complex is wide and unrelated to the P waves (Fig. 8-38).

ETIOLOGY: Degeneration of the AV node due to underlying heart disease or an acute MI. Blockage of the AV node is a side effect of some antidysrhythmic drugs.

PHYSIOLOGY: In third-degree, or complete, AV block no atrial impulses can conduct through the AV node to cause ventricular depolarization. The opportunity for conduction is optimal but does not occur. Ideally a junctional or ventricular focus depolarizes spontaneously at its intrinsic rate of 20 to 60 beats per minute and ventricular contraction continues. If not, asystole occurs, the pulse stops, and death results if intervention is not immediate.

TREATMENT: Complete heart block almost always requires use of a pacemaker. If patients are hemodynamically unstable, an isoproterenol (Isuprel) drip or external pacemaker can be used to maintain an adequate ventricular rate until a temporary transvenous pacemaker can be inserted.

Chest Radiography

The oldest noninvasive method for visualizing images of the heart, chest radiography, or chest x-ray, remains a frequently used and valuable diagnostic tool, providing information about cardiac anatomy and physiology with ease and safety at a relatively low cost.

Tissue densities

As x-rays travel through the chest from the emitting tube to the film plate, they are absorbed to a varying degree by the tissues through which they pass and consequently appear white, gray, or black on the x-ray film (Table 8-6).

1. The white areas are created by very dense tissue such as bone, which absorbs almost all the x-rays and leaves the film unexposed.
2. The gray areas result from moderately dense, blood-filled structures such as the heart, aorta, and the pulmonary vessels.
3. The black areas are caused by air. Air-filled lungs allow the greatest penetration of x-rays, resulting in fully exposed areas on the film.

Standard x-rays

In most institutions a standard radiographic examination of the heart and lungs consists of posterioanterior (PA) and lateral films. Ideally the chest radiograph is taken in the x-ray department with patients in an upright position; the film exposed during a deep, sustained inhalation; and the x-ray tube aimed horizontally 6 feet from the film. This is known as a *PA film* because the beam traverses the patient from posterior to anterior.

Portable x-rays

Because most patients in critical care units are too ill to go to the x-ray department, chest radiographs are obtained using a portable x-ray machine with patients either sitting upright or lying supine, depending on patients' clinical condition and the judgment of nurses. For a portable chest x-ray the film plate is placed behind patients' back and an anterioposterior (AP) projection, in which the x-ray beam enters from the front of the chest, is used.

Normal chest x-ray

When examining a PA or AP chest x-ray, nurses should be familiar with normal cardiac anatomy. The heart is rotated to the left in the chest so the right atrium and ventricle are the anterior chambers. The normal cardiothoracic structures are outlined in Figure 8-39, *A* and *B.* Additional information on chest x-ray interpretation is found in Chapter 11.

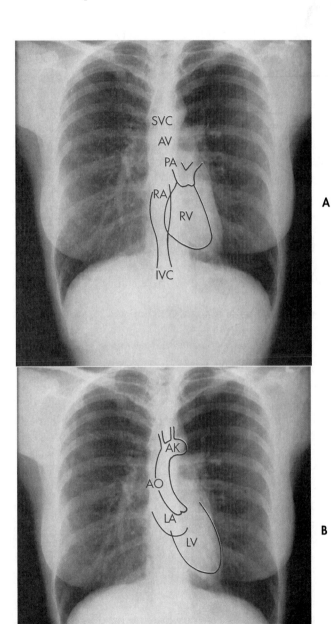

FIG. 8-39 Location of cardiac structures on a PA chest film. **A,** *AV,* Azygos vein; *SVC,* superior vena cava; *PA,* pulmonary artery; *RA,* right atrium; *RV,* right ventricle; *IVC,* inferior vena cava. **B,** *AO,* Aorta; *AK,* aortic knob; *LA,* left atrium; *LV,* left ventricle.

TABLE 8-6		
X-RAY DENSITIES OF INTRATHORACIC STRUCTURES		
METAL OR BONE (WHITE)	**FLUID (GRAY)**	**AIR (BLACK)**
Ribs, clavicle, sternum, spine	Blood	Lung
Calcium deposits	Heart	
Surgical wires or clips	Veins	
Prosthetic valves	Arteries	
Pacemaker wires	Edema	

Abnormal chest x-ray

Some cardiac abnormalities can be detected on the chest x-ray: for example, enlargement of the heart or great vessels and pulmonary congestion or edema.

Cardiothoracic ratio

The cardiothoracic ratio, often abbreviated as CT ratio, is a technique that estimates overall heart size from a chest x-ray, as shown in Figure 8-40. The maximum cardiac width is measured and compared with the maximum chest width at the level of the diaphragm. The CT ratio is considered abnormal if the cardiac diameter is greater than 50% of the total chest diameter.

Holter Monitoring

Indications

Ambulatory electrocardiography, often described as *Holter monitoring,* is a technique that records the ECG of patients while they perform their usual activities at home or work. It is designed to document abnormal cardiac electrical activity that occurs at random. Clinical indications include palpitations, dizziness, syncope, and pacemaker evaluation (Box 8-11).

Procedure

Holter monitoring is the oldest and most widely used continuous recording system. Patients wear five pregelled skin electrodes and carry a box that contains a specialized tape recorder. The Holter box has an event marker, which patients can press to indicate the onset of symptoms. In addition, patients are asked to keep a diary with times of activities, symptoms, and medications so ECG events can be correlated with clinical symptoms, activities, and drug side effects. The monitor measures about 4″ × 6″ and weighs less than 1 lb. Carried either by a shoulder strap or clipped to a belt or pocket, it is left on for 24 or 48 hours and then returned to the hospital or clinic for reading. When the tape is returned for reading, a technician places it in a machine that displays the tracing for review. Usually the tape is run at 60 to 120 times normal speed, allowing a 24-hour report to be read

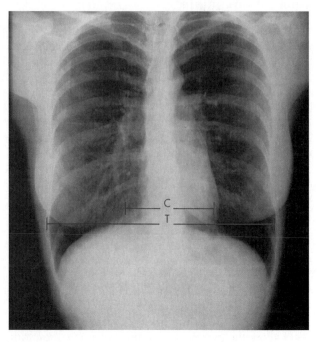

FIG. 8-40 Cardiothoracic (CT) ratio, a technique for estimating heart size on a PA chest film. Normally the cardiac diameter is 50% or less of the thoracic diameter when measured during full inhalation. *C,* Maximal cardiac diameter; *T,* maximal thoracic diameter measured to the inside of the ribs.

in 15 to 30 minutes. Printed reports are generated as the tape is read. Real-time printouts, at normal speed, can be run when any significant dysrhythmias are noted. A trend plot of heart rate, ST-segment level, or number of ectopics can also be printed.

PRECAUTIONS. The only activities that are restricted while wearing a Holter monitor are those that would get the chest electrodes or monitor wet, such as swimming and taking a shower or tub bath. Sponge baths are permitted as long as the chest electrodes are avoided.

Significance

The Holter ECG is interpreted in conjunction with the diary of symptoms using standard ECG interpretation techniques.

Transtelephonic Monitoring

Indications

Transtelephonic monitoring is an intermittent method of recording dysrhythmias. Many individuals have cardiac dysrhythmias that occur sporadically and unpredictably and may not occur during one 24-hour recording. A device that is only activated when there are symptoms is the most useful in these situations. When the symptoms occur, patients press a button to initiate the recording.

Procedure

The transtelephonic monitor consists of a small box, about 4″ × 2″, with four metal plates on the bottom. Patients carry the box at all times and also maintain a record of activities, events, and medications. Whenever they experience symptoms, patients place the four metal electrodes in firm contact with their skin and press a button to activate the recording, which lasts 1 to 2 minutes. The recording is stored until patients transmit it by telephone to the analysis facility, where it prints out as a real-time ECG. Patients are then advised if urgent medical attention is necessary. The center can contact patients' physicians or emergency medical personnel if the dysrhythmia is life threatening.

Significance

Standard ECG interpretation techniques are used.

Exercise Electrocardiography

Indications

Also referred to as *exercise tolerance testing* or *exercise stress test,* exercise electrocardiography consists of an ECG recorded during a period of stress on the heart muscle. The stress ECG helps evaluate the symptoms of coronary artery disease in both patients with known coronary heart disease and those initially seen with chest pain of unclear origin. Stress testing can evaluate the functional capacity of patients with or without heart disease and can be done serially to evaluate the effectiveness of medical or surgical therapy.

Procedure

Patients are asked to fast for 3 hours before the test, refrain from smoking for at least 2 hours before the test, and wear comfortable shoes and loose-fitting clothes. A resting 12-lead ECG is taken as a baseline. Most exercise stress tests are performed using a treadmill on which both speed and slope can be adjusted. A number of protocols have been developed using a treadmill. All reach virtually the same end point but at varying speeds. Two popular ones are the Bruce protocol, in which both grade and speed are varied every 3 minutes, and the Balke protocol, in which speed remains constant and grade is gradually increased every minute. A 12-lead ECG is recorded at rest before beginning the exercise protocol, and another 12-lead ECG is recorded on completion of the test. During the treadmill test the ECG is printed at 1-minute intervals as well as during symptoms, visible ECG changes, or dysrhythmias. Blood pressure is also measured and recorded every minute.

VITAL SIGNS. The treadmill test is terminated when the predicted maximum heart rate for that patient is achieved or when other symptoms, such as those listed in Table 8-7, develop.[19] Blood pressure is expected to rise during exercise, but a systolic blood pressure greater than 220 mm Hg or a diastolic blood pressure greater than 110 mm Hg is considered high enough to stop the test.

COMPLICATIONS. Complications are rare during exer-

TABLE 8-7
REASONS FOR STOPPING THE EXERCISE ECG

ABSOLUTE	RELATIVE
Acute MI	Marked ST or QRS changes
Severe angina	Increasing chest pain
Hypotension*	Fatigue and shortness of
Second- or third-degree AV	breath
block	Wheezing
Ventricular tachycardia	Leg cramps, claudication
Poor perfusion (pallor; cyanosis; cold, clammy skin)	Hypertension*
CNS symptoms (ataxia, vertigo, visual or gait disturbances, confusion)	Supraventricular tachycardia
Technical problems	
Patient's request	

cise testing, but they do occur. The mortality rate is 0.01% (1:10,000). The morbidity rate is 0.05% (5:10,000) and includes such adverse outcomes as myocardial infarction, cardiac arrest, and sustained ventricular tachycardia.[19] Cardiopulmonary resuscitation equipment must be readily available whenever exercise testing is performed. Nurses performing the test must be certain that emergency medications and a defibrillator are available in the test area and should be certified in advanced cardiac life support (ACLS). (See Appendix A for more details.)

Post-procedure

After completing the exercise test, patients rest in a supine position. A 12-lead ECG is recorded. The ECG, pulse rate, and blood pressure are monitored for at least 10 more minutes to detect dysrhythmias or signs of ischemia. Patients are instructed to rest for the next 30 to 60 minutes after release from the exercise laboratory.

Significance

A positive (abnormal) test result is indicated by ST-segment depression, either horizontal or downsloping, of 1 mm or more during or after exercise. Other criteria that strongly suggest a positive result are found in Table 8-8. For patients with cardiac symptoms, other more invasive tests may be prescribed if the exercise stress test is not diagnostic.

Signal-Averaged ECG

Indications

The signal-averaged ECG is a diagnostic study used when a risk of sudden cardiac death from life-threatening ventricular dysrhythmias exists. The results are combined

TABLE 8-8
CRITERIA FOR POSITIVE EXERCISE ECG TEST

DEFINITELY POSITIVE	STRONGLY SUGGESTIVE
Horizontal ST-segment depression of 1 mm or more during or after exercise	Horizontal or downsloping ST-segment depression of <1 mm during or after exercise
Downsloping ST-segment depression of 1 mm or more during or after exercise	Upsloping ST-segment depression of 2 mm or more beyond 0.08 sec from J-point during or after exercise
	Horizontal or upsloping ST-segment elevation of 1 mm or more during or after exercise
	ST-segment sagging 1 mm or more during or after exercise
	Hypotension
	Inverted U wave
	Frequent premature ventricular contractions (PVCs), multifocal PVCs, grouped PVCs, ventricular tachycardia provoked by mild exercise (70% or less of maximal heart rate)
	Exercise-induced typical angina, S_3, S_4, or heart murmur

with other studies (such as the 12-lead ECG and electrophysiologic study [EPS]) to reach a diagnosis.

Procedure

Patients assume a supine position and are asked to keep muscle movement to a minimum. Electrode leads are applied to the anterior and posterior chest wall, and the leads are connected to a signal-averaged ECG computer, which produces a high-resolution, high-magnification ECG signal. This "noise-free" ECG is then analyzed for both QRS duration and the presence, duration, and measurement of late myopotentials.[20] After computer analysis the signal-averaged ECG is described as either negative (normal) or positive (abnormal). A positive signal-averaged ECG is a predictor of increased risk for sudden cardiac death.

Significance

Damaged myocardium produces late-activating myopotentials that may cause reentry ventricular dysrhythmias. The 12-lead ECG is not sufficiently sensitive to detect these low amplitude, late potentials—hence the need for

a high-resolution signal. Many patients with a positive signal-averaged ECG (abnormal) will display a normal signal-averaged ECG when placed on antidysrhythmic medications. The signal-averaged ECG is not analyzed in isolation but used in conjunction with other cardiac diagnostic tests, including the electrophysiology study. It is a helpful adjunct to the EPS but does not replace it.

Thallium Scan

Indications

Developed as an adjunct to the exercise ECG stress test, the thallium scan determines whether there is a perfusion defect in cardiac muscle. A thallium scan is indicated for patients with chest pain and known or suspected coronary artery disease and for patients with a left bundle branch block (LBBB) or a permanent pacemaker, which may distort the QRS complex and cause difficulty in interpreting an ECG stress test.

THALLIUM ISOTOPE. A thallium scan involves the use of thallium-201 and a specialized perfusion-scanning camera. A low-energy radioactive isotope, thallium-201 is an analog of potassium that acts like potassium when injected into the bloodstream. Because thallium is similar to potassium, it is absorbed from the bloodstream by cardiac muscle cells as part of the sodium-potassium adenosine triphosphatase (ATPase) pump. Thallium uptake depends on two factors: (1) the patency of the coronary arteries and (2) the amount of healthy myocardium with a functional sodium-potassium ATPase pump. If an area of myocardium is infarcted (dead), it will not take up thallium.

Procedure

Before undergoing the thallium scan, patients receive a full explanation of the procedure, including a description of the equipment, which may overwhelm some patients. Patients are usually instructed to fast because a thallium scan involves vigorous exercise. A patent IV line is inserted before the test. The thallium test takes place in a specialized laboratory that contains ECG monitoring equipment, cardiovascular exercise equipment (treadmill or stationary bicycle), and an Anger gamma scintillation camera. Once in the laboratory, patients are asked to exercise vigorously for 1 minute or longer, or until angina or fatigue develops. At this point the thallium is injected into the bloodstream. After the injection patients are asked to exercise vigorously for another minute to stress the heart and circulate the thallium. As soon as possible after exercise (within 10 minutes), the patient is asked to lie on the examination table for the first perfusion scan by the scintillation camera to detect the areas of thallium concentration (uptake).

PHARMACOLOGIC THALLIUM TEST. Occasionally, patients who cannot physically tolerate a thallium/ECG stress test receive a pharmacologic thallium test in which dipyridamole (Persantine) is administered to increase coronary artery blood flow. The thallium scan is then performed without exercise.[21]

Significance

If no perfusion defect is seen, the test is complete. If a perfusion defect is noted (no thallium uptake), patients are asked to return for a repeat scan in 4 hours. If the perfusion defect is still present 4 hours later, the area is infarcted. If the perfusion defect has taken up thallium since the first test, the area is considered ischemic.[21]

Transthoracic Echocardiography

Indications

Echocardiography is used to detect cardiac abnormalities of the mitral or aortic valve and congenital heart defects. In the critical care unit echocardiography is used to evaluate acute valvular dysfunction, wall-motion abnormalities, and presence of pericardial effusions. An echocardiography study uses ultrasound waves to obtain and display images of cardiac structures.

Procedure

During the echocardiogram, patients assume either a supine or left lateral position. A transducer is placed on the skin between either the third or fourth intercostal space to the left of the sternum. Lubricant is placed between the skin and the transducer to improve contact and decrease artifact. The active element in the transducer is a piezoelectric crystal that transforms electrical energy into mechanical (sound) energy. The transducer emits ultrasound waves (more than 20,000 hertz [Hz]) and receives a signal from the reflected sound waves. Ultrasound is reflected best at interfaces between tissues that have different densities. In the heart these are the blood, cardiac valves, myocardium, and pericardium. Because all these structures differ in density, their borders can be seen on the echocardiogram.[22]

M-MODE ECHOCARDIOGRAM. In M-Mode (motion mode) echocardiography, a thin beam of ultrasound is directed through the heart (Fig. 8-41). Each interface is represented by a dot and when recorded over time each dot becomes a line on an oscilloscope. A strip-chart recording can be made of this tracing as the heart beats. The M-mode echocardiogram is particularly useful for measuring cardiac wall thickness and chamber size and evaluating valve motion.

TWO-DIMENSIONAL ECHOCARDIOGRAM. The Two-Dimensional echocardiogram uses numerous crystals in the transducer to create a cross-sectional imaging plane, which allows sections of the heart to be viewed from several different angles (Fig. 8-42). The picture is displayed on an oscilloscope, and photographs are taken to serve as a permanent record. The 2-D echocardiogram is superior to the M-mode echocardiogram because a whole "slice" of the heart is seen at once. Thus the location of cardiac structures and thickness of the wall in relation to the rest of the heart can be better appreciated.

PHONOCARDIOGRAM. Phonocardiography is frequently combined with echocardiography to evaluate valvular dysfunction. It provides a graphic display of the sounds that occur in the heart and great vessels. The transducer placed on the chest wall records cardiac sounds that correspond to auscultation with a stethoscope.

Significance

The M-mode and the 2-D echocardiograms complement each other. The 2-D echo provides a more general view of the heart, whereas the M-mode is able to focus on a specific muscle or valve segment.[23] Echocardiographic evidence of structural abnormalities such as pericardial effusion, mitral regurgitation, or decreased left ventricular wall motion allows treatment to be directed at the cause of patients' symptoms.

Doppler Echocardiography

Indications

Doppler echocardiography is used for patients with valvular and congenital heart disease. Both regurgitation and stenosis can be detected and severity estimated. A special kind of echocardiogram that assesses blood flow, it uses a pulsed or continuous wave of ultrasound to record frequency shifts of reflected sound waves, showing velocity and direction of blood flow relative to the transducer.

COLOR-FLOW DOPPLER. Doppler signals are now available in color. Known as *color-flow mapping* or *imaging*, this technique analyzes Doppler signals from multiple intracardiac sites simultaneously. The Doppler tracing for each site is displayed in a color-coded format superimposed on a real-time 2-D echocardiographic image. Flow toward the transducer is displayed in red, and flow away from the transducer is blue. Color mixes denote turbulent flow, and the brightness of the color is varied to signify varying flow velocities.

Significance

Most Doppler studies now include color-flow mapping because it enables abnormalities to be identified more rapidly. Mitral regurgitation is best evaluated with color-flow mapping because the Doppler probe can be placed very close to the location of the mitral valve, yielding a clear signal.[23]

Transesophageal Echocardiography (TEE)

Indications

The indications for transesophageal echocardiography (TEE) are identical to those for a transthoracic echocardiogram, but TEE is frequently used in the critical care unit because of the clarity of the TEE image.

Procedure

Prior to insertion of the TEE, the back of the throat is sprayed with a topical anesthetic and a sedative is often administered to minimize gagging. The TEE transducer (either M-mode, 2-D, color Doppler, or a combination of these) is mounted on a flexible shaft similar to a gastroscope. It is guided through the mouth into po-

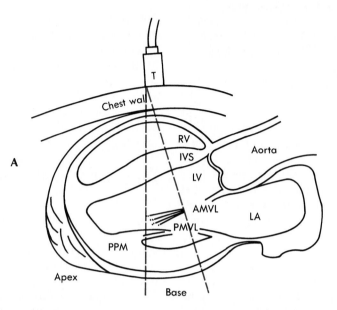

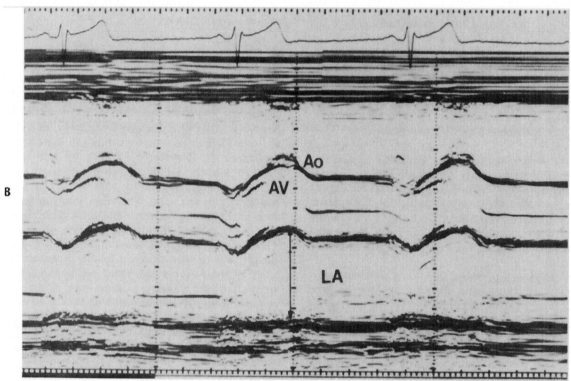

FIG. 8-41 A, Schematic presentation of cardiac structures transversed by two echobeams. **B,** Normal, M-mode echocardiogram at the level of the aorta, aortic valve leaflets, and left atrium. *RV,* right ventricle; *LV,* left ventricle; *IVS,* interventricular septum; *AMLV,* anterior mitral valve leaflet; *PMVL,* posterior mitral valve leaflet; *PPM,* posterior papillary muscle; *LA,* left atrium; *T,* transducer; *Ao,* aorta; *AV,* aortic valve. (**B** from Kinney M and others: *Comprehensive cardiac care,* ed 8, St Louis, 1996, Mosby.)

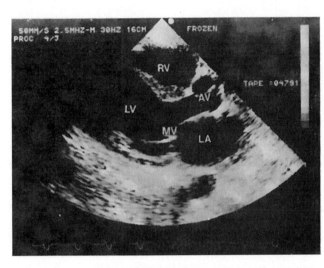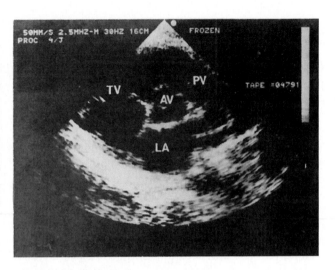

FIG. 8-42 Two-dimensional echocardiogram. Note that several sections of the heart can be viewed at one time, and it is easier to see the relationship of the chambers to one another. Abbreviations are as in Fig. 8-41, plus *TV,* tricuspid valve; *LV,* left ventricle. (From Kinney M and others: *Comprehensive cardiac care,* ed 8, St Louis, 1996, Mosby.)

sition in the esophagus and gently moved up and down and rotated to achieve the best image possible. Because of the close anatomic relationship between the heart and the esophagus, TEE produces high-quality images of intracardiac structures and the thoracic aorta without interference from the chest wall, bone, or air-filled lung.

COMPLICATIONS. The risk involved in TEE is surprisingly low, even in unstable critically ill patients. The overall incidence of complications is less than 1%.[24,25] However, TEE is somewhat uncomfortable, comparable to an upper GI endoscopy. Suction equipment should be available in the event that patients vomit or have difficulty handling oral secretions.

Significance

Because of the clarity of TEE images, clearly visualizing structural cardiac abnormalities is possible. It provides diagnostic information for valve disorders such as regurgitation or stenosis and is increasingly used to evaluate aortic disease and impending dissection. TEE can also be used to identify congenital heart disease in the adult and evaluate tumors and thrombi in the heart.[23]

Head-Up Tilt-Table Test

Indications

Patients who are being evaluated for unexplained loss of consciousness (syncope) may undergo a head-up tilt-table test (HUTT) in addition to an electrophysiology study and a complete neurologic examination. If the neurologic examination is normal and the EPS is negative for dysrhythmias, the cause of loss of consciousness may be vasodepressor syncope (VDS), which is evaluated by a HUTT. *VDS* describes transient syncope caused by hypotension secondary to parasympathetic vasodilatation and venous pooling.

Procedure

The HUTT is usually conducted in the radiology department. Patients lie supine on a table and are connected to an ECG monitor. A noninvasive blood pressure cuff is applied, and a peripheral IV line inserted. The table head is elevated to between 40 and 80 degrees, following a standard protocol. Blood pressure and heart rate measurements are taken frequently. A positive VDS response occurs if patients lose consciousness as the head of the table is raised. However, not all susceptible individuals experience syncope under resting conditions. In this situation drugs such as isoproterenol (Isuprel), 1 to 8 mcg/min, may be infused to increase heart rate and circulating catecholamines. If patients have a HUTT-induced syncopal episode, secondary ventricular dysrhythmias may occur.

COMPLICATIONS. Because ventricular dysrhythmias may occur following loss of consciousness due to VDS, ACLS qualified personnel must be in attendance with antidysrhythmic medications and a defibrillator.

Significance

If the HUTT causes a syncopal episode in patients with a normal EPS, it strongly suggests a diagnosis of VDS.

Electrophysiology Study

Indications

The **electrophysiology study** (EPS) is an invasive diagnostic tool used to record intracardiac electrical activity. An EPS is performed if patients have had unexplained syncope, sinus node or AV block, wide complex tachycardia, and other cardiac electrical problems not diagnosed by noninvasive diagnostic studies such as the 12-lead ECG, exercise stress test, signal-averaged ECG, or Holter monitoring.[26] The study is performed in a specialized cardiac catheterization laboratory.

Procedure

Before the electrophysiology study, patients and families receive written and verbal education to increase their knowledge and decrease stress and anxiety.[27] All antidysrhythmic medications are discontinued several days before the EPS so any ventricular dysrhythmias may be readily induced during the study. Patients fast 6 hours before the EPS and are premedicated to induce relaxation. Throughout the study, patients are conscious but receive sedation at regular intervals. A peripheral IV, radial arterial line, and surface ECG leads are placed. Electrophysiology catheters are then inserted into the femoral vein and advanced to the right side of the heart under fluoroscopy. These catheters, similar to pacing catheters, are placed at specific anatomic sites within the heart to record the earliest electrical activity. These sites include the sinoatrial (SA) node, the atrioventricular (AV) node, the coronary sinus, the bundle of His, the bundle branches, and other selected areas of myocardium. Once the catheters are in position, a pacing technique known as *programmed electrical stimulation* is used to trigger the dysrhythmia. This technique delivers pulses of two to four early ventricular pacing beats, via the catheter, to the selected area of myocardium. Once the dysrhythmia is induced, it can convert to normal sinus rhythm spontaneously or be converted by rapid atrial pacing, cardioversion, defibrillation, or IV antidysrhythmic medications. At the end of the study all of the electrophysiology catheters are removed before patients return to the nursing unit for ECG monitoring and care of the femoral area, where the catheters were inserted. Nursing care priorities are similar to those for patients following cardiac catheterization, as described in the following section.

Significance

During the EPS the electrophysiologist looks for a site of early electrical activation that stimulates the myocardium before the SA node. After the EPS diagnosis, medical management is prescribed. Many of the possible interventions necessitate a return to the electrophysiology laboratory to monitor the effectiveness of the treatment.

Cardiac Catheterization and Coronary Arteriography

Indications

Cardiac catheterization and coronary arteriography are invasive diagnostic procedures for patients with known or suspected heart disease. Clinical indications for cardiac catheterization include myocardial ischemia, unstable angina, evolving myocardial infarction, heart failure with a history that suggests coronary artery disease or valvular disease, and congenital heart disease. Cardiac catheterization is used to both confirm physical findings and provide a baseline for medical or surgical interventions.

Procedure

Before undergoing catheterization, patients meet with the cardiologist to discuss the purpose, benefit, and risks of the study. Patients fast for 6 hours before the procedure, ingesting only prescribed cardiac medications. They receive a light premedication. If patients have a history of allergy, an antihistamine or corticosteroid may be administered to prevent an anaphylactic reaction to the radiopaque contrast dye. Cardiac catheterization comprises pressure measurements and visualization of both the left and right sides of the heart. During catheterization of the left side of the heart, pressure measurements are taken in the aortic root, left ventricle, and left atrium. Radiopaque contrast (dye) is used to visualize the aorta, the left ventricle (ventriculogram), and the coronary arteries (arteriogram). A thermodilution pulmonary artery catheter is used to obtain hemodynamic pressure measurements on the right side of the heart. This includes measurements in the right atrium, right ventricle, pulmonary artery, and pulmonary artery wedge position, as well as the measurement of cardiac output, calculated hemodynamic values, oxygen saturations, and an angiogram of chambers on the right side of the heart, using radiopaque contrast. Throughout the cardiac catheterization, patients are awake, positioned on a hard table with a C- or U-shaped camera arm overhead or to the side. This arm can be moved so the heart may be viewed from several angles. Cardiac catheterization catheters, available in a variety of designs and sizes, are placed in the groin area after patients receive a local anesthetic. The femoral artery is used to gain access to the aorta, left side of the heart, and coronary arteries. The femoral vein is used to pass catheters to the right side of the heart. During the study patients receive heparin systematically to reduce the risk of emboli. Many patients also receive nitroglycerin to control chest pain, particularly when the coronary arteries are full of contrast material during the coronary arteriographic procedure. At this time patients may also experience bradycardia or hypotension. To move the contrast dye more quickly and minimize the vagal effect on heart rate and blood pressure, clinicians may ask patients to cough. If the bradycardia persists, atropine may be used. If hypotension continues, IV fluids are administered as a bolus. At the end of the study, protamine reverses the heparin effect. The catheters are removed, and pressure is applied to the groin area until bleeding has stopped.

Significance

The cardiologist interprets the cardiac catheterization films during and after the procedure. The cardiologist is able to identify blockages in the coronary arteries, see valvular stenosis or regurgitation, estimate left ventricular ejection fraction, and assess left ventricular wall movement. A valuable source of information about cardiovascular function, the results of cardiac catheterization are often used to confirm the need for a coronary interventional procedure (see pages 192 to 196) or cardiac surgery (see pages 185 to 190).

Nursing management

After cardiac catheterization, patients remain supine for 6 hours. **The priorities of nursing management involve assessing the femoral insertion site, monitoring pedal pulses, encouraging fluids, and educating patients and family.**

Assessing the femoral insertion site

The femoral site, where the arterial and venous catheters were inserted, is assessed frequently for evidence of bleeding or hematoma. Strategies to decrease bleeding include asking patients to lie supine (without moving and without bending at the hip) and placing a sandbag over the femoral site to decrease hematoma formation.

Monitoring pedal pulses

Pedal and posterior tibial pulses are assessed every 15 minutes for the first hour after the catheterization and every 30 minutes to 1 hour thereafter. The limb is assessed for changes in color, temperature, pain, or paresthesia—in other words, monitoring to detect early evidence of acute arterial occlusion.

Encouraging fluids

Because the radiopaque contrast acts as an osmotic diuretic, patients are encouraged to drink large amounts of clear liquids, and the IV fluid rate is increased to 100 ml/hour. Patients who have elevated blood urea nitrogen or creatinine levels before catheterization are at risk for renal failure from the dye. For these patients the quantity of contrast material injected during the procedure is reduced to preserve kidney function.

Educating patients and families

Following cardiac catheterization, education of patients and families is focused on current nursing care: the reasons for resting in bed for 6 hours, keeping the affected hip straight, drinking large amounts of fluids, and cooperating with assessment of pulses. Patients are also asked to report any other unusual symptoms, such as nausea or chest pain.

Bedside Hemodynamic Monitoring

Indications

Hemodynamic monitoring can be used for a wide range of medical diagnoses. Most of these medical diagnoses are linked by three nursing diagnoses: (1) *Alteration in Cardiac Output,* (2) *Alteration in Fluid Volume,* and (3) *Alteration in Tissue Perfusion.* These nursing diagnoses are based on pathophysiologic processes that alter one of the four hemodynamic mechanisms supporting normal car-

diovascular function: preload, afterload, heart rate, and contractility. Treatment of *Alterations in Cardiac Output, Fluid Volume,* and *Tissue Perfusion* will vary based on the precipitating cause and medical diagnosis, as discussed in the section on pulmonary artery catheters.

Hemodynamic monitoring equipment

A hemodynamic monitoring system has three component parts: (1) the invasive catheter and tubing connected to patients, (2) the transducer, which receives the physiologic signal from the catheter and converts it into electrical energy, and (3) the amplifier/recorder, which increases the volume of the electrical signal and displays it on both an oscilloscope and a digital scale read in millimeters of mercury (mm Hg). Although many different invasive catheters are inserted to monitor hemodynamic pressures, all catheters are connected to similar equipment: a bag of 0.9% normal saline solution, which usually contains 0.25 to 2 units of heparin per milliliter; a 300-mm Hg pressure infusion cuff; intravenous (IV) tubing; three-way stopcocks; and an in-line flush device for both continuous and manual fluid infusion. The addition of heparin to the IV setup is designed to maintain catheter patency. A multicenter nursing study has demonstrated that arterial monitoring lines maintained with a heparin flush solution are more likely to remain patent than lines maintained with nonheparinized solutions.[28] The tubing connects the invasive catheter to the transducer to avoid damping (flattening) of the waveform, which results in inaccurate pressure readings. The transducers most frequently used in clinical practice are disposable and use a silicon chip.

Calibration of equipment

For accurate hemodynamic pressure readings, two baseline measurements are necessary: (1) calibration of the system to atmospheric pressure, and (2) determination of the phlebostatic axis for transducer height placement. To calibrate the equipment, the three-way stopcock nearest to the transducer is turned simultaneously to open the transducer to air (atmospheric pressure) and close it to the patient and the flush system. The monitor is adjusted so that "0" is displayed, which equals atmospheric pressure. Then, the monitor is used to calibrate the upper scale limit while the system remains open to air. Standard scale limits for that monitor system are used. Finally the stopcock is returned to its original position to visualize the waveform and hemodynamic pressures.

Phlebostatic axis

The phlebostatic axis is a physical reference point on the chest that is used as a baseline for consistent transducer height placement. Obtaining the axis involves drawing a theoretic line from the fourth intercostal space, where it joins the sternum, to a midaxillary line on the side of the chest. The intersection of these lines approximates the level of the atria. The transducer air-reference stopcock is leveled with this reference point to obtain accurate patient hemodynamic pressures with head-of-bed positions up to 60 degrees of elevation.[29-32] Patients do not have to be supine to obtain accurate PA pressure readings. Error in measurement can occur if the transducer is placed *below* the phlebostatic axis because fluid in the system will weigh on the transducer and produce a false-high reading. If the transducer is placed *above* this atrial level, gravity and lack of fluid pressure will produce an erroneously low reading. If several clinicians will be taking measurements, the reference point can be marked on the side of patients' chests to ensure accurate measurements.

Intraarterial Pressure Monitoring

Indications

Intraarterial pressure monitoring is indicated for any medical or surgical condition that compromises cardiac output, tissue perfusion, or fluid volume status. The system is designed for continuous measurement of three blood pressure parameters—systole, diastole, and mean arterial blood pressure (MAP). In addition, direct arterial access is helpful in the management of patients with acute respiratory failure who require frequent arterial blood gas measurements.

Intraarterial catheters

The size of the catheter used is proportionate to the diameter of the cannulated artery. In small arteries—such as the radial or dorsalis pedis—a 20-gauge, 3.8 to 5.1 cm, nontapered Teflon catheter is most often used. If the larger femoral or axillary arteries are used, a 19- or 20-gauge, 16-cm Teflon catheter is used. Teflon catheters are preferred because of their lower risk of causing thrombosis.

Intraarterial catheter insertion

Catheter insertion is usually percutaneous, although technique varies with vessel size. Cannulas are most frequently inserted in the smaller arteries, using a "catheter-over-needle" unit in which the needle serves as a temporary guide for catheter placement. With this method, once the unit has been inserted into the artery, the needle is withdrawn, leaving the supple plastic cannula in place. Insertion of a cannula into the larger femoral artery usually necessitates use of the Seldinger technique. This procedure involves (1) entry into the artery using a needle, (2) passage of a supple guidewire through the needle into the artery, (3) removal of the needle, (4) passage of the catheter over the guidewire, and (5) removal of the guidewire, with the cannula left in the artery. If a cannula cannot be inserted into the artery using percutaneous methods, an arterial cutdown may be performed. Because it involves a skin incision that directly exposes the artery and is associated with a higher risk of infection, this procedure should be avoided unless it is absolutely necessary.

Arterial monitoring sites

Several major peripheral arteries are suitable for receiving a cannula and for long-term hemodynamic monitoring. The most frequently used site is the radial artery. If this artery is not available, the dorsalis pedis, femoral, axillary, or brachial arteries may be used. The major advantage of the radial artery is that collateral circulation to the hand is provided by the ulnar artery and palmar arch in most people; thus other avenues of circulation exist if the radial artery becomes blocked after catheter placement. Before radial artery cannulation, collateral circulation must be assessed by using either a Doppler flowmeter or the Allen test. In the Allen test the radial and ulnar arteries are compressed simultaneously. Patients are asked to clench and unclench one hand until it blanches. One of the arteries is then released, and the hand should immediately flush from that side. The same procedure is repeated for the remaining artery.

Nursing management

The priorities of nursing management of an intraarterial pressure monitoring system include monitoring arterial blood pressure, assessing the arterial pressure waveform, troubleshooting the arterial line, preventing complications, and educating patients and families.

Monitoring arterial blood pressure

Intraarterial blood pressure monitoring is designed for continuous assessment of arterial perfusion to the major organ systems of the body. MAP is the clinical parameter most frequently used to assess perfusion because it represents the perfusion pressure throughout the cardiac cycle. One third of the cardiac cycle is spent in systole and two thirds in diastole; thus the MAP calculation reflects the greater amount of time spent in diastole. The MAP formula when calculated by hand is as follows:

$$[(Diastole \times 2) \text{ plus } (Systole \times 1)] \div \text{ by } 3$$

Thus a blood pressure of 120/60 mm Hg has a MAP of 80 mm Hg. However, the bedside hemodynamic monitor may show a slightly different digital number because most computers calculate the area under the curve of the arterial line tracing (Table 8-9). A MAP greater than 60 mm Hg is necessary to perfuse the coronary arteries, brain, and kidneys. A MAP between 70 and 90 mm Hg is ideal to decrease LV work load for patients with cardiac disease. After a carotid endarterectomy or neurologic surgery, a MAP of 90 to 110 mm Hg may be more appropriate to increase cerebral perfusion pressure. Systolic and diastolic pressures are monitored in conjunction with the MAP as a further guide to the accuracy of perfusion. Should cardiac output decrease, the body will compensate by constricting peripheral vessels to maintain the blood pressure. In this situation the MAP may remain constant, but the pulse pressure (difference between systolic and diastolic pressures) will narrow. The following examples explain this point:

TABLE 8-9

SELECTED HEMODYNAMIC PRESSURES AND CALCULATED HEMODYNAMIC VALUES

HEMODYNAMIC PRESSURE	DEFINITION AND EXPLANATION	NORMAL RANGE*
Mean arterial pressure (MAP)	Average perfusion pressure created by arterial blood pressure during the complete cardiac cycle. The normal cardiac cycle is one-third systole and two-thirds diastole. These three components are divided by 3 to obtain the average perfusion pressure for the whole cardiac cycle.	70-100 mm Hg
Central venous pressure (CVP), also described as right atrial pressure (RAP)	Pressure created by volume in the right side of the heart. When the tricuspid valve is open, the CVP reflects filling pressures in the right ventricle. Clinically the CVP is often used as a guide to overall fluid balance.	2-5 mm Hg 3-8 cm water (H_2O)
Pulmonary artery pressure (PAP) (systolic, diastolic, mean) (PA systolic [PAS], PA diastolic [PAD], PAP mean [PAP_M])	Pulsatile pressure in the pulmonary artery, measured by an indwelling catheter.	PAS 20-30 mm Hg PAD 5-10 mm Hg PAP_M 10-15 mm Hg
Pulmonary capillary wedge pressure or pulmonary artery wedge pressure (PCW or PCWP or PAWP)	Pressure created by volume in the left side of the heart. When the mitral valve is open, the PAWP reflects filling pressures in the pulmonary vasculature, and pressures in the left side of the heart are transmitted back to the catheter "wedged" into a small pulmonary arteriole.	5-12 mm Hg
Cardiac output (CO)	The amount of blood pumped out by a ventricle. Clinically it can be measured using the thermodilution CO method, which calculates CO in liters per minute (L/min).	4-6 L/min (at rest)
Cardiac index (CI)	CO divided by body surface area (BSA), tailoring the CO to individual body size. A BSA conversion chart is necessary to calculate CI, which is considered more accurate than CO because it is individualized to height and weight. CI is measured in liters per minute per square meter BSA (L/min/m²).	2.2-4.0 L/min/m²
Stroke volume (SV)	Amount of blood ejected by the ventricle with each heartbeat. Hemodynamic monitoring systems calculate SV by dividing cardiac output (CO in L/min) by the heart rate (HR) then multiplying the answer by 1000 to change liters to milliliters (ml).	60-70 ml
Systemic vascular resistance (SVR)	Mean pressure difference across the systemic vascular bed, divided by blood flow. Clinically SVR represents the resistance against which the left ventricle must pump to eject its volume. This resistance is created by the systemic arteries and arterioles. As SVR increases, CO falls. SVR is measured by either units or dynes/sec/cm^{-5}. If the number of units is multiplied by 80, the value is converted to dynes/sec/cm^{-5}.	10-18 units or 800-1400 dynes/sec/cm^{-5}
Pulmonary vascular resistance (PVR)	Mean pressure difference across pulmonary vascular bed, divided by blood flow. Clinically PVR represents the resistance against which the right ventricle must pump to eject its volume. This resistance is created by the pulmonary arteries and arterioles. As PVR increases, the output from the right ventricle decreases. PVR is measured in either units or dynes/sec/cm^{-5}. PVR is normally one sixth of SVR.	1.2-3.0 units or 100-250 dynes/sec/cm^{-5}

*The formulas for these hemodynamic values are listed in Appendix B.

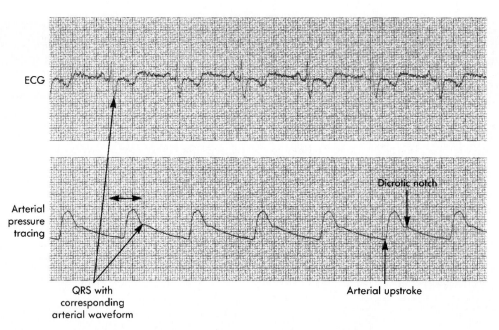

FIG. 8-43 Simultaneous ECG and arterial pressure tracings.

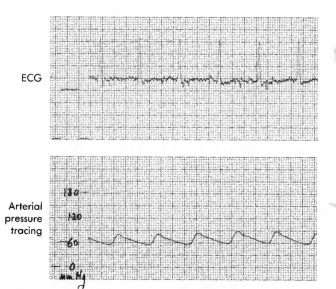

FIG. 8-44 Simultaneous ECG and arterial pressure tracings show a damped arterial pressure waveform.

Mr. A: BP, 90/70; MAP, 76 mm Hg

Mr. B: BP, 150/40; MAP, 76 mm Hg

Both of these patients have a perfusion pressure of 76 mm Hg, but clinically they are very different. Mr. A is peripherally vasoconstricted, as the narrow pulse pressure (90/70) demonstrates. His skin is cool to the touch, and he has weak peripheral pulses. Mr. B has a wide pulse pressure (150/40), warm skin, and normally palpable peripheral pulses. Thus nursing assessment of patients with an arterial line includes comparing current clinical findings with arterial line readings. Evaluating the trend of measurements over time is also important.

Assessing the arterial pressure waveform

The arterial pressure waveform represents the ejection phase of left ventricular systole. As the aortic valve opens, blood is ejected from the left ventricle and is recorded as an increase of pressure in the arterial system. The highest point recorded is called *systole*. After peak ejection (systole), force is decreased and pressure drops. A notch (the dicrotic notch) may be visible on the downstroke of this arterial waveform, representing closure of the aortic valve. The dicrotic notch signifies the beginning of diastole. The remainder of the downstroke represents diastolic runoff of blood flow into the arterial tree. The lowest point recorded is called *diastole*. A normal arterial pressure tracing is described in Figure 8-43.

Troubleshooting the arterial line

If air bubbles, clots, or kinks are in the system, the waveform will become damped, or flattened, and the troubleshooting methods described in Table 8-10 can be implemented. If the line is unreliable or becomes dislodged, a cuff pressure can be used as a reserve system.[33] A damped (flattened) arterial waveform is shown in Figure 8-44. Occurring when communication from the artery to the transducer is interrupted, damped arterial waveforms may be caused by a clot at the end of the catheter, kinks in the catheter or tubing, or air bubbles in the system. Troubleshooting techniques as described in Table 8-10 are used to find the origin of the problem and remove the cause of damping. If the arterial monitor shows a low blood pressure, nurses are responsible for determining whether it is a true patient problem or a problem with the equipment, as described in Table 8-10. A low arterial blood pressure waveform is shown in Figure 8-45. In this case the digital readout correlated with the patient's own cuff pressure, confirming that the patient was

TABLE 8-10

NURSING MEASURES TO ENSURE PATIENT SAFETY AND TO TROUBLESHOOT PROBLEMS WITH HEMODYNAMIC MONITORING EQUIPMENT

PROBLEM	PREVENTION	RATIONALE	TROUBLESHOOTING
Damping of waveform	Provide continuous infusion of solution containing heparin through an in-line flush device (1 unit of heparin for each millimeter of flush solution).	To ensure that recorded pressures and waveform are accurate because a damped waveform gives inaccurate readings.	Before insertion, completely flush the line and/or catheter. In a line attached to a patient, back flush through the system to clear bubbles from tubing or transducer.
Clot formation at end of catheter	Provide continuous infusion of solution containing heparin through an in-line flush device (1 unit of heparin for each millimeter of flush solution).	Any foreign object placed in the body can cause local activation of patients' coagulation system as a normal defense mechanism. The clots that are formed may be dangerous if they break off and travel to other parts of the body.	If a clot in the catheter is suspected because of a damped waveform or resistance to forward flush of the system, gently aspirate the line using a small syringe inserted into the proximal stopcock. Then flush the line again once the clot is removed and inspect the waveform. It should return to a normal pattern.
Hemorrhage	Use Luer-Lok (screw) connections in line setup. Close and cap stopcocks when not in use.	A loose connection or open stopcock will create a low-pressure sump effect, causing blood to back into the line and into the open air.	Once a blood leak is recognized, tighten all connections, flush the line, and estimate blood loss.
	Ensure that the catheter is either sutured or securely taped in position.	If a catheter is accidentally removed, the vessel can bleed profusely, especially with an arterial line or if the patient has abnormal coagulation factors (resulting from heparin in the line) or hypertension.	If the catheter has been inadvertently removed, put pressure on the cannulation site. When bleeding has stopped, apply a sterile dressing, estimate blood loss, and inform the physician. If patients are restless, an armboard may protect lines inserted in the arm.
Air emboli	Ensure that all air bubbles are purged from a new line setup before attachment to an indwelling catheter.	Air can be introduced at several times, including when central venous pressure (CVP) tubing comes apart, when a new line setup is attached, or when a new CVP or pulmonary artery (PA) line is inserted. During insertion of a CVP or PA line, patients may be asked to hold their breath at specific times to prevent drawing air into the chest during inhalation.	Because it is impossible to get the air back once it has been introduced into the bloodstream, prevention is the best cure.
	Ensure that the drip chamber from the bag of flush solution is more than half full before using the in-line, fast-flush system.	The in-line, fast-flush devices are designed to permit clearing of blood from the line after withdrawal of blood samples.	If any air bubbles are noted, they must be vented through the in-line stopcocks and the drip chamber must be filled.
	Some sources recommend removing all air from the bag of flush solution before assembling the system.	If the chamber of the IV tubing is too low or empty, the rapid flow of fluid will create turbulence and cause flushing of air bubbles into the system and into the bloodstream.	

Continued.

T A B L E   8 - 1 0

NURSING MEASURES TO ENSURE PATIENT SAFETY AND TO TROUBLESHOOT PROBLEMS WITH HEMODYNAMIC MONITORING EQUIPMENT—cont'd

PROBLEM	PREVENTION	RATIONALE	TROUBLESHOOTING
Normal waveform with *low* digital pressure	Ensure that the system is calibrated to atmospheric pressure. Ensure that the transducer is placed at the level of the phlebostatic axis.	To provide a 0 baseline relative to atmospheric pressure. If the transducer has been placed *higher* than the phlebostatic level, gravity and the lack of hydrostatic pressure will produce a false *low* reading.	Recalibrate the equipment if transducer drift has occurred. Reposition the transducer at the level of the phlebostatic axis. Misplacement can occur if patients move from the bed to the chair or if the bed is placed in a Trendelenburg position.
Normal waveform with *high* digital pressure	Ensure that the system is calibrated to atmospheric pressure. Ensure that the transducer is placed at the level of the phlebostatic axis.	To provide a 0 baseline relative to atmospheric pressure. If the transducer has been placed *lower* than the phlebostatic level, the weight of hydrostatic pressure on the transducer will produce a false *high* reading.	Recalibrate the equipment if transducer drift has occurred. Reposition the transducer at the level of the phlebostatic axis. This situation can occur if the head of the bed was raised and the transducer was not repositioned. Some centers require attachment of the transducer to the patient's chest to avoid this problem.
Loss of waveform	Always have the hemodynamic waveform monitored so that changes or loss can be quickly noted.	The catheter may be kinked, or a stopcock may be turned off.	Check the line setup to ensure that all stopcocks are turned in the correct position and that the tubing is not kinked. Sometimes the catheter migrates against a vessel wall, and having the patient change position will restore the waveform.
Infection	Change the bag of flush solution every 24 hours. Change the line setup and the disposable transducer every 72 hours. Change the catheter insertion site dressing every 24 hours, and inspect the cannulation site for signs of infections. Apply antiseptic ointment and a sterile dressing to the catheter site.	These recommendations are based on research studies with hemodynamic monitoring equipment and on reports of infectious complications. Note: Guidelines will vary for each hospital.	If local infection occurs, the catheter must be placed elsewhere by the physician, and the new insertion site must be dressed using antiseptic ointment and a sterile dressing. Sterile equipment must always be used, disposable equipment must not be reused, and nondisposable transducers must be sterilized after each patient usage. Hands should be washed before handling monitoring setup or dressings.

hypotensive. This arterial waveform is more rounded, without a dicrotic notch, when compared with the normal waveform in Figure 8-43. If the accuracy of the arterial waveform is in question, a cuff blood pressure reading should always be taken. As part of the routine nursing assessment, the cuff blood pressure is taken every shift and correlated with the intraarterial pressure.

Prevention of complications

The major complications of intraarterial pressure monitoring are hemorrhage, decreased perfusion to the distal extremity, and infection. Bleeding is probably the most frequent complication (Table 8-10).

1. The arterial pressure line and stopcocks are always visible (not covered by bed linen, for example) to prevent hemorrhage. All connections are secured by Luer Lok, and the catheter is securely taped or sutured in place. A radial artery catheter can also be stabilized by an arm board.

2. Whenever a catheter is inserted into an artery, circulation to the distal extremity may be compromised. Therefore nurses perform frequent neurovascular assessments. The extremity is compared with the other, noncannulated hand or leg, and color, temperature, pulse, paresthesia, and pain are assessed.

3. For the prevention of infection the guidelines specific to your institution should be followed

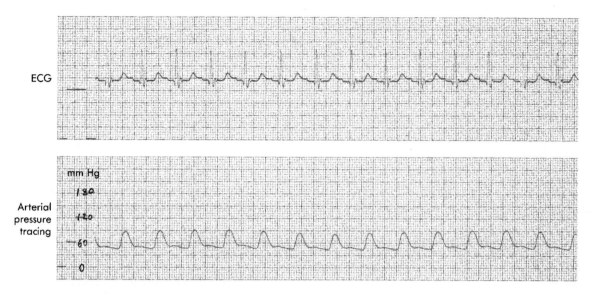

FIG. 8-45 Simultaneous ECG and arterial pressure tracings show a low arterial pressure waveform.

with the use of all invasive catheters (Table 8-10).

Educating patients and families

The focus of patient education is on safety. Radial artery catheters are small, often taped in place, and often not sutured. If patients are awake, nurses ask patients to keep the wrist with the catheter straight to prevent accidental dislodgement. Nurses should also explain the reasons for hemodynamic monitoring to decrease anxiety related to the lines and monitors.

Central Venous Pressure Monitoring

Indications

Central venous pressure (CVP) monitoring is indicated whenever patients have a significant alteration in fluid volume. In hypovolemic patients the CVP is used as a guide for fluid-volume replacement. For hypervolemic patients the CVP is used to assess the impact of diuresis after diuretic administration. In addition, when a major IV line is required for volume replacement, a central venous line is a good choice because large volumes of fluid can easily be delivered.

CVP catheters

CVP catheters are available as single-, double-, or triple-lumen infusion catheters, depending on the specific needs of patients, and are made from very soft and flexible polyvinylchloride.

CVP catheter insertion

Because many patients are awake and alert when a CVP catheter is inserted, a brief explanation about the procedure will minimize anxiety and increase cooperation during the insertion. This cooperation is important because catheter insertion is a sterile procedure and the Trendelenburg position may not be comfortable for many patients. The head is placed in a dependent position (Trendelenburg), which causes the internal jugular veins in the neck to become more prominent, facilitating line placement. To minimize the risk of air embolus during the procedure, clinicians should ask patients to take a deep breath and hold it any time the needle or catheter is open to air. CVP catheters are designed for placement by percutaneous insertion after preparation of skin and administration of a local anesthetic. The Seldinger technique, in which the vein is located by using a needle and syringe, is the preferred method of placement. A guidewire is passed through the needle, the needle is removed, and the catheter is passed over the guidewire. Once the catheter is correctly placed at the level of the right atrium, the guidewire is removed. Finally an IV setup is attached, and the catheter is sutured in place. After CVP catheter placement a chest radiograph may be obtained to verify placement and the absence of an iatrogenic hemothorax or pneumothorax.

CVP monitoring sites

The large veins of the upper thorax (subclavian or internal jugular) are most frequently used for percutaneous CVP line insertion. Other suitable insertion sites include the femoral and antecubital fossae veins.

CVP normal values

The CVP is used to measure the filling pressures of the right side of the heart. The central venous pressure is also known as the *right atrial (RA) pressure*. During diastole, when the tricuspid valve is open and blood is flowing from the right atrium to the right ventricle, the CVP will accurately reflect right ventricular end-diastolic pressure

(RVEDP). The normal CVP is 2 to 5 mm Hg (3 to 8 cm H₂O).

CVP measurement

In taking CVP measurements, clinicians have a choice of two methods: a mercury (mm Hg) system, using a transducer and a monitor; or a water (cm H_2O) manometer system. If patients change from one system to the other, the CVP value will also change because mercury is heavier than water and 1 mm Hg is equal to 1.36 cm H_2O. To convert water to mercury, clinicians divide the water value by 1.36 ($H_2O \div 1.36$). To convert mercury to water, they multiply the mercury value by 1.36 (mm Hg $\times$ 1.36). Accurate CVP measurements involve using the phlebostatic axis as a reference point on the body and ensuring that the transducer or water manometer zero is level with this point. If the phlebostatic axis is used and the transducer or water manometer is correctly aligned, any head-of-bed position of up to 45 degrees may be accurately used for CVP readings for most patients.[34] Elevating the head of the bed is especially helpful for patients with respiratory or cardiac problems who will not tolerate a flat position.

CVP monitoring limitations

The CVP monitors function of the right side of the heart. It is not, however, a reliable indicator of left ventricular dysfunction. LV dysfunction, which can occur after an acute myocardial infarction, will increase filling pressures on the left side of the heart. Because the CVP measures RVEDP, it will remain normal until the increase in pressure from the left side is reflected back through the pulmonary vasculature to the right ventricle. In this situation a pulmonary artery catheter that measures pressures on the left side is the monitoring method of choice.

Nursing management

The priorities of nursing management for patients with a CVP catheter include monitoring fluid volume, interpreting the CVP waveform, troubleshooting the CVP line, preventing CVP monitoring complications, and educating patients and families.

Monitoring fluid volume

The CVP is used in combination with the MAP and other clinical parameters to assess hemodynamic stability. In hypovolemic patients the CVP will fall before there is a significant fall in MAP because peripheral vasoconstriction will keep the MAP normal. Thus the CVP is an excellent early warning system for patients who are bleeding, vasodilating, or receiving diuretics.

Interpreting the CVP waveform

The normal RA or CVP waveform has three positive deflections—a, c, and v waves—that correspond to specific atrial events in the cardiac cycle (Fig. 8-46). Critical care nurses are responsible for assessing the waveform and troubleshooting problems that arise.

1. The a wave reflects atrial contraction and follows

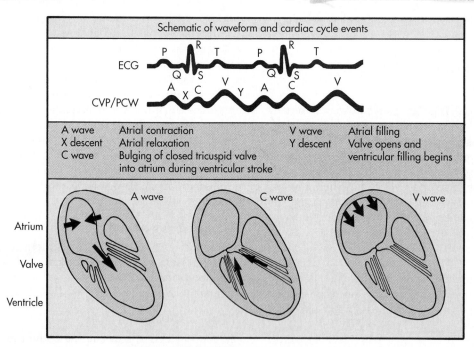

FIG. 8-46 Cardiac events that produce the CVP waveform with a, c, and v waves. The **a wave** represents atrial contraction. The **x descent** represents atrial relaxation. The **c wave** represents the bulging of the closed tricuspid valve into the right atrium during ventricular systole. The **v wave** represents atrial filling. The **y descent** represents opening of the tricuspid valve and filling of the ventricle.

the P wave seen on the ECG. The downslope of this wave is called the *x descent* and represents atrial relaxation.

2. The c wave reflects the bulging of the closed tricuspid valve into the right atrium during ventricular contraction. The c wave is small, not always visible, and corresponds to the QRS-T interval on the ECG.

3. The v wave represents atrial filling and pressure increase against the closed tricuspid valve in early diastole. The downslope of the v wave is named the *y descent* and represents the fall in pressure as the tricuspid valve opens and blood flows from the right atrium to the right ventricle.

Troubleshooting the CVP line

Air can enter the venous system during insertion because of a disconnected or broken CVP catheter or along the path of a removed catheter. Precautions to prevent an air embolism in a CVP line include using only Luer Lok (screw) connections, avoiding long loops of IV tubing, and using screw cap covers on three-way stopcocks.[35] If air bubbles, clots, or kinks are in the system, the waveform will become damped and the troubleshooting methods described in Table 8-10 may be implemented.

Preventing CVP monitoring complications

Three major complications that deserve specific attention include air embolus, hemorrhage, and infection.

AIR EMBOLUS. Air embolus is perhaps the most dangerous complication observed with a CVP line placed into a subclavian or jugular vein. Because patients are often sitting upright in bed, inspiratory respiratory efforts will pull the air into the venous system and into the right side of the heart by negative intrathoracic pressure if the CVP line becomes disconnected or open to air for any reason. If a large volume of air rapidly enters the venous system, it will become trapped in the RV outflow tract, stopping blood flow from the right side of the heart to the lungs. As a result, patients experience respiratory distress and cardiovascular collapse. Treatment involves administering 100% oxygen and placing the patient on the left side with the head downward (left lateral Trendelenburg position). This position displaces the air from the right ventricular outflow tract to the apex of the heart where it can be either reabsorbed or aspirated.

HEMORRHAGE. All patients with an invasive catheter are at risk for hemorrhage. If patients are supine, with high central venous pressures, blood will flow back toward the disconnection, leak, or open stopcock should the catheter be open to air. The risk of bleeding can be decreased by using Luer Lok (screw) connections and caps on all 3 way stopcocks.

INFECTION. Infection prevention guidelines specific to your institution should be followed when using all invasive catheters (Table 8-10). If patients develop symptoms of infection and the CVP is suspected as a possible cause, the line must be removed and the tip cultured.

Educating patients and families

Education of patients with a CVP line is ongoing, with the reason for CVP line placement explained prior to insertion. During insertion patients are asked to remain still and may be asked to hold their breath during parts of the procedure. The CVP waveform may be damped by patient movement, so patients with a CVP line in the IJ vein are asked not to turn their head to that side. Patients with a CVP line in the femoral vein are asked not to bend that leg at the hip. Also, patients are instructed to call immediately if they see blood in the line, if the line becomes disconnected, or for any other unusual signs or symptoms.

Pulmonary Artery Pressure Monitoring

Indications

When specific hemodynamic and intracardiac data are required for diagnostic and treatment purposes, a thermodilution pulmonary artery (PA) catheter may be inserted. This catheter is used for diagnosis and evaluation of heart disease, shock states, and medical conditions that compromise cardiac output or fluid volume. In addition, the PA catheter is used to evaluate patient response to treatment. A significant advantage of the PA catheter over the previously described methods of monitoring is that it simultaneously assesses several hemodynamic parameters—including pulmonary artery systolic and diastolic pressures, the pulmonary artery mean pressure, and the pulmonary artery wedge pressure (PAWP)—and is capable of measuring cardiac output and calculating additional parameters.

PA catheters

The traditional PA catheter, invented by Swan and Ganz, has four lumens for measurement of right atrial pressure or CVP, PA pressures, PAWP, and cardiac output (CO) (Fig. 8-47, *A*). The typical PA catheter is 110 cm in length and is made of polyvinylchloride. This supple material is ideal for flow-directional catheters. The most frequently used adult sizes are 7.0, 7.5, and 8.0 French (Fr). Each of the four lumens exits into the heart at a different point along the catheter length (Fig. 8-47, *A*). The proximal (CVP) lumen is situated in the RA and is used for IV infusion, CVP measurement, withdrawal of venous blood samples, and injection of fluid for cardiac output determinations. The distal (PA) lumen is used to record PA pressures. It is located at the end of the PA catheter and situated in the pulmonary artery. The third lumen opens into a latex balloon at the end of the catheter that can be inflated with 0.8 (7 Fr) to 1.5 (7.5 Fr) ml of air. Once the catheter reaches the right atrium, the balloon is inflated during catheter insertion to assist in forward flow of the catheter and minimize right ventricular ectopy from the catheter tip. It is also inflated to

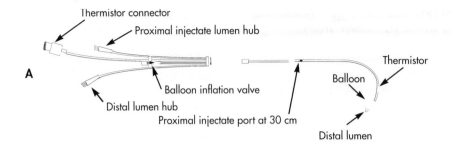

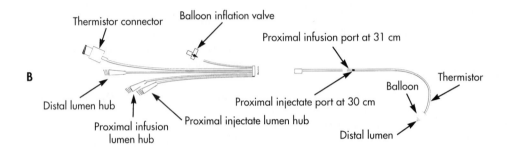

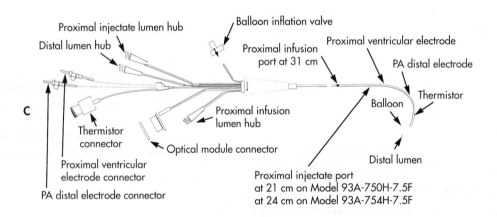

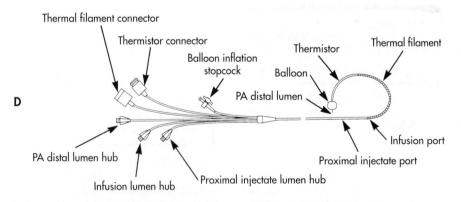

FIG. 8-47 Types of pulmonary artery catheters available for clinical use. **A,** Four-lumen catheter. **B,** Five-lumen catheter that includes an additional infusion lumen in the right atrium. **C,** Multifunction six-lumen catheter that combines an additional infusion lumen, right ventricular volume measurement, and continuous Svo$_2$ monitoring. **D,** Six-lumen catheter with continuous cardiac output capability. (Courtesy Baxter Healthcare Corporation, Edwards Critical Care Division.)

obtain PAWP measurements when the PA catheter is correctly positioned in the pulmonary artery. Located 4 cm from the catheter tip, the fourth lumen is a thermistor used to measure changes in blood temperature and thermodilution CO. The connector end of the lumen is attached directly to the CO computer.

Multifunction PA catheters

Multifunction PA catheters have extra lumens in addition to the four previously described—for example, an extra RA lumen for volume or drug infusion. If continuous Svo_2 is measured, the catheter has a fiberoptic lumen that exits at the tip of the catheter (Fig. 8-47, C). If cardiac pacing is used, two PA catheter methods are available. One type of catheter has three atrial and two ventricular pacing electrodes attached to the catheter so the patient can be connected to a temporary pacemaker and AV paced. The other catheter has an additional RV lumen through which a transvenous pacing wire can be inserted to provide ventricular pacing. A right ventricular volumetric PA catheter is available to measure RV stroke volume (Fig. 8-47, C).

PA catheter insertion

If a PA catheter is to be inserted into patients who are awake, nurses should briefly explain the procedure to ensure that patients understand what is going to happen. PA insertion sites are identical to those used for a CVP line. Before insertion of the PA catheter, a large introducer sheath (8.5 Fr) is placed in the vein, using the Seldinger technique as described in the section on CVP insertion. Introducer sheath length varies from 6 to 12 inches. An IV side-port lumen is frequently present, connected to an IV solution to maintain vein patency. The PA catheter will be threaded through the introducer. Before inserting the PA catheter into the introducer, physicians—using sterile technique—test the balloon for inflation and flush the catheter with normal saline solution to remove any air. The PA catheter is then attached to the bedside hemodynamic line setup and monitor, so the waveforms can be visualized while the catheter is advanced through the right side of the heart (Fig. 8-48). A thin plastic cuff is often placed on the outside of the catheter when it is inserted to maintain sterility of the part of the PA catheter that exits from the introducer. Following placement, the PA catheter can be repositioned if the catheter is not in the desired position or if it migrates out of position.

PA insertion waveforms

As the PA catheter is advanced through the right side of the heart, the specific waveform should be identified on the monitor.

RIGHT ATRIAL. The PA catheter is first advanced into the right atrium. An RA waveform should be visible on the monitor, with recognizable a, c, and v waves (Fig. 8-48). The normal mean pressure in the right atrium is 2 to 5 mm Hg. Before passage through the tricuspid valve the latex balloon is inflated to decrease the risk of ventricular dysrhythmias and permit the catheter to float with the flow of blood from the RV into the PA.

RIGHT VENTRICULAR. The right ventricular waveform has a saw-toothed pattern and is pulsatile, with distinct systolic and diastolic pressures. Normal right ventricular

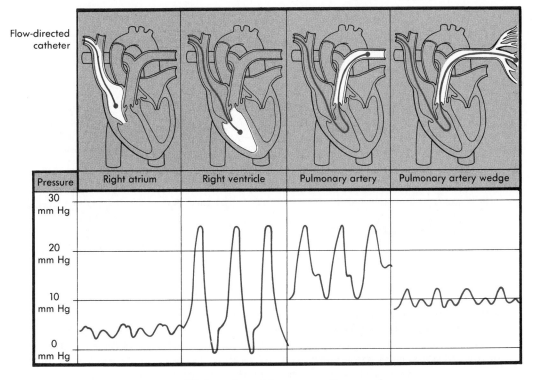

FIG. 8-48 PA insertion with corresponding waveforms.

pressures are 20-30/0-5 mm Hg. Even with the balloon inflated, the occurrence of ventricular ectopy during passage through the RV is not uncommon. All patients who have a PA catheter inserted must have simultaneous ECG monitoring, with defibrillator and emergency resuscitation equipment nearby.

PULMONARY ARTERY. As the catheter enters the pulmonary artery, the waveform changes and the diastolic pressure rises. Normal PA systolic and diastolic pressures are 20-30/10 mm Hg. A dicrotic notch, visible on the downslope of the waveform, represents closure of the pulmonic valve.

PULMONARY ARTERY WEDGE. While the balloon remains inflated, the catheter is advanced into the wedge position. Here the waveform decreases in size and is nonpulsatile—reflective of a normal left atrial tracing with a and v wave deflections. This phenomenon is described as a *wedge tracing* because the balloon is "wedged" into a small pulmonary vessel[36] (Fig. 8-48). The balloon occludes the pulmonary vessel so the PA lumen is exposed only to left atrial pressure and protected from the pulsatile influence of the PA. When the balloon is deflated, the catheter should spontaneously float back into the PA. When the balloon is reinflated, the wedge tracing should be visible. The normal PAWP ranges from 5 to 12 mm Hg.

PA CATHETER COMPLICATIONS. Insertion and use of PA catheters is not without risk. Potential cardiac complications include ventricular dysrhythmias, endocarditis, valvular damage, cardiac rupture, and tamponade. Potential pulmonary complications include rupture of a pulmonary artery, pulmonary artery thrombosis, embolism, hemorrhage, and infarction of a segment of lung. After insertion, a chest x-ray or fluoroscopy is used to verify PA catheter position and rule out pneumothorax or hemorrhagic complications. If the catheter is advanced too far into the pulmonary bed, patients are at risk for pulmonary infarction. If the catheter is not sufficiently advanced into the PA, it will not be useful for PAWP readings.

Nursing management

The nursing priorities when caring for patients with a PA catheter include monitoring the PA waveform, evaluating the PAD-PAWP relationship, recognizing PA waveform changes with respiration, assessing the impact of positive end-expiratory pressure (PEEP), removing PA catheters, and educating patients and families.

Monitoring the PA waveform

A significant component of the nursing assessment involves monitoring the PA waveform to ensure that the catheter has not migrated forward into the wedge position. A segment of lung can become infarcted if the catheter occludes an arteriole for a prolonged period.[37,38] If the PA catheter migrates backwards into the RV, the pressures are no longer reliable.

Evaluating the PAD-PAWP relationship

A major diagnostic advantage of the PA catheter compared with a CVP line is the ability to evaluate pressure

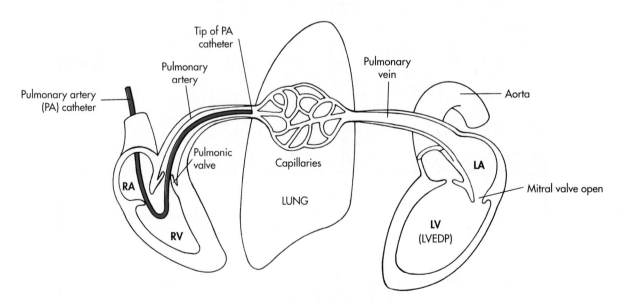

FIG. 8-49 Relationship of PAWP to LVEDP/preload. This diagram illustrates why the PAWP accurately reflects LVEDP or preload in the majority of clinical situations. During diastole, when the mitral valve is open, no other valves or obstructions exist between the tip of the catheter and the left ventricle. Thus the pressure exerted by the volume in the LV is reflected back through the left atrium through the pulmonary veins and to the pulmonary capillaries.

on the left side of the heart by use of the PAWP (Fig. 8-49). In addition to recognizing whether the PAWP is within the normal range, nurses can also evaluate the relationship between the pulmonary artery diastolic (PAD) pressure and the PAWP. Normally the PAD and the PAWP values are within 0 to 3 mm Hg. If the PAD-PAWP relationship is stable, patients may be monitored by PAD pressure, thereby decreasing possible trauma from repeated balloon inflations. However, in clinical conditions such as pulmonary hypertension or adult respiratory distress syndrome (ARDS), the gradient be-

tween the PAD and PAWP will widen, with significantly higher pulmonary pressures. In this situation the PAD does not accurately reflect LVEDP, and only the PAWP should be used.

Recognizing PA waveform changes with respiration

All PA and PAWP tracings are subject to respiratory interference, especially if patients are on a positive-pressure, volume-cycled ventilator. During inhalation the ventilator pushes up the PA tracing to produce an artificially high reading (Fig. 8-50, *A*). During spontaneous respi-

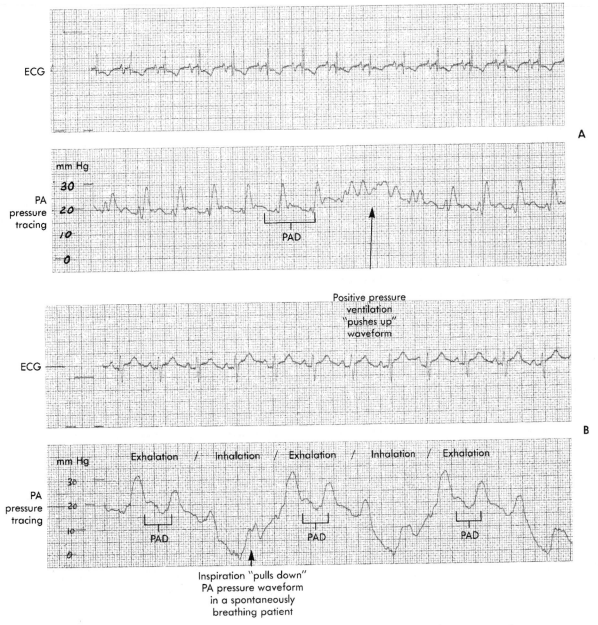

FIG. 8-50 PA waveforms that demonstrate the impact of ventilation of PA pressure readings. For accuracy, PA pressures should be read at end exhalation. **A,** Positive pressure ventilation: the increase in intrathoracic pressure during inhalation "pushes up" the PA pressure waveform, creating a false high reading. **B,** Spontaneous breathing: the decrease in intrathoracic pressure during normal inhalation "pulls down" the PA waveform, creating a false low reading.

ration, negative intrathoracic pressure pulls down the waveform and can produce an erroneously low measurement (Fig. 8-50, *B*). The PAD should be read at end expiration, the most stable point in the respiratory cycle, to minimize the impact of respiratory variation. If the digital number fluctuates with respiration, a paper readout can be obtained to verify true PAD.[39]

Assessing the impact of PEEP

Some clinical diagnoses, such as ARDS, require the use of high levels of PEEP to treat refractory hypoxemia. If PEEP greater than 10 cm H_2O is used, PAWP and PA pressure will be artificially elevated. Because of this tendency, patients in some critical care units were at one time taken off the ventilator to record PA pressure measurements. Research has since demonstrated that this practice decreases patients' oxygenation and may result in persistent hypoxemia.[32] Because patients remain on PEEP for treatment, they should remain on it during measurement of PA pressures. In this situation the trend of PA readings is more important than one individual measurement.

Removing PA catheters

PA catheters are routinely removed by critical care nurses without major complications. The most common incidents, ventricular dysrhythmias (5%), occur as the catheter is pulled through the RV.[40,41]

Educating patients and families

In explaining to patients and families the reasons for the use of a PA catheter, nurses should use uncomplicated language. Explanations are designed to decrease anxiety about the invasive lines and emphasize the need for limited movement.

Cardiac Output Measurement

CO method

The PA catheter measures CO with the bolus thermodilution method. This technique can be performed at the bedside and results in CO calculated in liters per minute. A known amount (5- or 10-ml bolus) of iced or room temperature normal saline solution is injected into the proximal lumen of the catheter. The injectant exits into the RA and travels with the flow of blood past the thermistor (temperature sensor) at the distal end of the catheter. This blood flow is diagrammatically represented as a CO curve in which temperature is plotted against time (Fig. 8-51, *A*).

Nursing management

Nursing management priorities include obtaining accurate CO measurements, evaluating the CO waveform, troubleshooting the CO system, and calculating hemodynamic profiles.

Obtaining accurate CO measurements

Generally three CO measurements within a 10% mean range are obtained and averaged to calculate CO. The CO is equally accurate whether iced or room temperature injectate is used.[42] An accurate reading requires that the difference between injectant temperature and body temperature is at least 10 degrees C and the injectant is delivered within 4 seconds, with minimal handling of the syringe to prevent warming of the solution. This safeguard is particularly important if iced injectate is used. The injectant should be delivered at the same point in the respiratory cycle, usually at end-exhalation. Reliable CO measurements can be obtained with patients in a supine position with the head of bed elevated up to 30 degrees.[30] Several options are available for clinical measurement of CO. These include single syringe CO measurements, closed injectate CO systems, and continuous CO measurement systems.

Evaluating the CO waveform

Most hemodynamic monitors display the CO curve. Critical care nurses evaluate the shape of the curve to determine whether the CO injection is valid. The normal curve has a smooth upstroke with a rounded peak and gradually tapering downslope. An uneven curve may indicate faulty injection technique, and the CO measurement should be repeated. Patient movement or coughing will also alter the CO, as shown in Fig. 8-51, *B*.

Troubleshooting the CO system

Sometimes the right atrial (proximal) port is clotted and not usable. Accurate COs can still be obtained using either a centrally placed introducer sheath,[43] an RA proximal infusion lumen,[44,45] or the right ventricular port of a specialized PA catheter.[46] Figure 8-47 provides detailed diagrams of the location of these additional lumens on the different PA catheters.

Calculating hemodynamic profiles

For patients with a thermodilution PA catheter in place, additional hemodynamic information can be calculated using routine vital signs, CO, and body surface area. These measurements are calculated using specific formulas that are indexed to patients' body size, using either the DuBois Body Surface Chart (Appendix B) or the computer program associated with the newer generation of hemodynamic monitors.[47]

Continuous Monitoring of Mixed Venous Oxygen Saturation (Svo_2)

Svo_2 indications

Continuous monitoring of mixed venous oxygen saturation, or Svo_2, is indicated for patients who may develop an imbalance between oxygen supply and metabolic tissue demand. Patients in shock and those with severe respiratory compromise, such as ARDS, are possible candidates. Continuous Svo_2 monitoring measures the balance achieved between arterial oxygen supply (Sao_2) and oxygen demand at the tissue level by sampling desaturated venous mixed blood from the pulmonary artery (Svo_2).[48] It is called *mixed venous blood* because it is a mixture of all of the venous blood saturations from many body tissues. Under normal conditions the cardiopulmonary system achieves a balance between oxygen supply and demand. The four factors that contribute to this balance include CO, hemoglobin (Hgb), Sao_2, and tissue metabolism (Vo_2). Three of these factors—CO, Hgb, and Sao_2—contribute to the supply of oxygen to the tissues. Vo_2 determines the quantity of oxygen extracted at tissue level or oxygen consumption and creates the demand for oxygen.

Assessment of Svo_2

If Svo_2 is within the normal range (60% to 80%) and patients are not clinically compromised, nurses may assume that oxygen supply and demand are balanced. The balance is disturbed when there is either a decrease in oxygen delivery because of changes in Sao_2, CO, or Hgb or an increase in oxygen demand. If Svo_2 falls below 60% and is sustained, clinicians must assume that oxygen supply is not equal to demand (Table 8-11). Assessing the cause of decreased Svo_2 in a logical sequence is helpful. To determine whether decreased Svo_2 is caused by decreased oxygen supply, clinicians verify the effectiveness of the ventilator or oxygen mask or check arterial oxygen saturation (Sao_2). To assess cardiac function, clinicians perform a CO measurement. To assess Hgb value, clinicians draw a blood sample for laboratory analysis. They should also determine whether decreased Svo_2 is caused by patient movement, nursing activities, or a change in the clinical condition. If Svo_2 falls below 40%, the oxygen supply/demand balance may not adequately meet tissue needs at the cellular level. The cells change from aerobic to anaerobic modes of metabolism, which results in the production of lactic acid and represents a shock state in which cellular injury or cell death may result. At this point every attempt should be made to determine the cause of the low Svo_2 and correct the oxygen supply/demand imbalance.[48]

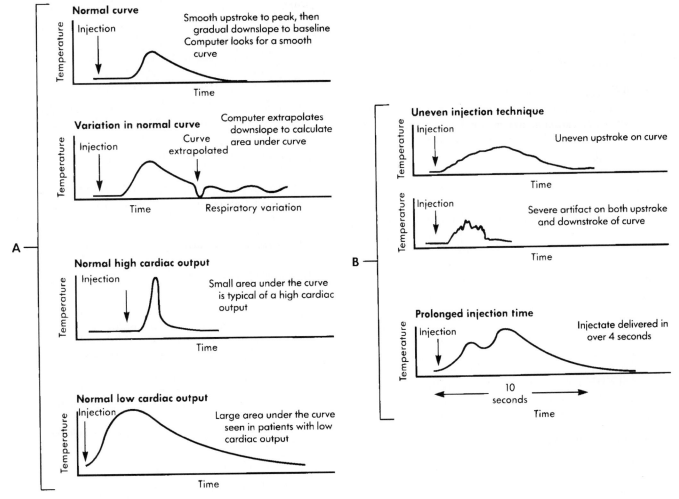

FIG. 8-51 **A,** Variations in the normal cardiac output curve. **B,** Abnormal cardiac output curves that will produce an erroneous cardiac output value.

T A B L E   8 - 1 1

CLINICAL INTERPRETATION OF SVO₂ MEASUREMENTS

SVO₂ MEASUREMENT	PHYSIOLOGIC BASIS FOR CHANGE IN SVO₂	CLINICAL DIAGNOSIS AND RATIONALE
High Svo₂ (80%-95%)	Increased oxygen supply	Patients receiving more oxygen than required by clinical condition
	Decreased oxygen demand	Anesthesia, which causes sedation and decreased muscle movement
		Hypothermia, which lowers metabolic demand (e.g., with cardiopulmonary bypass)
		Sepsis caused by decreased ability of tissues to use oxygen at a cellular level
		False high positive because PA catheter is wedged in a pulmonary capillary
Normal Svo₂ (60%-80%)	Normal oxygen supply and metabolic demand	Balanced oxygen supply and demand
Low Svo₂ (less than 60%)	Decreased oxygen supply caused by	
	Low hemoglobin (Hgb)	Anemia or bleeding with compromised cardiopulmonary system
	Low arterial saturation (Sao₂)	Hypoxemia resulting from decreased oxygen supply or lung disease
	Low cardiac output (CO)	Cardiogenic shock caused by left ventricular pump failure
	Increased oxygen consumption (Vo₂)	Metabolic demand exceeds oxygen supply in conditions that increase muscle movement and increase metabolic rate, including such physiologic states as shivering, seizures, and hyperthermia and such nursing interventions as obtaining bedscale weight and turning

Conclusion

The range of diagnostic tools available to bedside critical care nurses will continue to expand as we approach the end of the century. As the needs of critical care patients become more complex and the responsibilities of nurses increase, incorporation of appropriate diagnostic information into the nursing management plan will continue to gain importance.

References

1. Braunwald E, editor: *Heart disease: a textbook of cardiovascular medicine,* ed 4, Philadelphia, 1992, WB Saunders.
2. Anardi D: Assessment of right heart function, *J Cardiovasc Nurs* 6(1):12, 1991.
3. Willis P: Inspection of the neck veins, *Heart disease and stroke* 3(1):9-15, 1994.
4. Hurst J, editor: *The heart, arteries, and veins,* ed 7, New York, 1990, McGraw-Hill.
5. Blank C, Irwin G: Peripheral vascular disorders: assessment and interventions, *Nurs Clin North Am* 25(4):777, 1990.
6. Adolph, R: The value of bedside examination in an era of high technology: III, *Heart disease and stroke* 3(5):236-239, 1994.
7. Pierce CO: Acute post-MI pericarditis, *J Cardiovasc Nurs* 6(4):46, 1992.
8. Goldberger AL, Goldberger E: *Clinical electrocardiography: a simplified approach,* ed 4, St Louis, 1990, Mosby.
9. McLean, R: Magnesium and its therapeutic uses: a review, *Am J Med* 96(1):63-76, 1994.
10. Keller KB, Lemberg L: The importance of magnesium in cardiovascular disease, *Am J Crit Care* 2(4):348-50, 1993.
11. Henry JB: *Clinical diagnosis and management by laboratory methods,* ed 18, Philadelphia, 1991, WB Saunders.
12. Expert panel on detection, evaluation, and treatment of high blood cholesterol in adults: Summary of the second report of the National Cholesterol Education Program (NCEP) Expert Panel on detection, evaluation, and treatment of high blood cholesterol in adults (Adult Treatment Panel II), *JAMA* 269:3015, 1993.
13. LaRosa JH: An update from the National Cholesterol Education Program: implications for nurses, *J Cardiovasc Nurs* 5(2):1-9, 1991.
14. Drew B, Ide B, Sparacino P: Accuracy of bedside electrocardiographic monitoring: a report on current practices of critical care nurses, *Heart Lung* 20(6):597, 1991.
15. Drew B: Bedside electrocardiographic monitoring: state of the art for the 1990s, *Heart Lung* 20(6):610, 1991.

16. Sevenson AL, Meyer LT: Treatment of paroxysmol supraventricular tachycardia with adenosine: implications for nursing, *Heart Lung* 21(4):350, 1992.

17. Morganroth J: Pharmacologic management of ventricular arrhythmias after the CAST, *Am J Cardiol* 65(22):1497, 1990.

18. Wood D: Potentially lethal ventricular arrhythmias: minimizing the danger, *Postgrad Med* 88(6):65, 1990.

19. Froelicher V: *Exercise and the heart: clinical concepts,* ed 3, St Louis, 1993, Mosby.

20. Schactman M, Greene JS: Signal-averaged electrocardiography: a new technique for determining which patients may be at risk for sudden cardiac death, *Focus Crit Care* 18(3):202, 1991.

21. Brown KA: Prognostic value of thallium-201 myocardial perfusion imaging: a diagnostic tool comes of age, *Circulation* 83(2):363, 1991.

22. Jawad I: *A practical guide to echocardiography and cardiac Doppler ultrasound,* Boston, 1990, Little, Brown & Co.

23. Zabalgoitia M and others: Transesophageal echocardiography in the awake elderly patient: its role in the clinical decision-making process, *Am Heart J* 120(5):1147, 1990.

24. Matsuzaki M, Toma Y, Kusukawa R: Clinical applications of transesophageal echocardiography, *Circulation* 82(3):709, 1990.

25. Thompson E: Transesophageal echocardiography: a new window on the heart and great vessels, *Crit Care Nurs* 13(5):55, 1993.

26. ACC/AHA Task Force Report: Guidelines for clinical intracardiac electrophysiologic studies, *JACC* 14(7):1827, 1989.

27. Connelly AG: An examination of stressors in the patient undergoing cardiac electrophysiologic studies, *Heart Lung* 21(4):335, 1992.

28. American Association of Critical Care Nurses: Evaluation of the effects of heparinized and nonheparinized flush solutions on the patency of arterial pressure monitoring lines: the AACN Thunder Project, *Am J Crit Care* 2:3-15, 1993.

29. Lambert CW, Cason CL: Backrest elevation and pulmonary artery pressures: research analysis, *DCCN* 9(6):327, 1990.

30. Cline JK, Gurka AM: Effect of backrest position on pulmonary artery pressure and cardiac output measurements in critically ill patients, *Focus Crit Care* 18(5):383, 1991.

31. Dobbin K and others: Pulmonary artery pressure measurements in patients with elevated pressures: effect of backrest elevation and method of measurement, *Am J Crit Care* 1(2):61, 1992.

32. Bridges EJ, Woods SL: Pulmonary artery pressure measurement: state of the art, *Heart Lung* 22(2):99, 1993.

33. Hand HL: Direct or indirect blood pressure measurement for open heart surgery patients: an algorithm, *Crit Care Nurse* 12(6):52, 1992.

34. Cason CL, Lambert CW: Position and reference level of measuring right atrial pressure, *Crit Care Q* 12(4):77, 1990.

35. Thielen JB: Air emboli: a potentially lethal complication of central venous lines, *Focus Crit Care* 17(5):374, 1990.

36. Weed HG: Pulmonary "capillary" wedge pressure not the pressure in the pulmonary capillaries, *Chest* 100(4):1138, 1991.

37. Komodina KH and others: Interobserver variability in the interpretation of pulmonary artery catheter pressure tracings, *Chest* 100(6):1647, 1991.

38. Iberti TJ and others: A multicenter study of physicians' knowledge of the pulmonary artery catheter, *JAMA* 264(22):2928, 1990.

39. Levine-Silverman S, Johnson J: Pulmonary artery pressure measurements, *West J Nurs Res* 12(4):488, 1990.

40. Rountree WD: Removal of pulmonary artery catheters by registered nurses: a study in safety and complications, *Focus Crit Care* 18(4):313, 1991.

41. Biel MH, Stotts JR: The RN's role in manipulation of pulmonary artery catheters, *Crit Care Nurs* 15(1):30, 1995.

42. Groom L, Elliott M, Frisch S: Injectate temperature: effects on thermodilution CO measurements, *Crit Care Nurse* 10(5):112, 1990.

43. Hunn D and others: Thermodilution cardiac output values obtained by using a centrally placed introducer sheath and right atrial port of a pulmonary artery catheter, *Crit Care Med* 18(4):438, 1990.

44. Medley RS, DeLapp TD, Fisher DG: Comparability of the thermodilution cardiac output method: proximal injectate versus proximal infusion lumens, *Heart Lung* 21(1):12, 1992.

45. Pesola GR, Rostata HP, Carlon GC: Room temperature thermodilution cardiac output: central venous vs. right ventricular port, *Am J Crit Care* 1(1):76, 1992.

46. Pesola GR, Carlon GC: Thermodilution cardiac output: proximal lumen versus right ventricular port, *Crit Care Med* 19(4):563, 1991.

47. Ramsey JD, Tisdale LA: Use of ventricular stroke work index and ventricular function curves in assessing myocardial contractility, *Crit Care Nurs* 15(1):61, 1995.

48. White K: Using continuous Svo$_2$ to assess oxygen supply/demand balance in the critically ill patient, *AACN Clinical Issues in Critical Care Nursing* 4(1):134, 1993.

9

Cardiovascular Disorders

MIMI O'DONNELL

CHAPTER OBJECTIVES

- List the risk factors for coronary artery disease and peripheral vascular disease.
- Explain the electrocardiographic and physiologic changes expected with transmural myocardial infarction.

- Discuss important aspects of the diagnosis and management of patients with heart failure, endocarditis, cardiomyopathy, valvular heart disease, and peripheral vascular disease.

KEY TERMS

An understanding of the pathology of a disease, the areas of assessment on which to focus, and the usual medical management allows critical care nurses to anticipate and plan interventions with greater accuracy and precision. This chapter focuses on priority cardiovascular disorders that nurses commonly encounter in the critical care environment and important aspects of diagnosis and management.

Coronary Artery Disease

Description and Etiology

Cardiovascular disease remains the leading cause of death in the United States. It claims more than 900,000 lives annually and places a heavy emotional and financial burden on society.[1] In 1968 a massive public health campaign was initiated to increase awareness of the risk factors that contribute to the development of **coronary artery disease** (CAD). Since that time the mortality rate has steadily declined, a positive effect believed to result from changes in lifestyles.[2] Although the trend is encouraging, enthusiasm should be tempered by the recognition that the population is aging and cardiovascular disease is a progressive, degenerative process most prevalent in older people.

CAD has a long latent period.[3] Fatty streaks can appear within the aorta during childhood, but symptoms occur only when the atherosclerotic plaque occludes 75% of the vessel lumen, usually in late middle age. Epidemiologic data collected during the past 40 years have demonstrated an association between specific risk factors and the development of CAD. One of the most important epidemiologic studies is the Framingham Heart Study,[4] which began in 1948 and continues today with third and fourth generations of subjects. Blood cholesterol levels, smoking and activity level, blood pressure, and electrocardiographic results of participants in this study are checked regularly. As a result, researchers have identified specific factors associated with increased probability of CAD development. These lifestyle habits are referred to as *CAD risk factors.*

CAD risk factors

Factors that increase risk for CAD include age, gender, race, family history, elevated serum cholesterol levels, hypertension, cigarette smoking, abnormal glucose tolerance, sedentary lifestyle, stress, and type A behavior pattern. These factors are subdivided into nonmodifiable and modifiable CAD risk factors (Box 9-1).

AGE. The symptoms of CAD occur with age. In general, CAD is a disease of middle and old age.

GENDER. CAD occurs approximately 10 years later in women than it does in men. After menopause, women develop CAD at the same rate as men.

FAMILY HISTORY. A positive family history includes a close blood relative who had a myocardial infarction or stroke before the age of 60 years.

RACE. Nonwhite populations of both genders have higher CAD mortality rates than white populations.

CHOLESTEROL. Hyperlipidemia is a leading factor responsible for severe atherosclerosis and development of CAD.[5] Total serum cholesterol levels above 200 mg/dl are associated with a higher risk of CAD, and levels greater than 270 mg/dl carry a fourfold increase in risk.[6] Total cholesterol is subdivided into specific lipoproteins:

1. High density lipoprotein cholesterol (HDL-C)
2. Low density lipoprotein cholesterol (LDL-C)
3. Very low density lipoprotein cholesterol (VLDL-C)
4. Triglycerides

Elevated LDL-C, VLDL-C, and triglyceride levels are associated with an increased incidence of CAD. Low

---

BOX 9-1

CORONARY ARTERY DISEASE RISK FACTORS

NONMODIFIABLE

Age
Gender
Family history
Race

MODIFIABLE

Major

Elevated serum lipids
Hypertension
Cigarette smoking
Impaired glucose tolerance
Diet high in saturated fat, cholesterol, and calories
Physical inactivity

Minor

Psychologic stress
Personality type

HDL-C levels also increase CAD risk.[5] (More information on total cholesterol and the specific lipoproteins is described in Chapter 8.)

HYPERTENSION. In the context of CAD, hypertension is the elevation of either systolic blood pressure (SBP) or diastolic blood pressure (DBP). The higher the blood pressure, the greater the risk. CAD is reduced when the SBP and DBP are below 140/90 mm Hg.[7] Hypertension is a risk factor because it damages the endothelium of the vessel. Hypertension has many predisposing factors that overlap with CAD risk factors, including older age, high dietary sodium intake, obesity, sedentary lifestyle, excessive alcohol consumption, cocaine abuse, oral contraceptive use, African-American race, and the use of some medications that influence intrinsic mediators of blood pressure, such as the renin-angiotensin-aldosterone system and the sympathetic nervous system. Management of hypertension is initially directed toward lifestyle modifications such as weight loss, decreased dietary sodium chloride, increased physical activity, reduced alcohol consumption, and stress management. If these measures are not successful, hypertension may be managed by pharmacologic therapy.[7,8] Hypertensive emergencies are managed by IV antihypertensives and vasodilators (see Chapter 10).

CIGARETTE SMOKING. The greater the number of cigarettes smoked per day, the greater the CAD risk. Cigarette smoking unfavorably alters serum lipid levels, decreasing HDL-C levels and increasing LDL-C and triglyceride levels. Smoking results in cardiac electrical instability within cell membranes and impairs oxygen transport and use while increasing myocardial oxygen demand. Smoking is also thought to alter intimal endothelial permeability and foster platelet agglutination. Fortunately, the damage from smoking is not unalterable; after cessation the coronary risk falls.[6]

DIABETES MELLITUS. Individuals with diabetes mellitus have a higher incidence of CAD than the general population. In fact, diabetes triples or quadruples the risk of developing CAD.[9] Premenopausal women with diabetes are at increased risk of developing CAD compared with nondiabetic women of the same age because diabetes negates the protective effect of estrogen. CAD risk from diabetes also rises in the presence of increased serum cholesterol levels, hypertension, and cigarette smoking.[9]

ORAL CONTRACEPTIVES. Oral contraceptives increase women's risk of developing CAD, particularly women older than 35 years of age, because they (1) alter blood coagulation, (2) alter platelet function, (3) alter fibrinolytic activity, and (4) may adversely affect the integrity of vascular endothelium. Women who take oral contraceptives and smoke cigarettes further increase their risk.

OBESITY. Often associated with a sedentary lifestyle, obesity increases susceptibility to other risk factors, such as hypertension, impaired glucose tolerance, and hyperlipidemia, with increased LDL-C and decreased HDL-C levels.

PHYSICAL INACTIVITY. Accumulating evidence suggests that a sedentary lifestyle increases the risk for CAD. A 20-year follow-up of 16,936 Harvard alumni demonstrated that those subjects who burned less than 2000 calories per week beyond their basal (minimum) level had a 64% higher risk for CAD.[6] Physical inactivity is also associated with lower HDL levels, higher LDL-C lev-els, hypertension, obesity, increased glucose intolerance, and hyperlipidemia.[10]

STRESS AND ANXIETY. Type A behavior patterns such as time urgency, hostility, anger, and anxiety have also been associated with development of CAD.[4,11] The way stress and certain behaviors influence the development of CAD is not well understood, but stress is associated with increased circulating catecholamines, which may precipitate hypertension, alteration in platelet function, increased fatty acid mobilization, and a resultant elevation of free fatty acid levels.

MULTIFACTORIAL RISK. Researchers do not currently understand the reason a risk factor in one individual may result in serious consequences but not cause problems for another individual. Studies show that CAD is a multifactorial disease, and as the number of known risk factors increase, the risk of developing the disease increases exponentially rather than cumulatively.[6]

Pathophysiology

CAD is a progressive disorder of the coronary arteries that results in narrowing or complete occlusion. There are multiple causes for coronary artery narrowing, but **atherosclerosis** is the most prevalent, affecting the medium-sized arteries perfusing the heart, brain, kidneys, and large arteries branching off the aorta. Atherosclerotic lesions may take different forms depending on their anatomic location; the individual's age, genetic makeup, and physiologic status; and the number of risk factors present. Normal arterial walls are composed of three cellular layers: the intima (innermost endothelial layer), media (middle muscular layer), and adventitia

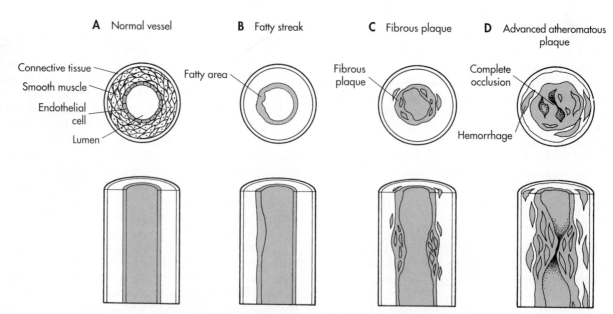

FIG. 9-1 The progression of atherosclerosis shown in both the longitudinal and the cross-sectional views. **A,** Normal vessel. **B,** First stage, fatty streaks. **C,** Second stage, fibrous plaque development. **D,** Third stage, advanced (complicated) lesions.

(outermost connective tissue layer). Three major elements are associated with atherosclerotic plaque development and luminal narrowing[12]: (1) proliferation of smooth muscle; (2) formation of a connective tissue matrix composed of collagen, elastic fibers, and proteoglycans; and (3) accumulation of lipids.

Stages of plaque development

Specific stages of atherosclerotic plaque development have been identified[3,12,13] (Fig. 9-1). In the first stage, fatty streaks develop. These are broad-based lesions composed of lipid-laden macrophages and smooth muscle cells. In the second stage the streaks develop into fatty plaques. Subsequently, collagen and dense connective tissue create atherosclerotic fibrous plaques. Finally, during the advanced or complicated lesion phase the fibrous plaque becomes vascularized, the core calcifies, and the surface ulcerates, resulting in hemorrhage and thromboembolic episodes. Furthermore the media may develop aneurysmal changes resulting from the decrease in smooth muscle cells.

CAD hemodynamic effects

The major hemodynamic effect of CAD is the disturbance of the delicate balance between myocardial oxygen supply and demand. Atherosclerosis alters the normal coronary artery's response to increased demand in two ways: (1) lesions that result in vessel-lumen occlusion of 75% or more restrict flow under resting conditions, and (2) vessels become stiff and lose the ability to dilate. The result is decreased driving pressure beyond the site of the lesion and less oxygenated blood available to the myocardial cells perfused by that vessel.[14] During ischemia (resulting from exercise or angina) the myocardium is forced to shift from aerobic metabolism to anaerobic metabolism, the consequences of which are (1) less efficient energy production, (2) lactic acid buildup, (3) intracellular hypokalemia, (4) intracellular acidosis, (5) intracellular hypernatremia, and (6) interference with the release of calcium from its storage sites in the sarcoplasmic reticulum.[3,14] Tissue hypoxia or ischemia is the end result of this process.

Assessment and Diagnosis

Angina

Angina, or chest pain caused by myocardial ischemia, is not a disease but a symptom of CAD. Angina has many characteristics (Box 9-2) and may occur anywhere in the chest, neck, arms, or back. The most commonly cited location is behind the sternum. The pain frequently radiates to the left arm but may also radiate to both arms, the mandible, and the neck (Fig. 9-2). Angina is classified as stable, unstable, and variant.

STABLE ANGINA. Stable angina is predictable and caused by consistent precipitating factors such as exercise, emotional upset, and tachycardia. Patients become used to the pattern of this angina and may describe it as "my usual chest pain." Rest and administration of a coronary artery vasodilator such as sublingual nitroglycerin may help control pain. Stable angina results from fixed lesions (blockages) of greater than 75%. Ischemia and chest pain occur when myocardial demand exceeds blood oxygen supply. Stable angina can be managed medically for long periods.

UNSTABLE ANGINA. *Unstable angina* is defined as a change in a previously established stable pattern or a new onset of severe angina. Usually more intense than stable

---

BOX 9-2

CHARACTERISTICS OF ANGINA PECTORIS

LOCATION

Beneath sternum, radiating to neck and jaw
Upper chest
Beneath sternum, radiating down left arm
Epigastric
Epigastric, radiating to neck, jaw, and arms
Neck and jaw
Left shoulder, inner aspect of both arms
Intrascapular

DURATION

0.5 to 30 minutes (stable)
Duration of longer than 30 minutes, without relief from rest or medication, indicating unstable or preinfarction symptoms

QUALITY

Sensation of pressure or heavy weight on the chest
Feeling of tightness, like a vise
Visceral quality (deep, heavy, squeezing, aching)
Burning sensation
Shortness of breath, with feeling of suffocation
Most severe pain ever experienced

RADIATION

Medial aspect of left arm
Jaw
Left shoulder
Right arm

PRECIPITATING FACTORS

Exertion/exercise
Cold weather
Exercising after a large, heavy meal
Walking against the wind
Emotional upset
Fright, anger
Coitus

MEDICATION RELIEF

Usually within 45 seconds to 5 minutes of sublingual nitroglycerin or nifedipine (Procardia) administration

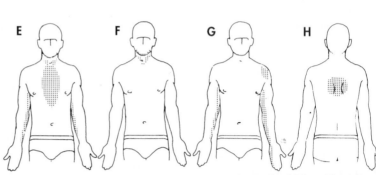

FIG. 9-2 Common sites for anginal pain. **A,** Upper part of chest. **B,** Beneath sternum radiating to neck and jaw. **C,** Beneath sternum radiating down left arm. **D,** Epigastric **E,** Epigastric radiating to neck, jaw, and arms. **F,** Neck and jaw. **G,** Left shoulder. **H,** Intrascapular.

angina, it may awaken patients, who may also find that nitrates alone no longer provide pain relief. A change in level or frequency of symptoms requires immediate medical evaluation.[15] Severe angina that persists for more than 20 minutes and is not relieved by three nitroglycerin tablets is called *preinfarction,* or *crescendo angina.* This is a medical emergency that requires immediate attention in a hospital emergency room. The pathology underlying the change from stable to unstable angina may be plaque hemorrhage or fissure that causes an increase in localized platelet agglutination and acute thrombosis.[15]

VARIANT ANGINA. Variant (Prinzmetal's) angina is caused by coronary artery spasm and believed to result from spasm, with or without atherosclerotic lesions. Variant angina frequently occurs at rest and can also be cyclic, occurring at the same time every day. It is usually associated with ST-segment elevation and occasionally transient abnormal Q waves.[14] Smoking tobacco and ingesting alcohol and cocaine may also precipitate spasm. Drugs of choice for the treatment of spasm are agents that vasodilate the coronary arteries (such as nitroglycerin) or calcium channel blockers such as nifedipine and diltiazem.

Silent ischemia

Silent ischemia is defined as objective ECG evidence of myocardial ischemia (ST-segment changes) without any symptoms of angina experienced by patients.[16] It is classified into three clinical types (Box 9-3). Although patients with type I ischemia experience no signs or symptoms of cardiovascular disease, continuous monitoring or stress testing demonstrates myocardial ischemia. These patients are frequently found to have multivessel CAD when later tested by coronary arteriography. Type II patients are those who have had an acute myocardial in-

CLINICAL CHARACTERISTICS OF SILENT ISCHEMIA

TYPE I

Objective evidence of myocardial ischemia without chest pain/symptoms

TYPE II

No anginal symptoms following a previous MI, but objective evidence of myocardial ischemia continues

TYPE III

Symptoms of angina with some episodes of ischemia, and asymptomatic with other ischemic events. May or may not have had a previous MI.

MI, Myocardial infarction.

farction and demonstrate active ischemia but have no anginal symptoms. Patients with type III ischemia have some ischemic episodes that are accompanied by chest pain and some without chest discomfort. Type III patients may or may not have had a prior infarction. Once identified, silent ischemia is usually treated in the same manner as classic angina—with nitrates, beta blockers, calcium channel blockers, and lifestyle changes.[17]

Medical Management

The major goals of medical therapy for CAD and angina are to (1) increase coronary artery perfusion, (2) decrease myocardial workload, (3) prevent MI disability or death, and (4) treat unstable angina. Specific medical management depends on the frequency, severity, duration, and hemodynamic consequences of the angina.

Myocardial supply-demand balance

Pharmacologic therapy such as oxygen, nitrates, and analgesics[18,19] are used to increase coronary artery perfusion and myocardial oxygen supply and treat symptoms of angina. Bed rest, beta blockers, and calcium channel blockers are used to decrease myocardial oxygen demand.[20,21]

MI prevention

CAD risk factors, such as hypertension and hyperlipidemia, are treated aggressively. A low-sodium, low-cholesterol diet may be recommended. Activity is restricted until episodes of angina are controlled.

Angina management

The change from stable to unstable angina represents a serious problem. Patients are usually admitted to a hospital and prescribed bed rest. Treating any identified precipitating problems is important. If the anginal pain continues, cardiac catheterization, intraaortic balloon support, thrombolytic therapy, percutaneous transluminal coronary angioplasty (PTCA), or coronary artery bypass surgery may be indicated.[12,19]

Nursing Management

Nursing management of the patient with CAD and angina incorporates a variety of nursing diagnoses (Box 9-4). **Nursing priorities are directed toward assessing chest pain, controlling chest pain, maintaining a calm environment, and educating patients and families.**

Assessing chest pain

Nurses should quickly evaluate complaints of chest discomfort. Chest pain in patients with known or suspected coronary disease may represent myocardial ischemia, which must be treated while it is still reversible. Nurses should ask patients to rate the intensity of their chest discomfort on a scale of 1 to 10. The words *chest pain* should not be used exclusively because some patients will use words such as *pressure* or *heaviness* to describe their angina. Chapter 10 contains a full discussion of the range of therapies available for the treatment of acute or preinfarction angina.[19] Documenting the characteristics of the pain, patients' heart rate and rhythm, the presence of ectopic beats or conduction defects, patients' mentation, and overall tissue perfusion is also important. Documentation should also include skin color, temperature, peripheral pulses, and urine output. A 12-lead ECG is taken to identify the area of ischemic myocardium.[22]

Controlling chest pain

In the critical care unit, angina is controlled by a combination of supplemental oxygen, nitrates, and analgesia.

BOX 9-4

NURSING DIAGNOSIS PRIORITIES

CORONARY ARTERY DISEASE/ANGINA

- *Acute Pain* related to transmission and perception of cutaneous, visceral, muscular, or ischemic impulses secondary to myocardial ischemia, p. 499
- *Activity Intolerance* related to decreased cardiac output and/or myocardial tissue perfusion alterations, p. 482
- *Anxiety* related to threat to biologic, psychologic, and/or social integrity, p. 464
- *Knowledge Deficit:* _____(Specify) related to lack of previous exposure to information, p. 455

OXYGEN. All patients with acute ischemic pain are administered supplemental oxygen to increase myocardial oxygenation. Those patients who develop symptoms of acute heart failure may require emergency intubation and mechanical ventilation to correct significant hypoxemia.[19]

NITRATES. A combination of intravenous and sublingual nitroglycerin is used to vasodilate the coronary arteries and control pain. After administering nitrates, nurses closely observe patients for relief of chest pain, return of the ST segment to baseline, and development of unwanted side effects such as hypotension and headache.

ANALGESIA. Because it both relieves pain and decreases fear and anxiety, morphine sulphate is the analgesic of choice for preinfarction angina. After administering the analgesic, critical care nurses assess patients for pain relief and unwanted side effects such as hypotension and respiratory depression.

Maintaining a calm environment

Critical care patients with acute angina experience extreme anxiety and fear of death. Critical care nurses are challenged to create a calm environment that alleviates fear and anxiety while remaining ready to respond to emergencies (such as cardiac arrest) or to assist with emergency intubation or insertion of hemodynamic monitoring catheters.

Educating patients and families

In the critical care unit the ability of patients to retain educational information is severely affected by stress and pain. Once the ischemic pain is controlled, nurses should educate patients and family members on risk factor modification, signs and symptoms of angina, appropriate reasons to call the physician, use of medication, and techniques for dealing with emotions and stress.[23] However, because the acute hospital length of stay for uncomplicated angina is usually less than 3 days, referral to a cardiac rehabilitation program for controlled exercise and risk factor modification after discharge is perhaps the most helpful teaching intervention critical care nurses can make.

Myocardial Infarction

Description and Etiology

Myocardial infarction (MI) is the term used to describe irreversible myocardial necrosis (cell death) that results from an abrupt decrease or total cessation of coronary blood flow to a specific area of the myocardium. Atherosclerosis is responsible for most myocardial infarctions because it causes luminal narrowing and reduced blood flow, resulting in decreased oxygen delivery to the myocardium. The three mechanisms primarily responsible for the acute reduction in oxygen delivery to the myocardium are (1) coronary artery thrombosis, (2) plaque fissure or hemorrhage, and (3) coronary artery spasm. Infarction is more prevalent in the left ventricle, with multivessel occlusions, and in myocardium distal to vessels that have not developed collateral flow.

Coronary artery thrombi

Thrombi are now known to be present in almost all acute coronary artery occlusions. These thrombi, usually composed of platelets, fibrin, erythrocytes, and leukocytes, may be superimposed on a plaque or may align adjacent to a plaque. They release thromboxane A_2, serotonin, and thrombin, all vasoconstricting substances that compound vessel narrowing and initiate a vicious cycle of recurrent occlusion. Scientists have not determined the cause of thrombus formation, but plaque fissure, hemorrhage, or both are thought to be predisposing events.[12,13]

Atherosclerotic plaques

Plaques are classified according to their composition. Hard plaques are heavily calcified and fibrotic, whereas soft plaques are composed of cholesterol esters and lipids. Coronary artery thrombosis has been associated with rupture or cracks of the plaques and release of the plaque material into the vascular lumen. Plaque rupture can induce thrombosis by (1) forming a platelet plug, (2) releasing tissue thromboplastin from the plaque material that activates the clotting cascade, and (3) obstructing the vessel lumen with plaque components. Coronary artery spasm is often present in acute occlusions.

Assessment and Diagnosis

Infarction

The area of cellular death and muscle necrosis in the myocardium is known as the *zone of infarction* (Fig. 9-3). On the ECG, evidence of this zone is seen by pathologic Q waves, which reflect a lack of depolarization from the cardiac surface involved in the myocardial infarction (Fig. 9-4, *D*). As healing takes place, scar tissue replaces the cells in this area.

Injury

The infarcted zone is surrounded by injured but still potentially viable tissue in an area known as the *zone of injury* (see Fig. 9-3). Cells in this area do not fully repolarize because of the deficient blood supply. This is recorded as elevation of the ST segment (Fig. 9-4, *C*).

Ischemia

The outer region, as illustrated in Fig. 9-3, is the zone of ischemia and is composed of viable cells. Repolarization in this zone is impaired but eventually restored to normal. Repolarization of the cells in this area manifests as T wave inversion (Fig. 9-4, *B*).

MI evolution

During the first 6 weeks after an infarction the damaged myocardium undergoes many changes. Approximately 6 hours after the infarction the muscle becomes distended, pale, and cyanotic. Over the next 2 days the myocardium becomes reddish purple, and an exudate may form on the epicardium. Leukocyte scavenger cells begin to infiltrate the muscle and carry away the necrotic debris, thereby thinning the necrotic wall. Approximately 3 to 4 weeks after the infarction, scar tissue begins to form and the affected wall becomes whiter and thicker.[14]

Transmural MI

MIs are classified according to their location on the myocardial surface and the muscle layers affected. A transmural MI involves all three muscle layers—the endocardium, the myocardium, and the epicardium—and produces significant ECG changes.

Non–Q wave MI

Nontransmural infarctions are classified as either subendocardial (involving the endocardium) or subepicardial (involving the epicardium). Some myocardium may be involved in a nontransmural MI, but it is not a full thickness. Generally, abnormal Q waves are not seen, so a nontransmural MI is frequently called a *non–Q wave MI*.

12-lead ECG changes

ECG changes produced by a transmural infarction demonstrate alteration in both myocardial depolarization (QRS complex) and repolarization (ST segment). The changes in repolarization are marked by the presence of new Q waves. These Q waves are deeper (greater than one-third the height of the corresponding R wave) and wider than normal (greater than 0.04 seconds or longer in duration).

MI location

The location of infarction is determined by correlating the ECG leads with Q waves and the ST segment T-wave abnormalities (Table 9-1). Infarction most commonly occurs in the left ventricle and the interventricular septum; however, close to 25% of all patients who sustain an inferior MI have some right ventricular damage.[19] The ECG manifestations used to diagnose an MI and

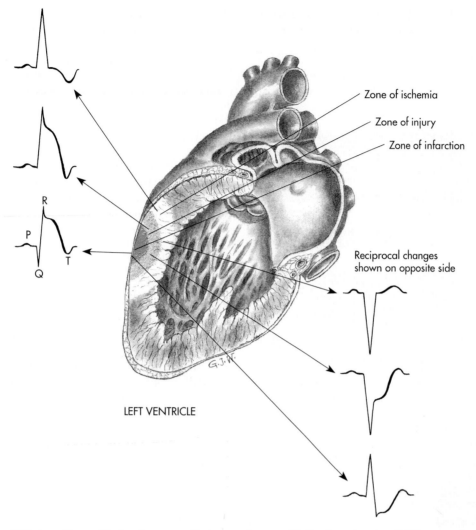

FIG. 9-3 Zone of ischemia, zone of injury, and zone of infarction, showing ECG waveforms and reciprocal waveforms corresponding to each zone.

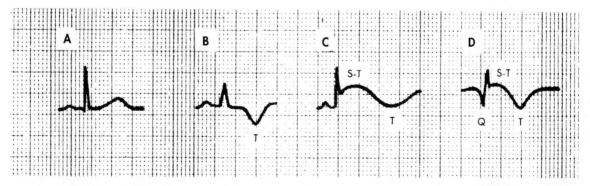

FIG. 9-4 ECG changes indicative of ischemia, injury, and infarction (necrosis) of the myocardium. **A,** Normal ECG. **B,** Ischemia indicated by inversion of the T wave. **C,** Ischemia and current of injury indicated by T-wave inversion and ST-segment elevation. The ST segment may be elevated above or depressed below the baseline, depending on whether the tracing is from a lead facing toward or away from the infarcted area and whether epicardial or endocardial injury occurs. Epicardial injury causes ST elevation in leads facing the epicardium. **D,** Ischemia, injury, and myocardial necrosis. The Q wave indicates necrosis of the myocardium. (From Kinney M and others: *Comprehensive cardiac care,* ed 8, St Louis, 1996, Mosby.)

pinpoint the area of damaged ventricle include inverted T waves, ST-segment elevation, and pathologic Q waves.[22]

Anterior wall infarction

Anterior wall infarction results from occlusion of the proximal left anterior descending (LAD) artery and may

TABLE 9-1		
CORRELATION AMONG VENTRICULAR SURFACES, ECG LEADS, AND CORONARY ARTERIES		
SURFACE OF LEFT VENTRICLE	**ECG LEADS**	**CORONARY ARTERY USUALLY INVOLVED**
Inferior	II, III, aVF	Right coronary
Lateral	I, aVL	Left circumflex
Anterior	V_2-V_4	Left anterior descending
Septal	V_1-V_2	Left anterior descending
Apical	V_5-V_6	Left anterior descending
Posterior	V_1-V_2 (reciprocal changes)	Left circumflex

From Price SA, Wilson LM: *Pathophysiology: clinical concepts of disease processes,* ed 4, St Louis, 1992, Mosby.

involve the left main artery. ST-segment elevation is expected in leads V_1 through V_4, and T-wave inversion may occur in leads I, aVL, and V_3 to V_5 (Fig. 9-5). There is a loss of positive R-wave progression in leads V_1 through V_6. A large anterior wall MI may be associated with left ventricular (LV) pump failure, cardiogenic shock, or death. Because the anterior surface is so large, it is frequently subdivided into true anterior, anteroseptal, and anterolateral sections.

Anteroseptal infarction

Anteroseptal infarctions result from an occlusion of the LAD. Leads V_1 through V_4 on the 12-lead ECG reflect the electrical activity of the anterior wall. There is a loss of R-wave progression in V_1 and V_2, leaving a QS complex. Q waves are seen in V_2 through V_4. Reciprocal changes are usually not seen with an anteroseptal MI.

Anterolateral infarction

Anterolateral infarction occurs as a result of occlusion of the circumflex coronary artery. On 12-lead ECG, Q waves and ST-T wave changes are seen in leads I and aV_L and in leads V_4, V_5, and V_6, which reflect lower lateral wall or left apical involvement. Reciprocal changes occur in the inferior leads II, III, and aV_F.

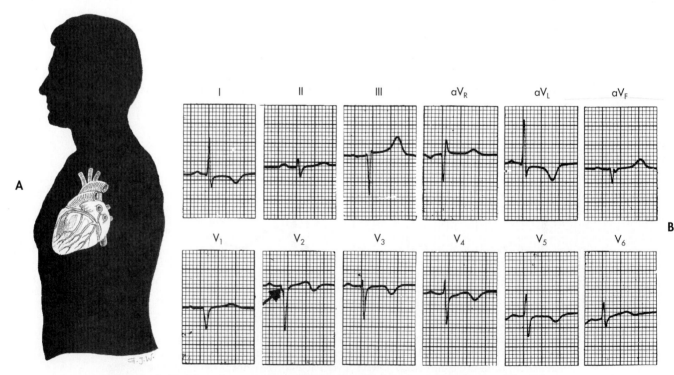

FIG. 9-5 **A,** Position of an anterior wall infarction. **B,** Anterior wall infarction. The QS complexes in leads V_1 and V_2 indicate anteroseptal infarction. There is also a characteristic notching *(arrow)* of the QS complex, often seen in infarctions. In addition, diffuse ischemic T-wave inversions are present in leads I, aV_L, and V_2 to V_5, indicating generalized anterior wall ischemia. (From Goldberger AL, Goldberger E: *Clinical electrocardiography: a simplified approach,* ed 5, St Louis, 1994, Mosby.)

Inferior wall infarction

Inferior wall infarction occurs with occlusion of the right coronary artery (RCA) and is manifested by ECG changes in leads II, III, and aV_F. Reciprocal changes occur in leads I and aV_L (Fig. 9-6). Because the RCA perfuses the sinoatrial (SA) node, the proximal bundle of His, and the atrioventricular (AV) node, conduction disturbances may appear with an inferior wall MI.

Posterior wall infarction

Posterior wall infarction occurs with occlusion of the circumflex branch of the left coronary artery. Because the standard 12-lead ECG does not directly record activity on the posterior surface, a posterior wall MI is documented by reciprocal changes seen as tall R waves and ST-segment depression in leads V_1 and V_2.

MI diagnosis

The definitive diagnosis of MI is based on a combination of patients' clinical symptoms, 12-lead ECG changes, and cardiac enzyme levels.[19] MI location can help predict risk. Anterior and anteroseptal infarctions are associated with twice the mortality rate of inferior wall infarctions.

Chest pain during MI

The most common clinical manifestation of infarction is prolonged, severe chest pain that is frequently associated with nausea, vomiting, and diaphoresis. This pain generally lasts 30 minutes or more and is usually located in the substernal or left precordial area. Unlike angina, which is often described as discomfort, the pain of infarction may be described as the most severe pain individuals have ever experienced. Patients may say that the pain is "like an elephant sitting on my chest," or of a viselike tightness. The pain may radiate to the back, neck, jaw, or left arm, particularly down the ulnar aspect.[24,25] Neither rest nor nitrates relieve the pain.

Cardiac enzymes during MI

Specific cardiac enzymes and isoenzymes are released in the presence of damaged or infarcted myocardial cells (see Chapter 8). Serum CK-MB isoenzymes are measured at 6-hour intervals for the first 24 hours and then daily to confirm the diagnosis of MI.[19] With a large anterior MI the CK-MB can rise to greater than 150 IU/L with a total CK of greater than 1000 IU/L.[19]

Complications

Many patients experience complications either early or late in the postinfarction course (Box 9-5). These complications may result from pumping or electrical dysfunctions. Pumping complications cause heart failure, pulmonary edema, and cardiogenic shock. Electrical dysfunctions include bradycardia, bundle branch blocks, and varying degrees of heart block.[19,26] Close to 95% of all patients who experience an MI will have dysrhythmias.

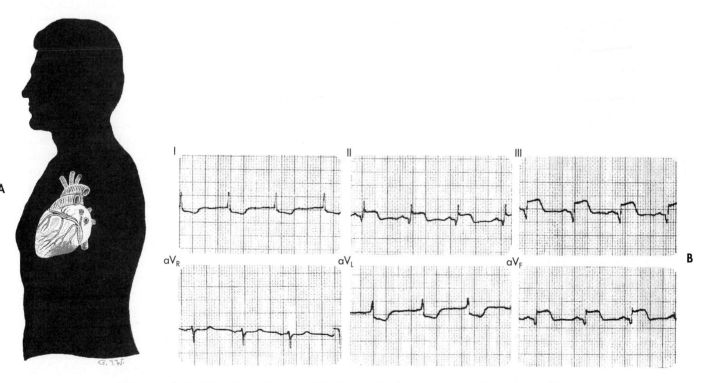

FIG. 9-6 A, Position of an inferior wall infarction. **B,** Acute inferior wall infarction. ST elevations in leads II, III, and aV_F with reciprocal ST depressions in leads I and aV_L are shown. Abnormal Q waves are also seen in leads II, III, and aV_F. (From Goldberger AL, Goldberger E: *Clinical electrocardiography: a simplified approach,* ed 5, St Louis, 1994, Mosby.)

BOX 9-5

COMPLICATIONS OF MYOCARDIAL INFARCTION

Dysrhythmias
Ventricular aneurysms
Ventricular septal defect
Papillary muscle rupture
Pericarditis

Cardiac rupture
Sudden death
Heart failure
Pulmonary edema
Cardiogenic shock

BOX 9-6

ETIOLOGY OF DYSRHYTHMIAS IN MYOCARDIAL INFARCTION

Tissue ischemia
Hypoxemia
Autonomic nervous system influences
Metabolic derangements
    Acid-base imbalances
Hemodynamic abnormalities
Drugs (especially digoxin toxicity)
Electrolyte imbalances (e.g., hypokalemia, hypomagnesemia)
Fiber stretch
    Chamber dilatation
    Cardiomyopathy

There are many potential causes as described in Box 9-6. Preserving cardiac output and tissue perfusion is the major goal of therapy for any dysrhythmia. Medications must be used with caution, particularly those that increase the cardiac workload or depress myocardial function.

Sinus rhythms during MI

Sinus bradycardia (heart rate less than 60 beats/min) occurs in approximately 40% of all patients who sustain an acute MI and is more prevalent with an inferior wall infarction. It is seen most frequently in the immediate postinfarction period. Symptomatic bradycardia with hypotension and low cardiac output is treated with atropine 0.5 mg IV push, repeated every 5 minutes to a maximum dose of 2 mg.[19] Sinus tachycardia (heart rate greater than 100 beats/min) occurs most often with anterior wall MIs. Anterior infarctions impair left ventricular pumping ability, thereby reducing the ejection fraction and stroke volume. In an attempt to maintain cardiac output, the heartrate increases. Sinus tachycardia must be corrected because it not only greatly increases myocardial oxygen consumption but also shortens diastolic filling time, thereby decreasing stroke volume, systemic perfusion, and coronary artery filling.

Atrial dysrhythmias during MI

Premature atrial contractions (PAC) occur in almost half of all patients who sustain acute infarction.[14] PACs are most commonly caused by cell irritability resulting from distention of the left atrium secondary to increased left ventricular end-diastolic pressure and volume. A common atrial dysrhythmia associated with acute MI, atrial fibrillation is more prevalent with an anterior wall infarction. It may occur spontaneously or follow PACs or atrial flutter. With atrial fibrillation there is loss of atrial contraction, and hence a loss of atrial kick and the extra stroke volume it carries. Cardiac output is estimated to decrease by 30% when atrial kick is lost.[14]

Ventricular dysrhythmias during MI

Premature ventricular contractions (PVCs) are seen in almost all patients within the first few hours after an MI. PVCs are controlled by administering oxygen to reduce myocardial hypoxia, correcting acid-base or electrolyte imbalances, and administration of an IV lidocaine bolus and infusion. In the setting of an acute MI, PVCs are treated if they are (1) frequent (greater than 6/min), (2) closely coupled (R on T phenomenon), (3) multiform, or (4) occurring in bursts of 3 or more.[19] PVCs and ventricular tachycardia (VT) occurring within the first few hours postinfarction are usually transient. However, when these same dysrhythmias occur late in the course, they tend tobe associated with high in-hospital mortality rates because they are usually related to the cumulative loss of myocardium.[26] Ventricular fibrillation (VF) is a life-threatening dysrhythmia associated with high mortality in acute MI.

AV heart block during MI

AV heart block usually follows an inferior wall MI. Because the right coronary artery perfuses the AV node in 90% of the population, RCA occlusion leads to ischemia and infarction of the cells of the AV node. Symptomatic AV block with hemodynamic compromise is treated by intravenous administration of atropine or by insertion of a temporary pacemaker.[19]

Ventricular aneurysm post-MI

A ventricular aneurysm (Fig. 9-7) is a noncontractile, thinned left ventricular wall that results in a reduction of the stroke volume. It occurs in approximately 12% to 15% of patients who survive acute transmural infarction.[14,26,27] The most common complications of a ventricular aneurysm are heart failure, systemic emboli, and VT. Treatment is directed toward management of these complications and surgical repair by left ventricular aneurysmectomy. The prognosis depends on the size of the aneurysm, overall left ventricular function, and the severity of coexisting CAD. Rupture of the aneurysm is rare—but nonetheless life threatening—and usually occurs only if there is reinfarction of the border of the aneurysm.

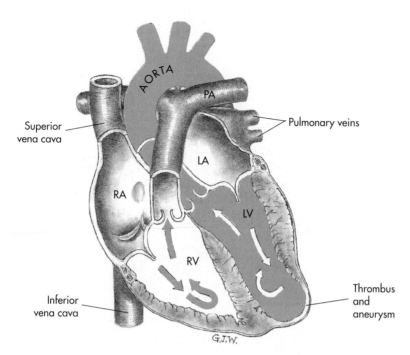

FIG. 9-7 Ventricular aneurysm after acute myocardial infarction.

Ventricular septal defect post-MI

Rupture of the ventricular septal wall (Fig. 9-8) affects approximately 1% to 3% of patients who sustain acute transmural MI.[27] The rupture is often followed by acute heart failure and shock. Ventricular septal defect manifests as severe chest pain, syncope, hypotension, and sudden hemodynamic deterioration caused by shunting of blood from the high-pressure left ventricle into the low-pressure right ventricle through the new septal opening. A holosystolic murmur (accompanied by a thrill) can be auscultated and is best heard along the left sternal border. A diagnosis of postinfarction VSD can be made at the bedside with use of a pulmonary artery catheter or by transesophageal echocardiogram. Rupture of the septum is a medical and surgical emergency. Patients' conditions are stabilized with vasodilators and an intraaortic balloon pump (IABP) to decrease afterload. The goal of afterload reduction in these patients is to decrease the amount of blood being shunted to the right side of the heart and to increase the forward flow of blood to the systemic circulation. Mortality rates exceed 80% with medical therapy alone; therefore most patients require emergency surgery to close the ventricular septum.

Papillary muscle rupture post-MI

Papillary muscle rupture can occur when the MI involves the area around the mitral valve. Infarction of the papillary muscles results in ineffective mitral valve closure and in blood being forced back into the low-pressure left atrium during ventricular systole. The rupture may be partial or complete. Complete rupture is catastrophic and precipitates severe acute mitral regurgi-

tation, shock, and death. Partial rupture (Fig. 9-9) also results in mitral regurgitation, but the condition can usually be stabilized with the IABP and vasodilators. Urgent surgical intervention is required to replace the mitral valve.[28]

Cardiac wall rupture post-MI

Of deaths after MI, 15% can be attributed to cardiac rupture, which often occurs in older patients who have systemic hypertension during the acute phase of their infarction. Rupture frequently occurs around 5 days after the infarction, when leukocyte scavenger cells remove necrotic debris, thus thinning the myocardial wall. The onset is sudden. Bleeding into the pericardial sac results in tamponade, cardiogenic shock, electromechanical dissociation, and death. Survival is rare, and emergency pericardiocentesis is required to relieve the tamponade until a surgical repair can be attempted.[27]

Pericarditis post-MI

An inflammation of the pericardial sac, pericarditis can occur after acute MI when the damage extends into the epicardial surface of the heart during a transmural MI. The damaged epicardium then becomes rough and tends to irritate and inflame the pericardium lying adjacent to it, precipitating pericarditis.[29] Pain is the most common symptom of pericarditis, and a pericardial friction rub the most common sign. Best heard at the sternal border, the friction rub is described as a grating, scraping, or leathery scratching. Pericarditis may result in a pericardial effusion. Once the effusion (fluid) occurs, the friction rub may disappear. Pericarditis is treated with aspirin or nonsteroidal antiinflammatory drugs.[29]

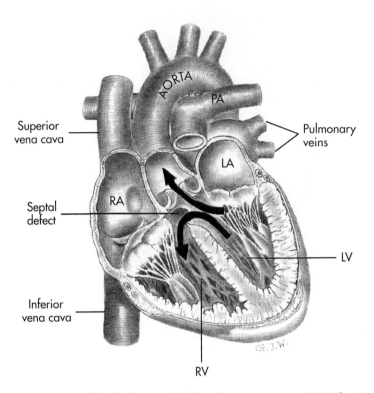

FIG. 9-8 Ventricular septal defect after acute myocardial infarction.

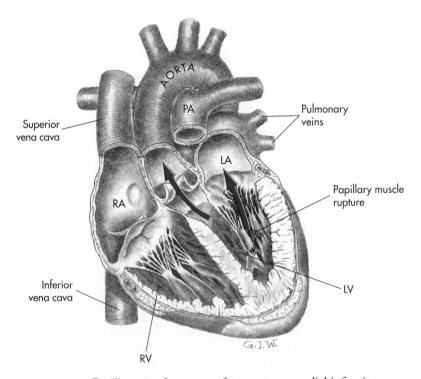

FIG. 9-9 Papillary muscle rupture after acute myocardial infarction.

Medical Management

The goals of medical management during MI include myocardial preservation, pain control, management of complications, and pharmacologic therapy.

Myocardial preservation

The first 6 hours after the onset of chest pain constitute the crucial period for salvage of the myocardium.[30] During this period, achieving reperfusion of the infarcting myocardium may be possible with either one or a combination of the following interventions[19]: (1) intravenous or intracoronary thrombolysis, (2) PTCA or coronary atherectomy, and (3) emergency coronary artery bypass surgery. (These therapies are discussed in detail in Chapter 10.) Studies show that myocardial tissue can be salvaged for at least 4 hours after the onset of symptoms, and in some patients this period may extend to 6 hours. Unfortunately, many people do not seek treatment until this phase has passed.[30]

Pain control

Pain control is a priority because continued pain is a symptom of ongoing ischemia, which places additional risk on noninfarcted myocardial tissue. Morphine, the analgesic of choice, decreases anxiety, restlessness, autonomic nervous system activity, and preload and thereby decreases myocardial oxygen demands. After infarction, oxygen is used for a minimum of 24 to 48 hours to prevent tissue hypoxia.

Management of complications

When complications occur, a pulmonary artery catheter is frequently inserted.[19] The pulmonary artery catheter allows correlation of chamber pressures to heart rate, blood pressure, cardiac output, and patients' clinical conditions. Thus pharmacologic and fluid-replacement decisions can be based on concrete parameters of ventricular function. The goal is to manage acute heart failure more effectively. The second most common complication of MI, heart failure is responsible for one third of the deaths of patients with an acute MI.

Pharmacologic therapy

The major goals of drug therapy are anticoagulation, reduction in myocardial workload, and analgesia. Anticoagulants are used to decrease the incidence of embolic complications from deep vein thrombosis and left ventricular thrombi, especially while bed rest is prescribed. Antiplatelet agents are used to decrease the release of thromboxane A_2 from platelets to prevent vasoconstriction and platelet aggregation. This therapy may be continued for an indefinite period; recent studies have documented the beneficial antiplatelet effect of low-dose prophylactic aspirin.[31] Beta-blocking agents are used to reduce infarct size by decreasing myocardial oxygen demand during the first few hours of infarction. However, beta blockers are contraindicated if there is left ventricular failure because they depress cardiac contractility.[19,21] Beta blockade is also used after the completed

infarction to lower the risks of reinfarction or death.[19] Calcium channel blockers are a diverse group of drugs used in conjunction with the other agents described to decrease coronary artery spasm and as antihypertensives.[19] (Cardiac medications are described in more detail in Chapter 10.)

Nursing Management

Nursing management of patients with an acute MI incorporates a variety of nursing diagnoses (Box 9-7). **Nursing priorities are directed toward assessing patients, controlling pain, achieving myocardial oxygen supply and demand balance, preventing complications, and educating patients and families.**

Assessing patients

Nurses spend a considerable portion of time monitoring patients for dysrhythmias; assessing vital signs for hemodynamic deterioration; assessing breath sounds for signs of pulmonary congestion and heart sounds for abnormalities, such as an S_3, S_4, or a murmur; and evaluating side effects from the medication regimen.[32,33] If left ventricular pump failure is present, the use of a pulmonary artery catheter is necessary for hemodynamic assessment.[19]

Controlling pain

Continued ischemic pain represents a myocardium at risk. Pain can be controlled by nitroglycerin and morphine, but thrombolytic therapy or emergency PTCA

BOX 9-7

NURSING DIAGNOSIS PRIORITIES

MYOCARDIAL INFARCTION AND COMPLICATIONS

- *Acute Pain* related to transmission and perception of cutaneous, visceral, muscular, or ischemic impulses, secondary to myocardial ischemia, p. 499
- *Decreased Cardiac Output* related to relative excess of preload and afterload secondary to impaired ventricular contractility, p. 473
- *Decreased Cardiac Output* related to supraventricular tachycardia, p. 472
- *Decreased Cardiac Output* related to ventricular tachycardia, p. 477
- *Decreased Cardiac Output* related to atrioventricular (AV) heart block, p. 474
- *Anxiety* related to threat to biologic, psychologic, and/or social integrity, p. 464
- *Knowledge Deficit:* activity restrictions, fluid restrictions, medication, reportable symptoms related to lack of previous exposure to information, p. 455

are the interventions of choice if patients are within the 4-hour window when the myocardium can be salvaged.

Achieving myocardial oxygen supply/demand balance

If there is severe myocardial damage in the acute period, myocardial oxygen supply is increased by using positive inotropic drugs such as dobutamine and dopamine and by avoiding negative inotropic agents such as beta blockers. Supplemental oxygen is administered to prevent tissue hypoxia. Bed rest with commode privileges is often prescribed during the first 24 to 48 hours to decrease cardiac work and myocardial oxygen consumption.

Preventing complications

For the first 24 hours, acute MI patients may be placed on a liquid or soft diet to decrease the risk of aspiration in case of cardiac arrest. During bed rest, patients remain in an upright or semi-Fowler's position to foster better lung expansion and decrease the risk of atelectasis. An upright position also decreases venous return, lowers preload, and decreases cardiac work. Stool softeners lessen the risk of constipation from analgesics and bed rest and decrease the risk of straining. Nurses should also control the critical care unit environment to decrease noise, diminish sensory overload, and allow adequate rest periods.

Educating patients and families

Patients who come into the emergency room within 4 hours of onset of chest pain immediately receive education about possible therapies to salvage the threatened myocardium, such as thrombolytic therapy and emergency PTCA. If patients arrive at the hospital too late to save the myocardium, they have had an MI and are admitted to the critical care unit. In this case, patients and families receive education on risk factor reduction, signs and symptoms of angina, times to call a physician or emergency services, medications, and resumption of physical and sexual activity. If possible, nurses should make a referral to a cardiac rehabilitation program so that this education can be reinforced outside the acute care hospital environment.[23]

Heart Failure

Description and Etiology

The National Heart Lung and Blood Institute[34] has estimated that more than 2 million Americans have **heart failure** and that about 400,000 new cases are diagnosed each year. The heart failure rate is higher in men than in women for all age groups, and the 5-year mortality rate in men is about 60%, whereas in women it is about 45%.[35] Responsible for one third of the deaths of patients with an acute MI, heart failure is the most common cause of in-hospital mortality for patients with cardiac disease.

Pathophysiology

Heart failure is a response to cardiac dysfunction in which the heart cannot pump blood at a volume required to meet the body's needs.[14,34] For many years heart failure was known as "congestive heart failure," but because pulmonary congestion does not always occur, the terms *acute heart failure* and *chronic heart failure* are increasingly used. The function of the heart is to transfer blood coming into the ventricles from the venous system into the arterial system. Impaired cardiac function results in failure to empty the venous system and reduced delivery of blood to the pulmonary and arterial circulations—hence, heart failure. Many precipitating causes of heart failure are listed in Box 9-8.

Assessment and Diagnosis

Heart failure can be described in many ways, including by the New York Heart Association (NYHA) classification and by whether primary ventricular involvement is right or left. However heart failure is classified, remembering that the ventricles do not function in isolation is important. The ventricles have a common septal wall and are encircled and bound together by continuous muscle fibers; thus any interruption or damage to one chamber will eventually affect all the chambers.

NYHA classification

A frequently used method to describe heart failure is the NYHA functional classification, which is based on patient symptoms (Box 9-9).

Failure of the right side of the heart

Failure of the right side of the heart is defined as ineffective right ventricular contractile function. Pure failure of the right side of the heart may result from an acute condition such as a pulmonary embolus or a right ventricular infarction, but most commonly it is caused by failure of the left side of the heart or the backing up of blood behind the left ventricle. Common manifestations of failure of the right side of the heart are weakness, periph-

---

BOX 9 - 8

PRECIPITATING CAUSES OF HEART FAILURE

Reduction or cessation of medication
Dysrhythmias
Systemic infection
Pulmonary embolism
Physical, environmental, and emotional stress
Pericarditis, myocarditis, and endocarditis
High ventricular output states
Development of serious systemic illness
Cardiac depressant or salt-retaining drugs
Development of a second form of heart disease

eral or sacral edema, jugular venous distention, hepatomegaly, jaundice, liver tenderness, and elevated central venous pressure. If peripheral perfusion is greatly compromised, cyanosis may be present. Gastrointestinal symptoms include anorexia, nausea, and a feeling of fullness[14] (Table 9-2).

Failure of the left side of the heart

Failure of the left side of the heart is defined as a disturbance of the contractile function of the left ventricle, resulting in pulmonary congestion and edema, decreased cardiac output, or both.[34] It most frequently occurs in patients with left ventricular infarctions, hypertension, and aortic and/or mitral valve disease. Classic clinical manifestations include decreased peripheral perfusion (such as weak or diminished pulses); cool, pale extremities; and peripheral cyanosis, as described in Table 9-2. As the disease progresses, the fluid accumulation behind the dysfunctional left ventricle produces dysfunction of the right ventricle, resulting in failure of the right side of the heart and its manifestations.

BOX 9-9

NEW YORK HEART ASSOCIATION FUNCTIONAL CLASSIFICATION*

Class I: Normal daily activity does not initiate symptoms.
Class II: Normal daily activities initiate onset of symptoms, but symptoms subside with rest.
Class III: Minimal activity initiates symptoms. Patients are usually symptom-free at rest.
Class IV: Any type of activity initiates symptoms, and symptoms are present at rest.

*Activity level that initiates onset of symptoms.

Acute versus chronic heart failure

Acute versus chronic heart failure refers to the rapidity with which the syndrome develops, the presence and activation of compensatory mechanisms, and the presence or absence of fluid accumulation in the interstitial space. Acute heart failure has a sudden onset, with no compensatory mechanisms. Patients may experience acute pulmonary edema, low cardiac output, or even cardiogenic shock. Patients with chronic heart failure are hypervolemic and have sodium and water retention and structural heart chamber changes such as dilatation or hypertrophy. Chronic heart failure is ongoing, with symptoms that may be made tolerable by medication, diet, and low activity level. A change to acute failure, however, can be precipitated by the onset of dysrhythmias, acute ischemia, and sudden illness or by cessation of medications. Acute failure may necessitate admission to a critical care unit.

Compensatory mechanisms in heart failure

When the heart begins to fail and cardiac output no longer meets the metabolic needs of the tissues, the body activates major compensatory mechanisms such as the adrenergic system, the renin-angiotensin-aldosterone system, sinus tachycardia, and the development of ventricular hypertrophy.

ADRENERGIC SYSTEM. Blood pressure is raised by the adrenergic compensatory mechanism. As a result of increased sympathetic activity, levels of circulating catecholamines are increased, resulting in peripheral vasoconstriction. This development leads to shunting of blood from nonvital organs such as the skin to vital organs such as the heart and brain.

RENIN-ANGIOTENSIN-ALDOSTERONE SYSTEM. The activation of the renin-angiotensin system promotes fluid retention. This system causes constriction of the renal arterioles, decreased glomerular filtration, and increased reabsorption of sodium from the proximal and distal tubules. In addition, diminished hepatic metabolism of

---

TABLE 9-2

CLINICAL MANIFESTATIONS OF FAILURE OF RIGHT AND LEFT SIDES OF HEART

LEFT VENTRICULAR FAILURE		RIGHT VENTRICULAR FAILURE	
SIGNS	**SYMPTOMS**	**SIGNS**	**SYMPTOMS**
Tachypnea	Fatigue	Peripheral edema	Weakness
Tachycardia	Dyspnea	Hepatomegaly	Anorexia
Cough	Orthopnea	Splenomegaly	Indigestion
Bibasilar crackles	Paroxysmal nocturnal dyspnea	Hepatojugular reflux	Weight gain
Gallop rhythms (S_3 and S_4)	Nocturia	Ascites	Mental changes
Increased pulmonary artery pressures		Jugular venous distention	
Hemoptysis		Increased central venous pressure	
Cyanosis		Pulmonary hypertension	
Pulmonary edema			

aldosterone increases the antidiuretic hormone level and enhances water retention.

SINUS TACHYCARDIA. Initially helpful as compensation in heart failure, sinus tachycardia may eventually become destructive because it increases myocardial oxygen demand while shortening the amount of time for coronary artery perfusion. This imbalance can lead to myocardial ischemia, which may decrease ventricular contraction, reduce ventricular filling, and necessitate a higher filling pressure. When heart failure progresses to the point at which tissue perfusion is inadequate to meet the body's needs, patients experience cardiogenic shock.

VENTRICULAR HYPERTROPHY. Because myocardial hypertrophy increases the force of contraction, hypertrophy helps the ventricle overcome an increase in afterload.[36]

Complications of Heart Failure

The clinical manifestations of HF result from tissue hypoperfusion and organ congestion (Table 9-2). The severity of clinical manifestations progresses as the heart failure worsens. Signs and symptoms initially appear only with exertion but eventually occur at rest (see Box 9-9).

Shortness of breath in heart failure

Breathlessness in heart failure is described by the following terms:

1. *Dyspnea* refers to the sensation of shortness of breath. It results from pulmonary vascular congestion and decreased lung compliance.

2. *Orthopnea* describes difficulty in breathing that results from an increase in venous return when patients are in the supine position.

3. *Paroxysmal nocturnal dyspnea* is a severe form of orthopnea in which the patient awakens from sleep gasping for air.

4. *Cardiac asthma* refers to dyspnea with wheezing, a nonproductive cough, and pulmonary crackles that progress to the gurgling sounds of pulmonary edema.

Pulmonary edema during heart failure

Pulmonary edema, or fluid in the alveoli (Fig. 9-10), inhibits gas exchange by impairing the diffusion pathway between the alveolus and capillary. Caused by increased left atrial and ventricular pressures, it results in an excessive accumulation of serous or serosanguineous fluid in the interstitial spaces and alveoli of the lungs. This fluid may be coughed up as a frothy pink sputum. Two stages mark the formation of pulmonary edema: Stage I is characterized by interstitial edema, engorgement of the perivascular and peribronchial spaces, and increased lymphatic flow; stage II is characterized by alveolar edema resulting from fluid moving into the alveoli from the interstitium. Eventually, blood plasma moves into the alveoli faster than the lymphatic system can clear it, interfering with diffusion of oxygen, depressing the arterial partial pressure of oxygen, and leading to tissue hypoxia.

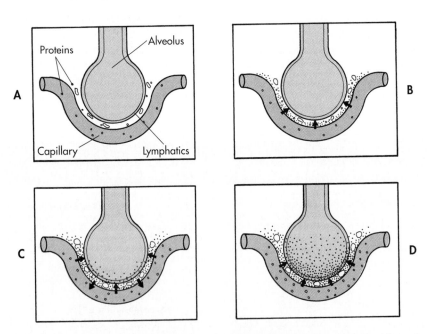

FIG. 9-10 As pulmonary edema progresses, it inhibits oxygen and carbon dioxide exchange at the alveolar capillary interface. **A,** Normal relationship. **B,** Increased pulmonary capillary hydrostatic pressure causes fluid to move from the vascular space into the pulmonary interstitial space. **C,** Lymphatic flow increases in an attempt to pull fluid back into the vascular or lymphatic space. **D,** Failure of lymphatic flow and worsening of left-sided heart failure results in further movement of fluid into the interstitial space and the alveoli.

Symptoms of pulmonary edema

With acute onset, patients experience breathlessness, anxiety, and a sensation of suffocation. They expectorate pink, frothy liquid and may feel as if they are drowning. They may sit bolt upright, gasp for breath, or move erratically. The respiratory rate is elevated, and patients' use of accessory muscles of ventilation manifests in flared nostrils and bulging neck muscles. Respirations are characterized by loud inspiratory and expiratory gurgling sounds. Diaphoresis is profuse, and the skin is cold, ashen, and cyanotic, reflecting low cardiac output, increased sympathetic stimulation, peripheral vasoconstriction, and desaturation of arterial blood.

Arterial blood gases in pulmonary edema

Arterial blood gas (ABG) values are variable. In the early stage of pulmonary edema, respiratory alkalosis may be present because of hyperventilation. As the pulmonary edema progresses and gas exchange becomes impaired, respiratory acidosis and hypoxemia ensue. The chest x-ray film usually confirms an enlarged cardiac silhouette, pulmonary venous congestion, and interstitial edema.

Medical Management

The goals for medical management of HF are to relieve symptoms and enhance cardiac performance and to identify and correct precipitating causes.

Relieve symptoms and enhance cardiac performance

In the acute phase, patients usually have a pulmonary artery catheter in place so that LV function can be followed closely. Control of symptoms involves managing fluid overload, improving cardiac output by decreasing systemic vascular resistance, and increasing contractility. Diuretics are administered to decrease preload and eliminate fluid from the body. If pulmonary edema develops, additional diuretics are used. Morphine is given to facilitate peripheral dilatation and decrease anxiety. Afterload is decreased by vasodilators such as sodium nitroprusside and nitroglycerin. Some patients also require an IABP. Digitalis and positive inotropic agents such as dopamine and dobutamine increase contractility. Angiotensin-converting enzyme inhibitors may alter chamber remodeling and slow the decline in contractility.[37,38]

Correct precipitating causes

Once symptoms of HF are controlled, diagnostic studies such as cardiac catheterization, echocardiogram, and thallium scan are undertaken to uncover its cause and potential treatment. Structural problems such as valvular disease may require surgical correction.

Nursing Management

Nursing management of patients with HF incorporates a variety of nursing diagnoses (Boxes 9-10 and 9-11). **Nursing priorities are directed toward assessing cardiopulmonary function, promoting rest, monitoring pharmacologic therapy, facilitating nutrition and skin integrity, and educating patients and families.**

Assessing cardiopulmonary function

The ECG is evaluated for any dysrhythmias that may be present or may develop as a result of drug toxicity or electrolyte imbalance. Patients in heart failure are prone to digoxin toxicity secondary to decreased renal perfusion as well as electrolyte imbalances. Breath sounds are auscultated frequently to determine adequacy of respiratory effort and assess for onset or worsening of congestion. Oxygen is administered through a nasal cannula to relieve dyspnea. Diuretics or vasodilators are used to decrease excessive preload and afterload.

BOX   9 - 1 0

NURSING DIAGNOSIS PRIORITIES

CHRONIC HEART FAILURE

- *Impaired Gas Exchange* related to ventilator perfusion mismatching or intrapulmonary shunting, p. 488
- *Decreased Cardiac Output* related to relative excess of preload and afterload secondary to impaired ventricular contractility, p. 473
- *Activity Intolerance* related to decreased cardiac output and/or myocardial tissue perfusion alterations, p. 482
- *Anxiety* related to threat to biologic, psychologic and/or social integrity, p. 464
- *Sleep Pattern Disturbance* related to fragmented sleep secondary to paroxysmal nocturnal dyspnea, p. 470

BOX   9 - 1 1

NURSING DIAGNOSIS PRIORITIES

ACUTE HEART FAILURE AND PULMONARY EDEMA

- *Impaired Gas Exchange* related to ventilation/perfusion mismatching or intrapulmonary shunting, p. 488
- *Decreased Cardiac Output* related to relative excess of preload and afterload secondary to impaired ventricular contractility, p. 473
- *Activity Intolerance* related to decreased cardiac output and/or myocardial tissue perfusion alterations, p. 482
- *Knowledge Deficit:* medications, fluid restrictions, activity restrictions, diet, reportable symptoms related to lack of previous exposure to information, p. 455

If patients are not hypotensive, morphine may be administered to decrease hyperventilation and anxiety. If the ventilatory status worsens, nurses must be prepared for endotracheal intubation and mechanical ventilation. Obtaining daily weights is important until the weight stabilizes at a "dry" weight. Generally the daily weight is used in fluid management, and a weekly weight is used for tracking body weight (e.g., muscle, fat).

Promoting rest

During periods of breathlessness, activity must be restricted; patients are usually prescribed bed rest and positioned with the head of the bed elevated to allow maximal lung expansion. The arms can be supported on pillows to prevent undue stress on the shoulder muscles. The legs may be placed in a dependent position to encourage venous pooling and thereby decrease venous return. Nurses should foster independence within the patients' activity prescription while ensuring that patients adhere to regularly scheduled rest periods.[39] Nurses should record patients' vital signs at the beginning and end of activities, documenting signs of activity intolerance such as dyspnea, fatigue, sustained increase in pulse, and onset of dysrhythmias and reporting them to physicians. Activity is gradually increased according to patient tolerance.

Monitoring pharmacologic therapy

Patients in acute heart failure require aggressive pharmacologic therapy.[40] Nurses must know the action, side effects, therapeutic levels, and toxic effects of diuretics, positive inotropic agents used to increase ventricular contractility, and vasodilators used to decrease preload. Patients' hemodynamic responses to these agents as well as diuretic therapy and fluid restrictions are closely monitored.[41]

Facilitating nutrition and skin integrity

Patients in heart failure frequently experience decreased appetite and nausea; therefore small, frequent meals may be more appropriate than the standard three large meals. Food should be as flavorful as possible; favorite foods and food from home may be worked into the diet as long as they are compatible with nutritional restrictions. Skin breakdown is a risk because of immobility, bed rest, inadequate nutrition, edema, and decreased perfusion to the skin and subcutaneous tissue. Frequent position changes are helpful in preventing this complication.

Educating patients and families

In planning activities and helping patients organize their daily schedule, nurses need to ensure that patients understand the importance of conserving their energy. Nurses initiate discussion of the importance of a low-salt diet and the multiple medications used to control the symptoms of HF.

Endocarditis

Description and Etiology

Infection by a microorganism of a platelet-fibrin vegetation on the endothelial surface of the heart results in infective **endocarditis**. Development of endocarditis depends on two factors: (1) a susceptible lesion in the vascular endothelium and (2) an organism to establish the infection.[42] The source of the organism may be unknown or traced to an invasive procedure such as a biopsy, cannulation of the veins or arteries, urogenital procedures, dental work, or intravenous drug use.[42-44] Almost any bacteria or fungus can infect a susceptible site. In western Europe and North America, streptococci and staphylococci account for 75% to 85% of all cases of endocarditis.

Pathophysiology

Endocarditis begins after the onset of bacteremia and the colonization of thrombotic vegetation. The bacteria is then encased in a platelet and fibrin shell that protects it from destruction by phagocytic neutrophils, leading to a zone of localized agranulocytosis. Because of this extensive protective mechanism, which restricts the body's normal response to infection, antibiotic therapy must be intensive and prolonged.

Assessment and Diagnosis

Endocarditis may be described as either acute or subacute. Acute infection develops on normal valves, progresses rapidly, causes severe destruction, and may be fatal if patients are not treated. Subacute infection occurs on damaged heart valves and progresses much more slowly. The term *subacute bacterial endocarditis* is not always accurate because although most infections are bacterial, some are caused by yeast or fungus. Classifying the disease according to causative microorganism is much more useful. In cases of prosthetic valve endocarditis, antibiotics are usually not sufficient and surgical replacement of the valve is required. Clinical manifestations of endocarditis are found in Box 9-12.

Medical Management

Treatment requires prolonged parenteral therapy with adequate doses of bactericidal antibiotics. An increasing number of patients are being discharged to continue the parenteral therapy at home via a surgically implanted line such as Port-A-Cath.

Nursing Management

Nursing management of patients with endocarditis incorporates a variety of nursing diagnoses (Box 9-13). **Nursing priorities are directed toward resolution of infection, prevention of complications, preserving mobility, and educating patients and families.**

B O X   9 - 1 2

CLINICAL MANIFESTATIONS OF ENDOCARDITIS

Fever
Splenomegaly
Hematuria
Petechiae
Cardiac murmurs
Easy fatigability
Osler's nodes (small, raised, tender areas most commonly found in pads of fingers and toes)
Splenic hemorrhages
Roth's spots (round or oval spots consisting of coagulated fibrin; appears in the retina and leads to hemorrhage)

Resolution of infection

Endocarditis requires a long course (usually 6 weeks) of intravenous antibiotics, beginning in the hospital and continuing at home with an indwelling central catheter. Nursing assessment includes monitoring for signs of worsening infection such as temperature elevation, malaise, weakness, easy fatigability, and night sweats.

Prevention of complications

Patients with infective endocarditis are at risk for embolic events, either cerebral or pulmonary. Therefore nurses should assess level of consciousness, checking for visual changes and headache. As valvular dysfunction accelerates, acute heart failure will develop. Cardiac assessment includes auscultation of heart sounds to detect the presence or change in a cardiac murmur. Shortness of breath or chest pain with hemoptysis must also be reported. These conditions could be caused by either pulmonary emboli or worsening heart failure.

Preserving mobility

During the most critical period, bed rest is prescribed for patients. Range-of-motion exercises maintain muscle tone, and frequent turning and repositioning prevent skin breakdown. Support and diversional activity are important at this time because depression related to a prolonged hospital stay is common.

Educating patients and families

Patients will need to know the signs and symptoms of infection, methods of taking an oral temperature, activities that increase risk of a recurrence of the endocarditis, and the importance of informing health care providers such as the dentist and podiatrist of the endocarditis history.[44] Nurses should also explain the way to obtain Medic Alert bracelets and cards if required.

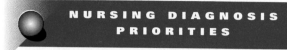

B O X   9 - 1 3

NURSING DIAGNOSIS PRIORITIES

ENDOCARDITIS

• *Activity Intolerance* related to decreased cardiac output and/or myocardial tissue alterations, p. 482
• *Risk for Infection* risk factor: invasive monitoring devices, p. 482

Cardiomyopathy

Description and Etiology

Cardiomyopathy is defined as a disease of the heart muscle: *cardio* means "heart," *myo* means "muscle," and *pathy* means "pathology." Cardiomyopathies are described as *primary* or *secondary* and further classified on the basis of associated structural abnormalities. These categories are hypertrophic, restrictive, and dilated cardiomyopathy (Fig. 9-11).

Primary cardiomyopathy

Primary, or *idiopathic, cardiomyopathy* is defined as a heart muscle disease, the cause of which is unknown, although both viral infections and autoimmune disorders have been implicated.

Secondary cardiomyopathy

Secondary cardiomyopathy is defined as heart muscle disease that results from some other systemic disease, such as coronary artery disease, valvular heart disease, severe hypertension, alcohol abuse, or known autoimmune disease.

Pathophysiology and Medical Management

Hypertrophic cardiomyopathy

Hypertrophic cardiomyopathy (HCM) is characterized by stiff, noncompliant myocardial muscle with left ventricular hypertrophy and bizarre cellular hypertrophy of the upper ventricular septum. This septal hypertrophy results in obstruction of the aortic valve outflow tract . (Fig 9-11) and also pulls the papillary muscle out of alignment, causing mitral regurgitation. This disorder used to be known as "idiopathic hypertrophic subaortic stenosis (IHSS)," but because IHSS described only 25% of affected patients, the more general term of *HCM* is now used.[45,46] Symptoms include exertional dyspnea, myocardial ischemia, supraventricular tachycardia, ventricular tachycardia, syncope, and heart failure. Sudden cardiac death occurs in 2% to 3% of adults with HCM per year.[45]

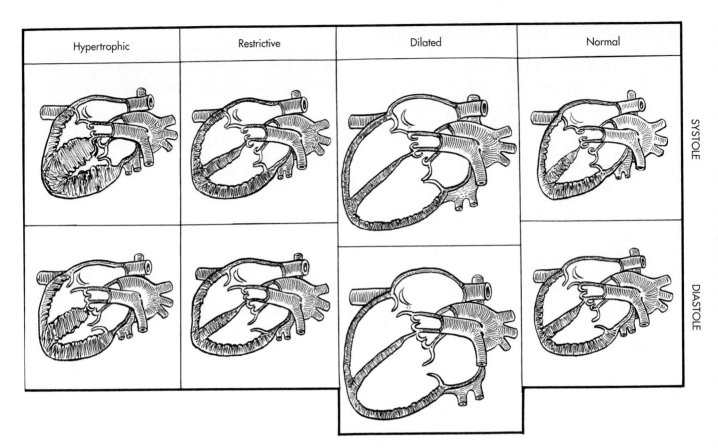

| Hypertrophic | Restrictive | Dilated | Normal |

SYSTOLE

DIASTOLE

FIG. 9-11 Types of cardiomyopathies compared with a normal heart.

Medical management includes limitation of physical activity, beta blockers, calcium channel blockers, antidysrhythmic therapy, and treatment of heart failure. For some patients an implantable cardioverter defibrillator, surgical myectomy, and mitral valve replacement are also treatment options.[45]

Dilated cardiomyopathy

Dilated cardiomyopathy is characterized by grossly dilated ventricles without muscle hypertrophy (Fig. 9-11). The muscle fibers contract poorly, resulting in global left ventricular dysfunction, low cardiac output, atrial and ventricular dysrhythmias, blood pooling that leads to ventricular clots and embolic episodes, and finally refractory heart failure and premature death.[47] The goals of medical management of dilated cardiomyopathy are improvement of pump function, removal of excess fluid, control of heart failure, and prevention of complications.

Restrictive cardiomyopathy

Characterized by abnormal diastolic function, restrictive cardiomyopathy (Fig. 9-11) is the least common form. Ventricular wall rigidity occurs as a consequence of myocardial fibrosis, the overall effect of which is to obstruct ventricular filling. Restrictive cardiomyopathy may be misdiagnosed as constrictive pericarditis. Heart failure, low cardiac output, dyspnea, orthopnea, and liver engorgement are the most common clinical manifestations of restrictive cardiomyopathy. Medical management is directed toward the improvement of pump function, removal of excess fluid, and a low-sodium diet.

Nursing Management

Nursing management of patients with cardiomyopathy incorporates a variety of nursing diagnoses (Box 9-14). **Nursing priorities are individualized according to the type of cardiomyopathy and are directed toward maintaining fluid balance, monitoring pharmacologic therapy, promoting mobility, and educating patients and families.**

Maintaining fluid balance

Patients are monitored for clinical manifestations of worsening heart failure, such as tissue edema, increased ventricular filling pressures, neck vein engorgement, pulmonary congestion, weight gain, increased fatigue, and onset of gallop rhythms. Daily weight readings and strict fluid restriction with accurate intake and output records are required.

Monitoring pharmacologic therapy

Patients with cardiomyopathy usually take a wide range of medications that includes diuretics, calcium-channel blockers, beta blockers, vasodilators, anticoagulant or antiplatelet agents, and antidysrhythmics. Often the transition from IV to oral administration is supervised by critical care nurses, who must be knowledgeable about appropriate and unwanted side effects. For example, patients with cardiomyopathy are prone to digoxin toxicity related to decreased excretion of the drug secondary to a decreased glomerular filtration rate.[45,46]

Promoting mobility

Nursing interventions are directed at maintaining patients' current levels of conditioning and collaborating with physical therapists to maintain or improve current functional levels. Activity plans need to reflect energy conservation, with clustered activities and frequent rest periods.

Educating patients and families

In educating patients and families, nurses should address all topics applicable to acute heart failure, incorporating assessment of patients' understanding of their illness, adaptive coping mechanisms, and support systems. Patients and families need to know what support services are available. Because most cardiomyopathies have only palliative treatments, patients need to be prepared for several possible outcomes, including heart transplantation, cardiac disability, and sudden cardiac death.

Valvular Heart Disease

Description and Etiology

Valvular heart disease describes structural and/or functional abnormalities of single or multiple cardiac valves resulting in alteration in blood flow across the valve. Two types of valvular lesions, stenotic and regurgitant, exist and are described with reference to the specific cardiac valves involved. At one time in the United States most

valvular lesions were rheumatic in origin; that is, damage was a direct result of group A beta-hemolytic streptococcal pharyngitis. With today's aging population, degenerative valve changes are equally important (Box 9-15).

Pathophysiology

Mitral valve stenosis

Mitral stenosis describes a progressive narrowing of the mitral valve orifice from the normal size of 4 to 6 cm to less than 1.5 cm. This narrowing is usually caused by aging valve tissue or by acute rheumatic valvulitis (Table 9-3). The diffuse valve leaflet fibrosis and fusion of one or both commissures reduce leaflet mobility. The chordae tendineae may be thickened, shortened, and fused, further contributing to the stenotic mitral orifice. As a result the mitral valve can no longer open and close passively in response to chamber pressure changes, and blood flow across the valve is impeded.

Mitral valve regurgitation

Mitral regurgitation may occur secondary to rheumatic disease or aging of the valve, or it can be caused by endocarditis, papillary muscle dysfunction, or a number of other events. In mitral valve regurgitation the valve annulus, leaflets, commissures, chordae tendineae, and papillary muscles may all be dysfunctional or the dysfunction may be isolated to just one component of the valve. Mitral valve regurgitation results in retrograde flow of blood into the left atrium with each ventricular contraction. The left atrium dilates to accommodate this additional volume, whereas the left ventricle hypertrophies as it tries to maintain forward flow and an adequate stroke volume. Acute mitral valve regurgitation, caused by papillary muscle rupture secondary to acute MI, is a medical emergency requiring aggressive medical therapy, which frequently includes use of an IABP, to stabilize patients' conditions. Once patients stabilize, surgical replacement of the incompetent valve is undertaken.[28]

Aortic valve stenosis

Aortic stenosis can result from aging, calcification of a congenital bicuspid valve, or rheumatic valvulitis (see

TABLE 9-3
VALVULAR DYSFUNCTION

PATHOPHYSIOLOGY	CLINICAL MANIFESTATIONS	PHYSICAL SIGNS
MITRAL VALVE STENOSIS		
Left atrium required to generate more pressure to propel blood beyond the lesion Rise in left atrial pressure and volume reflected retrograde into pulmonary vessels Right ventricular hypertrophy Right ventricular failure	Dyspnea on exertion Fatigue and weakness Pronounced respiratory symptoms—orthopnea, paroxysmal nocturnal dyspnea Mild hemoptysis with bronchial capillary rupture Susceptibility to pulmonary infections	Chest radiograph—pulmonary congestion, redistribution of blood flow to upper lobes ECG—atrial fibrillation and other atrial dysrhythmias Auscultation—diastolic murmur, accentuated S_1, opening snap Catheterization—elevated pressure gradient across valve; increased left atrial pressure, pulmonary artery wedge, pulmonary artery pressure; low cardiac output
MITRAL VALVE REGURGITATION		
Left ventricular dilatation and hypertrophy Left atrial dilatation and hypertrophy	Weakness and fatigue Exertional dyspnea Palpitations Severe symptoms precipitated by left ventricular failure, with consequent low output and pulmonary congestion	Chest radiograph—left atrial and left ventricular enlargement, variable pulmonary congestion ECG—P-mitrale, left ventricular hypertrophy, atrial fibrillation Auscultation—murmur throughout systole Catheterization—opacification of left atrium during left ventricular injection, V waves, increased left atrial and left ventricular pressures Variable elevations of pulmonary pressures
AORTIC VALVE STENOSIS		
Left ventricular hypertrophy Progressive failure of ventricular emptying Pulmonary congestion Failure of right side of heart, with systemic venous congestion Sudden death	Exertional dyspnea Exercise tolerance Syncope Angina Heart failure (left ventricular failure)	Chest radiograph—poststenotic aortic dilatation, calcification ECG—left ventricular hypertrophy Auscultation—systolic ejection murmur Catheterization—significant pressure gradient, increased left ventricular end-diastolic pressure
AORTIC VALVE REGURGITATION		
Increased volume load imposed on left ventricle Left ventricular dilatation and hypertrophy	Fatigue Dyspnea on exertion Palpitations	Chest radiograph—boot-shaped elongation of cardiac apex ECG—left ventricular hypertrophy Auscultation—diastolic murmur Catheterization—opacification of left ventricle during aortic injection Peripheral signs—hyperdynamic myocardial action and low peripheral resistance

PATHOPHYSIOLOGY	**CLINICAL MANIFESTATIONS**	**PHYSICAL SIGNS**

TABLE 9-3—cont'd

VALVULAR DYSFUNCTION

TRICUSPID VALVE STENOSIS

| Right atrium required to generate higher pressure to eject blood beyond the lesion
Right atrial dilatation
Systemic venous engorgement
Increased venous pressures | Venous distention
Peripheral edema
Ascites
Hepatic engorgement
Anorexia | Chest radiograph—right atrial enlargement
ECG—right atrial enlargement (P-pulmonale)
Auscultation—diastolic murmur
Catheterization—elevated right atrial pressure with large a waves, pressure gradient across the tricuspid valve |

TRICUSPID VALVE REGURGITATION

| Right ventricular hypertrophy and dilation | Decreased cardiac output
Neck vein distention
Hepatic engorgement
Ascites
Edema
Pleural effusions | Chest radiograph—right atrial and ventricular enlargement.
ECG—right ventricular hypertrophy and right atrial enlargement, atrial fibrillation
Auscultation—murmur throughout systole
Catheterization—elevated right atrial pressure and V waves |

Table 9-3). Whatever its cause the effect is to impede ejection of blood from the left ventricle into the aorta, resulting in increased left ventricular systolic pressure, left ventricular hypertrophy, and eventually, at end-stage disease, left ventricular dilatation. In addition, when the increase in volume and pressure is communicated back to the atrial and pulmonary vasculature, the result is an increase in left atrial pressure and volume, elevated pulmonary venous pressure, and pulmonary congestion.

Aortic valve regurgitation

Aortic regurgitation or insufficiency can occur as a result of rheumatic fever, systemic hypertension, Marfan's syndrome, syphilis, rheumatoid arthritis, aging valve tissue, or discrete subaortic stenosis (see Table 9-3). Aortic valve incompetence results in reflux of blood back into the left ventricle during ventricular diastole. To accommodate this extra volume, the left ventricle initially dilates and then hypertrophies in an attempt to empty more completely and meet the needs of the peripheral circulation.

Tricuspid valve stenosis

Rarely an isolated lesion, tricuspid stenosis frequently occurs in conjunction with mitral or aortic disease or both. Its origin is usually rheumatic fever (see Table 9-3). Tri-

cuspid stenosis increases the pressure work of the usually low-pressure right atrium, resulting in right atrial hypertrophy. In addition, the right atrium dilates in an attempt to accommodate the residual right atrial volume and the incoming venous return. As a result, systemic venous congestion occurs, the consequences of which include jugular venous congestion, liver failure, hepatomegaly, ascites, and peripheral edema.

Tricuspid valve regurgitation

Tricuspid regurgitation usually results from advanced failure of the left side of the heart or severe pulmonary hypertension (see Table 9-3).

Pulmonic valve disease

Usually related to congenital anomalies, pulmonic valve disease produces failure of the right side of the heart. If untreated, it can result in severe, irreversible pulmonary vascular changes.

Mixed valvular lesions

Many people have mixed lesions—that is, an element of both stenosis and regurgitation. Mixed lesions can accentuate the severity of a condition. For example, a combination of aortic stenosis and aortic regurgitation increases left ventricular volume and pressure, thereby multiplying the degree of left ventricular work.

Medical Management

Management of valvular disorders includes pharmacologic therapy to control symptoms of heart failure, balloon dilatation, and valve repair or replacement (see Chapter 10).

Nursing Management

Nursing management of patients with valvular disease incorporates a variety of nursing diagnoses (Box 9-16). **Nursing priorities are directed toward assessing cardiac output, managing fluid balance, and educating patients and families.**

Assessing cardiac output

Low cardiac output, which can occur because of decreased forward flow through a stenotic valve or bidirectional flow across an incompetent valve, is frequently found in patients with valvular heart disease. Vital signs and the effect of positive inotropic and afterload reducing agents are assessed and documented. If patients have hemodynamic catheters, cardiac output and hemodynamic parameters are measured and evaluated. Nurses should carefully plan patient care activities and provide adequate rest periods to prevent fatigue.

Managing fluid balance

Fluid status is assessed by auscultating breath and heart sounds. The appearance of pulmonary crackles or an S_3 may indicate volume overload. The jugular vein may be assessed for signs of increased distention. Diuretics and vasodilators are administered if required. Nurses should weigh patients daily and monitor and record fluid intake and output.

Educating patients and families

Nurses should provide information related to diet and fluid restrictions, actions and side effects of heart failure medications, need for prophylactic antibiotics before invasive procedures such as dental work,[42-44] and cues to call physicians about a change in cardiac status.

Diseases of the Aorta

Description and Etiology

Two conditions affect the aorta: aortic aneurysm and **aortic dissection.** An aortic aneurysm is a localized dilatation of the arterial wall that results in an alteration in vessel shape and blood flow. Figure 9-12 displays the four types of aneurysms. Abdominal aortic aneurysm is four times more common than thoracic aneurysm. The incidence of abdominal aortic aneurysm, which is higher in men than in women, is diagnosed most commonly after the fifth decade of life. Approximately 90% of patients with an aortic aneurysm have a history

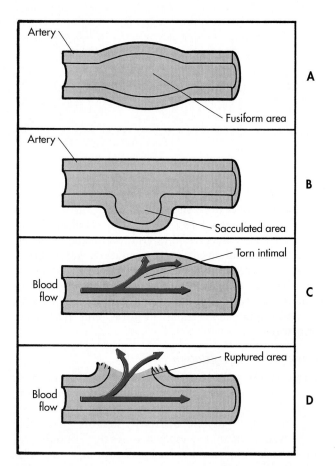

FIG. 9-12 Four types of aneurysms. **A,** Fusiform aneurysm, in which an entire segment of an artery is dilated, thus taking on a spindle or bulbous shape. Fusiform aneurysms occur most often in the abdominal aorta secondary to atherosclerosis. **B,** Sacculated aneurysm, which involves only one side of an artery and is usually located in the ascending aorta. **C,** Dissecting aneurysm, which occurs because of a tear in the intima, resulting in the shunting of blood between the intima and media of a vessel. **D,** Pseudoaneurysm, which results from a ruptured artery wall.

BOX 9-16

NURSING DIAGNOSIS PRIORITIES

VALVULAR HEART DISEASE

- *Decreased Cardiac Output* related to relative excess of preload and afterload secondary to impaired cardiac valvular function, p. 473
- *Activity Intolerance* related to decreased cardiac output and/or myocardial tissue perfusion alterations, p. 482
- *Knowledge Deficit:* medications, activity restrictions, and possible future interventions to correct valvular dysfunction related to lack of exposure to information, p. 455

of systemic hypertension. Other causes of aortic aneurysm include (1) atherosclerotic changes in the thoracic and abdominal aorta, (2) blunt trauma, (3) Marfan's syndrome, (4) pregnancy, and (5) iatrogenic injury or dissection. An aortic dissection occurs when vascular layers are separated by a column of blood. This column creates a false lumen, which communicates with the true lumen through a tear in the intima.[48]

Assessment and Diagnosis

An aortic aneurysm does not always cause symptoms. It may be detected during routine abdominal examination as a palpable, pulsatile mass located in the umbilical region of the abdomen to the left of midline. A thoracic aneurysm may be identified on a routine chest x-ray film. An aortic dissection is usually identified emergently by the onset of acute pain.

Aortic aneurysm

An aneurysm less than 4 cm in diameter can be managed on an outpatient basis with frequent monitoring of blood pressure and ultrasound testing to document any changes in size of the aneurysm. Patients are encouraged to lose weight if obesity is a factor and are treated for hypertension to decrease hemodynamic stress on the site. An aneurysm greater than 5 cm usually requires surgical intervention (Box 9-17). After surgery, patients may be admitted to the critical care unit.

Aortic dissection

Aortic dissections are classified according to site of the tear. There are two classification systems used in clinical practice, featuring either the letters *A* and *B* or numerals *I*, *II*, and *III* (Fig. 9-13). The classic clinical manifestation is the sudden onset of intense, severe, tearing pain, which may be localized initially in the chest, abdomen, or back. As dissection extends, pain radiates to the back or distally toward the lower extremities. Cardiovascular signs may include severe hypertension, acute neurologic deficits, fleeting peripheral pulses, and a new murmur indicative of aortic regurgitation. The location of the dissection may be established by the site of pain. A descending aortic dissection is usually accompanied by pain that radiates to the back, abdomen, or legs. An ascending dissection produces central chest pain. Invasive diagnostic procedures that may be performed include aortogram (with radiopaque contrast), magnetic resonance imaging (MRI), and computed tomographic scan using contrast.

Medical Management

Medical management of an aortic aneurysm involves controlling hypertension and educating patients about the need for corrective surgery if the aneurysm is greater than 5 cm in diameter. Medical management of acute aortic dissection involves control of hypertension with IV agents and control of pain with narcotics such as morphine sulphate. Progression of the dissection is evaluated by patients' reports of worsening or new pain. For dissections that involve the ascending aorta (including type A and type I and II dissections), surgery is usually performed to prevent death from cardiac tamponade. The surgical procedure includes resection of the affected area, followed by graft placement and restoration of blood flow to major branches of the aorta. Replacement of the aortic valve may be undertaken if the dissection involves the valve. Dissections that involve the descending aorta (type B or type III) do not always require surgery.

Nursing Management

Nursing management of patients with aortic aneurysm or dissection incorporates a variety of nursing diagnoses (Box 9-18). **Nursing priorities are directed toward controlling hypertension, decreasing pain, and educating patients and families.**

Controlling hypertension

Patients' cardiovascular status is assessed hourly, including monitoring blood pressure in both arms, checking peripheral pulses bilaterally, auscultating for an aortic murmur, and monitoring the ECG for ischemic changes or dysrhythmias. Patients usually require an arterial line and receive potent vasodilators such as labetalol and sodium nitroprusside.

BOX 9-17

INDICATIONS FOR ANEURYSM SURGERY

Aneurysm greater than 5 cm
Aneurysm progressively increasing in size
Impending rupture
Symptoms resulting from cerebral or coronary ischemia
Pericardial tamponade
Uncontrollable pain
Aortic insufficiency

BOX 9-18

NURSING DIAGNOSIS PRIORITIES

AORTIC DISEASE

- *Acute Pain* related to acute dissection of the aortic wall, p. 499
- *Anxiety* related to threat to biologic integrity, p. 464
- *Knowledge Deficit:* treatment of hypertension, activity restrictions and possible future surgical repair of aorta related to lack of exposure to information, p. 455

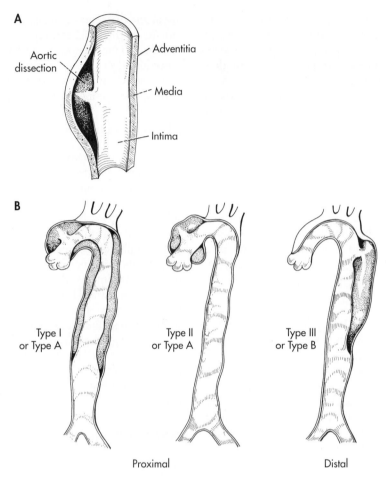

FIG. 9-13 Aortic dissection. **A,** Separation of vascular layers. **B,** Classification of aortic dissection. (Modified from Price SA, Wilson LM: *Pathophysiology: clinical concepts of disease processes,* ed 5, St Louis, 1996, Mosby.)

Decreasing pain

Acute pain is a classic sign of aortic dissection. Analgesics are given to control pain, decrease anxiety, and increase comfort. Because analgesics can mask the pain of further dissection, they are administered judiciously. Patients' neurovascular status is assessed hourly. Nurses should document the presence and distribution of pain, pallor, paresthesia, and paralysis and the absence of a pulse.

Educating patients and families

In the acute period, education is limited to an explanation of the critical care environment and the importance of blood pressure control. If additional procedures such as an aortogram, CT scan, and surgery are to be performed, critical care nurses assist with the explanations.

Peripheral Vascular Disease

Description and Etiology

Peripheral vascular disease (PVD) is divided into arterial and venous diseases of the peripheral vessels. Venous disease is a chronic condition that is managed on an out-patient basis and does not require admission to a critical care unit. In contrast, arterial PVD requires critical care admission for an acute thrombotic occlusion. PVD can occur in any peripheral vessel but is most frequently seen in the lower extremities. The following descriptions relate to arterial PVD.

Pathophysiology

It is estimated that 2.4 million persons are affected with PVD. Risk factors are the same as for CAD. As with CAD, atherosclerosis is the most common cause, and diabetes,[49] smoking, hypertension, and male gender all increase the risk.

Assessment and Diagnosis

Intermittent claudication

Arterial occlusion obstructs blood flow to the distal extremity. The lack of blood flow produces ischemic muscle pain or intermittent claudication.[50] This cramping, aching pain while walking is usually the first symptom of peripheral occlusive disease. The pain is relieved by rest and may remain stable in occurrence and intensity for many years. Symptoms do not occur until more than 75% of the vessel lumen is occluded. Arterial pulses are diminished, transiently present (vessel spasm), or absent distal to the site of occlusion.

Rest pain

As PVD progresses, 20% to 30% of patients develop pain during rest.[50] Pain at rest threatens the viability of the limb and requires immediate catheterization or surgical intervention to relieve the blockage and restore circulation to the extremity.

Acute occlusion

Acute occlusion from thrombosis presents with sudden onset of severe pain, loss of pulses, collapse of superficial veins, coldness, pallor, and impaired motor and sensory function. As with rest pain, it requires immediate intervention to open the artery.

Atrophic tissue changes

Skin changes include thickening of the nails and drying of the skin. Hair loss is common on the lower leg, dorsum of the feet, and toes. A temperature gradient is usually present as a line of demarcation between well-perfused and poorly perfused areas. Wasting of muscle or soft tissue may also occur. As the disease progresses, ulcerations and gangrene may result.

Medical Management

Medical therapy is geared toward controlling or eliminating risk factors, providing good foot care, and suggesting lifestyle alterations that promote rest and pain relief. Pharmacologic management may include the use of anticoagulants, vasodilators, or antiplatelet drugs. If these therapies do not produce positive results, percutaneous transluminal angioplasty (PTA) or surgery may be considered. PTA is effective if the lesion (blockage) is discrete and localized. However, if the arterial disease is diffuse, bypass surgery is usually undertaken. The presence of gangrene (cell death) necessitates limb or partial limb amputation.

Nursing Management

Nursing management of patients with peripheral arterial insufficiency incorporates a variety of nursing diagnoses (Box 9-19). **Nursing priorities are directed toward assessing arterial pulses, maintaining tissue integrity, controlling pain, and educating patients and families.**

Assessing arterial pulses

Assessment of peripheral pulses, color, and temperature are all critical in the evaluation of an ischemic limb. Many hospitals use a standard scale to improve documentation of pulses. If the pulse cannot be palpated, a Doppler scan may be used to assess flow.

BOX 9-19

NURSING DIAGNOSIS PRIORITIES

PERIPHERAL VASCULAR DISEASE

- *Acute Pain* related to transmission and perception of cutaneous, visceral, muscular, or ischemic impulses secondary to tissue ischemia, p. 499
- *Anxiety* related to threat to biologic integrity, p. 464
- *Risk for peripheral neurovascular dysfunction* related to decreased arterial perfusion to limb, p. 479
- *Knowledge deficit:* foot care, medications, reportable symptoms and possible surgical intervention for PVD related to lack of exposure to information, p. 455

Maintaining tissue integrity

Health care providers should be careful to protect the limb from injuries such as pressure sores. Poor blood flow or diabetes often impairs healing. Cotton or lamb's wool placed between the toes or use of a bed cradle may protect feet from injury. However, removal of the thrombus is the only treatment for an acute ischemic limb that will salvage tissue.

Controlling pain

The pain of intermittent claudication is managed by rest. However, because the pain of an acute ischemic limb is extreme, morphine sulphate is used for pain control.

Educating patients and families

Nurses should educate patients and family on risk factor modification, inspection of the feet and legs, foot care, and medications. If patients have a surgically implanted prosthetic bypass graft, they should receive information about bacterial endocarditis precautions.[42-44]

References

1. Alspach JG: The cost of cardiovascular disease: a life every 32 seconds, *Crit Care Nurse* 11(2):8,10, 1990.
2. Stovsky B: Nursing interventions for risk factor reduction, *Nurs Clin North Am* 27(1):257-270, 1992.
3. Teplitz L, Siwik DA: Cellular signals in atherosclerosis, *J Cardiovasc Nurs* 8(3):28-52, 1994.
4. Kannel WB and others: A general cardiovascular risk profile: the Framingham study, *Am J Cardiol* 38:46-51, 1976.
5. Expert Panel on Detection, Evaluation, and Treatment of High Blood Cholesterol in Adults: Summary of the second report of the National Cholesterol Education Program (Adult treatment panel II), *JAMA* 269:3015-3022, 1993.
6. McIntosh HD: Risk factors for cardiovascular disease and death: a clinical perspective, *J Am Coll Surg* 14:24, 1989.
7. National High Blood Pressure Education Program Working Group Report on Primary Prevention of Hypertension, *Arch Intern Med* 153:186-208, 1993.
8. Joint National Committee on Detection, Evaluation, and Treatment of High Blood Pressure: The fifth report of the

joint national committee on detection, evaluation, and treatment of high blood pressure, *Arch Intern Med* 153:154-183, 1993.

9. Stamler J and others: MRFIT 12 year follow-up: diabetes and mortality, *Diabetes Care* 16:434-444, 1993.

10. Paffenbarger RS and others: Physical activity as an index of heart attack risk in college alumni, *Am J Epidemiol* 108:161-175, 1978.

11. Kawachi I and others: Symptoms of anxiety and risk of coronary heart disease: the normative aging study, *Circulation* 90(5):2225-2229, 1994.

12. Fuster V and others: The pathogenesis of coronary artery disease and the acute coronary syndromes II, *N Engl J Med* 326(5):310-318, 1992.

13. Fuster V and others: The pathogenesis of coronary artery disease and the acute coronary syndromes I, *N Engl J Med* 326(4):242-250, 1992.

14. Braunwald E, editor: *Heart disease,* ed 4, Philadelphia, 1991, WB Saunders.

15. Braunwald E and others: Unstable angina: diagnosis and management: clinical practice guideline, Pub. No. 94-0602, Rockville, MD, 1994, Agency for Health Care Policy and Research and the National Heart, Lung and Blood Institute, Public Health Service, US Department of Health and Human Services.

16. Cohn PF: Silent ischemia, *Heart Disease Stroke* 1(5):295, 1992.

17. Creel CA: Silent myocardial ischemia and nursing implications, *Heart Lung* 23(3):218-227, 1994.

18. Kuhn M: Nitrates, *AACN Clin Issues in Crit Care Nurs* 3(2):409-422, 1992.

19. ACC/AHA Task Force Report: Guidelines for the early management of patients with acute myocardial infarction, *JACC* 16(2):249-292, 1990.

20. White P: Calcium channel blockers, *AACN Clin Issues Crit Care Nurs* 3(2):437-446, 1992.

21. Clark BC: Beta-adrenergic blocking agents: their current status, *AACN Clin Issues Crit Care Nurs* 3(2):447-460, 1992.

22. Hearns PA: Differentiating ischemia, injury, infarction: expanding the 12-lead electrocardiogram, *DCCN* 13(4):172-183, 1994.

23. Wang WWT: The educational needs of myocardial infarction patients, *Prog Cardiovasc Nurs* 9(4):28-39, 1994.

24. Martin JS and others: Early recognition and treatment of the patient suffering from acute myocardial infarction: a description of the myocardial infarction triage and intervention project, *Crit Care Nurs Clin North Am,* 2(4):681-688, 1990.

25. Jacavone J, Dostal M: A descriptive study of nursing judgment in the assessment and management of cardiac pain, *Adv Nurs Science* 15(1):54-63, 1992.

26. Mayberry-Toth B, Landron S: Complications associated with acute myocardial infarction, *Crit Care Nurs Q* 12(2):49-63, 1989.

27. Molchany CA: Ventricular septal and free wall rupture complicating acute MI, *J Cardiovasc Nurs* 6(4):38-45, 1992.

28. O'Sullivan CK: Mitral regurgitation as a complication of MI: pathophysiology and nursing implications, *J Cardiovasc Nurs* 6(4):26-37, 1992.

29. Pierce CD: Acute post-MI pericarditis, *J Cardiovasc Nurs* 6(4):46-56, 1992.

30. Funk M, Pooley-Richards RL: Predicting hospital mortality in persons with acute myocardial infarction, *Am J Crit Care* 3(3):168, 1990.

31. Antiplatelet Trialist's Collaboration: Collaborative overview of randomized trials of antiplatelet therapy: prevention of death, myocardial infarction and stroke by prolonged antiplatelet therapy in various categories of patients, *Br Med J* 308:81-106, 1994.

32. Stewart SL: Acute MI: a review of pathophysiology, treatment, and complications, *J Cardiovasc Nurs* 6(4):1-25, 1992.

33. Woo MA: Clinical management of the patient with an acute myocardial infarction, *Nurs Clin North Am* 27(1):189-203, 1992.

34. Konstam M and others: Heart failure: evaluation and care of patients with left-ventricular systolic dysfunction: clinical practice guideline Pub. No. 94-0612, Rockville, MD, 1994, Agency for Health Care Policy and Research and the National Heart, Lung and Blood Institute, Public Health Service, US Department of Health and Human Services.

35. Funk M: Epidemiology of heart failure, *Crit Care Nurs Clin North Am* 5(4):569-573, 1993.

36. Piano MR: Cellular and signaling mechanisms of cardiac hypertrophy, *J Cardiovasc Nurs* 8(4):1-26, 1994.

37. Braunwald E: ACE inhibitors—a cornerstone of the treatment of heart failure, *N Engl J Med* 325(5):351-353, 1991.

38. The SOLVD Investigators: Effect of enalapril on survival in patients with reduced left ventricular ejection fractions and congestive heart failure, *N Engl J Med* 325(5):293-302, 1991.

39. Schaefer KM, Polylycki MJS: Fatigue associated with congestive heart failure: use of Levine's conservation model, *J Adv Nurs* 18(2):260-268, 1993.

40. Whalen DA, Izzi G: Pharmacologic treatment of acute congestive heart failure resulting from left ventricular systolic and diastolic dysfunction, *Crit Care Nurs Clin North Am* 5(2):261-269, 1993.

41. Kennedy GT: Acute congestive heart failure: pharmacologic intervention, *Crit Care Nurs Clin North Am* 4(2):365-375, 1992.

42. Lukes AS and others: Diagnosis of infective endocarditis, *Infect Dis Clin North Am* 7(1):1-8, 1993.

43. Steckelberg JM, Wilson WR: Risk factors for infective endocarditis, *Infect Dis Clin North Am* 7(1):9-19, 1993.

44. Dajani AS and others: Prevention of bacterial endocarditis, *JAMA* 264:2919-2922, 1990.

45. Louie EK, Edwards LC: Hypertrophic cardiomyopathy, *Prog Cardiovasc Dis* 36(4):275-308, 1994.

46. Uszenski HJ and others: Hypertrophic cardiomyopathy: medical surgical and nursing management, *J Cardiovasc Nurs* 7(2):13-22, 1993.

47. Purcell JA: Advances in the treatment of dilated cardiomyopathy, *AACN Clin Issues Crit Care Nurs,* 1(1):31-45, 1990.

48. Buruss N: Aortic dissection: diagnosis and acute care management, *Cardiovasc Nurs* 29(6):41-51, 1993.

49. LoGerfo FW: Peripheral arterial occlusive disease and the diabetic: current clinical management, *Heart Disease Stroke* 1(6):395-397, 1992.

50. Emma LA: Chronic arterial occlusive disease, *J Cardiovasc Nurs* 7(1):14-24, 1992.

10

Cardiovascular Therapeutic Management

JONI DIRKS

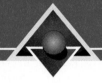

A wide variety of therapeutic interventions are employed in the management of patients with cardiovascular dysfunction. This chapter focuses on the priority interventions used to manage cardiac disorders in the critical care environment.

Temporary Pacemakers

Pacemakers are electronic devices used to initiate the heartbeat when the heart's intrinsic electrical system is unable to generate a rate adequate to support cardiac output. Pacemakers can be used temporarily until the condition responsible for the rate or conduction disturbance is resolved. Pacemakers can also be used on a permanent basis if the condition persists despite adequate therapy. This section emphasizes **temporary pacemakers** because they are used so frequently in critical care units. Critical care nurses are often responsible for preventing, assessing, and managing pacemaker malfunctions. Brief references are made to permanent pacemakers where appropriate.

Therapeutic Indications for Temporary Pacing

The clinical indications for instituting temporary pacemaker therapy are similar regardless of the cause of the rhythm disturbance necessitating the placement of a pacemaker (Box 10-1). Such causes range from drug toxicity and electrolyte imbalances to sequelae related to acute myocardial infarction or cardiac surgery.

1. Dysrhythmia management: Dysrhythmias that are unresponsive to drug therapy and result in compromised hemodynamic status are a primary indication. The goal of therapy in the case of a bradydysrhythmia is to increase the ventricular rate and thus enhance cardiac output. Alternately, "overdrive" pacing can be used to decrease the rate of a rapid supraventricular or ventricular rhythm. This rapid pacing of the heart, or over-

drive pacing, functions either to prevent the "breakthrough" ectopy that can result from a slow heart rate or to "capture" an ectopic focus and allow the heart's natural pacemaker to regain control.

2. Following cardiac surgery: After cardiac surgery temporary pacing is used to improve a transiently depressed, rate-dependent cardiac output. In addition, conduction disturbances that can occur after valvular surgery can be managed effectively with temporary pacing.

Diagnostic Indications for Temporary Pacing

Several diagnostic uses for temporary pacing have evolved over the past several years.

1. Electrophysiology studies (EPS): During an EPS special pacing electrodes are used to induce dysrhythmias in patients with recurrent symptomatic tachydysrhythmias. This allows physicians to closely evaluate the particular dysrhythmia and determine appropriate therapy.
2. Atrial electrogram (AEG): The AEG is simply an amplified recording of atrial activity that can be obtained through the use of atrial pacing wires and a standard electrocardiogram (ECG) machine. It is often used after cardiac surgery to facilitate the diagnosis of supraventricular dysrhythmias in patients with temporary atrial epicardial electrodes already in place.[1]

Pacemaker System

A pacemaker system is a simple electrical circuit consisting of a pacemaker generator and a pacing lead (an insulated electrical wire) with one or two electrodes.

Pacemaker Generator

The pacemaker pulse generator is designed to generate an electrical current that travels through the pacing lead and exits through an electrode (exposed portion of the wire) that is in direct contact with the heart. This electrical current initiates a myocardial depolarization. The current then returns by one of several ways to the pacemaker generator to complete the circuit. The power source for a temporary pacemaker is a standard 9-volt alkaline battery inserted into the generator. Implanted permanent pacemaker batteries are generally long-lived lithium cells.

Pacing Lead Systems

Temporary pacing leads may be either transvenous or epicardial. The lead used in transvenous pacing has two electrodes on one catheter (Fig. 10-1, *D*). The distal, or negative, electrode is at the tip of the pacing lead and in

---

BOX 10-1

INDICATIONS FOR TEMPORARY PACING

Bradydysrhythmias
　Sinus bradycardia and arrest
　Sick sinus syndrome
　Heart blocks
Tachydysrhythmias
　Supraventricular
　Ventricular
Permanent pacemaker failure
Support cardiac output after cardiac surgery
Diagnostic studies
　Electrophysiology studies (EPS)
　Atrial electrograms (AEG)

direct contact with the heart, usually inside the right atrium or ventricle. Approximately 1 cm above the negative electrode is a positive electrode. The negative electrode is attached to the negative terminal, and the positive electrode is attached to the positive terminal of the pulse generator, either directly or via a bridging cable (Fig. 10-1, *B*). The pacing impulse always flows from the negative electrode to the positive electrode.

Pacing Routes

Several routes are available for temporary cardiac pacing (Box 10-2). Permanent pacing is usually accomplished transvenously, although in situations in which a thoracotomy is otherwise indicated, such as cardiac surgery, physicians may elect to insert epicardial pacing wires.

Transcutaneous Cardiac Pacing

Transcutaneous cardiac pacing is an accepted emergency procedure involving the use of two large skin electrodes, one placed anteriorly and the other posteriorly on the chest, that are connected to an external pacemaker generator. A rapid, noninvasive procedure that nurses can perform emergently, it is increasing in use since improved technology has helped decrease the problems of painful muscle contractions and soft tissue burns.

Transthoracic Pacing

Transthoracic pacing is an emergency procedure involving the insertion of a pacing wire into the ventricle through a needle inserted through the chest wall. This technique may be associated with serious complications such as pneumothorax and cardiac tamponade.

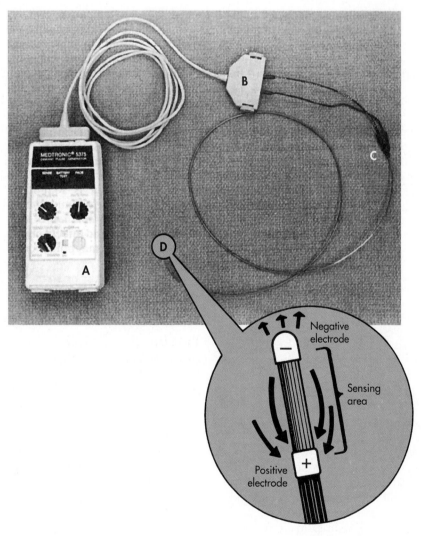

FIG. 10-1 The components of a temporary bipolar transvenous system. **A,** Single-chamber temporary (external) pulse generator. **B,** Bridging cable. **C,** Pacing lead. **D,** Enlarged view of the components. (Modified from Persons CB: *Critical care procedures and protocols: a nursing approach,* Philadelphia, 1987, JB Lippincott.)

BOX 10-2

ROUTES FOR TEMPORARY PACING

TRANSCUTANEOUS

Emergency pacing is achieved by depolarizing the heart through the chest by means of two large skin electrodes.

TRANSTHORACIC

A pacing wire is inserted emergently by threading it through a transthoracic needle into the right ventricle.

EPICARDIAL

Pacing electrodes are sewn to the epicardium during cardiac surgery.

TRANSVENOUS (ENDOCARDIAL)

The pacing electrode is advanced through a vein into the right atrium or right ventricle, or both.

BOX 10-3

PACEMAKER TERMINOLOGY

FIXED-RATE (ASYNCHRONOUS)

Delivers a pacing stimulus at a set (fixed) rate regardless of the occurrence of spontaneous myocardial depolarizations.

DEMAND (SYNCHRONOUS)

Delivers a pacing stimulus only when the heart's intrinsic pacemaker fails to function at a predetermined rate; the pacing stimulus will be either inhibited or triggered into the QRS complex when the intrinsic pacemaker functions.

ATRIOVENTRICULAR (AV) SEQUENTIAL (DUAL-CHAMBER PACING)

Delivers a pacing stimulus to both the atrium and ventricle in proper sequence with sufficient AV delay to permit adequate ventricular filling.

Temporary Epicardial Pacing

The insertion of temporary epicardial pacing wires is a routine procedure during most cardiac surgical cases. Ventricular, and in many cases atrial, pacing wires are loosely sewn to the epicardium. The terminal pins of these wires are pulled through the skin before the chest is closed. If both chambers have pacing wires attached, the atrial wires exit subcostally to the right of the sternum and the ventricular wires exit in the same region but to the left of the sternum.[1] Several days after the surgery these wires can be removed by gentle traction at the skin surface with minimal risk of bleeding.

Temporary Transvenous Endocardial Pacing

Temporary transvenous endocardial pacing is accomplished by advancing a pacing electrode wire through a vein, often the subclavian or internal jugular, into the right atrium or right ventricle. Insertion can be facilitated either through direct visualization with fluoroscopy or by the use of the standard ECG.

Five-Letter Pacemaker Code

In the 1960s pacemaker terminology was limited to "fixed-rate" and "demand" pacing, followed by the introduction of "AV sequential" pacing in the early 1970s. Although these terms are still useful today for understanding pacemaker function (Box 10-3), the continued expansion of pulse generators' capabilities made it necessary to develop a more precise classification system. Therefore in 1974 the Inter-Society Commission for Heart Disease (ICHD) adopted a three-letter code for describing the various pacing modalities available. The code has since undergone several revisions, including the addition of two more letters representing programming characteristics and antitachycardia functions. Table 10-1 provides a full description of the five-letter pacemaker code.[2]

Basic pacemaker function is described by the first three letters of the code (Table 10-2):

1. The first letter refers to the cardiac chamber that is paced.
2. The second letter refers to the cardiac chamber that is sensed.
3. The third letter indicates the response to the sensed event.

Temporary Pacemaker Settings

The controls on all external temporary pulse generators are similar (Fig. 10-2). Control functions should be thoroughly understood so pacing can be initiated quickly in an emergency situation and troubleshooting facilitated should problems with the pacemaker arise.

1. Pacemaker rate control: The rate control regulates the number of impulses that can be delivered to the heart per minute. The rate setting depends on the physiologic needs of patients, but it is generally maintained between 60 and 80 beats/min.
2. Pacemaker output control: The output control regulates the amount of electrical current (measured in milliamperes [mA]) that is delivered to the heart to initiate depolarization. The point at

TABLE 10-1
NASPE/BPEG GENERIC (NBG) CODE

POSITION I	II	III	IV	V
Chamber(s) paced	Chamber(s) sensed	Response to sensing	Programmability	Antitachydysrhythmia function(s)
0 = None	0 = None	0 = None	0 = None	0 = None
A = Atrium	A = Atrium	T = Triggered	P = Simple programmability (rate, output, sensitivity)	P = Pacing (antitachydysrhythmia)
V = Ventricle	V = Ventricle	I = Inhibited	M = Multiprogrammability	S = Shock
D = Dual (A + V)	D = Dual (A + V)	D = Dual (T + I)	C = Communicating	D = Dual (P + S)
			R = Rate modulation (rate responsive)	
S* = Single (A or V)	S = Single (A or V)			

Modified from Bernstein AD and others: The NASPE/BPEG generic pacemaker code for antibradycardia and adaptive rate pacing and antitachyarrhythmia devices, *PACE* 10:794, 1987.
*Used by manufacturer only.
NOTE: Positions I through III are used exclusively for antibradydysrhythmia function.
NASPE, North American Society of Pacing and Electrophysiology.
BPEG, British Pacing and Electrophysiology Group.
NBG, North American British Generic.

TABLE 10-2
EXAMPLES OF THREE-LETTER PACEMAKER CODE

PULSE GENERATOR	DESCRIPTION
AOO	Atrial fixed rate
	Atrial pacing, no sensing
VOO	Ventricular fixed rate
	Ventricular pacing, no sensing
DOO	AV sequential fixed rate
	Atrial and ventricular pacing, no sensing
VVI	Ventricular demand
	Ventricular pacing, ventricular sensing, inhibited response to sensing
VVT	Ventricular demand
	Ventricular pacing, ventricular sensing, triggered response to sensing
AAI	Atrial demand
	Atrial pacing, atrial sensing, inhibited response to sensing
AAT	Atrial demand
	Atrial pacing, atrial sensing, triggered response to sensing
VAT	AV synchronous
	Ventricular pacing, atrial sensing, triggered response to sensing. The ventricular pacing stimulus will fire at a set time after sensing of a spontaneous atrial depolarization.
DVI	AV sequential
	Atrial and ventricular pacing, ventricular sensing, inhibited response to sensing. Both atrial and ventricular pacing are inhibited if spontaneous ventricular depolarization is sensed; if no spontaneous ventricular activity is sensed, the atrium and ventricle will be paced sequentially.
VDD	Atrial synchronous, ventricular inhibited
	Ventricular pacing, atrial and ventricular sensing, inhibited response to sensing in the ventricle and triggered response to sensing in the atrium
DDD	Universal
	Both chambers are sensed and paced, inhibited response to sensing in the ventricle and triggered response to sensing in the atria

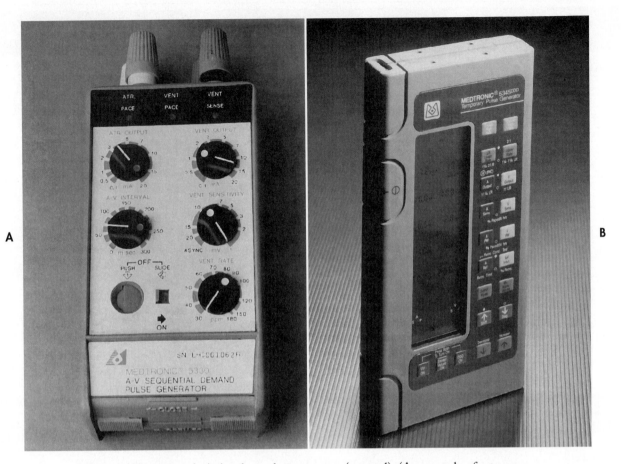

FIG. 10-2 Temporary dual-chamber pulse generators (external). (An example of a temporary single-chamber pulse generator is shown in Fig. 10-1.) **A,** AV sequential demand pulse generator. **B,** DDD pulse generator. (Courtesy Medtronic Inc., Minneapolis.)

which depolarization occurs is termed *threshold* and indicated by a myocardial response to the pacing stimulus (capture). Separate output controls for both the atrium and the ventricle are used with an AV sequential pulse generator.

3. Pacemaker sensitivity control: The sensitivity control regulates the ability of the pacemaker to detect the heart's intrinsic electrical activity. A sense indicator (often a light) on the pacemaker generator flashes each time it registers intrinsic cardiac electrical activity. The pacemaker's sensing ability can be quickly evaluated by observing this light flash and looking for ECG evidence of patients' intrinsic rhythm without pacemaker spikes.

4. Pacemaker AV interval: The AV interval control is available only on AV sequential pacers. It regulates the time interval in milliseconds (msec) between the atrial and ventricular pacing stimuli. Adjustment of this interval to between 150 and 250 msec preserves AV synchrony.

5. Pacemaker on/off safety switch: The on/off switch has a safety feature to prevent accidental termination of pacing.

6. Temporary DDD pacemakers: The new temporary DDD pacemakers have several other digital controls unique to this newer type of temporary pulse generator (Fig. 10-2, *B*). These include lower- and higher-rate pacing settings, and a programmable pulse width and atrial refractory period.

Pacing Artifacts

All patients with temporary pacemakers require continuous ECG monitoring. The pacing artifact is the spike seen on the ECG tracing as the pacing stimulus is delivered to the heart. A P wave should be visible after the pacing artifact if the atrium is being paced (Fig. 10-3, *A*). Similarly a QRS complex should follow a ventricular pacing artifact (Fig. 10-3, *B*). With dual chamber pacing a pacing artifact precedes both the P wave and the QRS complex (Fig. 10-3, *C*). The QRS of a ventricular paced beat is wide and bizarre and resembles a right ventricular PVC because the pacing electrode is usually in contact with the right ventricle.

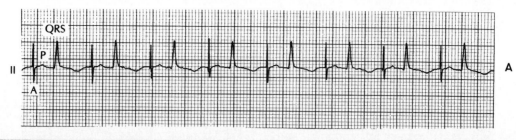

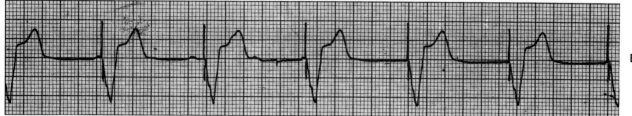

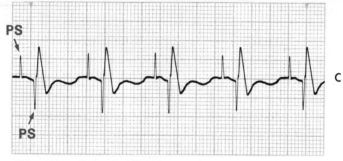

AV sequential pacemaker

FIG. 10-3 **A,** Atrial pacing. **B,** Ventricular pacing. **C,** Dual chamber pacing. (**A** from Goldberger AL, Goldberger E: *Clinical electrocardiography: a simplified approach,* ed 5, St Louis, 1994, Mosby; **B** from Conover MB: *Understanding electrocardiography: arrhythmias and the 12-lead ECG,* ed 6, St Louis, 1992, Mosby; **C** from Huszar RJ: *Basic dysrhythmias: interpretation and management,* ed 2, St Louis, 1993, Mosby.)

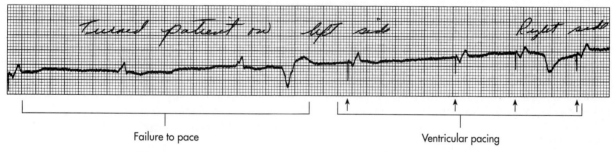

Failure to pace   Ventricular pacing

FIG. 10-4 Failure to pace. Pacemaker shows only intermittent ventricular pace spikes. Patient's heart rate is extremely low without pacemaker support. (From Kesten KS, Norton CK: *Pacemakers: patient care; troubleshooting, rhythm analysis,* 1985, Baltimore, Resource Applications, Inc.)

Pacemaker Complications

Most pacemaker complications that are recognized on ECG are categorized as abnormalities of either pacing or sensing.

Failure to fire

Failure of the pacemaker to deliver the pacing stimulus results in the disappearance of the pacing artifact, even though patients' intrinsic rate is less than the set rate on the pacer (Fig. 10-4). This can occur either intermittently or continuously and can be attributed to failure of the pulse generator, battery failure, a loose connection between the various components of the pacemaker system, broken lead wires, stimulus inhibition as a result of electromagnetic interference (EMI), or oversensing. Tightening connections, replacing the batteries or the pulse generator itself, removing the source of EMI, or adjusting the sensitivity control may restore pacemaker function.

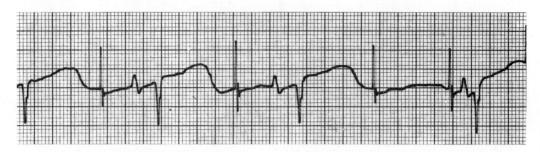

FIG. 10-5 Failure to capture. (From Conover MB: *Understanding electrocardiography: arrhythmias and the 12-lead ECG,* ed 6, St Louis, 1992, Mosby.)

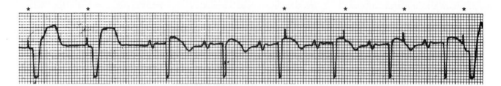

FIG. 10-6 Failure to sense. Notice that after the first two paced beats there is a series of sinus beats with first-degree AV block. Failure of the pacemaker unit to sense these intrinsic QRS complexes leads to inappropriate pacemaker spikes (*), which fall on T waves. Three of these spikes do not capture the ventricle because they occur during the refractory period of the cardiac cycle. (From Conover MB: *Understanding electrocardiography: arrhythmias and the 12-lead ECG,* ed 6, St Louis, 1992, Mosby.)

Failure to capture

If the pacing stimulus fires but fails to initiate a myocardial depolarization, a pacing artifact will be present but not followed by the expected P wave or QRS complex, depending on the chamber being paced (Fig. 10-5). This "loss of capture" can most often be attributed either to displacement of the pacing electrode or an increase in threshold (electrical stimulus necessary to elicit a myocardial depolarization) as a result of drugs, metabolic disorders, electrolyte imbalances, and fibrosis or myocardial ischemia at the site of electrode placement. Repositioning patients to the left side or increasing the output (milliamperes [mA]) may elicit capture.

Failure to sense

Failure to sense is the inability of the pacemaker to sense spontaneous myocardial depolarizations. This malfunction results in competition between paced complexes and the heart's intrinsic rhythm and is demonstrated on the ECG by pacing artifacts that follow too closely or in the middle of spontaneous QRS complexes (Fig. 10-6). Because the "R on T" phenomenon is a real danger with this type of pacer aberration, nurses must act quickly to determine the cause, which can often be attributed to an inadequate sensitivity threshold. This situation can be promptly remedied by increasing the sensitivity (moving the sensitivity dial toward its lowest setting). Other possible causes include lead displacement or fracture, pulse generator failure, or EMI-precipitated asynchronous pacing.

Oversensing

Oversensing results from the inappropriate sensing of extraneous electrical signals leading to unnecessary triggering or inhibiting of stimulus output, depending on the pacer mode. In the critical care environment the source of these electrical signals can range from the presence of tall, peaked T waves to EMI. Because most temporary pulse generators in use today are ventricular inhibited, oversensing results in unexplained pauses in the ECG tracing as the extraneous signals are sensed and inhibit ventricular pacing. Often, simply moving the sensitivity dial toward 20 mV stops the pauses.

Nursing Management

Nursing management of patients with a temporary pacemaker incorporates a variety of nursing diagnoses (Box 10-4). **Nursing priorities are directed toward detecting complications, preventing microshock, eliminating electromagnetic interference (EMI), securing pacemaker connections, and educating patients and families.**

Detecting complications

Continuous assessment of the ECG is required to detect problems with pacing or sensing, as previously discussed. Infection at the lead insertion site is another possible complication. During daily dressing changes the site is inspected for purulent drainage, erythema, or edema, and patients are observed for signs of systemic infection. Site

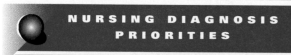

care must be performed according to the institution's policy and procedures. Although most infections remain localized, endocarditis can occur in patients with endocardial pacing leads. A rare complication associated with transvenous pacing leads is myocardial perforation, which can result in rhythmic hiccoughs or cardiac tamponade.

Preventing microshock

Because the pacing electrode is in intimate contact with the heart, nurses must take special care while handling the external components of the pacing system to avoid conducting stray electrical current from other equipment. Even a small amount of stray current could precipitate a lethal tachycardia. The possibility of microshock can be minimized by wearing rubber gloves when handling the pacing wires and properly insulating terminal pins of pacing wires when they are not in use. The latter can be accomplished by either using caps provided by the manufacturer or improvising with a needle cover or section of disposable rubber glove. The wires are then taped securely to patients' chest to avoid accidental electrode displacement. Additional safety measures include using a nonelectric or a properly grounded electric bed, keeping all electrical equipment away from the bed, and permitting the use of only rechargeable electric razors.

Eliminating EMI

It is important to be aware of all sources of EMI that could interfere with effective pacemaker function. Sources of EMI in the critical care area include electrocautery, defibrillation, radiation therapy, magnetic resonance imaging devices, and transcutaneous electrical nerve stimulation units. If EMI is suspected of precipitating pacemaker malfunction, converting to the asynchronous mode (fixed-rate) will in most cases maintain pacing until the cause of the EMI can be removed. If patients require defibrillation, the pulse generator should be temporarily turned off during delivery of the shock to prevent possible damage to the pacemaker circuitry.

Securing pacemaker connections

The temporary pacing lead and bridging cable should be taped to the body to prevent accidental displacement of the electrode, which can result in failure to pace or sense. The external pulse generator can be secured to patients' waists with a strap or placed in a telemetry bag for mobile patients. For patients on a regimen of bed rest the pulse generator can be suspended with twill tape from an intravenous (IV) pole. Nurses regularly inspect for loose connections between lead and pulse generator. In addition, replacement batteries and pulse generators must be available on the unit. Although the battery has an anticipated life span of 1 month, the policy for many units is to change the battery if the pacemaker has been operating continually for several days. The pulse generator should always be labeled with the date that the battery was replaced.

Educating patients and families

Education for patients with a temporary pacemaker emphasizes safety precautions. Patients are instructed to refrain from handling any exposed portion of the lead wires and notify nurses should the dressing over the insertion site become wet, soiled, or dislodged. Patients are also advised not to use any electrical devices brought from home that could interfere with pacemaker functioning. Furthermore, patients with temporary or permanent transvenous pacemakers are asked to restrict movement of the affected arm to prevent accidental lead displacement.

Cardiac Surgery

The nursing management of patients undergoing cardiac surgery is demanding, exciting work that requires the talents of an experienced team of critical care nurses. The following discussion introduces basic cardiac surgical techniques and principles of cardiopulmonary bypass and highlights key points about postoperative care of adult patients who require valve replacement or coronary artery revascularization.

Coronary Artery Bypass Surgery

Since its introduction more than 2 decades ago, **coronary artery bypass graft (CABG)** surgery has proved both safe and effective in relieving medically uncontrolled angina pectoris in most patients. Many patients now have the choice between undergoing open heart surgery or a catheter-based procedure such as angioplasty. However, CABG is still recommended for patients with left main or diffuse multivessel coronary artery disease. See Chapter 9 for a complete discussion of CAD and associated clinical complications. Myocardial revascularization involves the use of a conduit or channel designed to bypass an occluded coronary artery. Currently the two most successful conduits are the saphenous vein graft

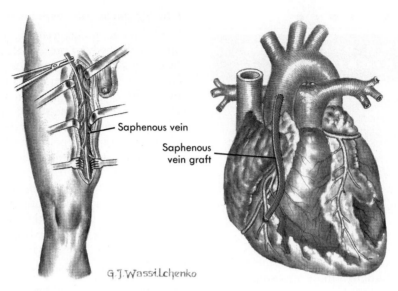

G.J.Wassilchenko

FIG. 10-7 Saphenous vein graft.

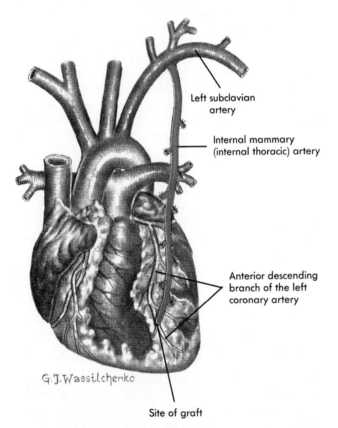

G.J.Wassilchenko

FIG. 10-8 Internal mammary artery graft.

(SVG) and the internal mammary artery graft (IMA). The SVG is taken from the leg and surgically anastomosed from the aorta to the coronary artery, bypassing the obstruction (Fig. 10-7). The IMA, which usually remains attached to its origin at the subclavian artery, is dissected free of connecting vessels, swung down, and anastomosed distal to the coronary artery occlusion (Fig. 10-8). Both the right IMA and left IMA may be used

as conduits. The IMA graft is the conduit of choice because it has demonstrated short-term and long-term patency rates superior to those of SVG.[3]

Valvular Surgery

Valvular disease results in various hemodynamic dysfunctions that can usually be managed medically for as long as patients remain free of symptoms. Clinicians are reluctant to intervene surgically early in the course of the disease because of the surgical risks and long-term complications associated with prosthetic valve replacement. This consequence, however, must be weighed against the possibility of irreversible deterioration in left ventricular function that may develop during the compensated asymptomatic phase. Chapter 9 contains a complete discussion of valvular heart disease. Surgical therapy for aortic valve disease is limited at this time to aortic valve replacement. However, three surgical procedures are available to treat mitral valve disease: commissurotomy, mitral valve repair, and mitral valve replacement. Commissurotomy is performed for mitral stenosis and involves incising fused leaflets to increase valve mobility. Mitral valve repair is indicated for mitral regurgitation. In addition, a ring or annulus is used to reduce the size of the dilated mitral valve. This procedure is called an *annuloplasty*. Both these forms of valve reconstruction avoid the complications associated with a prosthetic valve and may obviate the need for long-term anticoagulation.[4,5] The mitral valve is replaced if it cannot be repaired.

Prosthetic Valves

There are two categories of prosthetic valves: mechanical and biologic, or tissue valves. Mechanical valves are made from combinations of metal alloys, pyrolite carbon,

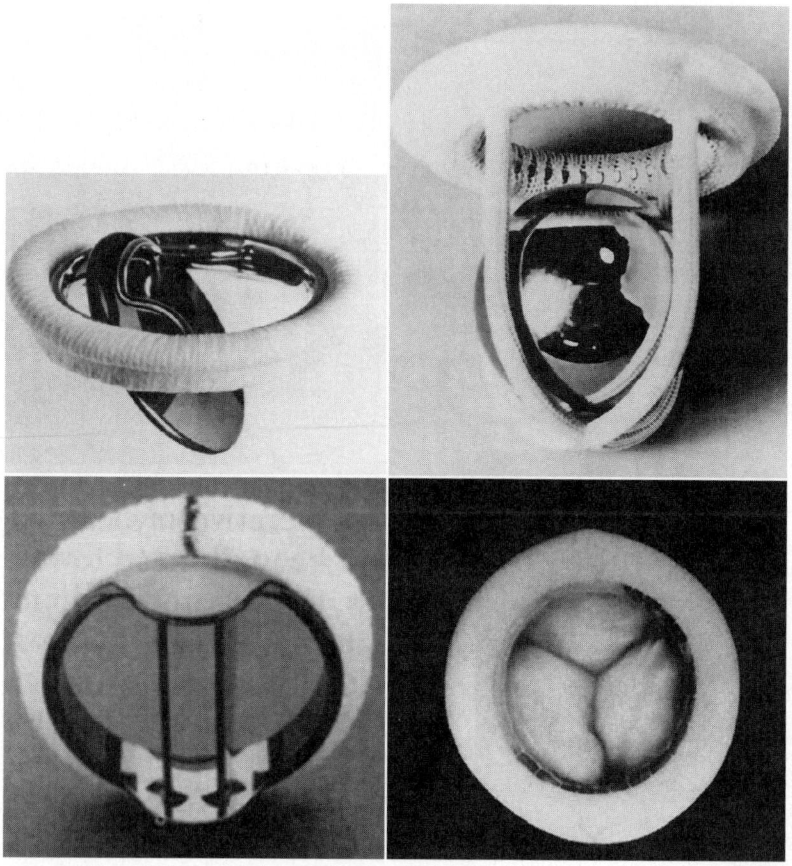

FIG. 10-9   Replacement Heart Valves. **A,** The Bjork-Shiley tilting disk valve with pyrolytic-carbon disk, stellite cage, and Teflon cloth sewing ring. The valve opens to 60 degrees. **B,** Starr-Edwards caged-ball valve with completely cloth-covered stellite cage and hollow stellite ball with specific gravity close to that of blood. **C,** St. Jude mechanical heart valve, a mechanical central flow disk. **D,** Hancock II porcine aortic valve. The flexible Derlin stent and sewing ring are covered in dacron cloth. (**A, B,** and **D** from Eagle K and others: *The practice of cardiology,* ed 2, Boston, 1989, Little, Brown & Co; **C** courtesy St. Jude Medical, Inc., Copyright 1993, St Paul, Minn.)

Dacron, and Teflon (Fig. 10-9, *A, B, C*). Their construction renders them highly durable, but all patients require anticoagulation to reduce the incidence of thromboembolism. Biologic, or tissue valves, are usually constructed from animal or human cardiac tissue, have low thrombogenicity, and offer patients freedom from therapeutic anticoagulation. Their durability, however, is limited by a tendency toward early calcification (Fig. 10-9, *D*). Box 10-5 describes various valvular prostheses.

Choice of Valve

The choice of a valvular prosthesis depends on many factors. For example, because mechanical valves are more durable, one may be chosen over a tissue valve for a young person whose expected life span is relatively long. Similarly, a bioprosthesis (tissue valve) may be chosen for a patient who is older than 65 years of age because the reduced longevity of the valve is consistent with the patient's decreased life expectancy. Patients with medical

contraindications to anticoagulation and patients whose past compliance with drug therapy has been questionable should receive tissue valves. Technical considerations such as the size of the annulus (anatomic ring in which the valve sits) also influence the choice of valve.

Cardiopulmonary Bypass

Cardiopulmonary bypass (CPB) is a mechanical means of circulating and oxygenating patients' blood while diverting most of the circulation from the heart and lungs during cardiac surgical procedures. The extracorporeal circuit consists of cannulas that drain off venous blood, an oxygenator that oxygenates the blood, and a pump that pumps the arterialized blood back to the aorta through a single cannula. Patients are systemically heparinized before initiation of bypass to prevent clotting within the bypass circuit. At the end of cardiopulmonary bypass the heparin effect is reversed with protamine sulphate.

CLASSIFICATION OF PROSTHETIC CARDIAC VALVES

MECHANICAL VALVES

Tilting-disk: a lens-shaped disk mounted onto a circular sewing ring
   Bjork-Shiley
   Omniscience (Lillehei-Kaster)
   Medtronic-Hall (Hall-Kaster)
Caged-ball: a ball moves freely within a three- or four-sided metallic cage mounted on a circular sewing ring
   Starr-Edwards
Bileaflet: two semicircular leaflets, mounted on a circular sewing ring, that open centrally
   St. Jude Medical

BIOLOGIC TISSUE VALVES (BIOPROSTHESES)

Porcine heterograft: a porcine aortic valve mounted on a semiflexible stent
   Hancock
   Carpentier-Edwards
Bovine pericardial heterograft: bovine pericardium fashioned into three identical cusps that are then mounted on a cloth-covered frame
   Ionescu-Shiley
Homograft: a human heart valve (aortic or pulmonic) harvested from a donated heart and cryopreserved; may or may not be mounted on a support ring

Hypothermia During CPB

Systemic hypothermia during bypass is induced to reduce tissue oxygen requirements to 50% of normal to protect major organs from ischemic injury. Lowering the body temperature to about 28 I SD C° (82.4 I SD F°) is accomplished through a heat exchanger in the pump. The blood is warmed back up to normal body temperature before bypass is discontinued (Table 10-3).

Hemodilution During CPB

Hemodilution is used to improve blood circulation during bypass. *Hemodilution* refers to the dilution of patients' blood with the isotonic crystalloid solution used to prime the pump. Capillary perfusion is enhanced by hemodilution because reduced blood viscosity (stickiness) decreases the possibility of microthrombi formation. At the completion of CPB the large quantities of "pump blood" that remain in the bypass circuit are collected and used for initial postoperative volume replacement.

Nursing Management

Nursing management of patients following cardiac surgery incorporates a variety of nursing diagnoses (Box 10-

TABLE 10-3
PHYSIOLOGIC EFFECTS OF CARDIOPULMONARY BYPASS (CPB)

EFFECTS	CAUSES
Intravascular fluid deficit (hypotension)	Third spacing
	Postoperative diuresis
	Sudden vasodilation (drugs, rewarming)
Third spacing (weight gain, edema)	Decreased plasma protein concentration
	Increased capillary permeability
Myocardial depression (decreased cardiac output)	Hypothermia
	Increased systemic vascular resistance
	Prolonged CPB pump run
	Preexisting heart disease
	Inadequate myocardial protection
Coagulopathy (bleeding)	Systemic heparinization
	Mechanical trauma to platelets
	Depressed release of clotting factors from liver as a result of hypothermia
Pulmonary dysfunction (decreased lung mechanics and impaired gas exchange)	Decreased surfactant production
	Pulmonary microemboli
	Interstitial fluid accumulation in lungs
Hemolysis (hemoglobinuria)	Red blood cells damaged in pump circuit
Hyperglycemia (rise in serum glucose)	Decreased insulin release
	Stimulation of glycogenolysis
Hypokalemia (low serum potassium) and	Intracellular shifts during bypass
Hypomagnesemia (low serum magnesium)	Postoperative diuresis secondary to hemodilution
Neurologic dysfunction (decreased level of consciousness, motor/sensory deficits)	Inadequate cerebral perfusion
	Microemboli to brain (air, plaque fragments, fat globules)
Hypertension (transient rise in blood pressure)	Catecholamine release and systemic hypothermia causing vasoconstriction

6). **Nursing priorities are directed toward optimizing cardiac output, controlling postoperative bleeding, preventing pulmonary complications, monitoring neurologic recovery, preserving renal function, preventing infection, and educating patients and families.**

Optimizing cardiac output

Many factors may contribute to a low cardiac output (CO) following open heart surgery, including preexisting heart disease, prolonged CPB run, and inadequate myocardial protection. Critical care nurses maximize cardiac output by adjusting heart rate, preload, afterload, and contractility.

HEART RATE AND CO. The heart rate can be regulated with temporary pacing or drug therapy. Temporary epicardial pacing is often used when the heart rate drops below 80 beats/min. Because ventricular ectopy can result from hypokalemia, serum potassium levels are maintained in the high normal range (4.5 to 5.0 mEq/L).

PRELOAD AND CO. Low preload is a frequent cause of postoperative low CO. To enhance preload, clinicians administer volume in the form of colloid, packed red cells, or crystalloid solutions. It is not uncommon to achieve greatest hemodynamic stability when filling pressures (PAWP) are in the range of 18 to 20 mm Hg (normal 5 to 12 mm Hg).

SYSTEMIC VASCULAR RESISTANCE (SVR) AND CO. High SVR, also described as *afterload* or *resistance to ventricular ejection*, occurs as a result of the vasoconstrictive effect of hypothermia during CPB. This phenomenon lowers cardiac output and predisposes patients to hypertension. Vasodilator therapy with intravenous sodium nitroprusside (Nipride) is used to reduce afterload, control hypertension, and improve cardiac output.

CONTRACTILITY AND CO. Myocardial contractility is enhanced with positive inotropic medications or in-traaortic balloon pumping (IABP) to augment circulation.

Controlling postoperative bleeding

Some postoperative bleeding from the mediastinal chest tubes is expected. Excessive bleeding is due to either a coagulopathy or surgical leak. Clotting factors are normalized by administration of fresh frozen plasma, platelets, and additional protamine to reverse the effect of heparin. Blood volume is replaced. If mediastinal bleeding persists despite normalization of clotting studies, patients usually return to the operating room for reexploration of the surgical site. Throughout the bleeding episode, critical care nurses are responsible for replacing intravascular volume to maintain the CO.

Preventing pulmonary complications

Extubating patients who have undergone cardiac surgery on the day of surgery is becoming common.[6] Extubation is achieved by use of short acting anesthetic agents and decreased use of narcotics. A shorter intubation decreases the incidence of postoperative pulmonary complications. Following extubation, supplemental oxygen is administered, and patients are medicated for postoperative chest pain so they will cough and breathe deeply to prevent atelectasis.

Monitoring neurologic recovery

The neurologic recovery of most patients following cardiac surgery and CPB is uneventful. However, transient confusion, especially in the elderly, is not uncommon, and a small percentage of patients experience coma or stroke from emboli or hypoperfusion.[7]

Preserving renal function

Because of the crystalloid prime solution used in CPB, most patients have a positive fluid balance following surgery. Diuretics such as furosemide (Lasix) are given to promote urine flow. Occasionally the urine may be red or pink following CPB. This change in color is caused by hemolysis of red blood cells during CPB. Diuretics are used to "flush the kidneys" at the end of surgery and prevent damage to renal tubules.

Preventing infection

Postoperative fever is common after CPB as part of the rewarming process. However, persistent temperature elevation above 101 I SD F° (37.8 I SD C°) requires investigation. Sternal wound infections and infective endocarditis are the most devastating infectious complications, but leg wound infection, pneumonia, and urinary tract infection can also occur.[8]

Educating patients and families

Before surgery patients and families must discuss all the risks and benefits of the surgery with the cardiovascular surgeon. Most hospitals also provide comprehensive education about the procedure, critical care unit, equipment such as the endotracheal tube and ventilator, and expected length of stay following the operation. In the hours immediately following the operation the educational focus is limited to brief explanations about the recovery from anesthesia and cardiopulmonary bypass. Once awake, extubated, and hemodynamically stable, patients are transferred from the critical care unit to a telemetry or medical-surgical unit. Education for discharge is focused on gradual resumption of normal activity, modification of cardiac risk factors, and cardiac medications. In the first 6 weeks following surgery patients are asked to avoid lifting any weight over 10 pounds to prevent strain on the sternum that might interfere with healing.

Implantable Cardioverter Defibrillator

Indications

Since 1980 when the first **implantable cardioverter defibrillator (ICD)** was used clinically, over 500,000 devices have been implanted worldwide.[9] Designed to identify and terminate life-threatening ventricular dysrhythmias, the ICD is indicated for patients who have survived a cardiac arrest or who have ventricular tachyrhythmias poorly controlled by antidysrhythmic drugs. The ICD system contains sensing electrodes to recognize the dysrhythmia, as well as defibrillation electrodes or patches that are in contact with the heart and can deliver a shock.[10] These electrodes are connected to a generator that is surgically placed in the subcutaneous tissue in the upper left abdominal quadrant (Fig. 10-10). The early model ICD generators could defibrillate or cardiovert only lethal dysrhythmias. Recent improvements in ICD design include the use of tiered therapy generators that incorporate antitachycardia pacing, bradycardia back-up pacing, low-energy cardioversion, and high-energy defibrillation options. With tiered therapy, antitachycardia pacing is used as the first line of treatment in many cases of ventricular tachycardia (VT). If the VT can be successfully pace-terminated, patients do not receive a shock from the generator and may not even realize that the ICD terminated the dysrhythmia. If programmed bursts of pacing do not terminate the VT, the ICD will cardiovert the rhythm. If the dysrhythmia deteriorates into ventricular fibrillation (VF), the ICD is programmed to defibrillate at a higher energy. Should the dysrhythmia terminate spontaneously, the device will not discharge[10] (Fig. 10-10, *C*). Occasionally the electrical rhythm may deteriorate to asystole or a slow idioventricular rhythm. In such cases the bradycardia backup pacing function is activated. With the most recent technology the ICD battery will last about 4 years before a replacement is necessary.

ICD Insertion

The ICD has progressed not only in the area of programmable functions but also in the insertion design. Initially all ICDs were implanted during open heart surgery, with electrode patches sewn directly onto the epicardium, or by means of a thoracotomy incision, with the patches attached to the outside of the pericardium. Currently, several new devices render a thoracic surgical intervention unnecessary. Transvenous electrode leads are inserted into the subclavian vein and advanced into the right side of the heart, where contact with the heart endocardium is achieved. An additional subcutaneous patch may be placed with some models to improve defibrillation efficacy. The endocardial leads are used for sensing, pacing, cardioversion, and defibrillation and are connected to the generator by tunneling through the subcutaneous tissue rather than performing surgery. The endocardial lead system offers several advantages: it is less invasive and costly, requires only an overnight hospital stay, and is less traumatic to patients and family. As ICDs become smaller, some have been placed in the pectoral position, similar to a permanent pacemaker implant.[11]

Nursing Management

Nurses should know what type of ICD was implanted, how the device functions, and whether it is activated (on) (Box 10-7). **The priorities of nursing care for patients with an ICD include monitoring dysrhythmias, recognizing complications, and educating patients and families.**

Monitoring dysrhythmias

Most patients who have an ICD implant continue to take antidysrhythmic medications, although the dosages may be lower than before the ICD implant. The medications decrease the frequency of life-threatening VT or VF and thus prolong battery life. Patients with new ICDs have continuous ECG monitoring to detect correct ICD func-

BOX 10-7

NURSING DIAGNOSIS PRIORITIES

IMPLANTABLE CARDIOVERTER DEFIBRILLATOR

- *Decreased Cardiac Output* related to ventricular tachycardia, p. 477
- Acute *Pain* related to transmission and perception of ischemic impulses secondary to ICD generator discharge, p. 499
- *Body Image Disturbance* related to actual change in body structure and appearance secondary to implant of ICD generator and lead system, p. 458
- *Knowledge Deficit:* Preimplant and Postimplant Teaching, What ICD Does, and What Generator "Shock" Feels Like related to no previous exposure, p. 455

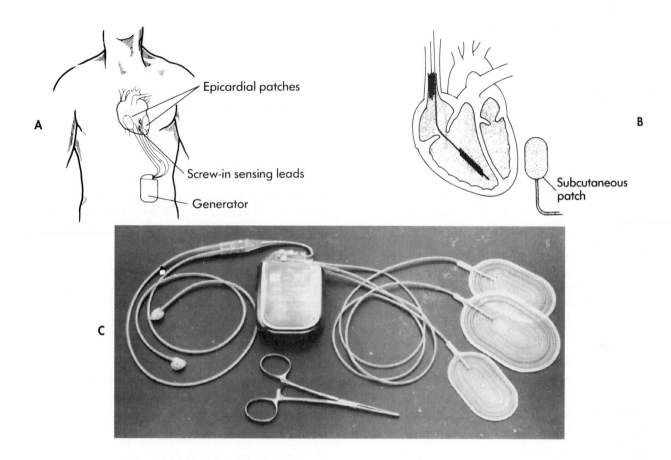

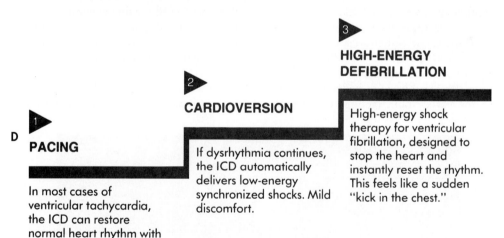

FIG. 10-10 **A,** Placement of an implantable cardioverter defibrillator (ICD) and epicardial lead system. The generator is placed in a subcutaneous "pocket" in the left upper abdominal quadrant. The epicardial screw-in sensing leads monitor the heart rhythm and connect to the generator. If a life-threatening dysrhythmia is sensed, the generator can pace-terminate the dysrhythmia or deliver electrical cardioversion or defibrillation through the epicardial patches. With this system the leads/patches must be placed during open-chest (sternal or thoracotomy) surgery. **B,** In the transvenous lead system, open-chest surgery is not required. The pacing/cardioversion/defibrillation functions are all contained in a lead (or leads) inserted into the right atrium and ventricle. A subcutaneous patch may be placed under the skin. **C,** An example of an ICD tiered therapy generator (Medtronic PCD) with epicardial screw-in sensing leads and patches. **D,** Tiered therapy is designed to use increasing levels of intensity to terminate ventricular dysrhythmias. (Courtesy Medtronic Inc., Minneapolis.)

tion in the event of a dysrhythmia. During an episode of VT or VF nurses monitor the ECG to ensure that the device terminates the dysrhythmia successfully.

Recognizing complications

Complications associated with the ICD include infection of the implanted system, broken leads, and inappropriate sensing of supraventricular tachydysrhythmias, resulting in unneeded discharges.[10,12]

Educating patients and family

Education of patients and families facilitates a positive psychologic adjustment to the ICD. Many centers have successfully used family support groups to assist patients following the ICD implant. Nurses explain that while the ICD is programmed to terminate a lethal arrhythmia, it will not cure the underlying heart disease that causes the arrhythmias. Many patients have severe heart failure from either cardiomyopathy or a previous MI, and the ICD will not lessen the symptoms caused by these disorders.

Catheter Interventions for Coronary Artery Disease

Percutaneous Transluminal Coronary Angioplasty (PTCA)

PTCA

Percutaneous transluminal coronary angioplasty (PTCA), often referred to simply as **angioplasty,** involves the use of a balloon-tipped catheter that, when advanced through an atherosclerotic coronary lesion, can be inflated intermittently to dilate the stenotic area and improve blood flow through it (Fig. 10-11). The high balloon inflation pressure stretches the vessel wall, fractures the plaque, and enlarges the vessel lumen. PTCA provides an alternative to both traditional medical management of atherosclerotic heart disease and CABG surgery.

Indications

Indications for PTCA have broadened considerably. Whereas once only patients with single-vessel disease were considered for PTCA, now patients with multivessel disease—even those who have previously undergone saphenous vein and internal mammary artery grafting—may be eligible for this procedure. Because complications such as abrupt closure may arise during angioplasty, the availability of cardiac surgical services on site is necessary. However, urgent bypass surgery is required in less than 3% of cases.

PTCA procedure

PTCA is performed in the cardiac catheterization laboratory by means of fluoroscopy. Introducer sheaths are inserted percutaneously into the femoral artery and vein. The venous sheath can be used to perform a right ventricular catheterization with a pulmonary artery (PA) catheter or to insert a pacing catheter. Patients are systemically heparinized to prevent clots from forming on or in any of the catheters. A special guiding catheter designed to engage the coronary ostia is inserted through the femoral arterial sheath and advanced retrograde through the aorta. Nitroglycerin or calcium channel blockers may be given at this time to prevent coronary artery spasm and maximize coronary vasodilation during the procedure. A guidewire is then advanced down the coronary artery across the occluding atheroma. The balloon catheter is advanced over this guidewire and positioned across the lesion. The balloon is inflated and deflated repetitively (each inflation not to exceed 90 seconds) until evidence of dilatation is demonstrated on an-

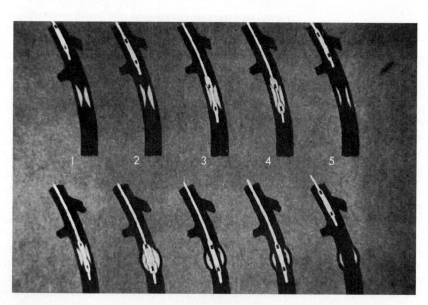

FIG. 10-11 Balloon compression of an atherosclerotic lesion. (From Kinney M and others: *Comprehensive cardiac care,* ed 7, St Louis, 1991, Mosby.)

giogram. In cases that require prolonged balloon inflations, an autoperfusion angioplasty catheter, which has side holes that allow blood flow through the central lumen to the distal coronary artery, is used.

Atherectomy, Stents, and Lasers

Coronary atherectomy, placement of endovascular prostheses (stents), and laser angioplasty are newer interventional technologies developed to address the problems of acute closure and restenosis associated with PTCA.[13]

Atherectomy

Atherectomy is the excision and removal of the atherosclerotic plaque by cutting, shaving, or grinding; specialized coronary catheters are used to achieve a more controlled mechanism of injury, with the hope of fewer complications.[14] Three atherectomy devices are described in Table 10-4: Directional Coronary Atherectomy (Fig. 10-12), Rotoblader,[15] and Transluminal Extraction Catheter. All three devices are FDA approved for use in coronary and peripheral arteries.

Coronary stent

Another major coronary technology that has recently evolved is the coronary stent. The stent is introduced into the coronary artery over a guidewire, into a region that has been previously dilated with PTCA. It is used to prevent abrupt closure and obtain a larger vessel lumen diameter.[16,17] Once the stent is positioned at the target side, it is expanded and the catheter removed. Several types of stents are available. As shown in Fig. 10-13, stents have either thermal memory (Fig. 10-13, *A*) or are self-expanding (Fig. 10-13, *B*) or balloon expandable (Fig. 10-13, *C*). At present, stents are not a routine procedure but are used when angioplasty or atherectomy has failed.

Anticoagulation with a stent

Because the stent is a foreign object (generally made of stainless steel) the stent's presence in the coronary artery activates the coagulation cascade. Patients are anticoagulated with IV heparin both during and after the procedure to prevent acute thrombosis of the stent. The efficacy of anticoagulation is assessed by the partial thromboplastin time (PTT) or activated clotting time (ACT) every 4 to 6 hours. Subsequently warfarin sodium (Coumadin) is used to make the transition to oral anticoagulation. Bleeding is the major risk factor after a stent is placed. **Nursing priorities are directed toward prevention of bleeding complications,** especially when the introducer sheaths are removed. Other drugs used to decrease platelet adhesiveness include IV Dextran infusion and oral low-dose aspirin. Conventional medications for treatment of coronary artery disease, such as IV nitroglycerin and calcium channel blockers, are also prescribed. The average hospital stay for a stent procedure is 5 to 7 days because of the intensive anticoagulation required. Within 3 to 6 weeks the stent surface is covered by endothelium, and anticoagulation is no longer required.

Laser

Laser is an acronym for *Light Amplification by Stimulated Emission of Radiation.* Laser plaque ablation in coronary arteries, using the Excimer laser, is currently undergoing clinical trials. The Excimer laser is a contact cutter, meaning that it only ablates tissue it touches. The catheter is advanced by a guidewire system similar to that used in angioplasty. The Excimer laser (sometimes de-

---

TABLE 10-4
ATHERECTOMY DEVICES

DEVICE	DESIGN	USES
Directional atherectomy (Simpson Atherocath)	Rotating cup-shaped cutter within a windowed cylindric housing; plaque that protrudes into window is shaved off and collected within nose cone of cutter housing	Ostial lesions SVG Eccentric lesions in large vessels Proximal, discrete lesions
Rotational ablation (Rotablator)	A high-speed rotating diamond-studded bur; "sanding effect"; generates microparticles that pass distally into microcirculation	Distal lesions Long, diffuse lesions Tortuous vessels Calcified lesions Eccentric lesions Ostial lesions Small vessels
Transluminal extraction catheter (TEC)	Motorized cutting head with triangular blades; excised plaque removed by suction	Diffuse disease SVG

SVG, Saphenous venous graft.

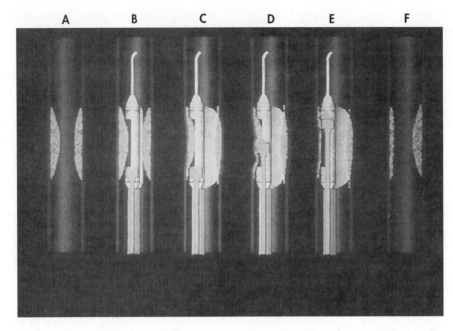

FIG. 10-12 Directional coronary atherectomy: **A,** Atheroma (plaque) in vessel lumen; **B,** Simpson atherocath (DCA device) in position; **C,** Inflation of low-pressure support balloon that pushes the plaque into the "window" of the device (the ability to turn the atherocath in different directions within the artery explains the name of the DCA device); **D,** The cutter begins to shear away plaque; **E,** The plaque is pushed into the nose cone (collection chamber) of the atherocath; **F,** Vessel lumen shows decreased plaque after removal of catheter.

scribed as a *cold laser*) uses high-energy, pulsed ultraviolet light to vaporize plaque and is particularly suited for distal disease and occluded SVG.[16]

Complications

Early complications

Serious complications can result from PTCA, atherectomy, stent, and laser that necessitate emergency CABG surgery. These complications include persistent coronary artery spasm, myocardial infarction, and acute coronary occlusion. Other complications that can occur in the period immediately after the procedure include bleeding and hematoma formation at the site of vascular cannulation, compromised blood flow to the involved extremity, allergic reaction to radiopaque contrast dye, dysrhythmias, and vasovagal response (hypotension, bradycardia, and diaphoresis) during manipulation or removal of introducer sheaths.

Late complications

Restenosis can occur up to 6 months after PTCA, atherectomy, or stent; however, this late complication is typically amenable to a repeat procedure. The mechanism involved in restenosis is thought to be related to intimal hyperplasia and platelet deposition. For this reason patients are prescribed antiplatelet drugs, usually low dose aspirin.

BOX 10-8

NURSING DIAGNOSIS PRIORITIES

Post PTCA, Coronary Atherectomy, or Stent

- *Altered Myocardial Tissue Perfusion* related to acute myocardial ischemia, p. 480
- Acute *Pain* related to transmission and perception of ischemic impulses secondary to abrupt coronary artery closure, p. 499
- *Fluid Volume Deficit* related to active blood loss, p. 503
- *Risk for Peripheral Neurovascular Dysfunction* risk factor, p. 479
- *Knowledge deficit:* related to medications, CAD risk factor modification, activity restrictions, and reportable symptoms related to no previous exposure, p. 455

Nursing Management

Following angioplasty, atherectomy, or stent patients are transferred to a specialized critical care unit. Nursing management of patients following a catheter interventional procedure incorporates a variety of nursing diagnoses (Box 10-8). **Nursing priorities are directed to-**

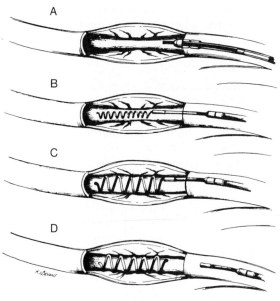

A. Stent is cooled with ice and straightened in catheter for placement.
B. Exposed to blood temperature, coil begins to expand.
C. Coil expands to full size in coronary artery.
D. Stent is released from delivery device and supports vessel. Catheter is removed from coronary artery.

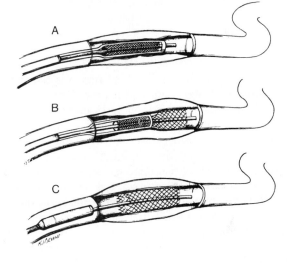

A. Stent is constricted in constraining catheter.
B. Stent is released from catheter.
C. Stent is fully expanded to support vessel. Catheter is removed from coronary artery.

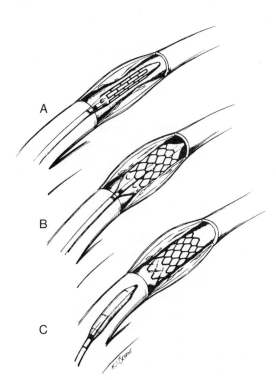

A. Stent is crimped onto balloon catheter for placement.
B. Stent is expanded against vessel wall.
C. Stent is supporting the vessel wall. Balloon catheter is withdrawn from coronary artery.

FIG. 10-13 Intracoronary stents. **Top,** Nitinol stent (heat sensitive). **Middle,** Medinvent stent (self-expanding). **Bottom,** Palmaz-Schatz stent (balloon expandable). (Modified from Bevans M, McLimore E: *J Cardiovasc Nurs* 7(1):34, 1992.)

ward managing the introducer sheaths, monitoring for recurrent chest pain, preventing limb ischemia, and educating patients and families.

Managing the introducer sheaths

The introducer sheaths are left in place for 6 to 24 hours for two reasons. (1) The IV infusion of heparin is continued to prevent clot formation on the roughened endothelium within the coronary artery. The sheaths cannot be removed during this time because of the risk of bleeding at the femoral insertion site. (2) Presence of the sheath allows for rapid vascular access should reintervention become necessary. The arterial sheath is attached to a continuous heparinized saline flush, and intravenous fluids are infused through the venous sheath to maintain luminal patency. If patients' postprocedure course is uneventful, the sheaths are removed within 24 hours. Following PTCA, atherectomy, and laser, patients may be discharged to home 6 to 12 hours after sheath removal and ambulation. The hospital stay is longer for patients who are treated with stents because of the prolonged anticoagulation.

Monitoring for recurrent chest pain

Observing patients for recurrent angina is essential. The occurrence of angina during the procedure is expected at the time of balloon inflation and caused by the temporary interruption of blood flow through the involved artery. It should subside, however, with deflation or removal of the balloon and the administration of nitroglycerin. Angina after a coronary interventional procedure may result from coronary vasospasm, thrombosis, or dissection within the coronary artery. Nurses must act quickly to obtain a 12-lead ECG, titrate IV nitroglycerin to alleviate chest pain, and inform physicians because patients may need to return to the cardiac catheterization laboratory for redilation or the operating room for emergency CABG surgery.

Controlling bleeding

While the femoral sheaths are in place or after their removal, bleeding or hematoma at the sheath insertion site may occur as a result of the effects of heparin. Nurses observe patients for bleeding or swelling at the puncture site and frequently assess adequacy of circulation to the involved extremity. Nurses also assess patients for back pain, which can indicate retroperitoneal bleeding from oozing femoral puncture sites. Patients are instructed to keep the involved leg straight and not to elevate the head of the bed any more than 30 degrees to prevent dislodgment of the sheath and bleeding. After sheath removal, direct pressure is applied to the puncture site for 15 to 30 minutes; a sandbag may be ordered if direct pressure is inadequate for hemostasis. Patients are usually allowed to resume ambulation 6 to 8 hours later, depending on institutional protocol. Excessive bleeding or hematoma formation can become a serious problem because it may result in hypotension or compromised blood flow to the involved extremity, or both, thus necessitating surgical intervention in rare cases.

Preventing limb ischemia

A potential complication of the introducer sheath in the femoral artery is ischemia of the distal limb, which may occur secondary to arterial occlusion by the sheath itself or by emboli from thrombus formation. Therefore the peripheral pulses distal to the catheter insertion site are assessed frequently for pulsation quality, color, temperature, and capillary refill. Doppler localization of peripheral pulses is required if pulses are difficult to palpate on the cannulated limb. Signs of diminished perfusion must be reported immediately. Nursing interventions to avoid kinking or clotting of the arterial sheath include elevating the head of the bed no more than 30 degrees and avoiding any flexion of the involved hip.

Educating patients and families

All of these interventional catheter-based procedures are palliative, not curative. Therefore patients need education in risk-factor modification. During the hospital stay nurses identify the offending risk factors and initiate basic instruction. (Chapter 8 provides more information on risk-factor modification.) Patients should also be referred to a local cardiac rehabilitation center for more extensive teaching and lifestyle changes. Nurses assess patients' knowledge deficit related to discharge medications. Patients are frequently sent home on a regimen of antiplatelet drugs, nitrates, and calcium channel blockers. Clearly understanding the rationale for therapy and potential side effects of each drug is essential for patients. Further information on cardiac drugs is described on pages 203-209.

Balloon Valvuloplasty

After the development of percutaneous balloon angioplasty for coronary artery disease, considering adaptation of this technique as a nonsurgical intervention for stenotic cardiac valves became reasonable. Although long-term results are not promising at this point, balloon valvuloplasty can provide palliation and short-term symptomatic relief in selected patient populations[18,19] (Box 10-9).

Balloon Valvuloplasty Procedure

Performed in the cardiac catheterization laboratory, balloon valvuloplasty is similar to a routine cardiac catheterization, which also involves cannulation of the femoral artery and vein with percutaneous introducer sheaths. The balloon dilatation catheter is then threaded over a guidewire across the stenotic valve opening. The valves may be approached either retrograde via the aorta or antegrade across the interatrial septum. In the antegrade transseptal approach the balloon catheter is passed across the interatrial septum, which results in the creation of a small, atrial septal defect.[20] Subsequent inflations of the balloon increase the valve opening by separating fused commissures, cracking calcified leaflets, and stretching valve structures. Inflations are continued until the balloon "waist" disappears, which indicates full inflation. Regurgitant flow can result, particularly after mitral valvuloplasty. The risks of balloon valvuloplasty include but are not limited to cardiac perforation, thromboembolic events, dysrhythmias, hypotension, and bleeding.[20] **Nursing priorities are similar to other catheter-based interventional cardiology procedures, such as PTCA or atherectomy, and include managing the introducer sheaths, recognition and control of chest pain, control of bleeding, prevention of limb** ischemia, **and education of patients and families.** The nursing management section in the previous section provides more information.

Thrombolytic Therapy

Thrombolytic therapy is an important clinical intervention for patients experiencing acute myocardial infarction (AMI). Before the introduction of **thrombolytics,** the medical management of AMI focused on decreasing myocardial oxygen demands in an effort to minimize myocardial necrosis. Today, efforts to limit the size of infarction are directed toward early reperfusion of the jeopardized myocardium. The use of thrombolytic therapy is based on the premise that the stimulus in most transmural infarctions is the rupture of an atherosclerotic plaque with thrombus (clot) formation.[21] The administration of a thrombolytic agent results in the lysis of the acute thrombus, thus opening the obstructed coronary artery and restoring blood flow to the affected myocardium (Table 10-5). Thrombolytics are different from anticoagulants because they lyse, or dissolve, existing thrombus but do not prevent new clots from forming. Anticoagulants do not affect existing thrombus but prevent the formation of new clot.[22]

Streptokinase

Streptokinase (SK) is a thrombolytic agent derived from beta-hemolytic streptococci, which, when combined with plasminogen, catalyzes the conversion of plasminogen to plasmin, the enzyme responsible for clot dissolution in the body. SK can be administered either intravenously or by an intracoronary approach during cardiac catheterization. The three major problems associated with the use of SK are its systemic lytic effects coupled with a long half-life, its potential for allergic reaction, and its ten-

---

BOX 10-9

INDICATIONS FOR BALLOON VALVULOPLASTY

AORTIC

High risk for nonsurgical candidates with incapacitating symptoms

Patients with aortic stenosis who require urgent noncardiac surgery

Patients with severe heart failure or cardiogenic shock because of aortic stenosis whose conditions need to be stabilized until valve replacement is deemed safer

Patients with poor left ventricular function, low cardiac output, and small gradient across a stenotic aortic valve whose need for aortic valve replacement requires assessment

MITRAL

As an alternative to open mitral commissurotomy

TABLE 10-5

THROMBOLYTIC AGENTS APPROVED BY THE FDA FOR USE IN ACUTE MYOCARDIAL INFARCTION

	STREPTOKINASE*	ANISTREPLASE (APSAC)	ALTEPLASE (T-PA)
Fibrin-selective	No	Semiselective	Yes
Half-life	20-25 min (intermediate)	90 min (long)	5-10 min (short)
Dose	1.5 MU	30 units	100 mg
Duration of infusion	60 min constant infusion	2-5 min bolus	180 min complex infusion
Hypotension	+	+/−	−
Allergic reactions	+	+	−
Cost	Low	Moderately high	High

*Also approved for intracoronary use.

NOTE: Urokinase—approved only for intracoronary administration. Because the area of thrombolytic therapy is rapidly evolving, drug dose ranges and regimens are subject to change when research findings are updated.

+ = Present; − = not present; +/− = may be present.

dency to cause hypotension. The recommended dosage is 1,500,000 IU administered intravenously over 60 minutes to achieve clot lysis. Patients then undergo IV heparinization to prevent early rethrombosis.[23]

Urokinase

Urokinase (UK) is an enzymatic protein secreted by the parenchyma of the human kidney. Its thrombolytic effect results from the direct activation of plasminogen to form plasmin. However, because it is difficult and expensive to produce, systemic use is rare. Usually intracoronary UK is administered in conjunction with PTCA or atherectomy to lyse a thrombus.[24]

Tissue Plasminogen Activator

Another mode of thrombolytic therapy is tissue plasminogen activator (t-PA). Marketed under the name *Activase*, t-PA is a naturally occurring, nonallergenic, clot-specific enzyme with a very short half-life (5 to 10 minutes). It converts plasminogen to plasmin after binding to the fibrin-containing clot. Researchers once hoped that this characteristic of t-PA would prevent the induction of the systemic lytic state that occurs with SK therapy. However, the results of recent studies comparing the adverse effects of SK and t-PA show similar incidence of bleeding after administration. The total dose of t-PA is 100 mg, with 60 mg administered over 1 hour (10 mg of which is administered as a bolus) to rapidly recanalize the infarct-related coronary artery. The remaining 40 mg is given over the next 2 hours, followed by a heparin drip to maintain patency of the recanalized artery and to prevent rethrombosis.

APSAC

Anisoylated plasminogen-streptokinase activator complex (APSAC, Eminase) is another thrombolytic used in the treatment of AMI. Often referred to as a *second-generation streptokinase*, it has certain advantages over SK related specifically to duration of action, ease of administration, and fibrin selectivity. Compared with SK, the duration of action has been quadrupled and the time of administration reduced from 60 minutes to 2 to 5 minutes. Its disadvantages, similar to those of SK, include the potential for allergic reactions and hypotension.

Thrombolytic Eligibility Criteria

Patients with recent onset of chest pain (less than 6 hours) are candidates for thrombolytic therapy. Research suggests that the earlier the treatment is instituted, the higher the likelihood of successful reperfusion. However, there are selection criteria, as described in Box 10-10.

BOX 10-10

THROMBOLYTIC THERAPY SELECTION CRITERIA

- No more than 6 hours from onset of chest pain and less if possible
- ST segment elevation on ECG
- Ischemic chest pain of 30 minutes' duration
- Chest pain unresponsive to sublingual nitroglycerin or nifedipine
- No conditions that might cause a predisposition to hemorrhage

---

BOX 10-11

NURSING DIAGNOSIS PRIORITIES

POST-THROMBOLYTIC THERAPY

- *Altered Myocardial Tissue Perfusion* related to acute myocardial ischemia (p. 480) and reperfusion dysrhythmias, p. 477
- *Knowledge deficit:* medications, CAD risk factor modification, activity restrictions and reportable symptoms related to no prior exposure, p. 455
- *Fluid Volume Deficit* related to active blood loss, p. 503
- Acute *Pain* related to transmission and perception of ischemic impulses secondary to abrupt coronary artery closure, p. 499

Nursing Management

Nursing management of patients receiving thrombolytic therapy incorporates a variety of nursing diagnoses (Box 10-11). **Nursing priorities are directed toward monitoring reperfusion, controlling bleeding, and educating patients and families.**

Monitoring reperfusion

Critical care nurses monitor several criteria to assess for reperfusion of an artery that was previously occluded by a thrombus. These include

1. Relief from chest pain as blood flow is restored.
2. Reperfusion dysrhythmias such as PVCs, bradycardias, or heart block.
3. Elevated ST segments returning to baseline.
   Prior to initiation of thrombolytic therapy, nurses select a monitoring lead that demonstrates the

ST elevation.[25] Chapter 9 provides a description of ST segment changes during acute MI.

4. Serum creatine kinase (CK) and its associated myocardial isoenzyme (CK-MB) peak earlier than would be expected with an MI. This is termed *washout*. CK-MB washout results from the rapid return of cardiac enzymes into the circulation after restoration of blood flow to the unperfused areas of the heart. Chapter 8 contains additional information on cardiac enzymes.

Controlling bleeding

Bleeding is the most common complication related to thrombolysis, occurring not only as a result of the thrombolytic therapy but also because of anticoagulation therapy designed to minimize the possibility of rethrombosis. Therefore nurses must continually monitor for clinical manifestations of bleeding. Mild gingival bleeding and oozing around venipuncture sites are common and not cause for concern. Should serious internal bleeding occur, all fibrinolytic and heparin therapy is discontinued and volume expanders or coagulation factors or both are administered.

Educating patients and families

Nurses should explain to patients and families the reasons for thrombolytic therapy. Bleeding is the major side effect that is discussed. Nurses should also emphasize that although thrombolytic therapy may prevent a myocardial infarction at this time, it is not a cure for coronary artery disease; risk factor reduction is important.

Mechanical Circulatory Assist Devices

Intraaortic Balloon Pump (IABP)

IABP indications

The **intraaortic balloon pump** (IABP) is the most widely employed temporary mechanical circulatory assist device used to support failing circulation (Box 10-12). Its therapeutic effects are based on the hemodynamic principles of diastolic augmentation and afterload reduction.

IABP catheter

The intraaortic balloon catheter consists of a single, sausage-shaped, polyurethane balloon positioned in the descending thoracic aorta just below the takeoff of the left subclavian artery. It is usually inserted into the aorta via the femoral artery, either through an introducer sheath or percutaneously.

IABP pump

When attached to a bedside pumping console and properly synchronized to patients' ECG pattern, the intraaor-

---

> **BOX 10-12**
>
> ### INDICATIONS FOR THE USE OF INTRAAORTIC BALLOON PUMP
>
> Left ventricular failure after cardiac surgery
> Unstable angina refractory to medications
> Recurrent angina after AMI
> Complications of AMI
>   Cardiogenic shock
>   Papillary muscle dysfunction/rupture with mitral regurgitation
>   Ventricular septal defect
>   Refractory ventricular dysrhythmias

AMI, acute myocardial infarction.

tic balloon will inflate during diastole and deflate just before systole.[26]

IABP timing

Balloon inflation is timed to occur during diastole, following aortic valve closure. Once the balloon inflates, the blood in the aortic arch is displaced retrograde (backward) toward the aortic root to perfuse the coronary arteries and increase myocardial oxygen supply (Fig. 10-14, *A*). The blood volume in the aorta below the level of the balloon is propelled forward to perfuse the peripheral vascular system. Balloon deflation is timed to occur during systole, just before the opening of the aortic valve (Fig. 10-14, *B*). Diastolic counterpulsation creates a space or vacuum in the aorta that decreases resistance to left ventricular ejection, facilitating ventricular emptying and reducing myocardial oxygen demand.[27] Contraindications to balloon pumping include aortic aneurysm, aortic valve insufficiency, and severe peripheral vascular disease.

Nursing Management

Nursing management of patients with an IABP incorporates a variety of nursing diagnoses (Box 10-13). **Nursing priorities are directed toward managing dysrhythmias, preventing limb ischemia, monitoring thrombocytopenia, preventing infection, weaning patients from the IABP, and educating patients and families.**

Managing dysrhythmias

The ECG and arterial pressure tracing are constantly monitored to verify the timing and effect of balloon counterpulsations (Fig. 10-15). Dysrhythmias can adversely affect the timing of balloon inflation and deflation; thus rhythm disturbances are detected and treated promptly. Ideally, mean arterial pressure is maintained at about 80 mm Hg with adequate pumping.

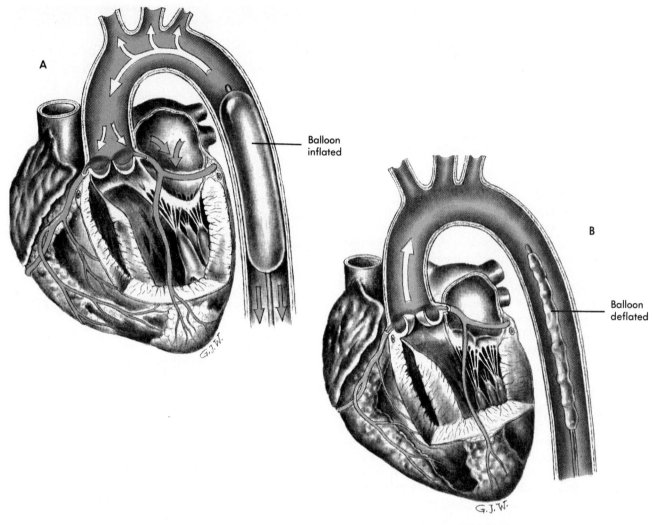

FIG. 10-14 Mechanisms of action of intraaortic balloon pump. **A,** Diastolic balloon inflation augments coronary blood flow. **B,** Systolic balloon deflation decreases afterload.

Balloon inflated

Balloon deflated

BOX 10-13

NURSING DIAGNOSIS PRIORITIES

INTRAAORTIC BALLOON PUMP

- *Altered Tissue Perfusion: Myocardial:* related to AMI, p. 480
- *Risk for Peripheral Neurovascular Dysfunction* risk factor, p. 479
- *Risk For Infection* risk factors: invasive monitoring devices, p. 482
- *Knowledge Deficit:* mobility and position restrictions related to lack of previous exposure to information, p. 455

Preventing limb ischemia

A major complication of IABP is ischemia of the involved limb secondary to occlusion of the femoral artery either by the catheter itself or emboli from thrombus formation on the balloon. Consequently the peripheral pulses distal to the catheter insertion site are assessed frequently for pulsation quality, plus color, temperature, and capillary refill of the involved extremity. Doppler localization of peripheral pulses may be required if pulses are difficult to palpate on the cannulated limb. Signs of diminished perfusion must be reported immediately. Other vascular complications of IABP include acute aortic dissection and the development of pseudoaneurysms. In addition, the balloon catheter may migrate proximally, occluding the left subclavian artery, or distally compromising renal circulation. Therefore careful assessment of the left radial pulse and urinary output is essential. Measures to avoid accidental displacement of the balloon catheter include ensuring that patients observe complete bed rest,

Counterpulsation started

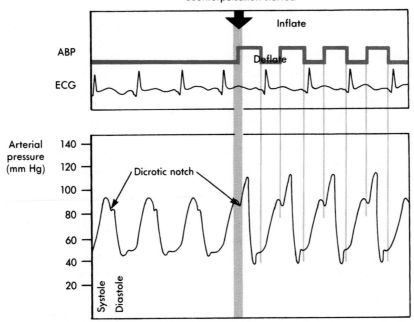

FIG. 10-15 The timing and effect of balloon counterpulsations. Timing is adjusted by synchronizing balloon inflation with the dicrotic notch on the arterial waveform resulting in an elevated diastolic pressure. Inflation continues until the next R wave serves as a stimulus for balloon deflation. The arterial waveform exhibits a reduced systolic pressure during counterpulsation. (From Guzzetta CE, Dossey BM: *Cardiovascular nursing: holistic practice,* St Louis, 1992, Mosby.)

elevating the head of the bed no more than 30 degrees, and preventing flexion of the involved hip.

Monitoring thrombocytopenia

Thrombocytopenia may occur as a result of mechanical destruction of the platelets by the pumping action of the balloon. Therefore platelet counts are closely monitored, and nurses observe patients for evidence of bleeding.

Preventing infection

Because the groin insertion site is at risk for contamination, a daily regimen of aseptic dressing changes is strictly followed.

Weaning patients from the IABP

Weaning patients from the balloon pump is attempted when hemodynamic stability has been achieved with only minimal pharmacologic support. Weaning may involve decreasing the IABP support from every beat to 1:2 or 1:3 or decreasing the balloon catheter volume. To prevent thrombus formation on the balloon surface, the catheter should never be left immobile inside patients. Dependence on the IABP for over 48 hours, indicative of severe cardiac dysfunction, may indicate a poor prognosis.

Educating patients and families

Nurses should explain the reason for the use of the IABP to patients and families. Many of the IABP companies provide helpful family education booklets written in uncomplicated terms. The importance of not bending at the hip and using the log-rolling technique for turning is emphasized, as well as the critical nature of the illness and the need for continuous nursing care.

Ventricular Assist Devices (VAD)

VAD Indications

The **ventricular assist device** (VAD) is designed to support a failing heart by flow assistance and is used for patients in cardiogenic shock, patients awaiting heart transplantation, and patients who are unable to successfully come off cardiopulmonary bypass after heart surgery. Patients placed on a VAD are further described by their potential to regain normal heart function:

1. Patients who despite aggressive medical therapy continue to demonstrate persistent acute heart failure but who have the potential for regaining normal heart function if the heart is given time to rest.[28]

2. Bridge-to-transplant patients who need circulatory support until heart transplantation can be performed.[28]

There are several types of VAD, but some general principles apply. The VAD diverts varying amounts of systemic blood flow around a failing ventricle by means of an extracorporeal pump.[29] The pump reduces cardiac workload while maintaining circulation. A VAD can also maintain adequate perfusion during periods of cardiac arrest.[29] The left ventricular assist device (LVAD) is used most commonly because LV failure occurs more frequently than RV failure. However, use of biventricular support (bi-VAD) is becoming more common because RV failure often follows LVAD placement.[30] VAD flow rates between 1 and 6 L/min are used to maintain adequate cardiac output.

VAD Insertion

Outflow cannulas that divert blood from the heart to the pump for LVAD are surgically placed in either the left atrium or LV apex, depending on the indication for the device. For example, if patients are expected to recover full cardiac function, preservation of LV function mandates left atrial cannulation. The right atrium is cannulated for outflow for right ventricular support. Inflow back to the heart from the pump is accomplished by cannulation of the aorta or femoral artery for the LVAD and pulmonary artery for the RVAD. Device selection is based on individual VAD capabilities and institutional preference. Differences between different VAD systems are described in Table 10-6.

Nursing Management

Nursing management of patients with a VAD incorporates a variety of nursing diagnoses (Box 10-14). **Nursing priorities are directed toward ensuring adequacy of pumping, monitoring for bleeding or thrombi, optimizing cardiac output, preventing infection, weaning patients from the VAD, and educating patients and families.**

Ensuring adequacy of pumping
VAD design varies considerably, and troubleshooting methods for the pump are unique to each device.

TABLE 10-6
VENTRICULAR ASSIST DEVICES

TYPE	EXAMPLE	USE	DESCRIPTION	INSERTION
Centrifugal	Biomedicus	Univentricular or biventricular support	Blood is diverted to a cone-shaped pump head where blades rotate and spin blood back through return cannula	Cannulate LA and aorta for LVAD Cannulate RA and PA for RVAD
Rotary	Hemopump	LV support	A propeller housed in the LV cannula draws blood from LV and propels it into the aorta	Via femoral artery, across aortic valve, and into LV
Pneumatic	Thoratec	Univentricular or bi-VAD support	External pulsatile pump that uses a pressurized air sac to eject blood through outflow cannula	Inflow through LA or RA and outflow to PA or aorta Inflow through ventricular apex when cardiotomy is expected
	TCI Heart-Mate	LVAD	A pneumatically driven, totally implantable pump with external drive console	Inflow from LV apex with outflow to aorta via graft
Electric	Novacor	LVAD	An electrically driven pulsatile pump that is implanted in an upper abdominal quadrant	Via LV apex and ascending aorta
Cardiopulmonary support	Bard CPS	Emergency resuscitation (e.g., supported angioplasty)	Femoral-femoral bypass; venous blood delivered to centrifugal pump that passes through normothermic heat exchanger to membrane oxygenator and back to patients	Percutaneous or cutdown insertion of catheters into femoral vein and femoral artery

LA, Left atrium; *RA*, right atrium; *RVAD*, right ventricular assist device.

Monitoring for bleeding or thrombi

The requirement for anticoagulation varies with different VADs, different flow rates, and between hospitals. If patients are anticoagulated with heparin, nurses are responsible for maintaining the activated clotting time (ACT) within a therapeutic range and monitoring for complications of bleeding. For example, with a centrifugal VAD no heparin is given if flow is consistently above 3L/minute. If flow is between 2 and 3 L/minute, an ACT of 100 to 200 seconds is maintained via constant heparin infusion.[31] If patients are not anticoagulated, the risk of thrombi obstructing a VAD cannula increases, as does the risk of an embolic event.

Optimizing cardiac output

Patients placed on a VAD are in cardiogenic shock with a cardiac index below 2.0 $L/min/m^2$. The strategies described on page 189 to optimize cardiac output following cardiac surgery also apply to care of patients with a VAD.

Preventing infection

Patients with a VAD in place have considerable opportunity to develop an infection. The most common infection is pneumonia secondary to immobility and need for ventilatory support. Other infectious risks come from invasive monitoring catheters and the surgically implanted VAD. Infection is monitored by taking patients' temperature, visualizing insertion sites or surgical wounds, and performing daily leukocyte counts. The risk of infection is reduced by frequent hand washing, strict aseptic technique for all dressing or line changes, and early removal of invasive catheters as soon as patients are hemodynamically stable. Early extubation and aggressive pulmonary hygiene are used to prevent pneumonia.

Weaning patients from the VAD

Clinicians wean patients from the VAD by gradually decreasing flow rates to allow the ventricle to contribute more to total blood flow. Anticoagulation is controversial; however, when weaning VAD flow rates below 2 L/min, ACT should be maintained between 160 and 480 seconds with heparin, depending on institutional protocols. Heparin minimizes the potential for thrombus formation in the extracorporeal circuit during weaning but increases the risk of bleeding.

Educating patients and families

The rapid and acute nature of cardiogenic shock limits nurses' ability to prepare patients and families for VAD insertion. Despite the critical nature of the illness, nurses should explain to patients and families the reason for use of the VAD and provide information about the critical care environment and equipment.

Cardiovascular Drugs

Critically ill cardiovascular patients receive multiple medications. Critical care nurses are responsible for preparing and administering these drugs and are often required to titrate the dose on the basis of patients' hemodynamic response. The medications used to treat cardiovascular disease are rapidly changing and expanding as researchers discover more about the pathophysiology of cardiac disease, and pharmaceutical companies improve formulas. With an understanding of the mechanism of action of the various drug classifications, critical care nurses can readily apply this knowledge to new drugs within the same classification. The following discussion provides a concise review of drugs commonly administered to support cardiovascular function in the critical care setting. The emphasis is on intravenously administered medications that are used for the acute rather than the chronic management of cardiovascular conditions.

Antidysrhythmic Drugs

Antidysrhythmic drugs make up a diverse category of pharmacologic agents used to terminate or prevent an array of abnormal cardiac rhythms. These drugs are commonly classified according to their primary effect on the action potential of the cardiac cell. The classification shown in Table 10-7 is the most commonly used system. Classification of newer agents becomes more complex because some of these agents have characteristics of more than one class and others have no characteristics of the current system.[32]

Class I drugs

Class I antidysrhythmic agents are sodium channel blockers that decrease the influx of sodium ions through "fast" channels during phase 0 depolarization. Class I drugs can be further subdivided into three groups, ac-

TABLE 10-7
CLASSIFICATION OF ANTIDYSRHYTHMIC AGENTS

CLASS	ACTION	DRUGS
I	Blocks sodium channels ("stabilizes" cell membrane)	
IA	Blocks sodium channels and delays repolarization, thus lengthening the duration of the action potential	quinidine procainamide disopyramide
IB	Blocks sodium channels and accelerates repolarization, thus shortening the duration of the action potential	lidocaine mexiletine tocainide
IC	Blocks sodium channels and slows conduction through the His-Purkinje system, thus prolonging the QRS duration	flecainide encainide propafenone
II	Blocks beta receptors	acebutolol esmolol propranolol
III	Prolongs the duration of the action potential	amiodarone bretylium sotalol
IV	Blocks calcium channels	verapamil

cording to their potency as sodium channel inhibitors and their effect on phase 3 repolarization.[32]

1. Class IA: Examples of Class IA drugs include quinidine, procainamide, and disopyramide, which block not only the fast sodium channels but also phase 3 repolarization, thereby prolonging the action potential duration. Clinically this effect may result in measurable increases in the QRS duration and the QT interval.[32]
2. Class IB: This category comprises lidocaine, mexiletine, and tocainide. These drugs have only a moderate effect on sodium channels and actually accelerate phase 3 repolarization to shorten the action potential duration.
3. Class IC: This category contains encainide, flecainide, and propafenone, which increase both the PR and the QRS intervals. The use of these agents in clinical practice has decreased since the *Cardiac Arrhythmia Suppression Trial* (CAST) demonstrated that treatment with encainide or flecainide was associated with increased mortality.[33]

Class II drugs

Class II drugs are beta-adrenergic blockers (beta blockers), which inhibit dysrhythmias mediated by the sympathetic nervous system by competing with endogenous catecholamines for available receptor sites. Drugs in this class can be further subdivided into cardioselective (those that block only beta$_1$) and noncardioselective (those that block both beta$_1$ and beta$_2$ receptors). Knowing the effects of adrenergic-receptor stimulation allows clinicians to anticipate not only the therapeutic responses brought about by beta blockade but also the potential adverse effects of these agents (Table 10-8). For example, bronchospasm can be precipitated by noncardioselective beta blockers in patients with chronic obstructive pulmonary disease secondary to blocking the effects of beta$_2$ receptors in the lungs. Beta blockers are also negative inotropes and should be used cautiously in patients with severe left ventricular dysfunction.[34] Although numerous beta blockers are available, only acebutolol, propranolol, and esmolol are approved for the treatment of dysrhythmias. Esmolol (Brevibloc) offers advantages to critically ill patients because of its short half-life (approximately 9 minutes). It is used in the treatment of SVTs such as atrial fibrillation and atrial flutter.

Class III drugs

Class III agents include amiodarone, bretylium, and sotalol. These agents markedly slow the rate of phase 3 repolarization, increasing the effective refractory period and the action potential duration. Although their effect on the action potential is similar, these drugs differ greatly in their mechanism of action and their side effects. Bretylium, the only drug in this classification approved for intravenous use, is used clinically in treating ventricular tachycardia that is refractory to other antidysrhythmic agents, such as lidocaine and procainamide.[35]

Class IV drugs

Class IV agents are calcium channel blockers that inhibit the influx of calcium through slow calcium channels during the plateau phase (phase 2). This effect occurs primarily in the sinus and atrioventricular (AV) nodes and atrial tissue. Verapamil (Calan, Isoptin) was the first drug in this category approved for use as an antidysrhythmic. It depresses sinus and AV node conduction and is effective in terminating SVT caused by AV nodal reentry.[33] Recently diltiazem (Cardizem) has become available in IV form. Initial studies suggest that diltiazem may be as effective as verapamil in converting SVT, with fewer hypotensive side effects.[36]

Adenosine

Adenosine (Adenocard) is an antidysrhythmic agent that remains unclassified under the current system. Adenosine occurs endogenously in the body as a building block of adenosine triphosphate. Administered in intravenous boluses, adenosine slows conduction through the AV node, causing transient AV block. It is used clinically to convert supraventricular tachycardias and facilitate differential diagnosis of rapid dysrhythmias. Side effects are transient because the drug is rapidly taken up by the cells and cleared from the body within 10 seconds.[37]

TABLE 10-8
PHARMACOLOGY OF SELECTED ANTIDYSRHYTHMIC AGENTS

DRUG	INDICATIONS	DOSAGE	MAJOR SIDE EFFECTS
Adenosine	Paroxysmal SVT	6 mg IV rapid push, repeat with 12 mg over 1-2 sec; follow with IV fluid (NS or D_5W)	Transient: flushing, dyspnea, hypotension
Lidocaine	Ventricular ectopy; PVC prophylaxis in AMI	50-100 mg bolus followed by continuous infusion of 1-4 mg/min	CNS toxicity
Procainamide	Ventricular ectopy resistant to lidocaine	50 mg IV q 1 min up to 1 g followed by infusion of 1-4 mg/min	Hypotension GI effects Widening of QRS and QT interval Drug-induced lupus syndrome
Propranolol	Supraventricular tachycardia	1-3 mg IV q 5 min not to exceed 0.1 mg/kg	Bradycardia Heart failure Heart block
Amiodarone	Life-threatening ventricular dysrhythmias	5-10 mg/kg slowly IV followed by an infusion of 10 mg/kg/day for 3-5 days	Corneal deposits Slate-gray or bluish skin Photosensitivity Pulmonary fibrosis Thyroid dysfunction
Bretylium	Refractory ventricular fibrillation	5 mg/kg IV bolus followed by 10 mg/kg dosages repeated at 15-30 min intervals for total of 30 mg/kg	Initially: hypertension, tachycardia, PVCs
	Ventricular tachycardia (second-line agent)	500 mg in 50 ml D_5W to infuse over 8-10 min, then continuous infusion at 1-2 mg/min	Subsequently: hypotension, bradycardia, nausea and vomiting
Verapamil	Supraventricular tachycardia	5-10 mg IV over 2 min followed 10 mg in 30 min if needed	Heart failure AV block Bradycardia Dizziness Peripheral edema
Esmolol	SVT	Loading dosage of 500 μg/kg/min over 1 min followed by infusion of 50 μg/kg/min for 4 min; repeat procedure q 5 min, increasing infusion by 25-50 μg/kg/min to maximum of 200 μg/kg/min	Hypotension Nausea

AMI, acute myocardial infarction; *CNS*, central nervous system; *D_5W*, 5% dextrose in water; *GI*, gastrointestinal; *NS*, normal saline; *PVC*, premature ventricular contraction.

Antidysrhythmic Drug Side Effects

Antidysrhythmic drugs carry the risk of serious side effects, some of which may be life threatening. The major side effects of the intravenous antidysrhythmic agents are listed in Table 10-8. The most severe complication is the potential for a "prodysrhythmic" effect, which may result in worsening of the underlying dysrhythmia, occurrence of a new dysrhythmia, or development of a bradydysrhythmia. Torsades de pointes is a dysrhythmia that can be caused by class IA agents.[38] The development of drug-induced dysrhythmia is unpredictable, and nurses play an important role in evaluating ECG changes, monitoring drug levels, and assessing patient symptoms. Chapter 8 discusses the prodysrhythmic effects of a prolonged QT interval in detail.

Inotropic Drugs

Critically ill patients with compromised cardiac function frequently require medications to enhance myocardial contractility. These medications are termed *positive inotropes*. Clinically available inotropes include cardiac glycosides, sympathomimetics, and phosphodiesterase inhibitors. These agents increase myocardial contractility,

TABLE 10-9
EFFECTS OF ADRENERGIC RECEPTORS

RECEPTOR	LOCATION	RESPONSE TO STIMULATION
alpha	Vessels of skin, muscles, kidneys, and intestines	Vasoconstriction of peripheral arterioles
beta$_1$	Cardiac tissue	Increased heart rate Increased conduction Increased contractility
beta$_2$	Vascular and bronchial smooth muscle	Vasodilation of peripheral arterioles Bronchodilation

resulting in improved cardiac output, more complete emptying of the ventricles, and decreased filling pressures.

Cardiac glycosides

This class of drugs includes digitalis and its derivatives. Used for centuries, these drugs have a slow onset of action and low risk of toxicity, benefits that make them appropriate for the management of chronic heart failure.[39] Because digoxin causes slowing of the sinus rate and a decrease in AV conduction, it is administered in the critical care unit to control supraventricular dysrhythmias.

Sympathomimetic agents

These drugs stimulate adrenergic receptors, thereby simulating the effects of sympathetic nerve stimulation. Included in this category are naturally occurring catecholamines (epinephrine, dopamine, and norepinephrine), as well as synthetic catecholamines (dobutamine and isoproterenol). The cardiovascular effects of these drugs, which vary according to their selectivity for specific receptor sites, may be dose-dependent as well.[40] Table 10-9 describes the effects of specific adrenergic receptors.

Dopamine

One of the most widely used drugs in the critical care setting, dopamine hydrochloride (Intropin) is a chemical precursor of norepinephrine, which, in addition to both alpha and beta receptor stimulation, can activate dopaminergic receptors in the renal and mesenteric blood vessels. The actions of this drug are entirely dose-related.[35]

1. Low-dose dopamine (less than 3 micrograms/kg/min) stimulates dopaminergic receptors, causing renal and mesenteric vasodilation. The resultant increase in renal perfusion increases urinary output.

2. Moderate dopamine dosages result in stimulation of beta$_1$ receptors to increase myocardial contractility and improve cardiac output.
3. High-dose dopamine (greater than 10 micrograms/kg/min) stimulates alpha receptors, resulting in vasoconstriction that often negates both the beta-adrenergic and dopaminergic effects.

Dobutamine

Dobutamine hydrochloride (Dobutrex) is a synthetic catecholamine with predominantly beta$_1$ effects. It also produces some beta$_2$ stimulation, resulting in a mild vasodilation. Dobutamine is useful in the treatment of heart failure, especially in hypotensive patients who cannot tolerate vasodilator therapy.[35] The usual dosage range is 2.5 to 20 micrograms/kg/min, titrated on the basis of hemodynamic parameters.

Epinephrine

Epinephrine (Adrenalin) is produced by the adrenal gland as part of the body's response to stress. This agent has the ability to stimulate both alpha and beta receptors, depending on the dose administered. At doses of 1 to 2 milligrams/min, epinephrine bonds with beta receptors to increase heart rate, cardiac conduction, contractility, and vasodilation, thereby increasing cardiac output. At higher dosages, alpha receptors are stimulated, resulting in increased vascular resistance and blood pressure.

Norepinephrine

Norepinephrine (Levophed) is similar to epinephrine in its ability to stimulate beta$_1$ and alpha receptors, but it lacks the beta$_2$ effects. At low infusion rates beta$_1$ receptors are activated to produce increased contractility and thus augment cardiac output. At higher doses the inotropic effects are limited by marked vasoconstriction mediated by alpha receptors. Clinically, norepinephrine is used most frequently as a vasopressor to elevate blood pressure in shock states.

Isoproterenol

Isoproterenol hydrochloride (Isuprel) is a pure beta receptor stimulant with no alpha effects that produces dramatic increases in heart rate, conduction, and contractility via beta$_1$ stimulation and vasodilation via beta$_2$ stimulation. Isoproterenol also produces vasodilation of the pulmonary arteries and bronchodilation. Its most common use is as a temporary treatment for symptomatic bradycardia until a pacemaker is available.

Amrinone

Phosphodiesterase inhibitors are a new group of inotropic agents that are also potent vasodilators. Drugs in this classification inhibit the enzyme phosphodiesterase, resulting in increased levels of cyclic adenosine monophosphate (AMP) and intracellular calcium. Amrinone (Inocor) is the first of these agents approved for use in the United States. Increases in cardiac output occur as a re-

TABLE 10-10

CHARACTERISTICS OF SELECTED VASODILATORS

| CLASSIFICATION/DRUG | DOSAGE | EFFECT (↓) | | SIDE EFFECTS |
		PRELOAD	AFTERLOAD	
DIRECT SMOOTH MUSCLE RELAXANTS				
Sodium nitroprusside (Nipride)	0.25-6 μg/kg/min IV infusion	Moderate	Strong	Hypotension, reflex tachycardia, thiocyanate toxicity
Nitroglycerin (Tridil)	5-300 μg/min IV infusion	Strong	Mild	Headache, reflex tachycardia, hypotension
Hydralazine (Apresoline)	5-10 mg IV q 4 hr	None to mild	Moderate	Reflex tachycardia
CALCIUM CHANNEL BLOCKERS				
Nifedipine (Procardia)	10-30 mg SL	None	Strong	Hypotension, headache, reflex tachycardia
ACE INHIBITORS				
Captopril (Capoten)	6.25-100 mg PO q 8-12 hr	Moderate	Moderate	Hypotension, chronic cough, neutropenia
Enalapril (Vasotec)	0.625 mg IV over 5 min, then q 6 hr	Moderate	Moderate	Hypotension, elevation of liver enzymes
ALPHA-ADRENERGIC BLOCKERS				
Labetalol (Normodyne)	20-80 mg IV bolus q 10 min, then 1-2 mg/min infusion	Moderate	Moderate	Orthostatic hypotension, bronchospasm, AV block
Phentolamine (Regitine)	1-2 mg/min infusion	Moderate	Moderate	Hypotension, tachycardia

ACE, Angiotensin-converting enzyme; *SL*, sublingual.

sult of increased contractility (inotropic effects) and decreased afterload (vasodilative effects). A loading dose of 0.75 mg/kg is given slowly over 2 to 3 minutes and followed by a continuous infusion of 5 to 10 mg/kg/min. Because thrombocytopenia has occurred in a small percentage of patients receiving amrinone, platelet counts are monitored and patients observed for hemorrhagic complications.[40]

Vasodilator Drugs

Vasodilators are pharmacologic agents that improve cardiac performance by arterial or venous dilatation, or both. SVR or afterload reduction is accomplished by vasodilation of arterial vessels. This results in decreased resistance to left ventricular ejection and may improve cardiac output without increasing myocardial oxygen demands. Reduction of preload is accomplished by dilating venous vessels to increase capacitance, which results in decreased filling pressures for a failing heart. These drugs may be classified into four groups on the basis of their mechanism of action (Table 10-10).

Sodium nitroprusside (SNP)

SNP (Nipride) is a potent, rapidly acting venous and arterial smooth muscle vasodilator, particularly suitable for rapid reduction of blood pressure. It is also effective for afterload reduction in the setting of severe heart failure. SNP is administered by continuous IV infusion, with the dosage titrated to maintain the desired blood pressure and SVR. Prolonged administration can result in thiocyanate toxicity, manifested by nausea, confusion, and tinnitus.[40]

Nitroglycerin

Nitroglycerin (Tridil) acts directly on the vessel smooth muscle to cause both arterial and venous vasodilation, but its venous effect is more pronounced. It is used in the critical care setting for the treatment of acute heart failure because it reduces cardiac filling pressures, relieves pulmonary congestion, decreases cardiac workload, and reduces myocardial oxygen consumption. In addition, nitroglycerin dilates the coronary arteries and is used in the treatment of unstable angina and acute MI. The initial dosage is 10 micrograms/min, and the infusion is titrated upward to achieve the desired clinical effect: reduced or eliminated chest pain, decreased PAWP, or decreased blood pressure. Nitroglycerin is also administered prophylactically to prevent coronary vasospasm after coronary angioplasty and atherectomy. The most common side effects of this drug include hypotension, flushing, and headache.[41,43]

TABLE 10-11

PHYSIOLOGIC EFFECTS OF CALCIUM CHANNEL BLOCKERS

DRUG	HEART RATE	CONDUCTION	CONTRACTILITY	PERIPHERAL DILATATION	CORONARY DILATATION
Nifedipine (Procardia)	0/↑	0/↑	0	↑↑↑	↑↑↑
Verapamil (Calan, Isoptin)	↓↓	↓↓↓	↓↓	↑	↑↑
Diltiazem (Cardizem)	↓	↓↓	↓	↑	↑↑

0, No change; ↓, decrease; ↑, increase.

Hydralazine

Hydralazine (Apresoline) is a potent arterial vasodilator, seldom given as a continuous infusion but rather in intravenously administered dosages of 5 to 10 mg every 4 to 8 hours. The major side effect is reflex tachycardia mediated by the sympathetic nervous system.

Calcium Channel Blockers

Calcium channel blockers are a chemically diverse group of drugs with differing pharmacologic effects, as described in Table 10-11.

Nifedipine

Nifedipine (Procardia) and other dihydropyridines are used primarily as arterial vasodilators. Used in the critical care setting to treat hypertension, nifedipine reduces the influx of calcium in the coronary and peripheral arteries. Although it is available only in an oral form, it is frequently prescribed sublingually.[42-44] Side effects of nifedipine are related to vasodilation and include hypotension, reflex tachycardia, flushing, headache, and ankle edema.

Verapamil

Verapamil (Calan, Isoptin) and diltiazem (Cardizem) dilate the coronary arteries but have little effect on the peripheral vasculature. They are used in the treatment of angina, especially types that have a vasospastic component, and as an antidysrhythmic in the treatment of SVT.

ACE Inhibitors

Angiotensin-converting enzyme (ACE)

ACE inhibitors produce vasodilation by blocking the conversion of angiotensin I to angiotensin II. Because angiotensin is a potent vasoconstrictor, limiting its production decreases peripheral vascular resistance. In contrast to the direct vasodilators and nifedipine, ACE inhibitors do not cause reflex tachycardia or induce sodium and water retention. These drugs may cause a profound fall in blood pressure, especially in patients who are volume-depleted. Blood pressure should be monitored carefully during initiation of therapy.[45]

Captopril (Capoten) and enalapril (Vasotec)

These drugs are used to decrease SVR (afterload) and pulmonary capillary wedge pressure (preload) in patients with heart failure. Captopril is available only in an oral form, but it has a relatively rapid onset of action (approximately 1 hour). Enalapril is available in an intravenous form and may be used to decrease afterload in more emergent situations.

Alpha-adrenergic Blockers

Peripheral adrenergic blockers block alpha receptors in arteries and veins, resulting in vasodilation. Orthostatic hypotension is a common side effect and may result in syncope.[41]

Labetalol

A combined alpha and beta blocker, labetalol (Normodyne) is used in the treatment of hypertensive emergencies. Because the blockade of beta₁ receptors permits the decrease of blood pressure without the risk of reflexive tachycardia and increased cardiac output, this drug is useful in the treatment of acute aortic dissection.

Phentolamine

Phentolamine (Regitine) is a peripheral alpha blocker that causes decreased afterload via arterial vasodilation. It is given as a continuous infusion at a rate of 1 to 2 mg/min and titrated to achieve the required reduction in blood pressure and SVR.[40] This drug is also used to treat the extravasation of dopamine. If this occurs, 5 to 10 mg is diluted in 10 ml normal saline and administered intradermally into the infiltrated area.

Vasopressors

Vasopressors are sympathomimetic agents that mediate peripheral vasoconstriction through stimulation of alpha receptors. This results in increased systemic vascular resistance and elevated blood pressure. Vasopressors are not widely used in the treatment of critically ill cardiac patients because the dramatic increase in afterload taxes a damaged heart. Vasopressors may occasionally be used to maintain organ perfusion in shock states. For example, phenylephrine hydrochloride (Neo-Synephrine) or norepinephrine (Levophed) may be administered as a continuous intravenous infusion to maintain organ perfusion by increasing peripheral vascular resistance in the warm phase of septic shock.

References

1. Manion PA: Temporary epicardial pacing in the postoperative cardiac surgical patient, *Crit Care Nurs* 13(2):30, 1993.
2. Bernstein AD and others: The NASPE/BPEG generic pacemaker code for antibradycardia and adaptive rate pacing and antitachyarrhythmia devices, *PACE* 10:794, 1987.
3. Edwards FH, Clark RE, Schwartz M: Impact of internal mammary conduits on operative mortality in coronary revascularization, *Ann Thorac Surg* 57(1):27, 1994.
4. Livesay JJ, Talledo OJ: The current preference for mitral valve reconstruction, *Tex Heart Inst J* 18(2):87, 1991.
5. Duran CMG, Gometza B, Devol EB: Valve repair in rheumatic mitral disease, *Circulation* 84(suppl 3):125, 1991.
6. Shinn JA: Rapid recovery from CABG surgery, *Prog Cardiovasc Nurs* 9(1):47, 1994.
7. Leahy NM: Neurologic complications of open heart surgery, *J Cardiovasc Nurs* 7(2):41, 1993.
8. Vaska PL: Sternal wound infections, *AACN Clin Issues Crit Care Nurs* 4(3):475, 1993.
9. Nisam S and others: AICD℠ Automatic Cardioverter Defibrillator Clinical update: 14 years experience in over 34,000 patients, *PACE* 18 (part II):142-147, 1995.
10. Jordaens L and others: A new transvenous internal cardioverter-defibrillator: implantation technique, complications, and short-term follow-up, *Am Heart J* 129(2):251-258, 1995.
11. Akhtar M and others: Role of implantable cardioverter defibrillator therapy in the management of high-risk patients, *Circulation* 85 (suppl 1):I131, 1992.
12. Burke LR, Rodgers BL, Jenkins LS: Living with recurrent ventricular dysrhythmias, *Focus Crit Care* 19(1):60, 1992.
13. Ryan TJ and others: Guidelines for Percutaneous transluminal coronary angioplasty, *JACC* 22(7):2033, 1993.
14. Safien RD and others: Coronary atherectomy—clinical, angiographic, and histological findings and observations regarding potential mechanisms, *Circulation* 82(1):69, 1990.
15. Deelstra MH: Coronary rotational ablation: an overview with related nursing interventions, *Am J Crit Care* 2(1):16, 1993.
16. Albert NM: Laser angioplasty and intracoronary stents: going beyond the balloon, *AACN Clin Issues in Crit Care Nurs* 5(1):15, 1994.
17. Bevans M, McLimore E: Intracoronary stents: a new approach to coronary artery dilation, *J Cardiovasc Nurs* 7(1):34, 1992.
18. Ferguson JJ and others: Balloon aortic valvuloplasty, *Tex Heart Inst J* 17(1):23, 1990.
19. Barden C and others: Balloon aortic valvuloplasty: nursing care implications, *Crit Care Nurse* 10(6):22, 1990.
20. Kawaniski DT, Rahimtoola SH: Catheter balloon commissurotomy for mitral stenosis: complications and results, *JACC* 19(1):192, 1992.
21. Tiefenbrunn AJ: Clinical benefits of thrombolytic therapy in acute myocardial infarction, *Am J Cardiol* 69(2):3A, 1992.
22. Workman ML: Anticoagulants and thrombolytics: what's the difference? *AACN Clin Issues in Crit Care Nurs* 5(1):26, 1994.
23. Stein B, Roberts R: Current status of thrombolytic therapy in acute myocardial infarction, *Tex Heart Inst J* 18(4):250, 1991.
24. Schieman G and others: Intracoronary urokinase for intracoronary thrombus accumulation complicating PTCA in acute ischemic syndromes, *Circulation* 82(6):2052, 1990.
25. Drew BJ and Tisdale LA: ST segment monitoring for coronary artery reocclusion following thrombolytic therapy and coronary angioplasty: identification of optimal bedside monitoring leads, *Am J Crit Care* 2(4):280, 1993.
26. Wojner AW: Assessing the five points of the intraaortic balloon pump waveform, *Crit Care Nurse* 14(3):48, 1994.
27. Shoulders-Odom B: Managing the challenge of IABP therapy, *Crit Care Nurse* 11(2):60, 1991.
28. Smith RG, Cleavinger M: Current perspectives on the use of circulatory assist devices, *AACN Clin Issues Crit Care Nurs* 2(3):488, 1991.
29. Moroney DA, Reedy JE: Understanding ventricular assist devices: a self study guide, *Cardiovasc Nurs* 8(2):1, 1994.
30. Emery RW, Joyce LD: Directions in cardiac assistance, *J Cardiac Surg* 6(3):400, 1991.
31. Quaal SJ: Centrifugal assist devices, *AACN Clin Issues Crit Care Nurs* 2(3):515, 1991.
32. Stier F: Antidysrhythmic agents, *AACN Clin Issues Crit Care Nurs* 3(2):483, 1992.
33. Bennett B, Singh S: Management of ventricular arrhythmias: then and now, *Am J Crit Care* 1(3):107, 1992.
34. Weiner B: Hemodynamic effects of antidysrhythmic drugs, *J Cardiovasc Nurs* 5(4):39, 1991.
35. American Heart Association: *Textbook of advanced cardiac life support*, Dallas, 1994, The American Heart Association.
36. Peitz TJ: Intravenous diltiazem hydrochloride rather than verapamil for resistant paroxysmal supraventricular tachycardia, *West J Med* 19(5):598, 1993.
37. McNulty SA: Pharmacological interventional testing for myocardial perfusion: a new application for adenosine, *Cardiovasc Nurs* 28(4):24, 1992.
38. Lefor N, Cardello FP, Felicetta JV: Recognizing and treating torsades de pointes, *Crit Care Nurs* 12(6):23, 1992.
39. Notterdam DA: Inotropic agents: catecholamines, digoxin, amrinone, *Crit Care Clin* 7(3):583, 1991.
40. Clements JV: Sympathomimetics, inotropics, and vasodilators, *AACN Clin Issues Crit Care Nurs* 3(2):395, 1992.
41. Deglin JH, Deglin S: Hypertension: current trends and choices in pharmacotherapeutics, *AACN Clin Issues Crit Care Nurs* 3(2):507, 1992.
42. Kuhn M: Nitrates, *AACN Clin Issues Crit Care Nurs* 3(2):409, 1992.
43. Schumann D: Sublingual nifedipine controversy in drug delivery, *DCCN* 10(6):314, 1991.
44. Hilleman DE, Banakar UV: Issues in contemporary drug delivery: part VI: advanced cardiac drug formulations, *J Pharmacy Technology* 8(5):203, 1992.
45. Kuhn M: Angiotensin-converting enzyme inhibitors, *AACN Clin Issues Crit Care Nurs* 3(2):461, 1992.

Pulmonary Alterations

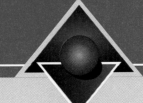

11

Pulmonary Assessment and Diagnostic Procedures

KATHLEEN M. STACY

CHAPTER OBJECTIVES

- Explain the contents of a complete pulmonary history.
- Discuss inspection, palpation, percussion, and auscultation of patients with pulmonary dysfunction.
- Describe the assessment findings associated with various pulmonary disorders.

- Outline the steps in analyzing an arterial blood gas.
- Identify key diagnostic procedures used in assessment of patients with pulmonary dysfunction.
- Discuss the nursing management of patients undergoing pulmonary diagnostic procedures.

KEY TERMS

Assessment of critical care patients with pulmonary dysfunction is a systematic process that incorporates a history and physical examination. The purpose of the assessment is twofold: (1) to recognize changes in pulmonary status that necessitate nursing or medical intervention and (2) determine the ways in which pulmonary dysfunction is interfering with self-care activities. To complete the assessment, nurses must review patients' laboratory studies and diagnostic tests. This chapter focuses on priority clinical assessments, laboratory studies, and diagnostic procedures currently used in the critical care setting.

Clinical Assessment

History

Patients' initial presentation determines the rapidity and direction of the interview. For patients in acute distress, the history should be curtailed to just a few questions about their chief complaint and precipitating events. For patients in no obvious distress the history should focus on the following areas: (1) review of their present illness, (2) overview of their general respiratory status, (3) examination of their general health status, and (4) survey of their lifestyle.[1,2] Questions to be included in the interview are outlined in Box 11-1.

Nurses should also obtain a description of patients' current symptoms. Symptoms that are common in pulmonary patients include dyspnea, cough, wheezing, edema, palpitations, fatigue, and chest pain.[3] Nurses should elicit information about the location, onset and duration, characteristics, setting, aggravating and alleviating factors, associated symptoms[3], and efforts to treat symptoms.[4] If the cough is productive, patients should be asked about the color, amount, odor, and consistency of the sputum.[5]

Physical Examination

Inspection

Inspection of patients should focus on three priorities: (1) observation of the tongue and sublingual area, (2) assessment of chest wall configuration, and (3) evaluation of respiratory effort. If possible, patients should be positioned upright, with their arms resting at their sides.[2]

OBSERVATION OF THE TONGUE AND SUBLINGUAL AREA. The tongue and sublingual area should be observed for a blue, gray, or dark purple tint or discoloration indicating the presence of central **cyanosis.** Cyanosis is a sign of hypoxemia, or inadequate oxygenation of the blood, and is considered to be life threatening. The fingers and toes may also appear discolored, an indication of peripheral cyanosis.[6]

ASSESSMENT OF CHEST WALL CONFIGURATION. The size and shape of the chest wall should be assessed. Normally the ratio of anteroposterior (AP) diameter to lateral di-

---

BOX 11-1

PULMONARY HISTORY QUESTIONS

PRESENT ILLNESS

What brought you to the hospital?
What were the precipitating events?
When did the problem start?

RESPIRATORY STATUS

Do you currently have a chronic lung disease, such as asthma, bronchitis, and emphysema?
Do you have a history of any lung disease, such as chronic respiratory infections and tuberculosis?
Have you had any chest surgery?

GENERAL HEALTH STATUS

Do you have any other chronic disease or illness?
Do you have a history of any other disease, illness, or surgery?
Are you currently taking any medications, prescription or nonprescription?

LIFESTYLE

Do you smoke, or have you smoked in the past?
Have you been exposed to secondhand smoke?
Have you ever been exposed to lung irritants or cancer-causing agents, such as asbestos, chemicals, fumes, beryllium, coal or stone quarry dust, and Agent Orange?

---

ameter ranges from 1:2 to 5:7.[7] An increase in the AP diameter suggests chronic obstructive pulmonary disease (COPD). Nurses should inspect the chest for any structural deviations. Some of the most common abnormalities are pectus excavatum, pectus carinatum, barrel chest, and spinal deformities. In pectus excavatum (funnel chest) the sternum and lower ribs are displaced posteriorly, creating a funnel- or pit-shaped depression in the chest. This deformity causes a decrease in the AP diameter of the chest and may interfere with respiratory function. In pectus carinatum (pigeon breast) the sternum projects forward, causing an increase in the AP diameter of the chest. The barrel chest is characterized by displacement of the sternum forward and the ribs outward—another cause for increased AP diameter of the chest. Spinal deformities such as kyphosis, lordosis, and scoliosis may also be present and can interfere with respiratory function.[7,8]

EVALUATION OF RESPIRATORY EFFORT. Nurses should assess patients' **respiratory effort** for rate, rhythm, symmetry, and quality of ventilatory movements. Normal breathing at rest is effortless and regular, occurring at a rate of 12 to 20 breaths per minute.[2] Some of the more common patterns in patients with pulmonary dysfunction are tachypnea, hyperventilation, and obstructive breathing. Tachypnea is manifested by an increase in rate and decrease in depth of ventilation. Hyperventilation is manifested by an increase in both rate and depth of ventilation. Patients with COPD often experience obstructive breathing. As they breathe, air becomes trapped in the lungs and ventilations become progressively shallower until they actively and forcefully exhale.[9]

ADDITIONAL ASSESSMENT AREAS. Other areas that should be assessed are patient position, effort to breathe, use of accessory muscles, presence of intercostal retractions, unequal movement of the chest wall, nasal flaring, and midsentence pauses for breath.[7] The presence of other iatrogenic features, such as chest tubes, central venous lines, artificial airways, and nasogastric tubes, should be noted because they may affect assessment findings.

Palpation

Palpation of patients should focus on three priorities: (1) confirmation of tracheal position, (2) assessment of respiratory excursion, and (3) evaluation of fremitus. In addition, the thorax should be assessed for any areas of tenderness, lumps, or bony deformities. The anterior, posterior, and lateral areas of the chest should be evaluated in a systematic fashion.[8]

CONFIRMATION OF TRACHEAL POSITION. Nurses should verify that the position of the **trachea** is midline. The trachea is assessed by placing the fingers in the suprasternal notch and moving upward. Deviation of the trachea to either side can indicate a pneumothorax, unilateral pneumonia, diffuse pulmonary fibrosis, a large pleural effusion, or severe atelectasis. With atelectasis the trachea shifts to the same side as the problem; with a pneumothorax the trachea shifts to the opposite side of the problem.[8]

ASSESSMENT OF RESPIRATORY EXCURSION. Assessment of respiratory excursion involves measuring the degree and symmetry of respiratory movement. Nurses should place their hands on the anterolateral part of the chest with the thumbs extended along the costal margin, pointing to the xiphoid process, or on the posterolateral part of the chest with the thumbs on either side of the spine at the level of the tenth rib. The patient is instructed to take a few normal breaths and then a few deep breaths. Chest movement is assessed for equality, or symmetry of thoracic expansion.[2,7,8] Asymmetry is an abnormal finding that can occur with pneumothorax, pneumonia, or other disorders that interfere with lung inflation. The degree of chest movement is felt to ascertain the extent of lung expansion. The thumbs should separate 3 to 5 cm during deep inhalation.[8] Lung expansion of a hyperinflated chest is less than that of a normal one.[3]

EVALUATION OF FREMITUS. Nurses assess tactile fremitus to identify, describe, and localize any areas of increased or decreased fremitus. *Fremitus* refers to the palpable vibrations felt through the chest wall when a patient speaks. It is assessed by placing the palms against opposite sides of the chest wall while the patient repeats

the word "ninety-nine."[7,8] Fremitus varies among individuals and depends on the pitch and intensity of the voice. Fremitus is described as *normal, decreased,* or *increased.* With normal fremitus, vibrations can be felt over the trachea but are barely palpable over the periphery. With decreased fremitus, interference occurs with the transmission of vibrations. Examples of disorders that decrease fremitus include pleural effusion, pneumothorax, bronchial obstruction, pleural thickening, and emphysema. With increased fremitus, the transmission of vibrations increases. Examples of disorders that increase fremitus include pneumonia, lung cancer, and pulmonary fibrosis.[2]

Percussion

Percussion of patients should focus on two priorities: (1) evaluation of the underlying lung structure and (2) assessment of diaphragmatic excursion. Although not in frequent use, percussion is a useful method for confirming suspected abnormalities.

EVALUATION OF UNDERLYING LUNG STRUCTURE. Nurses evaluate the underlying lung structure to estimate the amounts of air, liquid, or solid material present by placing the middle finger of the nondominant hand on the chest wall and then striking the distal portion (between the last joint and the nailbed) with the middle finger of their dominant hand. They move their hands from side to side systematically around the thorax, comparing similar areas, until the anterior, posterior, and both lateral areas have been assessed. Tones elicited can be described by five terms: resonance, hyperresonance, tympany, dullness, and flatness. These tones are distinguished by differences in intensity, pitch, duration, and quality. Table 11-1 describes the different percussion tones and their associated conditions.[9]

ASSESSMENT OF DIAPHRAGMATIC EXCURSION. Diaphragmatic excursion is assessed by measuring the difference in the level of the diaphragm during inhalation and exhalation. Nurses instruct the patient to inhale and hold a breath. The posterior chest is percussed downward over the intercostal spaces until the dull sound produced by the diaphragm is heard. The spot is marked, and the patient is instructed to take a few breaths, exhale completely, and hold a breath. Nurses percuss the posterior chest again and locate and mark the new area of dullness over the diaphragm, measuring and noting the difference between the two spots. Normal diaphragmatic excursion is 3 to 5 cm.[8] It may be decreased by ascites, pregnancy, hepatomegaly, and emphysema or increased by pleural effusion or disorders that elevate the diaphragm, such as atelectasis or paralysis.[3]

Auscultation

Auscultation of patients should focus on three priorities: (1) evaluation of normal breath sounds, (2) identification of abnormal breath sounds, and (3) assessment of voice sounds. Auscultation requires a quiet environment, proper positioning of the patient, and a bare

TABLE 11-1

PERCUSSION TONES AND THEIR ASSOCIATED CONDITIONS

TONE	DESCRIPTION	CONDITION
Resonance	Intensity–loud Pitch–low Duration–long Quality–hollow	Normal lung Bronchitis
Hyperresonance	Intensity–very loud Pitch–very low Duration–long Quality–booming	Asthma Emphysema Pneumothorax

Tympany	Intensity–loud
	Pitch–musical
	Duration–medium
	Quality–drumlike
		Large
		  pneumothorax
		Emphysematous
		  blebs

Dullness	Intensity–medium Pitch–medium-high Duration–medium Quality–thudlike	Atelectasis Pleural effusion Pulmonary edema Pneumonia Lung mass

Flatness	Intensity–soft
	Pitch–high
	Duration–short
	Quality–extremely
	  dull
		Massive
		  atelectasis
		Pneumonectomy

chest.[10] **Breath sounds** are best heard with the patient in the upright position.[8]

EVALUATION OF NORMAL BREATH SOUNDS. Evaluation of normal breath sounds is performed to assess air movement through the pulmonary system and identify the presence of abnormal sounds. Nurses place the diaphragm of the stethoscope against the chest wall and instruct the patient to breathe in and out slowly, with the mouth open. Both the inhalation and exhalation phases should be assessed. Auscultation should be done in a systematic sequence—side to side, top to bottom, anteriorly, laterally, and posteriorly (Fig. 11-1).[9]

DESCRIPTION OF NORMAL SOUNDS. Normal breath sounds differ according to their location and are classified in three categories: bronchial, bronchovesicular, and vesicular. Vesicular sounds are soft and low pitched and heard over most of the lung field. Bronchovesicular sounds are medium pitched and heard over the main bronchus area and the right upper-posterior lung fields. Bronchial sounds are heard only over the trachea and are high in pitch.[2,9,10]

IDENTIFICATION OF ABNORMAL BREATH SOUNDS. Abnormal breath sounds can be identified once the normal breath sounds have been clearly delineated. There are three categories of abnormal breath sounds: absent or di-

minished, displaced bronchial, and adventitious. Table 11-2 describes the various abnormal breath sounds and their associated conditions.[2,10]

DESCRIPTION OF ABNORMAL SOUNDS. An absent or diminished breath sound indicates that there is little or no airflow to a particular portion of the lung (either a small segment or an entire lung). Displaced bronchial breath sounds are normal bronchial sounds heard in the peripheral lung fields instead of over the trachea. This condition usually indicates fluid or exudate in the alveoli.[10] Classified as crackles, wheezes, and friction rubs, adventitious breath sounds occur in addition to the sounds already discussed. Crackles (also called *rales*) are short, discrete, popping or crackling sounds produced by fluid in the small airways or alveoli and mainly heard on inhalation.[10] Crackles can be further classified as *fine, medium,* or *coarse,* depending on pitch.[2] Wheezes are coarse, rumbling sounds produced by airflow over secretions in the larger airways or narrowing of the large airways. They are mainly heard on exhalation and can sometimes be cleared with coughing. Wheezes can be further classified as sibilant or sonorous (also called *rhonchi),* depending on the characteristics of the sound.[5] A pleural friction rub is a creaking, leathery, loud, dry, coarse sound produced by irritated pleural surfaces rubbing together. It is usually heard best in the lower anterolateral chest area during both inhalation and exhalation. Pleural friction rubs are caused by inflammation of the pleura.[2,5,7,8]

ASSESSMENT OF VOICE SOUNDS. Assessment of **voice sounds** is particularly useful in detecting lung consolidation or lung compression. Three abnormal types of voice sounds are bronchophony, whispering pectoriloquy, and egophony.[10]

DESCRIPTION OF VOICE SOUNDS. *Bronchophony* describes a condition in which the spoken voice is heard on auscultation with higher intensity and clarity than usual. Normally the spoken word is muffled when heard through the stethoscope. Nurses assess bronchophony by placing the diaphragm of the stethoscope against the posterior side of the patient's chest and instructing the patient to say "ninety-nine." Bronchophony is present when the sound is clear, distinct, and loud. *Whispering pectoriloquy* describes a condition of unusually clear transmission of the whispered voice on auscultation—normally the whispered word is unintelligible when heard through the stethoscope. Nurses assess whispering pectoriloquy by placing the stethoscope against the posterior side of the chest and instructing the patient to whisper "one, two, three." Whispering pectoriloquy is present when the sound is clear and distinct. *Egophony* describes a condition in which the voice sounds increase in intensity and develop a nasal, bleating quality on auscultation. Nurses assess egophony by placing the stethoscope against the posterior side of the chest and instructing the patient to say "e-e-e." Egophony is present when the "e" sound changes to an "a" sound.[8,10]

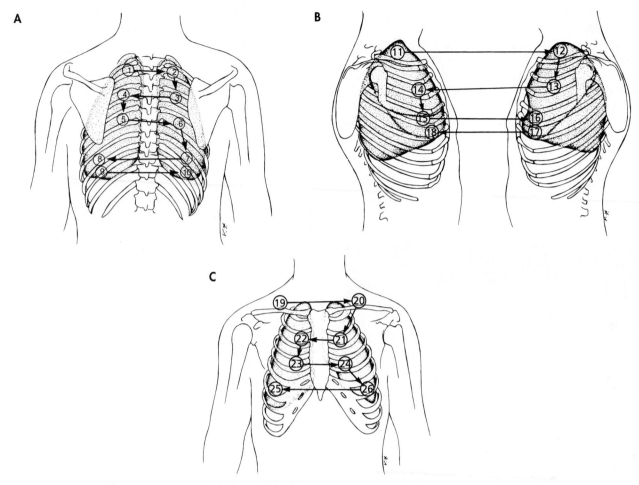

FIG. 11-1 Auscultation sequence. **A,** Posterior. **B,** Lateral. **C,** Anterior. (From Perry AG, Potter PA: *Clinical nursing skills and techniques,* ed 3, St Louis, 1994, Mosby.)

Laboratory Studies

Arterial Blood Gases

Interpreting arterial blood gases (ABGs) can be difficult, especially when nurses are under pressure to do it quickly and accurately. Following the same steps of interpretation each time can help ensure accuracy when analyzing arterial blood gas levels. A specific method to be used each time blood gas values are interpreted is presented here (Box 11-2).

Step 1

Nurses observe the PaO_2 level and answer the question, "Does the PaO_2 show hypoxemia?" The PaO_2 is a measure of the partial pressure of oxygen dissolved in arterial blood plasma, with "P" standing for "partial pressure" and "a" standing for "arterial." Sometimes PaO_2 is shortened to PO_2. It is reported in millimeters of mercury (mm Hg).

The normal range of PaO_2 for people breathing room air at sea level is 80 to 100 mm Hg. However, the normal range varies in infants and individuals 60 years of age and older. The normal level for infants breathing room air is 40 to 70 mm Hg. The normal level for people

60 years of age and older decreases with age because changes occur in the ventilation/perfusion (V/Q) matching in the aging lung. The correct PaO_2 for older people can be calculated as follows: 80 mm Hg (the lowest normal value) minus 1 mm Hg for every year that the person's age exceeds 60. This formula demonstrates that a 65-year-old individual can have a PaO_2 as low as 75 mm Hg and still be within the normal range (5 years over 60 years of age: 80 mm Hg − 5 mm Hg = 75 mm Hg). An acceptable range for an 80-year-old person is 60 mm Hg (20 years over the age of 60: 80 mm Hg − 20 mm Hg = 60 mm Hg). At any age, a PaO_2 lower than 40 mm Hg represents a life-threatening situation that requires immediate action. In addition, a PaO_2 less than the predicted lowest value indicates **hypoxemia**, which means that a lower-than-normal amount of oxygen is dissolved in plasma.[11]

Step 2

Nurses observe the pH level and answer the question, "Is the pH on the acid or alkaline side of 7.40?" The pH is the hydrogen ion (H^+) concentration of plasma. Calculation of pH is accomplished by using the partial pressure of carbon dioxide ($Paco_2$) and the plasma bicarbonate level (Hco_3^-).

The normal pH of arterial blood is 7.35 to 7.45, with the mean being 7.40. If the pH is less than 7.40, it is on the acid side of the mean. A pH less than 7.35 indicates acidemia, and the overall condition is called *acidosis.* If the pH is greater than 7.40, it is on the alkaline side of the mean. A pH greater than 7.45 indicates alkalemia, and the overall condition is called *alkalosis.*[2,12]

Step 3

Nurses observe the $Paco_2$ level and answer the question, "Does the $Paco_2$ show respiratory acidosis, alkalosis, or

normalcy?" The $Paco_2$ is a measure of the partial pressure of carbon dioxide dissolved in arterial blood plasma and is reported in mm Hg. The acid-base component reflects the effectiveness of ventilation in relation to the metabolic rate.[11] In other words, the $Paco_2$ value indicates whether patients can ventilate well enough to rid the body of the carbon dioxide produced as a consequence of metabolism.[13]

The normal range for $Paco_2$ is 35 to 45 mm Hg. This range does not change as people age. A $Paco_2$ of greater than 45 mm Hg indicates **respiratory acidosis,** which is caused by alveolar hypoventilation. Hypoventilation can result from COPD, oversedation, head trauma, anesthesia, drug overdose, neuromuscular disease, or hypoventilation with mechanical ventilation. A $Paco_2$ value less than 35 mm Hg represents **respiratory alkalosis,** which is caused by alveolar hyperventilation. Hyperventilation can result from hypoxia, anxiety, pulmonary embolism, pregnancy, and hyperventilation with mechanical ventilation.[12-14]

Step 4

Nurses observe the Hco_3^- level and answer the question, "Does the Hco_3^- show metabolic acidosis, alkalosis, or normalcy?" The bicarbonate (Hco_3^-) is the acid-base component that reflects kidney function. The bicarbonate is reduced or increased in the plasma by renal mechanisms. The normal range is 22 to 26 mEq/L. A bicarbonate level of less than 22 mEq/L represents

TABLE 11-2 ABNORMAL BREATH SOUNDS AND THEIR ASSOCIATED CONDITIONS		
ABNORMAL SOUND	**DESCRIPTION**	**CONDITION**
Absent breath sounds	No airflow to particular portion of lung	Pneumothorax Pneumonectomy Emphysematous blebs Pleural effusion Lung mass Massive atelectasis Complete airway obstruction
Diminished breath sounds	Little airflow to particular portion of lung	Emphysema Pleural effusion Pleurisy Atelectasis Pulmonary fibrosis
Displaced bronchial sounds	Bronchial sounds heard in peripheral lung fields	Atelectasis with secretions Lung mass with exudate Pneumonia Pleural effusion Pulmonary edema
Crackles (rales)	Short, discrete, popping or crackling sounds	Pulmonary edema Pneumonia Pulmonary fibrosis Atelectasis Bronchiectasis
Sonorous wheezes (rhonchi)	Coarse, rumbling, low-pitched sounds	Pneumonia Asthma Bronchitis Bronchospasm
Sibilant wheezes	High-pitched, squeaking, whistling sounds	Asthma Bronchospasm
Pleural friction rub	Creaking, leathery, loud, dry, coarse sounds	Pleural effusion Pleurisy

---

BOX 11-2

STEPS FOR INTERPRETATION OF BLOOD GAS LEVELS

STEP 1

Look at the Pao_2 level and answer the question, *"Does the Pao_2 level show hypoxemia?"*

STEP 2

Look at the pH level and answer the question, *"Is the pH level on the acid or alkaline side of 7.40?"*

STEP 3

Look at the $Paco_2$ level and answer the question, *"Does the $Paco_2$ level show respiratory acidosis, alkalosis, or normalcy?"*

STEP 4

Look at the Hco_3 level and answer the question, *"Does the Hco_3 level show metabolic acidosis, alkalosis, or normalcy?"*

STEP 5

Look back at the pH level and answer the question, *"Does the pH show a compensated or an uncompensated condition?"*

metabolic acidosis, which can result from ketoacidosis, lactic acidosis, renal failure, or diarrhea. A bicarbonate level greater than 26 mEq/L indicates **metabolic alkalosis,** which can result from fluid loss from the upper GI tract (vomiting or nasogastric suction), diuretic therapy, severe hypokalemia, alkali administration, or steroid therapy.[12-14]

Step 5

Nurses observe the pH level again and answer the question, "Does the pH show a compensated or an uncompensated condition?" If the pH level is abnormal (less than 7.35 or greater than 7.45), the $Paco_2$, the Hco_3^-, or both will also be abnormal. This is an uncompensated condition because the body has not had enough time to return the pH to its normal range (Box 11-3). If the pH is within normal limits and both the $Paco_2$ and the Hco_3^- are abnormal, the condition is compensated because there has been enough time for the body to restore the pH to within its normal range. Differentiating the primary disorder from the compensatory response can be difficult. The primary disorder is the abnormality that caused the pH to shift initially; thus, on whichever side of 7.40 the pH occurs is considered the primary disorder. The body will not fully compensate for the primary acid-base disturbance (Box 11-4).[11,13,14] Partial compensation may also be present and is evidenced by an abnormal pH, $Paco_2$, and Hco_3^-, indications that the body is attempting to return the pH to its normal range.[12]

Table 11-3 summarizes the changes in the acid-base components accompanying various acid-base disorders.[11-14] In addition to the parameters discussed, a number of other factors should be considered during review of patients' ABGs. These factors include oxygen saturation and content, expected Pao_2, and base excess and deficit.

Oxygen saturation (Sao₂)

Oxygen saturation is a measure of the amount of oxygen bound to hemoglobin, compared with hemoglobin's maximal capability for binding oxygen. It is reported as a percentage or decimal, with normal being greater than 95% on room air.[14] The Sao_2 level cannot reach 100% (on room air) because of the normal physiologic shunting.[15] However, when supplemental oxygen is administered, the Sao_2 level may be so close to 100% that it is reported as 100%.

Proper evaluation of the Sao_2 level is vital. For example, an Sao_2 of 97% means that 97% of the available hemoglobin is bound with oxygen. The word *available* is essential to evaluating the Sao_2 level because the hemoglobin level is not always within normal limits and oxygen can bind only with what is available. A 97% saturation level associated with 10 g of hemoglobin does not deliver as much oxygen to the tissues as does a 97% saturation level associated with 15 g of hemoglobin. Thus, assessing only the Sao_2 level and finding it within normal limits should not lead nurses to believe that patients' oxygenation status is normal. The hemoglobin level must also be evaluated before a decision on oxygenation status can be made.[16]

Arterial oxygen content (Cao₂)

Arterial oxygen content (Cao_2) is a measure of the total amount of oxygen carried in the arterial blood, including the amount dissolved in plasma (measured by the Pao_2) and the amount bound to the hemoglobin molecule (measured by the Sao_2). Cao_2 is reported in milliliters (ml) of oxygen carried per 100 ml of blood. The normal value is 20 ml of oxygen per 100 ml of blood. The Pao_2, Sao_2, and hemoglobin level are used to calculate the oxygen content (see Appendix B). A change in any of these parameters will affect the Cao_2.[15]

BOX 11-3

EXAMPLES OF UNCOMPENSATED ABGs

UNCOMPENSATED RESPIRATORY ACIDOSIS

Pao_2: 90 mm Hg
pH: 7.25
$Paco_2$: 50 mm Hg
Hco_3^-: 22 mEq/L

UNCOMPENSATED METABOLIC ACIDOSIS

Pao_2: 90 mm Hg
pH: 7.25
$Paco_2$: 40 mm Hg
Hco_3^-: 17 mEq/L

BOX 11-4

EXAMPLES OF COMPENSATED ABGs

COMPENSATED RESPIRATORY ACIDOSIS WITH METABOLIC ALKALOSIS

Pao_2: 90 mm Hg
pH: 7.37
$Paco_2$: 60 mm Hg
Hco_3^-: 38 mEq/L

In this example the acidosis is considered the main disorder and the alkalosis the compensating disorder because the pH is on the acid side of 7.40.

COMPENSATED METABOLIC ALKALOSIS WITH RESPIRATORY ACIDOSIS

Pao_2: 90 mm Hg
pH: 7.42
$Paco_2$: 48 mm Hg
Hco_3^-: 35 mEq/L

In this example the alkalosis is considered the main disorder and the acidosis the compensating disorder because the pH is on the alkaline side of 7.40.

TABLE 11-3
SUMMARY OF ARTERIAL BLOOD GAS ASSESSMENT

DISORDER	pH	Paco$_3$	Hco$_3$−
Respiratory Acidosis			
Uncompensated	< 7.35	> 45 mm Hg	22 - 26 mEq/L
Partially compensated	< 7.35	> 45 mm Hg	> 26 mEq/L
Compensated	7.35 - 7.39	> 45 mm Hg	> 26 mEq/L
Respiratory Alkalosis			
Uncompensated	> 7.45	< 35 mm Hg	22 - 26 mEq/L
Partially compensated	> 7.45	< 35 mm Hg	< 22 mEq/L
Compensated	7.41 - 7.45	< 35 mm Hg	< 22 mEq/L
Metabolic Acidosis			
Uncompensated	< 7.35	35 - 45 mm Hg	< 22 mEq/L
Partially compensated	< 7.35	< 35 mm Hg	< 22 mEq/L
Compensated	7.35 - 7.39	< 35 mm Hg	< 22 mEq/L
Metabolic Alkalosis			
Uncompensated	> 7.45	35 - 45 mm Hg	> 26 mEq/L
Partially compensated	> 7.45	> 45 mm Hg	> 26 mEq/L
Compensated	7.41 - 7.45	> 45 mm Hg	> 26 mEq/L
Combined Respiratory and Metabolic Acidosis	< 7.35	> 45 mm Hg	< 22 mEq/L
Combined Respiratory and Metabolic Alkalosis	> 7.45	< 35 mm Hg	> 26 mEq/L

Expected Pao$_2$

When patients receive supplemental oxygen, their Pao$_2$ level is expected to rise. Knowing the level to which the Pao$_2$ should rise in normal subjects on a given FIo$_2$ and comparing that with the level to which the Pao$_2$ actually does rise in patients with pulmonary disease has value because it illustrates how well the lung is functioning. Nurses calculate the expected Pao$_2$ by multiplying the FIo$_2$ value by 5.[11] Thus the expected Pao$_2$ on an FIo$_2$ of 30% should be at least 150 mm Hg (30 × 5), whereas the expected Pao$_2$ on an FIo$_2$ of 50% should be 250 mm Hg (50 × 5). These expected Pao$_2$ values represent the oxygen level achievable with healthy lungs. Pulmonary disease can radically decrease the expected Pao$_2$ level. Applying the "FIo$_2$ value × 5" rule to achieve the expected Pao$_2$ value is impossible when patients are on a system that delivers oxygen by liters per minute. In these situations the liter flow must be converted to a percentage of oxygen (Table 11-4).

Base excess and base deficit

Base excess and base deficit reflect the nonrespiratory contribution to acid-base balance and are reported in milliequivalents per liter above or below the normal range of −2 mEq/L to +2 mEq/L. A negative base level is reported as a base deficit, which correlates with metabolic acidosis, whereas a positive base level is reported as a base excess, which correlates with metabolic alkalosis.[2,13]

Intrapulmonary Shunt Equation

The efficiency of oxygenation can be measured using the intrapulmonary shunt (Qs/Qt) equation (see Appendix B). This formula measures the percentage of cardiac output being returned to the left side of the heart without participating in gas exchange.[11] An intrapulmonary shunt greater than 10% is considered abnormal and indicative of a shunt-producing disorder.[17] The major limitation to using this formula is that it requires information from both an arterial and a mixed venous blood gas to complete. Although a number of other methods exist for estimating intrapulmonary shunting, they have been found unreliable in critically ill patients.[11]

Deadspace Equation

The efficiency of ventilation can be measured using the clinical deadspace (Vd/Vt) equation (see Appendix B). The formula measures the fraction of tidal volume not participating in gas exchange. Deadspace greater than 0.6 indicates a deadspace-producing disorder and is considered abnormal. According to Shapiro, Peruzzi, and Kozelowski-Templin, the major limitations to using this formula are that it requires the measurement of exhaled carbon dioxide to complete and that the work of breathing by patients must remain stable during the collection.[11]

TABLE 11-4 GUIDELINES FOR ESTIMATING FIo₂ WITH LOW-FLOW OXYGEN DEVICES	
100% O₂ FLOW RATE (L)	**FIo₂ (%)**
NASAL CANNULA OR CATHETER	
1	24
2	28
3	32
4	36
5	40
6	44
OXYGEN MASK	
5-6	40
6-7	50
7-8	60
MASK WITH RESERVOIR BAG	
6	60
7	70
8	80
9	90
10	99+

From Shapiro BA, Peruzzi WT, Kozelowski-Templin R: *Clinical application of blood gases*, ed 5, St Louis, 1994. Mosby.
NOTE: Normal ventilatory pattern assumed.

Sputum Studies

Careful analysis of sputum specimens is crucial for the rapid identification and treatment of pulmonary infections. The most difficult aspect of sputum examination is proper collection of the specimen.

Procedure

In general, collection of a good sputum sample requires conscious, cooperative, sufficiently hydrated patients.[18] When patients have difficulty producing sputum, heated, nebulized saline may help to loosen secretions for expectoration. A combination of chest physiotherapy and nebulization improves the success rate. Collection of a sputum specimen is preferably accomplished in the morning because a greater volume of secretions are present as a result of nighttime pooling.[4] Because many critically ill patients cannot cough effectively, sputum collection by other means is required. These methods include tracheobronchial aspiration, transtracheal aspiration, and the use of a fiberoptic bronchoscopy with a protected brush catheter. Because each method has its own benefits and risks, the clinical condition of patients determines the appropriate technique.[19]

TABLE 11-5 SPUTUM CHARACTERISTICS SEEN IN VARIOUS PULMONARY DISORDERS	
APPEARANCE	**POTENTIAL CAUSE**
Pink-salmon	*Staphylococcus* pneumonia
Rusty	*Streptococcus* pneumonia
Green	*Pseudomonas* pneumonia
Currant	*Klebsiella* pneumonia
Blood-tinged	Pulmonary embolism
	Lung cancer
Frothy, clear	Early pulmonary edema
Frothy, copious, pink	Late pulmonary edema

Significance

Once a sputum specimen is obtained, it is examined for volume, physical properties, mucopurulence, and color. Table 11-5 describes the sputum characteristics of various pulmonary disorders.[5] A microscopic examination is performed next to identify the source of the specimen. If a bacterial infection is suspected, a Gram stain followed by a culture and sensitivity (C&S) is performed.[18] The Gram stain should be performed first to evaluate whether the specimen is contaminated with oropharyngeal secretions.[19]

Diagnostic Procedures

Fiberoptic Bronchoscopy

Fiberoptic bronchoscopy is a relatively safe procedure most often used as both a diagnostic and therapeutic tool. Diagnostic indications include inspection of the lower airways for secretions, burns, abscesses, lesions, injury, or hemorrhage and inspection of the upper airways for laryngeal edema or burns.[20,21] Therapeutic indications include the removal of foreign bodies or excessive secretions, atelectasis, hemoptysis, difficult intubation, and resection of small, benign growths from the airway.[20,22]

Procedure

Patients should receive nothing by mouth for at least 3 to 6 hours before the procedure or as ordered by the physician.[3] Prior to the bronchoscopy, antisialagogues, narcotics, anxiolytics, topical anesthetics, and oxygen are usually administered. An antisialagogue such as atropine, glycopyrrolate (Robinul), or scopolamine is usually given 1 hour before the procedure to reduce secretions. Narcotics such as meperidine (Demerol) or codeine may also be given to depress laryngeal reflexes, induce slower and deeper respirations, and prevent coughing during the procedure. Although a topical anesthesic can be used alone, it is generally supplemented by an intravenous anxiolytic agent. Diazepam (Valium) and midazolam (Versed) are two agents frequently administered intravenously during the procedure to provide sedation.[22] Oxygen is administered before and during the procedure. The bronchoscopy is accomplished using a flexible fiberoptic bronchoscope inserted via the mouth, nose, or endotracheal tube (if present) into the lungs. The scope contains four channels: one for viewing, two that provide light, and one that is open. The open channel may be used for administering oxygen, suctioning, lavaging, or obtaining samples.[4,22]

COMPLICATIONS. Complications during the procedure may be related to the procedure itself, the anesthetic, or an ancillary procedure. Minor complications include laryngospasm, epistaxis, fever, pulmonary infiltrates, altered pulmonary mechanics, and hemodynamic instability. Major complications include anaphylaxis, hypotension, cardiac dysrhythmias, bronchospasm, pneumothorax, hemorrhage, hypoxemia, and cardiopulmonary arrest.[21,22]

Significance

Any specimens obtained during the procedure are sent to the laboratory for further cytologic or bacteriologic examination. The results are used to guide further therapy.[22]

Thoracentesis

Thoracentesis is a usually uncomplicated procedure for the removal of fluid or air from the pleural space. Most frequently used as a diagnostic measure, it may in rare circumstances be performed therapeutically, as in drainage of a pleural effusion or empyema.[23] No absolute contraindications to thoracentesis exist, but it does require cooperative patients. The procedure should be used with caution in patients who have bleeding disorders or who are anticoagulated.[24]

Procedure

Patients are placed in a sitting position with legs over the side of the bed and hands and arms supported by a padded overbed table. If the condition of patients precludes them from sitting (e.g., patients on ventilators), they should be placed in the lateral decubitus position with the affected side down. Patients should be cautioned not to move or cough during the procedure.[24] The site of the needle insertion is usually determined by previous chest x-ray examination, CT scan, or chest percussion. A local anesthetic is used to minimize discomfort during insertion of the thoracentesis needle.[23] Nurses monitor patients by using a pulse oximeter and administer supplemental oxygen. Atropine should be available in case patients experience a vasovagal response and become bradycardic. A chest x-ray should follow the procedure to rule out complications.[24]

COMPLICATIONS. Complications associated with thoracentesis include pain, pleural infection, hemothorax,

laceration of the liver or spleen, pneumothorax, and reexpansion pulmonary edema.[24] Reexpansion pulmonary edema can occur when a large amount of effusion fluid is removed from the pleural space. Removal of the fluid increases the negative intrapleural pressure, which can lead to edema when the lung does not reexpand to fill the space. Patients may experience severe coughing and shortness of breath, symptoms indicating that thoracentesis should be discontinued. The major complication of thoracentesis is pneumothorax, the risk of which can be reduced by using a small gauge needle, ultrasonography with small effusions to guide the procedure, and a needle catheter system with large effusions.[24]

Significance

Any specimens obtained during the procedure are sent to the laboratory to determine if the fluid is transudative or exudative in nature. Transudative effusions occur with disorders that disrupt capillary or plasma oncotic pressure (e.g., congestive heart failure) and force fluid into the pleural space. Exudative effusions occur with disorders that alter the permeability of the pleural membrane (e.g., empyema) and allow fluid to enter the pleural space.[24]

Pulmonary Function Tests

An essential component of a thorough pulmonary evaluation, pulmonary function tests (PFTs) are designed to quantify respiratory function. PFTs are used for a variety of purposes, including preoperative assessment, evaluation of lung mechanics, and diagnosis and tracking of pulmonary diseases. Variations in the normal pulmonary function occur with age, gender, and body size.[4]

Types of tests

Many different types of pulmonary function tests exist. The following discussion is an overview of some of the tests that may be performed for critically ill patients.

STATIC LUNG VOLUMES. Measurements can be taken to evaluate the various properties of the lung-thorax system. Static lung volumes provide a basic assessment of ventilatory function and are altered by abnormalities of the respiratory muscles, chest wall, lung parenchyma, and airways. These tests include measurement of tidal volume, inspiratory reserve volume, inspiratory capacity, expiratory reserve volume, vital capacity, residual volume, functional residual capacity, and total lung capacity (Box 11-5).[25]

STATIC AND DYNAMIC COMPLIANCE. Pulmonary mechanics, the elastic properties of the lungs and chest wall, can be evaluated through measurement of static and dynamic compliance (see Appendix B). Static compliance measures lung compliance, whereas dynamic compliance measures both lung and airway resistance. Normal static compliance is approximately 50 ml/cm H_2O. It decreases with any decrease in lung compliance, such as occurs with pneumothorax, atelectasis, pneumonia, pulmonary edema, and chest wall restrictions. Normal dynamic compliance is approximately 40 to 50 ml/cm H_2O. It decreases with any decrease in lung compliance or increase in airway resistance, such as occurs with bronchospasms and retained secretions. If both static and dynamic compliance change, lung compliance has also changed. If static compliance remains the same while dynamic compliance changes, airway resistance has changed.[26]

DYNAMIC PULMONARY FUNCTION TESTS. Dynamic pulmonary function tests evaluate the function of the respiratory muscles, thorax, and lungs.[27] These tests are timed breathing studies that reflect the ease of ventilation and include forced vital capacity (FVC), forced expiratory flow at midpoint of vital capacity (FEF$_{25\%-75\%}$), forced expiratory flow at 1 and 3 seconds (FEV$_1$ and FEV$_3$), and maximal voluntary ventilation (MVV).[3]

Procedure

PFTs are usually performed at the bedside of critically ill patients, using spirometry. These tests can be performed for intubated or nonintubated patients. For intubated patients, the spirometer is attached to the end of the endotracheal tube. For nonintubated patients, a nose clip is attached and patients are instructed to breathe through a spirometer tube. Patients should be seated on the side of the bed if possible.[4]

Significance

The spirometer can be used to measure both static and dynamic lung parameters, with the exception of residual volume and functional residual capacity. Bedside PFTs usually include respiratory rate, tidal volume, minute ventilation, MVV, and FVC. Additional flow and pressure parameters that can be obtained include maximal inspiratory pressure, maximal expiratory pressure, and peak expiratory flow rate, FEF$_{25\%-75\%}$, FEV$_1$, and FEV$_3$. Table 11-6 provides a description of each of these parameters.[4]

Ventilation/Perfusion Scan

Ventilation/perfusion (V/Q) scanning is indicated when a serious alteration of the normal ventilation/perfusion relationship is suspected. V/Q studies are most frequently ordered to diagnose and follow a suspected pulmonary embolus. V/Q scanning is approximately 90% accurate in determining this diagnosis. Comparing the perfusion scan with the results of a chest x-ray examination may improve these percentages somewhat.[28]

BOX 11-5

LUNG VOLUMES AND CAPACITIES

Tidal volume (VT): The volume of air exhaled after a normal resting inhalation. VT × respiratory rate = minute ventilation. Normal is 500 ml.

Inspiratory reserve volume (IRV): The amount of additional air that can be taken in after a normal inhalation. Normal is 3000-3100 ml.

Inspiratory capacity (IC): The maximal amount of air that can be inhaled after a normal exhalation. Normal is 3500-3600 ml.

Expiratory reserve volume (ERV): The additional amount of air that can be exhaled after a normal resting exhalation. Normal is 1100-1200 ml.

Vital capacity (VC): The maximal amount of air that can be exhaled after a maximal inhalation. Normal is 4600-4800 ml.

Residual volume (RV): The amount of air left in the lung after maximal exhalation. Normal is 1200-1300 ml.

Functional residual capacity (FRC): The amount of air left in the lung after a normal exhalation. The total of the ERV and RV. Normal is 2300-2400 ml.

Total lung capacity (TLC): The maximal volume of air in the lung after a maximal inspiration. The total of all lung volumes. Normal is 5800-6000 ml.

TABLE 11-6

BEDSIDE PULMONARY FUNCTION TESTS

TEST	DESCRIPTION
Respiratory rate (f)	Number of breaths per minute
Tidal volume (VT)	Volume of air exhaled after a normal resting inhalation
Minute ventilation (VE)	Volume of air expired per minute (tidal volume × respiratory rate = minute ventilation)
Maximal voluntary ventilation (MVV)	Maximal amount of air that can moved into and out of the lungs in 1 minute
Forced vital capacity (FVC)	Maximal amount of air that can be forcefully exhaled from the lungs after maximal inhalation
Maximal inspiratory pressure (MIP)	Maximal negative pressure generated on inhalation
Maximal expiratory pressure (MEP)	Maximal positive pressure generated on exhalation
Peak expiratory flow rate (PEFR)	Maximal flow rate achieved during forced exhalation
Forced expiratory flow at midpoint of vital capacity (FEF$_{25\%-75\%}$)	Measure of the average flow rate during the middle 50% of exhalation
Forced expiratory flow at 1 and 3 seconds (FEV$_1$ and FEV$_3$)	Volume of air exhaled in first and third seconds of forced exhalation

Procedure

The V/Q scan consists of a ventilation scan and perfusion scan. In the ventilation scan patients inhale a radiolabeled gas and air mixture through a mask or endotracheal tube. The perfusion scan is performed by intravenously injecting patients with a radioisotope. Scintillation cameras record the gamma radiation images produced by the isotope as it is breathed or perfused into the lung. When the isotope's flow into an area of the lung is obstructed, the diminished radioactivity will be reflected in the camera image of that zone.[28]

Significance

While most pulmonary diseases cause abnormalities in both the ventilation and the perfusion scan (known as a matched defect), a pulmonary embolus causes an abnormality in the perfusion scan only (known as a mismatched defect). The results are usually reported in terms of the probability of a pulmonary embolus. Low probability indicates a 10% to 20% chance, intermediate probability indicates a 30% to 50% chance, and high probability indicates an 80% to 90% chance.[29]

Chest Radiography

Chest radiography is an important diagnostic procedure for critically ill patients. **Chest x-ray examinations** aid in the diagnosis of various disorders and complications and assist in the evaluation of treatment.[30] Chapter 9 provides a discussion of the basic principles and techniques of chest radiography. The interpretation of a chest x-ray film relies upon a systematic method of viewing (Box 11-6). Areas of the film that should be assessed include bones, mediastinum, diaphragm, pleural space, and lung tissue. (Fig. 11-2 depicts a normal chest x-ray film.)

Bones

The clavicles, ribs, thoracic and cervical spine, and scapulae should be assessed. The clavicles should be symmetric, and the ribs should be an equal distance apart. The thoracic and cervical spine should reveal no signs of curvature. The scapulae usually appear as areas of added density in the upper lung fields. No evidence of fractures, calcification and lesions (increased density), or demineralization (decreased density) should be present.[31-33]

Mediastinum

The structures in the mediastinal area that should be assessed are the cardiac silhouette and the trachea. The trachea should be midline with a slight deviation to the right as it approaches the carina.[31-33] Shifting of the mediastinal structures can occur with atelectasis (toward the area of involvement), pneumothorax (away from the area of involvement), pleural effusion, tumors, and removal of all or a portion of a lung.[32,33]

BOX 11-6

STEPS FOR INTERPRETATION OF A CHEST X-RAY FILM

STEP 1

Look at the different densities (black, gray, and white) and answer the question, *"What is air, fluid, tissue, and bone?"*

STEP 2

Look at the shape or form of each density and answer the question, *"What normal anatomic structure is this?"*

STEP 3

Look at both right and left sides and answer the question, *"Are the findings the same on both sides or are there differences (both physiologic and pathophysiologic)?"*

STEP 4

Look at all the structures (bones, mediastinum, diaphragm, pleural space, and lung tissue) and answer the question, *"Are there any abnormalities present?"*

STEP 5

Look for all tubes, wires, and lines and answer the question, *"Are the tubes, wires, and lines in the proper place?"*

Diaphragm

The diaphragm should be clearly visible with sharp costophrenic angles (where the chest wall and the tapered edges of the diaphragm meet).[32,33] The dome of the diaphragm (on deep inspiration) should appear at the level of the sixth rib, with the right side slightly higher than the left.[31-33] A gastric air bubble may be found under the left side of the diaphragm.[33] An elevated diaphragm is sometimes seen with pregnancy, obesity, conditions that cause air or fluid to accumulate in the peritoneal space, intestinal obstruction, and splitting. An elevated hemidiaphragm is associated with a number of conditions, including phrenic nerve injury, previous chest surgery, subphrenic abscess, trauma, stroke, tumor, pneumonia, and radiation therapy.[31] Flattening of the diaphragm can signal increased air in the lungs, such as occurs with COPD.[32] Obliteration or "blunting" of the costophrenic angle can occur with pleural effusion, atelectasis, or pneumothorax.[31,32]

Pleural space

Identification of the pleural space on a chest x-ray film is abnormal. The pleural space is not visible unless air (pneumothorax) or fluid enters it (pleural effusion). As fluid accumulates in the pleural space, it surrounds the lung and eventually compresses it. With a pleural effu-

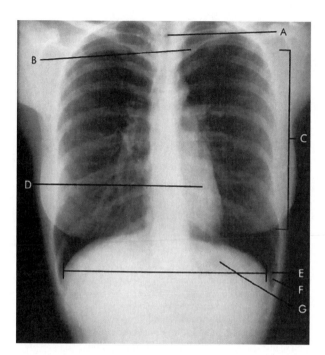

FIG. 11-2 Location of structures on normal PA chest film. **A,** Trachea. **B,** Clavicle. **C,** Ribs. **D,** Cardiac silhouette. **E,** Diaphragm. **F,** Costophrenic angle. **G,** Gastric air bubble.

<table>
<tr><td colspan="3">B O X 1 1 - 7</td></tr>
</table>

MANIFESTATIONS OF RESPIRATORY DECOMPENSATION

INADEQUATE AIRWAY

Stridor
Noisy respirations
Supraclavicular and intercostal retractions
Flaring of nares
Labored breathing with use of accessory muscles

INADEQUATE VENTILATION

Absence of air exchange at nose and mouth (breathlessness)
Minimal/absent chest wall motion
Manifestations of obstructed airway
Central cyanosis
Decreased or absent breath sounds (bilateral, unilateral)
Restlessness, anxiety, confusion
Paradoxical motion involving significant portion of chest wall
Decreased Pao_2, increased $Paco_2$, decreased pH

INADEQUATE GAS EXCHANGE

Tachypnea
Decreased Pao_2
Increased dead space
Central cyanosis
Chest infiltrates on x-ray evaluation

---

sion, blunting of the costophrenic angle may be evident first, with flattening of the diaphragm and obscuring of the heart borders occurring as the effusion grows.[30,32] With a pneumothorax the pleural edges become evident through and between the images of the ribs on the film. A thin line appears just parallel to the chest wall, indicating where the lung markings have pulled away from the chest wall.[31] In addition, the collapsed lung will appear as an area of increased density separated by an area of radiolucency (blackness).[32]

Lung tissue

The lung tissue should be assessed for any areas of increased density or increased radiolucency that could indicate an abnormality. Increased density can result from accumulated fluid in the lungs (e.g., water, pus, blood, edema fluid) or collapsed lung tissue (as occurs with atelectasis or pneumothorax). Increased radiolucency is caused by increased air in the lungs, as may occur with COPD. In some patients a fine line may be present on the right side at about the level of the sixth rib in the midlung field. This normal finding represents the horizontal fissure, which separates the right upper lobe from the right middle lobe.[31]

Tubes, wires, and lines

The chest x-ray film should also be assessed for proper placement of all tubes, wires, and lines. When properly positioned, an endotracheal tube should be 2 to 4 cm above the carina. The nasogastric tube should run the length of the esophagus with the tip in the stomach. The

pulmonary artery catheter should run through the right atrium and right ventricle into the pulmonary artery.[32] Additional items that may be present include temporary or permanent pacing wires, permanent pacing generator, automatic implantable cardioverter defibrillator, chest tubes (pleural or mediastinal), central venous pressure line, peripherally inserted central catheter, intraaortic balloon pump catheter, electrocardiograph electrodes, and surgical markers and clips.

Nursing Management

The nursing management of patients undergoing a diagnostic procedure involves a variety of interventions. **Priorities are directed toward preparing patients psychologically and physically for the procedure, monitoring patients' responses to the procedure, and assessing patients after the procedure.** Preparing patients includes teaching them about the procedure, answering any questions, and positioning them for the procedure. Monitoring patients' responses to the procedure includes observing them for signs of pain, anxiety, or respiratory decompensation (Box 11-7) and monitoring vital signs, breath sounds, and oxygen saturation. Assessing patients after the procedure includes observing for complications of the procedure and medicating patients for any post-procedure discomfort.[3] **Any evidence of respiratory decompensation should be immediately reported to the physician, and emergency measures to maintain airway and breathing must be initiated.**

References

1. Gehring PE: Physical assessment begins with a history, *RN* 54(11):26, 1991.
2. Brenner M, Welliver J: Pulmonary and acid-base assessment, *Nurs Clin North Am* 25:761, 1990.
3. Dettenmeier PA: *Pulmonary nursing care*, St Louis, 1992, Mosby.
4. Wilson SF, Thompson JM: *Respiratory disorders*, St Louis, 1990, Mosby.
5. Stiesmeyer JK: A four-step approach to pulmonary assessment, *Am J Nurs* 93(8):22, 1993.
6. Carpenter KD: A comprehensive review of cyanosis, *Crit Care Nurse* 13(4):66, 1993.
7. Kuhn KW, McGovern M: Respiratory assessment of the elderly, *J Gerontologic Nurs* (5):40, 1992.
8. Malasanos L, Barkauskas V, Stoltenberg-Allen K: *Health assessment*, ed 4, St Louis, 1990, Mosby.
9. Seidel HM and others: *Mosby's guide to physical examination*, ed 2, St Louis, 1991, Mosby.
10. Boyda EK and others: *Pulmonary auscultation*, St Paul, 1987, 3M Health Care Group.
11. Shapiro BA, Peruzzi WT, Kozelowski-Templin R: *Clinical application of blood gases*, St Louis, ed 5, 1994, Mosby.
12. Haber RJ: A practical approach to acid-base balance, *West J Med* 155:146, 1991.
13. Tasota FJ, Wesmiller SW: Assessing A.B.G.s: maintaining the delicate balance, *Nursing* 24(5):34, 1994.
14. Mims BC: Interpreting ABGs, *RN* 50(3):42, 1991.
15. Carpenter KD: Oxygen transport in the blood, *Crit Care Nurse* 11(9):20, 1991.
16. Reischman RR: Impaired gas exchange related to intrapulmonary shunting, *Crit Care Nurse* 8(8):35, 1988.
17. Grundberg E: Methods used and errors encountered in estimating intrapulmonary shunt, *Can J Resp Ther* 28:183, 1992.
18. Lekas NJ: *Clinical microbiology: nosocomial infections and microbiologic procedures.* In Victor LD, editor: *Manual of critical care procedures*, Rockville, Md, 1989, Aspen.
19. Chodosh S: *Sputum examination.* In Fishman AP, editor: *Pulmonary diseases and disorders*, ed 2, New York, 1988, McGraw-Hill.
20. Krell WS: *Bronchoscopy in the critically ill.* In Victor LD, editor: *Manual of critical care procedures*, Rockville, Md, 1989, Aspen.
21. Turner JS and others: Fiberoptic bronchoscopy in the intensive care unit: a prospective study of 147 procedures in 107 patients, *Crit Care Med* 22:259, 1994.
22. Arzueto A, Levine SM, Jenkinson SG: The technique of fiberoptic bronchoscopy, *J Crit Ill* 7:1657, 1992.
23. Talamonti WJ: *Thoracentesis and chest tube insertion.* In Victor LD, editor: *Manual of critical care procedures*, Rockville, Md, 1989, Aspen.
24. Qureshi N, Momin ZA, Brandstetter RD: Thoracentesis in clinical practice, *Heart Lung* 23:376, 1994.
25. Baum G, Wolinsky E: *Textbook of pulmonary disease*, ed 4, Boston, 1989, Little, Brown.
26. Mims BC: *Mechanical ventilation: process and practice*, Lewisville, Tex, 1989, Barbara Clark Mims Associates.
27. Williams D, Cugell D: Pulmonary function tests: indications and interpretation, *Hosp Med* 24(5):23, 1988.
28. Stratton MB: Ventilation-perfusion scintigraphy in diagnosis of pulmonary thromboembolism, *Focus Crit Care* 17:287, 1990.
29. Davis LP, Fink-Bennett D: Nuclear medicine in the acutely ill patient-I, *Crit Care Clin* 10:365, 1994.
30. Cascade PN, Kazerooni EA: Aspects of chest imaging in the intensive care unit, *Crit Care Clin* 10:247, 1994.
31. Sheldon RL, Dunbar RD: *Systematic analysis of the chest radiograph.* In Scalon CL, Spearman CB, Sheldon RL, editors: *Egan's fundamentals of respiratory care*, ed 6, St Louis, 1994, Mosby.
32. Dettenmeier PA: *Radiographic assessment for nurses*, St Louis, 1995, Mosby.
33. Krone KD, Weiner SA: How to read chest x-rays, *Hosp Med* 28(7):79, 1992.

12

Pulmonary Disorders

KATHLEEN M. STACY

Understanding the pathology of a disease, the areas of assessment on which to focus, and the usual medical management allows critical care nurses to anticipate and plan nursing interventions with greater accuracy. This chapter focuses on priority pulmonary disorders that nurses commonly encounter in the critical care environment.

Acute Respiratory Failure

Description and Etiology

Acute respiratory failure (ARF) is a clinical condition in which the pulmonary system fails to maintain adequate gas exchange.[1] Probably the most prevalent problem in critical care today,[2,3] ARF can be classified as *hypoxemic*

TABLE 12-1
ETIOLOGIES OF ACUTE RESPIRATORY FAILURE

AFFECTED AREA	DISORDERS
EXTRAPULMONARY	
Brain	Drug overdose
	Central alveolar hypoventilation syndrome
	Brain trauma or lesion
	Postoperative anesthesia depression
Spinal cord	Guillain-Barré syndrome
	Poliomyelitis
	Amyotrophic lateral sclerosis
	Spinal cord trauma or lesion
Neuromuscular system	Myasthenia gravis
	Multiple sclerosis
	Neuromuscular–blocking antibiotics
	Organophosphate poisoning
	Muscular dystrophy
Thorax	Massive obesity
	Chest trauma
Pleura	Pleural effusion
	Pneumothorax
Upper airways	Sleep apnea
	Tracheal obstruction
	Epiglottitis
INTRAPULMONARY	
Lower airways and alveoli	Chronic obstructive pulmonary disease (COPD)
	Asthma
	Bronchiolitis
	Cystic fibrosis
	Pneumonia
Pulmonary circulation	Pulmonary emboli
Alveolar-capillary membrane	Pulmonary edema
	Adult respiratory distress syndrome (ARDS)
	Inhalation of toxic gases
	Near-drowning

*Not an inclusive list.

normocapnic respiratory failure (Type I) or *hypoxemic hypercapnic respiratory failure* (Type II), depending on patients' arterial blood gases (ABGs).[2,3]

Caused by a deficiency in the performance of the pulmonary system,[2,3] ARF usually occurs secondary to another disorder that has affected some portion of the system.[4] The cause of ARF is classified as *extrapulmonary* or *intrapulmonary*, depending on the affected component of the respiratory system. Table 12-1 lists the etiologies of ARF and their associated disorders.[5]

Pathophysiology

The hallmark of acute respiratory failure, **hypoxemia** is the result of impaired gas exchange. Hypercapnia may be present, depending on the underlying cause of the problem. Causes of hypoxemia include alveolar hypoventilation, intrapulmonary shunting, and ventilation/perfusion mismatching.[6]

Alveolar hypoventilation

Alveolar hypoventilation occurs when the amount of oxygen being brought into the alveoli is insufficient to meet the metabolic needs of the body.[5] A decrease in ventilation results in a decrease of oxygen available for gas exchange.[4,6] Hypoxemia caused by alveolar hypoventilation is often associated with hypercapnia and commonly results from extrapulmonary disorders.[5]

Ventilation/perfusion mismatching

Ventilation/perfusion (V/Q) mismatching occurs when ventilation and blood flow are mismatched in various regions of the lung to an abnormal degree. Blood passes through alveoli that are underventilated for the given amount of perfusion. The blood leaving these areas has a lower than normal amount of oxygen.[5,6] V/Q mismatching is usually the result of alveoli that are partially collapsed or partially filled with fluid.

Intrapulmonary shunting

The extreme form of V/Q mismatching, **intrapulmonary shunting** occurs when blood reaches the arterial system without participating in gas exchange. The mixing of unoxygenated (shunted) blood and oxygenated blood lowers the average level of oxygen present in the blood.[5,6] Intrapulmonary shunting occurs when blood passes through a portion of a lung that is not ventilated, which may be the result of alveolar collapse (e.g., atelectasis), alveolar consolidation (e.g., pneumonia), or excessive mucus accumulation (e.g., chronic bronchitis).[5]

Complications

If allowed to progress, hypoxemia can result in a deficit of oxygen at the cellular level.[4] As the tissue demands for oxygen continue and the supply diminishes, an oxygen supply/demand imbalance occurs and tissue hypoxia develops. Decreased oxygen to the cells contributes to impaired tissue perfusion and the development of lactic acidosis.[1]

Assessment and Diagnosis

Patients with ARF may experience a variety of clinical manifestations, depending on the underlying cause and the extent of tissue hypoxia. The clinical manifestations are related to the development of hypoxemia, hypercapnia, acidosis, and activation of compensatory mechanisms. Table 12-2 lists the clinical manifestations of ARF. Because the clinical symptoms are so varied, they

<table>
T A B L E 1 2 - 2
CLINICAL MANIFESTATIONS OF ACUTE RESPIRATORY FAILURE
</table>

ORGAN SYSTEM	CLINICAL MANIFESTATIONS
Neurologic	Restlessness
	Agitation
	Headache
	Disorientation
	Seizures
	Decreased level of consciousness
Cardiovascular	Increased heart rate
	Hypertension (early)
	Hypotension (late)
	Chest pain
	Dysrhythmias
Pulmonary	Increased respiratory rate
	Increased respiratory depth
	Increased respiratory effort
Renal	Decreased urine output
	Edema
Gastrointestinal	Decreased bowel sounds
	Nausea and vomiting
	Abdominal distention
	Bleeding
Integumentary	Cool, clammy, pale skin
	Decreased capillary refill

are not considered reliable in predicting the degree of hypoxemia or hypercapnia.[4,7]

Diagnosing and following the course of respiratory failure is best accomplished by ABG analysis, which confirms the level of $Paco_2$, Pao_2, and blood pH. In both types of respiratory failure patients have a Pao_2 level lower than 50 mm Hg. In Type I respiratory failure the $Paco_2$ level is within normal range, whereas in Type II respiratory failure the $Paco_2$ is above 50 mm Hg.[2,3] In patients with chronically elevated $Paco_2$ levels, these criteria must be broadened to include a pH lower than 7.35.[8]

Medical Management

Medical management is aimed at treating the underlying cause, promoting adequate gas exchange, and monitoring for complications. Medical interventions for promoting gas exchange include improving oxygenation and ventilation.

Oxygenation

Actions to improve **oxygenation** include supplemental oxygen administration and the use of positive pressure. The goal of **oxygen therapy** is to correct hypoxemia. Although the absolute level of hypoxemia varies with each patient, most treatment approaches aim to keep the oxygen saturation at 90% or above. The goal is to satisfy the needs of tissues without producing carbon dioxide narcosis or oxygen toxicity.[2,6] Supplemental oxygen administration effectively treats hypoxemia related to alveolar hypoventilation and V/Q mismatching.[5] When intrapulmonary shunting exists, supplemental oxygen alone is ineffective.[5] In this situation positive pressure—in the form of constant positive airway pressure (CPAP) or positive end-expiratory pressure (PEEP)—is necessary to open collapsed alveoli and facilitate their participation in gas exchange. Because positive pressure is generally delivered via ventilator, patients who need positive pressure must usually be intubated and ventilated.[9]

Ventilation

Interventions to improve **ventilation** include **intubation** and **mechanical ventilation.** Intubation can be accomplished either orally, nasally, or via tracheostomy.[6] Once intubated, the patient is placed on a positive-pressure ventilator. The selection of mode and settings depends on the patient's underlying condition, severity of respiratory failure, and body size.[10] In a patient with chronic hypercapnia, settings should be adjusted to maintain a normal pH level as opposed to $Paco_2$ level.[8]

Medications

Medications to facilitate removal of secretions and dilate airways may also benefit patients with ARF. Mucolytics administered via nebulizer help liquefy secretions, which facilitates their removal. Bronchodilators aid in smooth muscle relaxation and are of particular benefit to patients with airflow limitations.[7,8] Many patients require sedation to maintain adequate ventilation. Sedation can be used to comfort patients and decrease the work of breathing, particularly when patients struggle against the ventilator.[4,6] Nurses should administer analgesics for pain control. In some patients sedation does not decrease spontaneous respiratory efforts enough to allow adequate ventilation; neuromuscular paralysis may be necessary in this situation.[10] Paralysis may also be necessary to decrease oxygen consumption in severely compromised patients.[11]

Nursing Management

Nursing management of patients with acute respiratory failure incorporates a variety of nursing diagnoses (Box 12-1). **Nursing priorities are directed toward optimizing oxygenation and ventilation, facilitating nutritional support, and educating patients and families.**

Optimizing oxygenation and ventilation

Nursing interventions to optimize oxygenation and ventilation include positioning, preventing desaturation during procedures, promoting secretion clearance, and administering medications as ordered (see Pharmacology section on page 262).[12,13]

POSITIONING. Positioning of patients with ARF depends on the type of lung injury. The goal of positioning is to facilitate or optimize V/Q matching and thereby help alleviate hypoxemia. Patients with unilateral lung disease should be positioned with the good lung down.[12-14] Patients with diffuse lung disease should be positioned prone, with the right lung down, and should be continuously turned. Some patients benefit from non-recumbent positions such as sitting or lying in a semierect position.[12,13] Although not in frequent use, the prone position has also been shown to increase oxygenation in patients with severe respiratory failure.[14] Nurses should reposition patients at least every 2 hours.[13]

PREVENTING DESATURATION. A number of activities can prevent desaturation from occurring during a procedure. These include performing the procedure only as needed, hyperoxygenating and hyperventilating patients before pulmonary toilet, and providing adequate rest and recovery time between various procedures. During procedures, patients should be continuously monitored with a pulse oximeter for signs of desaturation.[13,15]

PROMOTING SECRETION CLEARANCE. Interventions to promote secretion clearance include those that prevent secretion retention and those that facilitate secretion removal. Actions to prevent secretion retention include providing adequate systemic hydration, humidifying supplemental oxygen, and preventing hypoventilation. Actions to facilitate secretion removal include suctioning (endotracheal or nasotracheal) and chest physical therapy (percussion, vibration, postural drainage, and coughing).[15]

Facilitating nutritional support

Nutritional support is of utmost importance in the management of patients with ARF. The goals of nutritional support are to improve patients' overall nutritional status, enhance their immune system, and promote respiratory muscle function.[6,7] Chapter 6 contains a detailed discussion of nutrition.

Educating patients and family

Educating patients and families includes teaching them about ARF and its management, answering their questions, and preparing them for discharge. Upon discharge, patients should learn how respiratory failure develops, interventions to prevent it from recurring, adaptive breathing and energy-saving techniques, and the importance of taking prescribed medications.[16]

Adult Respiratory Distress Syndrome

Description and Etiology

Adult respiratory distress syndrome (ARDS) is a form of ARF that occurs secondary to another event. ARDS can be described as an "acute lung injury occurring in patients with identified risk factors to ARDS, characterized by the presence of refractory hypoxemia, diminished pulmonary compliance, radiographic evidence of pulmonary edema, and normal pulmonary capillary wedge pressure."[17] Mortality rates for ARDS range from 60% to 95%, depending on the initiating event and subsequent complications.[18] A wide variety of clinical conditions are associated with the development of ARDS (Box 12-2). They can be divided into direct and indirect injuries, depending on the primary event or site of injury.[18,19]

BOX 12-1

NURSING DIAGNOSIS PRIORITIES

ACUTE RESPIRATORY FAILURE

- *Impaired Gas Exchange* related to alveolar hypoventilation, p. 488
- *Impaired Gas Exchange* related to ventilation/perfusion mismatching and intrapulmonary shunting p. 488
- *Inability to Sustain Spontaneous Ventilation* related to respiratory muscle fatigue and metabolic factors, p. 487
- *Altered Nutrition: Less Than Body Requirements* related to lack of exogenous nutrients and increased metabolic demand, p. 506
- *Powerlessness* related to health care environment or illness-related regimen, p. 460

BOX 12-2

CONDITIONS LEADING TO ARDS

DIRECT PULMONARY INJURY

Aspiration of gastric contents or other toxic substances
Near-drowning
Inhalation of toxic substances
Pneumonia
Chest trauma
Embolism
Oxygen toxicity
Radiation pneumonitis

INDIRECT PULMONARY INJURY

Sepsis—especially gram-negative
Severe pancreatitis
Multiple blood transfusions
Multiple trauma
Disseminated intravascular coagulation (DIC)
Shock states
Nonpulmonary systemic diseases
Cardiopulmonary bypass
Anaphylaxis
Narcotic drug abuse

Pathophysiology

Recent studies are inconclusive on the sequence of events in the development of ARDS. Stimulation of the inflammatory-immune system is generally believed to initiate a systemic response that includes the sequestering of neutrophils in the lungs. Direct injury, complement activation, and stimulation of tissue macrophages and other mediators all play a role in attracting neutrophils to the lung interstitium. Once activated, the neutrophils release a variety of biochemical, humoral, and cellular mediators, which results in injury to the capillary endothelium.[18,20-22]

Increased capillary membrane permeability

The cumulative effect of the mediators is increased capillary membrane permeability. Injury to the alveolar-capillary endothelium allows increased amounts of fluid and proteins to leak into the pulmonary interstitium. As the fluids accumulate in the interstitium, normal local controlling factors (e.g., oncotic pressure, capillary hydrostatic pressure, lymphatic drainage) are overwhelmed. Eventually, fluid and proteins enter the alveoli and damage the type II cells, resulting in impaired surfactant production. The alveoli collapse as a result of interstitial-intraalveolar edema and the loss of surfactant. Collapse of the alveoli results in intrapulmonary shunting, decreased functional residual capacity (FRC), and decreased lung compliance.[18,22]

Other effects

In addition to increasing capillary permeability, the mediators cause bronchoconstriction, destruction of the elastin and collagen fibers of the lung parenchyma, pulmonary microemboli formation, and pulmonary artery vasoconstriction. Bronchoconstriction results in increased airway resistance, decreased lung compliance, and V/Q mismatching. Destruction of the lung parenchyma results in decreased lung compliance and diffusion defects. Pulmonary microemboli and pulmonary artery vasoconstriction result in pulmonary hypertension, increased pulmonary edema, and increased alveolar dead space. Hypoxic vasoconstriction also contributes to pulmonary hypertension. Combined with the effects of atelectasis, all of these consequences lead to an increase in work of breathing and hypoxemia. Increased work of breathing leads to fatigue and hypoventilation, which further heighten hypoxemia.[18,22,23]

Complications

ARDS is associated with many complications, including sepsis, nosocomial pneumonia, airway trauma, gastrointestinal hemorrhage, and multiple organ dysfunction syndrome (MODS).[18] MODS is the primary cause of death in patients with ARDS.[24] A number of theories postulate that ARDS is merely part of a multisystem response to injury. Organ failure was once believed to be related to impaired gas exchange from the pulmonary consequences of the disease; new theories indicate that organ failure starts from the same inflammatory–immune–mediated response that initiated the ARDS. It is theorized that ARDS appears first because of the immediate nature of impaired gas exchange.[20,24]

Assessment and Diagnosis

Patients with ARDS may have a variety of presenting symptoms, depending on the precipitating event. Clinical manifestations may be acute pulmonary edema, ARF, or gradually increasing respiratory insufficiency. Clinical manifestations generally include dyspnea, tachypnea, tachycardia, labored breathing, and change in mental status. As the disease progresses, diffuse fine crackles and wheezes may be heard.[18,23,25,26]

Analysis of ABGs reveals a low PaO_2 level, despite increases in supplemental oxygen administration (refractory hypoxemia). The $PaCO_2$ level is low at first, as a result of compensatory hyperventilation. Eventually the $PaCO_2$ level increases as patients become fatigued. The pH is high initially but decreases as acidosis develops.[26]

The actual diagnosis of ARDS is based on clinical, laboratory, and radiologic criteria. Clinical criteria include the history of a precipitating event associated with ARDS and presence of dyspnea, tachycardia, and tachypnea. Radiologic criteria include diffuse bilateral alveolar infiltrates on the chest x-ray film.[27] As the disease progresses, widespread pulmonary opacification ("whiteout") occurs. In addition, decreased volumes and atelectasis becomes evident.[28] Laboratory criteria include evidence of hypoxemia, including a PaO_2 level below 60 mm Hg on an FIO_2 of 40% and a shunt level above 20%. Pulmonary function studies reveal a decrease in static and dynamic compliance, decrease in FRC, decrease in vital capacity, and increase in minute ventilation. In addition, patients should have a pulmonary artery wedge pressure (PAWP) of less than 18 to rule out pulmonary edema of cardiac origin.[26]

Medical Management

Medical management of patients with ARDS involves a multifaceted approach that includes treating the underlying cause, promoting gas exchange, supporting tissue oxygenation, and monitoring for complications. Medical interventions to promote gas exchange include supplemental oxygen administration, PEEP, intubation, and mechanical ventilation.[22,29]

Supplemental oxygen administration

Oxygen should be administered at the lowest level possible to support tissue oxygenation. Continued exposure to high levels of oxygen can lead to oxygen toxicity, which perpetuates the entire process. The goal is to maintain a PaO_2 level of 60 mm Hg with an FIO_2 of below 60.[18] Because the hypoxemia that develops with ARDS is often refractory to oxygen therapy, facilitating oxygenation with PEEP is usually necessary.[29]

PEEP

The positive effects of PEEP on the lungs include recruiting collapsed alveoli, increasing FRC, and redistributing fluid from the intraalveolar space to the interstitial space.[29,30] PEEP thereby decreases intrapulmonary shunting and V/Q mismatching, increases compliance, and improves gas exchange. PEEP also has several negative effects. These include a decrease in cardiac output (CO) caused by decreasing venous return, ventricular dysfunction as a result of increasing pulmonary vascular resistance, and barotrauma. The amount of PEEP patients require is determined by considering both Pa_{O_2} levels and CO.[29]

Intubation and mechanical ventilation

Intubation and mechanical ventilation are required to facilitate ventilation, particularly as fatigue develops and ventilatory failure occurs. During the acute phase of ARDS, patients should receive complete ventilator support. Because the ventilator does the majority of the work of breathing, the patient can rest. Ventilator support is provided by a variety of modes, including assist-control (also called continuous mandatory ventilation), synchronized intermittent mandatory ventilation, and pressure control ventilation.[18,29] Other ventilatory modes available are high-frequency jet ventilation (HFJV) and inverse ratio ventilation (IRV), but these modes are usually employed when conventional ventilatory strategies are not working.[22,29]

HIGH-FREQUENCY JET VENTILATION. HFJV uses small tidal volumes delivered at high rates to decrease inflation pressures. The advantage is decreased airway pressures, resulting in less hemodynamic compromise and a decreased risk of barotrauma. Recent studies indicate that HFJV does not improve oxygenation and is no better than conventional ventilation modes.[22,29]

INVERSE RATIO VENTILATION. IRV is another newer mode, one that shows more promise in the treatment of ARDS than HFJV. IRV prolongs the inspiratory (I) time and shortens the expiratory (E) time, thus reversing the normal I:E ratio. The effect is intentional air trapping, which increases FRC and alveolar recruitment while maintaining lower airway pressures. Disadvantages to IRV include the development of excessive auto-PEEP, which can cause hemodynamic compromise and worsening gas exchange. In addition, patients on IRV usually require neuromuscular blockade and sedation to prevent them from fighting the ventilator.[22,29]

Tissue perfusion

Interventions to support **tissue perfusion** include fluid administration, blood administration, and maintenance of CO. Fluid therapy is aimed at maintaining adequate intravascular volume to optimize preload and CO but minimize contribution to lung edema. Hemodynamic monitoring is an accurate way to assess fluid needs. A PAWP in the range of 10 to 12 mm Hg is desired, and the use of fluid challenges (or diuretics, depending on the direction of the pressure alteration) should be used to achieve this range. The type of fluid depends on patients' underlying condition and severity of ARDS.[26] When hemoglobin is low, blood administration helps maximize oxygen-carrying capacity.[18] Vasoactive and inotropic agents may be necessary to maintain an adequate CO.[25]

Investigational treatments

A number of investigational studies of other therapies for the treatment of ARDS are underway. These therapies include drugs to block or neutralize the various mediators released as part of the inflammatory–immune response and methods to limit the damage to the lungs. A number of drugs are being tested, including nonsteroidal antiinflammatory drugs, oxygen-free radical scavengers, platelet activation factor antagonists, and prostaglandin E_1. Methods to limit damage to the lungs include surfactant replacement and extracorporeal carbon dioxide removal.[18] Inhaled nitric oxide is also being investigated to help reverse pulmonary vasoconstriction and improve perfusion of ventilated regions of the lungs.[31]

Nursing Management

Nursing management of patients with ARDS incorporates a variety of nursing diagnoses (Box 12-3). **Nursing priorities are directed toward optimizing oxygenation and ventilation, administering fluids and vasoactive medications, facilitating nutritional support, and educating patients and families.**

Optimizing oxygenation and ventilation

Nursing interventions to optimize oxygenation and ventilation include positioning, preventing desaturation during procedures, promoting secretion clearance, and administering medications as ordered.[12,13] (For further dis-

---

BOX 12-3

NURSING DIAGNOSIS PRIORITIES

ADULT RESPIRATORY DISTRESS SYNDROME

- *Impaired Gas Exchange* related to ventilation/perfusion, mismatching and intrapulmonary shunting, p. 488
- Inability to Sustain Spontaneous Ventilation related to respiratory muscle fatigue and metabolic factors, p. 487
- *Altered Nutrition: Less Than Body Requirements* related to lack of exogenous nutrients and increased metabolic demand, p. 506
- *Anxiety* related to threat to biologic, psychologic, and/or social integrity, p. 464

cussion of these interventions, refer to the Nursing Management section on acute respiratory failure.)

ADMINISTERING NEUROMUSCULAR BLOCKING AGENTS. Nursing management of patients receiving a neuromuscular-blocking agent should incorporate a number of additional interventions. Because paralytic agents only halt muscle movement and do not inhibit pain or awareness, they should be administered with a sedative or anxiolytic agent. Pain medication should also be administered if patients are suspected of being in pain. Reorienting patients and explaining all procedures is critical because patients can still hear, although they cannot move or see. Patients are also at risk for developing complications associated with immobility. Interventions related to the prevention of skin breakdown, atelectasis, and deep vein thrombosis should be implemented. Because patients cannot react to their environment, special precautions should be taken to protect them at all times.[10,11]

Administering fluids and vasoactive medications

Adequate tissue perfusion depends on an adequate supply of oxygen being transported to the tissues. An adequate CO and hemoglobin level are critical to oxygen transport. CO depends on heart rate, preload, afterload, and contractility. A variety of fluids and medications are used to manipulate these parameters. Types of fluids used include both crystalloids and colloids. Types of medications include vasoconstrictors, vasodilators, positive inotropes, and antidysrhythmic agents.[25] Chapter 10 contains further information on this subject.

Facilitating nutritional support

The initiation of nutritional support is of utmost importance in the management of the patient with ARDS. The goals of nutritional support are to improve the patient's overall nutritional status, enhance the immune system and promote respiratory muscle function. Chapter 6 provides more information about nutritional needs of critical care patients.

Educating patients and families

Educating patients and families includes teaching them about ARDS and its management, answering their questions, and preparing them for discharge. Subjects for discharge education include how respiratory failure develops, interventions to prevent it from recurring and the importance of taking prescribed medications.[16]

Pneumonia

Description and Etiology

Once the leading cause of death, pneumonia continues to be a major health problem.[32] A number of conditions predispose patients to develop pneumonia, including depressed gag and cough reflexes, decreased ciliary activity, increased secretions, decreased lymphatic flow, **atelectasis,** fluid in the alveoli, abnormal phagocytosis and hu-

moral activity, and impaired alveolar macrophages.[33] Table 12-3 lists these conditions and their causes.

Pneumonias can be classified as *community-acquired* or *hospital-acquired* (nosocomial) infections. The most frequently seen community-acquired pneumonia is *S. pneumoniea.* Other organisms commonly seen are *Legionella spp* viruses, *M. pneumoniae,* and *H. influenzae.*[32] Nosocomial pneumonias are generally caused by gram-negative enteric bacteria. *Klebsiella pneumoniae, Enterobacter* species, *Escherichia coli, Proteus, Serratia, Pseudomonas aeruginosa,* and *Staphylococcus aureus* are those most frequently encountered.[34] Pneumocystis carinii is the predominant cause of pulmonary infection in patients with AIDS.[35] Often, institutions have their own resident flora that predominate in nosocomial infections.

Pathophysiology

Development of acute pneumonia implies a defect in host defenses, a particularly virulent organism, or an overwhelming inoculation event. Bacterial invasion of the lower respiratory tract can occur by inhalation, aspiration, migration from adjacent sites or colonization, direct inoculation, and hematogenous seeding. The most com-

TABLE 12-3
PREDISPOSING CONDITIONS

CONDITION	ETIOLOGIES
Depressed epiglottal and cough reflexes	Unconsciousness, neurologic disease, endotracheal or tracheal tubes, anesthesia, aging
Decreased cilia activity	Smoke inhalation—smoking history, oxygen toxicity, hypoventilation, intubation, viral infections, aging, COPD
Increased secretion	COPD, viral infections, bronchiectasis, general anesthesia, endotracheal intubation, smoking
Atelectasis	Trauma, foreign body obstruction, tumor, splinting, shallow ventilations, general anesthesia
Decreased lymphatic flow	CHF, tumor
Fluid in alveoli	CHF, aspiration, trauma
Abnormal phagocytosis and humoral activity	Neutropenia, immunocompetent disorders, such as AIDS, patients receiving chemotherapy
Impaired alveolar macrophages	Hypoxemia, metabolic acidosis, cigarette smoking history, hypoxia, alcohol use, viral infections, aging

COPD, chronic obstructive pulmonary disease; *CHF,* congestive heart failure.

mon method of infection appears to be microaspiration of bacteria colonized in the upper airway.[34,36]

The oropharynx has a stable population of resident flora that may be anaerobic or aerobic. When stress occurs—such as with illness, surgery, or a viral infection—pathogenic organisms replace normal resident flora. Previous antibiotic therapy affects the resident flora population, making replacement by pathologic organisms more likely. The pathogens are then able to invade the sterile lower respiratory tract. Researchers have demonstrated that 57% of critically ill patients have gram-negative bacteria present in the oropharynx. Disruption of the gag and cough reflexes, altered consciousness, abnormal swallowing, and artificial airways all predispose patients to aspiration and colonization of the lungs and subsequent infection.[34]

Infection results in pulmonary inflammation with or without significant exudates. V/Q mismatching and intrapulmonary shunting occur, resulting in hypoxemia as lung consolidation progresses. Untreated pneumonia can result in acute respiratory failure and initiation of the systemic inflammatory response.[34]

Assessment and Diagnosis

Pneumonia is diagnosed on the basis of clinical manifestations, radiologic changes, and microbiologic data. Dyspnea is the primary symptom experienced in diffuse pneumonia. Coughing and wheezing with sputum production may be present. Patients often complain of fever or chills, although these may occur less frequently in elderly and immunosuppressed patients. Pleuritic pain may be a prominent feature.[32]

Clinical examination reveals hyperpnea or tachypnea, possibly accompanied by crackles and wheezes over the area of involvement. Initially the crackles may be coarse and heard during midinspiration. As the pneumonia resolves, the crackles become fine and are heard toward the end of inspiration.[37] Chest x-ray evaluation may show infiltrates, depending on the length of illness and absence of other lung problems. An elevated leukocyte count appears in bacterial pneumonias. Because of the difficulty involved with sputum collection and culture, the causative agent may not be identified. A Gram stain is very useful because the results are immediately available and can indicate the probable bacteria.[32]

Medical Management

Medical management includes **antibiotic therapy,** oxygen therapy for hypoxemia, mechanical ventilation (if acute respiratory failure develops), fluid management for hydration, and treatment of associated medical problems and complications. Mucolytics and therapeutic bronchoscopy may be necessary if patients have difficulty mobilizing secretions.[34]

Antibiotic therapy

Although bacteria-specific antibiotic therapy is the goal, it may not always be possible when patients' conditions are serious and identifying the organism is difficult. The time spent obtaining bacterial specimens should be balanced against the need to begin treatment based on patient condition. Empiric therapy has become a generally acceptable approach. In this approach, choice of antibiotic treatment is based on the most likely etiologic organism, while avoiding drug toxicity or superinfection. If available, gram-stain results should be used to guide the choice of antibiotics.[34]

Nursing Management

Nursing management of patients with pneumonia incorporates a variety of nursing diagnoses (Box 12-4). **Nursing priorities are directed toward optimizing oxygenation and ventilation, preventing the spread of infection, and educating patients and families.**

Optimizing oxygenation and ventilation

Nursing interventions to optimize oxygenation and ventilation include positioning, preventing desaturation during procedures, promoting secretion clearance, and administering medications as ordered.[12,13] The Nursing Management section on acute respiratory failure (Unit X) discusses these interventions more thoroughly.

Preventing the spread of infection

Prevention should be directed at eradicating pathogens from the environment and interrupting the spread of organisms between individuals. Significant progress has been made in removing contaminants from the patient environment through proper disinfection of respiratory equipment and increased use of disposable supplies. Other possible environmental sources of pathogens include suctioning equipment and indwelling lines. These invasive tools must be given proper aseptic care. Proper

BOX 12-4

NURSING DIAGNOSIS PRIORITIES

PNEUMONIA

- *Ineffective Airway Clearance* related to excessive secretions or abnormal viscosity of mucus, p. 484
- *Impaired Gas Exchange* related to alveolar hypoventilation secondary to (specify), p. 488
- *Impaired Gas Exchange* related to ventilation/perfusion mismatching and intrapulmonary shunting, p. 488
- *Anxiety* related to threat to biologic, psychologic, and/or social integrity, p. 464

hand-washing technique is the single most important measure available to prevent the spread of bacteria between individuals.[36]

Educating patients and families

Educating patients and families includes teaching them about pneumonia and its management, answering their questions, and preparing for discharge. Upon patients' discharge, nurses should discuss how pneumonia develops, interventions to prevent it from recurring, adaptive breathing and energy-saving techniques, and the importance of taking prescribed medications.[16]

Aspiration Lung Disorder

Description and Etiology

The presence of abnormal substances in the airways and alveoli as a result of aspiration is usually called *aspiration pneumonia.* This term is misleading because the aspiration of toxic substances into the lung may not involve an infection. *Aspiration lung disorder* is a more accurate title because injury to the lung can result from the chemical, mechanical, and bacterial characteristics of the aspirate.[38]

Aspiration has been recorded in as many as 77% of critically ill patients with artificial airways in place.[38] A number of factors have been identified that place patients at risk for aspiration (Box 12-5).[39] Some common causes of aspiration lung disorder in critically ill patients are inert fluids, foreign bodies, oropharyngeal bacteria, and gastric contents. Table 12-4 describes the specific clinical entity each cause produces.

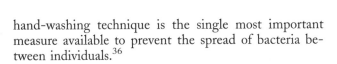

BOX 12-5

RISK FACTORS ASSOCIATED WITH ASPIRATION

Impaired consciousness
Compromised glottal closure
Compromised cough reflex
Ileus or gastric dilation
Nasogastric feeding tubes (large or small bore)
Artificial airways
Disorders affecting pharyngeal or esophageal motility
Tracheoesophageal fistulas
General anesthesia
Cardiopulmonary resuscitation
Improper patient positioning during tube feeding
Esophageal strictures

TABLE 12-4
CLINICAL ENTITIES ASSOCIATED WITH ASPIRATION LUNG DISORDER

INOCULUM	PULMONARY SEQUELAE	CLINICAL FEATURES	THERAPY
Acid	Chemical pneumonitis, late bacterial infection possible	Acute shortness of breath, tachypnea, tachycardia; hypoxemia, bronchospasm, fever; sputum: pink, frothy; x-ray film: infiltrates in one or both lower lobes	Correct hypoxemia, administer intravenous fluids, monitor blood gases, administer antibiotics for associated bacterial infections
Oropharyngeal bacteria	Bacterial infection, lung abscess, empyema	Usually insidious onset, cough, fever, purulent sputum, leukocytosis; x-ray film: infiltrate involving dependent pulmonary segment or lobe ± cavitation	Antibiotics
Inert fluids (water, blood, barium)	Airway obstruction, reflex airway closure	Acute shortness of breath, cyanosis ± apnea, pulmonary edema, hypoxemia	Tracheal suctioning during or immediately after aspiration event, correct hypoxemia
Particulate matter, foreign bodies	Airway obstruction	Depends on level of obstruction: ranges from acute apnea and rapid death to irritating chronic cough ± recurrent infections	Extraction of large particulate matter via bronchoscopy, antibiotics for infections

From Baum G, Wolinsky E: *Textbook of pulmonary disease,* ed 4, Boston, 1989, Little & Brown.

Pathophysiology

A number of factors, including the quality of the aspirate and the status of the patient's respiratory defense mechanisms, determine the type of lung injury that develops after aspiration. Aspirate qualities to be considered include volume and pH level, and presence of bile, particulate matter, food, and bacteria.[40] Aspiration of inert liquids and large foreign bodies may produce an airway obstruction. Smaller foreign bodies may block a portion of the lung, causing atelectasis, bronchospasm, or pneumonia. Aspiration of oropharyngeal secretions carries bacteria into the lower respiratory tract and can cause pneumonia.

Aspiration of gastric contents results in the development of chemical pneumonitis. Aspirates with a pH level lower than 2.5, a volume of 0.4 to 1.0 ml/kg,[38] or with food, particulate antacid, or fecal material increase the chance of damage to the lungs.[41] Initially, bronchospasm may occur secondary to reflex airway closure. Damage to the alveolar capillary membrane results in massive fluid leaks into the alveoli and the development of noncardiogenic pulmonary edema. The fluid decreases surfactant production, which results in atelectasis.[40,41] In addition, hypoxemia results from the intrapulmonary shunting and V/Q mismatching. Acute respiratory distress can develop in minutes. One third of affected patients develop overwhelming pneumonia or ARDS.[41]

Assessment and Diagnosis

Patients have presenting signs of respiratory distress. Initially, patients may have shortness of breath, coughing, or wheezing, depending on their level of consciousness. Tachypnea, tachycardia, hypotension, fever, and crackles are also present. Copious amounts of sputum are produced as pulmonary edema develops.[42]

ABGs reflect hypoxemia, and an increased FIO_2 is necessary to maintain satisfactory oxygenation. If bacterial infection becomes established, the white blood cell count may become elevated and sputum cultures positive. The validity of the chest x-ray examination in diagnosing aspiration lung disorder is related to the prior status of patients. Patients with underlying lung involvement may already have significant pulmonary infiltrates present on the chest x-ray film, clouding the interpretation. With aspiration of a foreign body, any number of radiologic findings may be present, including hyperinflation, atelectasis, pneumonia, and the presence of a foreign body. Generally the right lower lobe is most often affected due to gravity and the shape of the bronchial tree. In massive aspiration, diffuse bilateral infiltrates suggest the presence of pulmonary edema, whereas lesser aspirations show atelectasis in the early period.[42] Improvement usually occurs in 1 to 2 days.[28]

Medical Management

Management of patients with aspiration lung disorder includes both immediate and follow-up treatment.

Immediate treatment

When aspiration is witnessed, emergency treatment should be initiated to secure the airway and minimize pulmonary damage. Patients should be placed in a slight Trendelenburg's position (head lowered 6 to 8 inches) and turned to the right lateral decubitus position to aid drainage and avoid involvement of other lung areas. Oropharyngeal suctioning should follow immediately. Direct visualization by bronchoscopy is indicated when large, particulate aspirate blocks airways. Bronchial and pulmonary lavage is not recommended because this practice disseminates the aspirate in lungs and increases damage.[40]

Follow-up treatment

After airway clearance, nurses should attend to supporting oxygenation and hemodynamics. Hemodynamic changes result from fluid shifts that can occur after massive aspirations, causing noncardiogenic pulmonary edema. Monitoring intravascular volume is essential, and judicious amounts of replacement fluids should be administered to maintain adequate urinary output and vital signs. Hypoxemia should be corrected with supplemental oxygen or mechanical ventilation with PEEP, if necessary.[40]

Nursing Management

Nursing management of patients with aspiration lung disorder incorporates a variety of nursing diagnoses (Box 12-6). **Nursing priorities are directed toward optimizing oxygenation and ventilation, preventing further aspiration events, and educating patients and families.**

Optimizing oxygenation and ventilation

Nursing interventions to optimize oxygenation and ventilation include positioning, preventing desaturation during procedures, promoting secretion clearance, and administering medications as ordered.[12,13] The Nursing

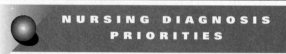

BOX 12-6

NURSING DIAGNOSIS PRIORITIES

ASPIRATION LUNG DISORDER

- *Impaired Gas Exchange* related to ventilation/perfusion mismatching and intrapulmonary shunting, p. 488
- *Ineffective Airway Clearance* related to excessive secretions or abnormal viscosity of mucus, p. 484
- Risk for Aspiration, p. 489
- *Anxiety* related to threat to biologic, psychologic, and/or social integrity, p. 464

Management section on acute respiratory failure (Unit X) contains further information.

Preventing further aspiration events

Interventions to prevent further aspiration events include careful monitoring of patients receiving tube feedings, maintaining elevation of the head of the bed, and frequent suctioning of the oropharynx of intubated patients to prevent secretions from pooling above the cuff of the tube.[39] Meticulous oral care is critical in decreasing the bacterial colonization of the oropharynx.[35]

Educating patients and families

Educating patients and families includes teaching them about aspiration lung disorder and its management, answering their questions, and preparing for discharge. Upon patients' discharge, nurses should inform them how aspiration develops and how to prevent it from recurring. Nurses should also remind them of the importance of taking prescribed medications.[16]

Pulmonary Embolus

Description and Etiology

A pulmonary embolus (PE) occurs when clots (thrombotic emboli) or other matter (nonthrombotic emboli) lodge in the pulmonary artery (PA), disrupting the blood flow to a region of the lungs. The majority of thrombotic emboli arise from the venous system, with 90% to 95% coming from the deep leg veins and the rest from the right ventricle, upper extremities, and renal, hepatic, and pelvic veins.[43,44] Nonthrombotic emboli arise from fat, amniotic fluid, air, and foreign bodies.[45]

A number of predisposing factors and precipitating conditions put patients at risk for developing a thromboembolism (Box 12-7).[44,46] Of the three predisposing factors (i.e., hypercoagulability, injury to vascular endothelium, and venous stasis [Virchow's triad]), venous stasis appears to be the most significant.[44]

Pathophysiology

A massive PE occurs with the blockage of a lobar or larger artery, resulting in occlusion of more than 50% of the pulmonary vascular bed. A submassive PE involves several smaller emboli that block the more distal branches of pulmonary circulation.[46] Blockage of the PA system has both pulmonary and hemodynamic consequences. The effects on the pulmonary system are an increase in alveolar dead space, pneumoconstriction, and loss of surfactant. The hemodynamic effects include an increase in pulmonary vascular resistance and right ventricular workload.[43,46]

Increase in alveolar dead space

Alveolar dead space increases because an area of the lung is receiving ventilation without being perfused. Ventila-

tion to this area is known as *wasted ventilation* because it does not participate in gas exchange. This effect leads to alveolar dead-space ventilation and an increase in the work of breathing. To limit the amount of dead-space ventilation, pneumoconstriction of the airways occurs in the area involved.[43,46]

Pneumoconstriction

Pneumoconstriction develops as a result of bronchoalveolar hypocarbia, hypoxia, and the release of humoral, cellular, and biochemical mediators. Bronchoalveolar hypocarbia occurs as a consequence of decreased carbon dioxide in the affected area and leads to constriction of the

---

BOX 12-7

RISK FACTORS FOR PULMONARY THROMBOEMBOLISM

PREDISPOSING FACTORS

Venous stasis
  Atrial fibrillation
  Decreased cardiac output (CO)
  Immobility
Injury to vascular endothelium
  Local vessel injury
  Infection
  Incision
  Atherosclerosis
Hypercoagulability
  Polycythemia

PRECIPITATING CONDITIONS

Previous pulmonary embolus
Cardiovascular disease
  Congestive heart failure
  Right ventricular infarction
  Cardiomyopathy
  Cor pulmonale
Surgery
  Orthopedic
  Vascular
  Abdominal
Cancer
  Ovarian
  Pancreatic
  Stomach
  Extrahepatic bile duct system
Trauma (injury or burns)
  Lower extremities
  Pelvis
  Hips
Gynecologic status
  Pregnancy
  Postpartum
  Birth control pills
  Estrogen replacement therapy

local airways, increased airway resistance, and redistribution of ventilation to perfused areas of the lungs. A variety of mediators are released from the site of the injury, either from the clot or the surrounding lung tissue, which causes further constriction of the airways.[43,46]

Loss of surfactant

Surfactant, which serves to keep the alveoli from collapsing, decreases in the affected area. Loss of surfactant leads to the development of atelectasis and transudation of interstitial fluid into the alveoli.[43,46]

Secondary effects

Dyspnea and hypoxemia develop secondary to these pathophysiologic responses. Dyspnea is thought to occur when fluid in the alveoli stimulates the J receptors (juxtacapillary receptors, which are located in the walls of alveoli near the capillaries).[47] In addition, the increase in work of breathing needed to maintain adequate gas exchange adds to the sensation of dyspnea. Hypoxemia occurs as a result of V/Q mismatching.[43]

Hemodynamic consequences

The major hemodynamic consequence of a PE is the development of pulmonary hypertension, which is part of the effect of a mechanical obstruction when more than 50% of the vascular bed is occluded. In addition, the mediators released at the injury site and the development of hypoxia cause pulmonary vasoconstriction, which further exacerbates pulmonary hypertension. As the pulmonary vascular resistance increases, so does the work load of the right ventricle, as reflected by a rise in PA pressures. Consequently, right ventricular failure occurs, which can lead to shock and decreases in left ventricular preload, CO, and blood pressure.[43-46]

Assessment and Diagnosis

Patients with a PE may have any number of presenting clinical manifestations. Common symptoms include dyspnea, chest pain, apprehension, anxiety, cough, hemoptysis, diaphoresis, and syncope.[44,45,47] The chest pain is pleuritic in nature, with an abrupt onset, and aggravated by deep breathing. The presence of hemoptysis usually indicates pulmonary infarction or atelectasis. Syncope is thought to occur secondary to the decrease in CO and blood pressure.[44]

Common signs include an increase in tachypnea, tachycardia, crackles, decreased breath sounds over the affected side, wheezing,[45,46] and low-grade fever.[45,47] If right ventricular failure occurs, distended neck veins and an S_3 on auscultation may be present.[44,45] Additional signs that indicate right ventricular decompensation are fixed splitting of the second heart sound (P_2), resulting from delayed closure of the pulmonic valve,[44,46] and a diastolic murmur, caused by pulmonic insufficiency.[44]

Initial laboratory studies that may be done are ABG analysis, electrocardiogram (ECG), and chest radiography. ABGs may show a low Pao_2 level, indicating hypoxemia; a low $Paco_2$ level, indicating hypocarbia; and a high pH, indicating respiratory alkalosis. Hypocarbia with resulting respiratory alkalosis is caused by tachypnea.[48] Common ECG changes are transient ST-T wave changes and sinus tachycardia. The classic findings of P-pulmonale, S wave in lead I, and Q wave with inverted T wave in lead III are associated with right ventricular failure and are seen in less than 20% of the patients.[43,44,48] Chest x-ray film findings vary from normal to abnormal with elevated hemidiaphragm, parenchymal infiltrates, and atelectasis.[43,44]

Differentiating a PE from other illnesses can be difficult because many of its clinical manifestations are found in a variety of other disorders.[48] Thus a variety of other tests may be necessary, including a V/Q scan, pulmonary angiogram, and deep vein thrombosis (DVT) studies. A definitive diagnosis of a PE requires confirmation by a high probability V/Q scan, positive pulmonary angiogram, or strong clinical suspicion coupled with abnormal findings on lower extremity DVT studies.[47]

Medical Management

Medical management includes prophylactic and definitive measures, reversal of the hemodynamic consequences, and correction of the hypoxemia.

Prophylactic measures

Prophylactic interventions are focused on preventing the recurrence of a PE and include the administration of heparin and warfarin (Coumadin) and interruption of the inferior vena cava. Heparin is administered to prevent further clots from forming, but it has no effect on the existing clot. Heparinization should continue for 5 days, with warfarin given simultaneously. Patients should remain on warfarin for 3 to 6 months.[44,47] Interruption of the inferior vena cava is reserved for patients in whom anticoagulation is contraindicated.[48] The procedure involves the placement of a multichanneled clip or an umbrella filter device in the vena cava. Neither device is completely effective in preventing the recurrence of a PE.[46]

Definitive measures

Definitive actions are directed at treating the current PE and include the administration of thrombolytic agents and surgery to remove the clot. Measures to correct the hypoxemia include supplemental oxygen administration, intubation, and mechanical ventilation. The administration of thrombolytic agents in the treatment of PE has had limited success. Currently thrombolytic therapy is reserved for use in patients with a massive PE and concomitant hemodynamic instability. Tissue plasminogen activator (tPA) is the thrombolytic agent of choice.[44] However, one recent study has demonstrated that a concentrated dose of urokinase given over 2 hours is as effective as tPA.[49] Surgical embolectomy is considered a last-resort measure wherein the embolus is extracted from the pulmonary arterial system. This procedure has an operative mortality rate of approximately 25%[44] and is reserved for patients with a massive PE refractory to all other measures.

Reversal of hemodynamic consequences

Additional measures may be taken to reverse the hemodynamic effects of pulmonary hypertension, including the administration of vasodilator and inotropic agents. Vasodilator agents have no effect on hypertension created by mechanical obstruction, but they do reverse the vasoconstrictor effects of mediators and hypoxia. Inotropic agents increase contractility to facilitate an increase in CO.[44]

Correction of hypoxemia

Measures to correct hypoxemia include supplemental oxygen administration, intubation, and mechanical ventilation.

Prevention

Prevention of PE is the first line of treatment for the disorder. In one study the prophylactic use of low-dose subcutaneous heparin in surgical patients demonstrated a 66% reduction in deep vein thrombosis and a 50% reduction of PE. Patients at risk for PE should receive 3500 U subcutaneously every 8 hours, with the dose adjusted to maintain a partial thromboplastin time in the high-to-normal range.[47]

Nursing Management

Nursing management of patients with a PE incorporates a variety of nursing diagnoses (Box 12-8). **Nursing priorities are directed toward optimizing oxygenation and ventilation, facilitating pain management, and educating patients and families.**

Optimizing oxygenation and ventilation

Nursing interventions to optimize oxygenation and ventilation include positioning, preventing desaturation during procedures, promoting secretion clearance, and administering medications as ordered.[12,13] The Nursing Management section on acute respiratory failure (Unit X) contains further discussion of these interventions.

Facilitating pain management

Pain management should incorporate reassurance, relaxation, and analgesia.[46]

Educating patients and families

Educating patients and families includes teaching them about PE and its management, answering their questions, and preparing them for discharge. Upon discharge, patients should be taught how a PE develops, interventions to prevent it from recurring, and the importance of taking prescribed medications. Medication teaching is critical for patients who will continue to take warfarin after discharge.[16]

Prevention

Prevention of PE should be a major nursing focus because the majority of critically ill patients are at risk for this disorder. Nursing actions are aimed at preventing the development of DVT, a major complication of immobility and a leading cause of PE. These measures include the use of antiembolic stockings and/or pneumatic compression stockings, active/passive range of motion, and progressive ambulation. Patients at risk should be routinely assessed for signs of a DVT, specifically, deep calf pain (Homan's sign) (see Chapter 8).[46]

Pneumothorax

Description and Etiology

The presence of air in the pleural space is known as a *pneumothorax*. A pneumothorax is referred to as *open* when there is a hole in the chest wall and *closed* when there is no opening to the outside. In a tension pneumothorax the air in the pleural space is under pressure.[50]

The three main causes of a pneumothorax are a perforation of the chest wall and parietal pleura allowing air to enter from the outside, perforation of the visceral pleura allowing air to enter from within the lung,[50,51] and formation of gas within the pleural space.[50] An open pneumothorax can be caused by a stab wound or gunshot wound to the chest. A closed pneumothorax can be caused by a wide variety of factors, including mechanical ventilation, blunt chest trauma, ruptured emphysematous bullae, chest wall defects, and central line insertions. Gas can form in the pleural space as the result of an infection or empyema.[50]

Pathophysiology

An open pneumothorax occurs when a defect in the chest wall allows air to enter the pleural space from the outside. Immediately after the chest wall is opened, the pres-

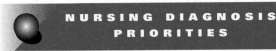

BOX 12-8

NURSING DIAGNOSIS PRIORITIES

PULMONARY EMBOLISM

- *Impaired Gas Exchange* related to ventilation/perfusion mismatching and intrapulmonary shunting, p. 488
- Acute *Pain* related to transmission and perception of cutaneous, visceral, muscular, or ischemic impulses, p. 499
- *Anxiety* related to threat to biologic, physiologic, and/or social integrity, p. 464

sure inside and outside the chest equilibrates. As air enters the chest, the lung collapses. If the defect is greater than two thirds of the diameter of the trachea, air is sucked into the chest with each breath instead of the trachea.[50,51] This condition is often referred to as a *sucking chest wound.*[51]

A closed pneumothorax occurs when a defect in the visceral pleura allows air to enter the pleural space. As air accumulates in the space, it compresses the surrounding lung tissue, resulting in its collapse. A spontaneous pneumothorax is a form of closed pneumothorax that occurs without an inciting event such as trauma or a central line insertion.[50]

A tension pneumothorax develops when air enters the pleural space from either the lung or the chest wall on inhalation and cannot escape on exhalation. A "one-way valve" effect is created, and the pressure inside the pleural space builds, collapsing the lung. The mediastinum and trachea are eventually displaced to the opposite side. This displacement results in decreased venous return and compression of the opposite lung.[50,51]

Regardless of the underlying cause, once air enters the pleural space, the affected lung collapses. The collapsed lung, although not ventilated, is still perfused, resulting in intrapulmonary shunting. If the pneumothorax is large, hypoxemia and ARF can quickly develop.[51]

Assessment and Diagnosis

The clinical manifestations of a pneumothorax depend on the degree of lung collapse and type of pneumothorax. When a pneumothorax is large, decreased respiratory excursion on the affected side may be noticed, along with bulging intercostal muscles. The trachea may deviate away from the affected side. Percussion reveals hyperresonance with decreased or absent breath sounds over the affected area. As air escapes from the lung, it may leak into the surrounding tissue, and subcutaneous emphysema develops. Patients should be assessed for crepitus, which indicates subcutaneous emphysema. Patients may complain of dyspnea and chest pain. A tension pneumothorax may produce distended neck veins as a result of rising intrathoracic pressure.[50] The pneumothorax is confirmed with a chest x-ray examination.[50,51]

Medical Management

A pneumothorax of less than 15% requires no treatment unless complications occur or underlying lung disease or injury is present.[50] A tension pneumothorax is an emergency that requires immediate relief. A large-bore needle is inserted into the second intercostal space in the midclavicular line of the affected side to relieve pressure within the chest. Sucking chest wounds require immediate treatment to prevent hypoxemia. The defect in the chest wall should be dressed with a sterile, occlusive dressing that allows air to escape on inhalation.[50,51]

Once stabilized, all tension pneumothoraces, open pneumothoraces, and pneumothoraces greater than 15% require intervention to evacuate the air from the pleural space and facilitate reexpansion of the collapsed lung. Interventions include aspiration of the air with a needle, placement of a percutaneous catheter attached to a Heimlich valve, insertion of a thoracic vent, and insertion of a chest tube with underwater seal suction drainage. A small one-way valve device that is easily secured to a catheter placed in the chest, the Heimlich valve allows air to escape from the pleural space but not enter it.[50,52] A thoracic vent is similar to a Heimlich valve in that it is a one-way valve, but it comes attached to the catheter.[53] Chest tubes are usually inserted in the fourth or fifth intercostal space on the midaxillary line.[52] Once the tubes are inserted and connected to an underwater chest drainage system with at least 20 cm of suction, a chest x-ray examination should be performed to confirm reexpansion of the lung.[51]

Nursing Management

Nursing management of patients with a pneumothorax incorporates a variety of nursing diagnoses (Box 12-9). **Nursing priorities are directed toward optimizing oxygenation and ventilation, maintaining the chest tube system, and educating patients and families.**

Optimizing oxygenation and ventilation

Nursing interventions to optimize oxygenation and ventilation include positioning, preventing desaturation during procedures, promoting secretion clearance, and administering medications as ordered.[12,13] The Nursing Management section on acute respiratory failure (Unit X) contains further discussion of these interventions.

Maintaining the chest tube system

Maintaining the chest tube system involves careful attention to the suction applied and to preservation of un-

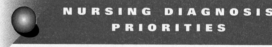

BOX 12-9

NURSING DIAGNOSIS PRIORITIES

PNEUMOTHORAX

- *Ineffective Breathing Pattern* related to decreased lung expansion, p. 485
- *Impaired Gas Exchange* related to ventilator/perfusion mismatching and intrapulmonary shunting, p. 488
- *Anxiety* related to threat to biologic, psychologic, and/or social integrity, p. 464

obstructed drainage tubes. Kinks and large loops of tubing should be prevented because they impede drainage and air evacuation, which may prevent timely lung reexpansion or result in a tension pneumothorax.

Educating patients and family

Educating patients and families includes teaching them about pneumothorax and its management, answering their questions, and preparing them for discharge. Upon discharge, patients should be taught how pneumothorax develops, interventions to prevent it from recurring, and the importance of taking prescribed medications.[16]

Thoracic Surgery

Types of Surgery

Thoracic surgery refers to a number of surgical procedures that involve opening the thoracic cavity (thoracotomy) and/or the organs of respiration. Indications for thoracic surgery range from tumors and abscesses to repair of the esophagus and thoracic vessels.[54] Table 12-5 describes a variety of thoracic surgical procedures and their indications. This discussion focuses only on the surgical procedures that involve removal of lung tissue.

Preoperative Care

Before surgery, clinicians complete an evaluation of patients to determine the appropriateness of surgery as a treatment and whether lung tissue can be removed without jeopardizing respiratory function. This step is especially important when a lobectomy or pneumonectomy is being considered. When resection is selected for tumor treatment, preoperative care includes evaluation of the type and extent of tumor and the physical condition of patients. The evaluation of patients' physical status should focus on the adequacy of cardiopulmonary function. The preoperative evaluation should include pulmonary function tests to determine patients' ability to lose lung tissue. Cardiac function should also be evaluated. Uncontrolled dysrhythmias, acute myocardial infarction, severe congestive heart failure, and unstable angina are all contraindications to surgery.[55,56]

Surgical Considerations

Patients are usually placed in a lateral decubitus position during surgery to provide adequate surgical exposure for a lung resection (pneumonectomy and lobectomy). A posterolateral incision permits upward displacement of the scapula. When a pneumonectomy or upper lobectomy is planned, an incision is generally made in the area of the fifth or sixth rib bed. When a lower lobectomy is planned, approach through the seventh rib area is more usual. Removing a rib and entering the thorax through the rib bed is preferred because a tighter air seal is pos-

sible at closure.[55] Special care is taken to avoid drainage of blood or secretions into the unaffected lung during surgery because such an occurrence could cause hypoxemia and cardiac dysfunction. A double-lumen endotracheal tube is used during surgery to protect the unaffected lung from secretions and necrotic tumor fragments. In addition, the deflated lung is suctioned and ventilated every 20 to 30 minutes during the procedure.[57]

After the pneumonectomy the mediastinal position requires evaluation. This is done after closure of the operative site and involves manometric measurement and a chest x-ray examination. With patients lying in the supine position, pressure in the empty chest cavity should be −4 to −6 cm of H_2O pressure. When the pressure is abnormal, air or fluid can be added or withdrawn. If the abnormality is not corrected, a mediastinal shift can occur, resulting in hemodynamic compromise and cardiac dysfunction. A chest x-ray examination will show the location of the mediastinum.[55] Careful, regular evaluation of the mediastinal position is also required in the postoperative period. The mediastinal position can be determined by palpating for tracheal deviation, palpating and auscultating the position of the apex of the heart, and performing a chest x-ray examination. If a mediastinal shift occurs, it should be corrected by injecting or withdrawing air or fluid.[58]

Complications and Medical Management

A number of complications are associated with a lung resection, including ARF, bronchopleural fistula, hemorrhage, and cardiovascular disturbances.

Acute respiratory failure

In the postoperative period, ARF may result from atelectasis, pneumonia, and/or ARDS. Atelectasis can occur as a result of anesthesia, the surgical procedure, immobilization, and pain. Treatment should be aimed at correcting the underlying problems and supporting gas exchange. Supplemental oxygen and mechanical ventilation with PEEP may be necessary.[58,59]

Bronchopleural fistula

The chief cause of mortality after a lung resection,[58] a postoperative bronchopleural fistula develops when the suture line fails to secure occlusion of the bronchial stump and an opening develops. This can result from an imperfect stump closure, perforation of the stump (e.g., with a suction catheter), or high pressure within the airways (e.g., caused by mechanical ventilation).[60] During surgery, careful attention is given to isolating and closing the bronchus in an attempt to secure a lasting seal with subsequent stump healing.[58] In addition, early extubation is encouraged to eliminate the possibility of perforation of the stump and high airway pressures.[60] Clinical manifestations of a bronchopleural fistula include fever, purulent sputum, and massive bubbling of air

THORACIC PROCEDURE	DEFINITION	INDICATIONS
Segmental resection	Removal of segment of pulmonary lobe	Chronic, localized pyogenic lung abscess Congenital cyst or bleb Benign tumor Segment infected with pulmonary tuberculosis or bronchiectasis
Wedge resection	Excision of small peripheral section of lobe	Small masses that are close to pleural surface of lung, e.g., subpleural granulomas, small peripheral tumors (benign primary tumors)
Lobectomy	Excision of one or more lobes of lung tissue	Cancer Infections such as tuberculosis Miscellaneous benign tumors
Pneumonectomy	Removal of entire lung	Malignant neoplasms Lung almost entirely infected Extensive chronic abscess Selected unilateral lesions
Decortication of lung	Removal of fibrinous, reactive membrane covering visceral and parietal pleura	Restrictive fibrinous membrane lining visceral and parietal pleura that limits ventilatory excursion; "trapped lung"
Thoracoplasty	Surgical collapse of portion of chest wall by multiple rib resections to intentionally decrease volume in hemithorax	Closure of chronic cavitary lesions and empyema spaces Closure of recurrent air leaks Reduction of open thoracic "dead space" after large resection
Thymectomy	Removal of thymus gland	Primary thymic neoplasm or myasthenia
Correction of pectus excavatum ("funnel chest")	Depression of sternum and costal cartilage corrected by moving sternum outward and realigning cartilage-sternal junction	Cosmesis and relief of cardiopulmonary compromise
Repair of penetrating thoracic wounds, drainage of hemothorax	Drainage of pleural cavity and control of hemorrhage	Hemorrhage produced by injury to thoracic vessels that causes blood loss, as well as compression of lung tissue and mediastinum, resulting in cardiopulmonary compromise
Excision of mediastinal masses	Removal of masses and cysts in upper anterior and posterior mediastinum	Mediastinal tumors (benign or malignant) Cysts Abscesses
Tracheal resection	Resection of portion of trachea, followed by primary end-to-end reanastomosis of trachea	Significant stenosis of tracheal orifice, usually related to mechanical pressure of cuffed tracheal tube; pressure produces tracheal wall ischemia, inflammation, and ulceration; these effects lead to formation of granulation tissue and fibrosis, which narrow tracheal orifice Tumors
Esophagogastrectomy	Resection of part of esophagus and at least cardial portion of stomach with primary anastomosis of proximal esophagus to remaining stomach	Carcinoma of esophagus anywhere from neck to esophagogastric junction Severe reflux esophagitis producing hemorrhage Extensive alkali burns of esophagus
Bullectomy	Removal by excision of cysts or pockets in lung, which result from confluence of many alveoli	Failure of medical therapy, such as antibiotics, and chest physiotherapy to control infection associated with such cysts or pockets Severe compression of tissue adjacent to pulmonary cysts or pockets
Closed thoracostomy	Insertion of chest tube through intercostal space into pleural space; chest tube is attached to water seal system, with or without suction	Provision of continuous aspiration of fluid from pleural cavity Prevention of accumulation of air in chest from leaks in lung or tracheobronchial tree
Open thoracostomy	Partial resection of selected rib or ribs, with insertion of chest tube into infected material to provide for continuous drainage	Drainage of empyemas when pleural space is fixed

From Johanson BC and others: *Standards for critical care*, ed 3, St. Louis, 1988, Mosby.

through the chest tube system. The diagnosis is confirmed by bronchoscopy. Antibiotics should be prescribed if an infection is suspected. The fistula may close on its own, but occasionally surgery is necessary. The development of a bronchopleural fistula in patients with a pneumonectomy can be life threatening. The disruption of the suture line can result in flooding of the remaining lung, with fluid from the residual space producing aspiration. If this occurs, patients should be placed with the operative side down (remaining lung up) and a chest tube inserted to drain the residual space.[58]

Hemorrhage

Hemorrhage is an early, life-threatening complication that can occur after a lung resection. It can result from bronchial or intercostal artery bleeding or disruption of a suture or clip around a pulmonary vessel.[60] In all patients except those with a pneumonectomy, an increase in chest tube drainage can signal excessive bleeding. During the immediate postoperative period, chest tube drainage should be measured every 15 minutes and this frequency decreased as the patient stabilizes. If chest tube loss is greater than 100 ml/hour, fresh blood is noted, or a sudden increase in drainage occurs, hemorrhage should be suspected.[57,58]

Cardiovascular disturbances

Cardiovascular complications after thoracic surgery include dysrhythmias and pulmonary edema. A rise in central venous pressure may follow resections of a large lung area or a pneumonectomy. With the loss of one lung the right ventricle must empty its stroke volume into a vascular bed that has been reduced by 50%, creating a higher pressure system, which increases right ventricular work load and precipitates right ventricular failure. Depending on previous heart function, acute decompensation of both ventricles can result. Measures are aimed at supporting cardiac function and avoiding intravascular volume excess. These measures include optimizing preload, afterload, and contractility with vasoactive agents.[58,60]

Postoperative Nursing Management

Nursing care of patients with thoracic surgery incorporates a number of nursing diagnoses (Box 12-10). **Nursing priorities are directed toward optimizing oxygenation and ventilation, preventing atelectasis, monitoring chest tubes, assisting patients with return to an adequate activity level, and educating patients and families.**

Optimizing oxygenation and ventilation

Nursing interventions to optimize oxygenation and ventilation include positioning and preventing desaturation during procedures, preventing hypovention, promoting secretion clearance, and administering medications as ordered.[12,13] The Nursing Management section on acute

---

BOX 12-10

NURSING DIAGNOSIS PRIORITIES

THORACIC SURGERY

- *Ineffective Breathing Pattern* related to decreased lung expansion, p. 485
- *Impaired Gas Exchange* related to ventilation/perfusion mismatching and intrapulmonary shunting, p. 488
- *Acute Pain* related to transmission and perception of cutaneous, visceral, muscular, or ischemic impulses, p. 499
- *Anxiety* related to threat to biologic, psychologic, and/or social integrity, p. 464

---

respiratory failure contains further discussion of these interventions.

Preventing atelectasis

Nursing interventions to prevent atelectasis include proper patient positioning and early ambulation, deep breathing and incentive spirometry, and pain management. The goal is to promote maximal lung ventilation and prevent hypoventilation.

PATIENT POSITIONING AND EARLY AMBULATION. Nurses should consider the surgical incision site and type of surgery when positioning patients. After a lobectomy, patients should be turned onto the nonoperative side to promote V/Q matching. When the good lung is dependent, blood flow is greater to the area with better ventilation and V/Q matching is better. V/Q mismatching results when the affected lung is positioned down because of the increase in blood flow to an area with less ventilation. Patients should be turned frequently to promote secretion removal but should have the affected lung dependent as little as possible.[60] Patients who have had a pneumonectomy should be positioned supine or on the operative side during the initial period. Turning onto the nonoperative side can result in disruption of the suture line and shifting of the mediastinum, which may compress the good lung. Tilting patients slightly toward the unaffected side is possible, but the surgeon should indicate when free side-to-side positioning is safe.[55,57,61] When sitting at the bedside or moving, patients must be encouraged to keep the thorax in straight alignment while they breathe deeply. This position best accommodates diaphragmatic descent and intercostal muscle action. The sitting or standing position provides enhanced ventilation to areas of the lung that are dependent in the supine position, thus accommodating maximal inflation and promoting gas exchange.[12,13] Ambulation is essential in restoring lung function and should be initiated as soon as possible.[58]

DEEP BREATHING AND INCENTIVE SPIROMETRY. Deep breathing exercises and incentive spirometry should be performed regularly by patients who have undergone a thoracotomy. Deep breathing involves taking a deep breath and holding it for approximately 3 seconds or longer. Incentive spirometry involves taking at least 10 deep, effective breaths per hour using an incentive spirometer. These activities help reexpand collapsed lung tissue, thus promoting early resolution of the pneumothorax in patients with partial lung resections. The chest should be auscultated during inflation to ensure that all dependent parts of the lung are well ventilated and to help patients understand the depth of breath necessary for optimal effect. Coughing, which should be encouraged only when secretions are present, assists in mobilizing secretions for removal. Because of intraoperative positioning and preoperative and perioperative medications, atelectasis and secretion pooling are common during the postoperative period. Furthermore, as a result of postoperative pain patients' ventilations may be shallow, thereby encouraging the development of atelectasis and secretion stasis. Respiratory infections can occur from retained secretions and incomplete lung expansion.[55,57-59]

PAIN MANAGEMENT. Pain can be a major problem after thoracic surgery, increasing the work load of the heart, precipitating hypoventilation, and inhibiting mobilization of secretions. Clinical manifestations of pain include tachypnea, tachycardia, elevated blood pressure, facial grimacing, splinting of the incision, hypoventilation, moaning, and restlessness. There are several alternatives for pain management after thoracic surgery. The two most common methods are systemic narcotic administration and epidural narcotic administration. Systemic narcotics can be administered intravenously, intramuscularly, or via patient-controlled analgesia method.[60] In addition, patients should be assisted with splinting the incision with a pillow or blanket when deep breathing and coughing. Splinting stabilizes the area and reduces pain when moving, deep breathing, or coughing.[61]

Monitoring the chest tubes

Chest tubes are inserted after all thoracic surgery procedures (except a pneumonectomy) to remove air and fluid. Initially bloody, the drainage becomes serosanguinous and then serous over the first 2 to 3 days after surgery. Approximately 100 to 300 ml of drainage occurs during the first 2 hours after surgery. Drainage decreases to less than 50 ml/hour over the next several hours. If clots are present, the chest tubes should be gently stripped or milked to facilitate patency.[61]

During auscultation of the lungs, air leaks should be evaluated. In the early phase an air leak is commonly heard over the affected area because the pleura is not yet tightly sealed. As healing occurs, this leak should disappear. An increase in an air leak or appearance of a new air leak should prompt investigation of the chest drainage system to determine whether air is leaking into the system from outside or whether the leak is originating from the incision. A significant air leak can result in a tension pneumothorax. Increased air leaks not related to the thoracic drainage system may indicate disruption of sutures.[56,57,61]

Assisting patients with return to adequate activity level

Within a few days after surgery, patients should be able to perform range of motion to the shoulder on the operative side. Patients frequently splint the operative side and avoid shoulder movement because of pain. If immobility is allowed, the shoulder joint may stiffen. This tendency is referred to as *frozen shoulder* and may require physical therapy and rehabilitation if satisfactory range of motion of the shoulder joint is to be regained.[57] On the day after surgery, patients are usually able to sit in a chair. Activity should be systematically increased, in accordance with patients' activity tolerance. With adequate pulmonary function before surgery and a surgical approach designed to preserve respiratory function, full return to previous activity levels is possible. This may take as long as 6 months to 1 year, depending on the tissue resected and patients' general condition.[56]

Educating patients and families

Educating patients and families includes teaching them about the postoperative management plan, answering their questions, and preparing them for discharge. Upon discharge, patients should receive information regarding activity and lifting, wound management, symptoms to report to their physicians, and the importance of taking prescribed medications.[16]

References

1. Shapiro BA and others: *Clinical application of respiratory care*, ed 4, St Louis, 1991, Mosby.
2. Bone RC: *Acute respiratory failure*. In Burton GG, Hodgkin JE, Ward JJ, editors: *Respiratory care: a guide to clinical practice*, ed 3, Philadelphia, 1991, JB Lippincott.
3. Balk R, Bone RC: Classification of acute respiratory failure, *Med Clin North Am* 67:551, 1983.
4. Norton LC: *Respiratory failure*. In Sexton DL, editor: *Nursing care of the respiratory patient*, Norwalk, Conn, 1990, Appleton & Lange.
5. Pratter MR, Irwin RS: Extrapulmonary causes of respiratory failure, *J Intens Care Med* 1:197, 1986.
6. Green KE, Peter JI: Pathophysiology of acute respiratory failure, *Clin Chest Med* 15:1, 1994.
7. Vaughan P: Acute respiratory failure in the patient with chronic obstructive lung disease, *Crit Care Nurse* 1(6):46, 1981.
8. Rosen RL: Acute respiratory failure and chronic obstructive lung disease, *Med Clin North Am* 70:895, 1986.
9. Popovich J: The physiology of mechanical ventilation and the mechanical zoo: IPPB, PEEP, CPAP, *Med Clin North Am* 67:621, 1983.
10. Halloran T: Use of sedation and neuromuscular paralysis during mechanical ventilation, *Crit Care Nurs Clin North Am* 3:651, 1991.

11. Davidson JE: Neuromuscular blockade, *Focus Crit Care* 18:513, 1991.
12. Castro MS, Everett B, deBolsblanc BP: Positioning patients with hypoxemia, *Crit Care Rep* 1:234, 1990.
13. Norton LC, Conforti C: The effect of body position on oxygenation, *Heart Lung* 14:45, 1985.
14. Doering LV: The effect of positioning on hemodynamics and gas exchange in the critically ill: a review, *Am J Crit Care* 2:208, 1993.
15. Cosenza JJ, Norton LC: Secretion clearance: state-of-the-art from a nursing perspective, *Crit Care Nurse* 6(4):23, 1986.
16. Wilson SF, Thompson, JM: *Respiratory disorders*, St Louis, 1990, Mosby.
17. Murray J and others: An expanded definition of the adult respiratory distress syndrome, *Am Rev Respir Dis* 138:720, 1988.
18. Vaughan P, Brooks C: Adult respiratory distress syndrome: a complication of shock, *Crit Care Nurs Clin North Am* 2:235, 1990.
19. Mattay MA: The adult respiratory distress syndrome: definition and prognosis, *Clin Chest Med* 11:575, 1990.
20. Rinaldo JE, Heyman SJ: ARDS: a multisystem disease with pulmonary manifestations, *Crit Care Rep* 1:174, 1990.
21. Rinaldo JE, Christman JW: Mechanisms and mediators of the adult respiratory distress syndrome, *Clin Chest Med* 11:621, 1990.
22. Atkins P, Egloff ME, Wilms DC: Respiratory consequences of multisystem crisis: the adult respiratory distress syndrome, *Crit Care Nurs Q* 16:27, 1994.
23. Bradley RB: Adult respiratory distress syndrome, *Focus Crit Care* 14(5):48, 1987.
24. Dorinsky PM, Gadek JE: Multiple organ failure, *Clin Chest Med* 11:581, 1990.
25. Idell S: The deadly danger of ARDS, *Emerg Med* 21(7):67, 1989.
26. Roberts S: High-permeability pulmonary edema: nursing assessment, diagnosis, and interventions, *Heart Lung* 19:287, 1990.
27. Aberle DR, Brown K: Radiologic considerations in the adult respiratory distress syndrome, *Clin Chest Med* 11:737, 1990.
28. Cascade PN, Kazerooni EA: Aspects of chest imaging in the intensive care unit, *Crit Care Clin* 10:247, 1994.
29. Stoller JK, Kacmarek RM: Ventilatory strategies in the management of the adult respiratory distress syndrome, *Clin Chest Med* 11:755, 1990.
30. Gattinone L and others: Regional effects and mechanisms of positive end-expiratory pressure in early adult respiratory distress syndrome, *JAMA* 269:2122, 1993.
31. Rossaine R and others: Inhaled nitric oxide for the adult respiratory distress syndrome, *N Eng J Med* 328:399, 1993.
32. Campbell GD: Overview of community-acquired pneumonia, *Med Clin North Am* 78:1035, 1994.
33. Skerrett SJ: Host defenses against respiratory infection, *Med Clin North Am* 78:941, 1994.
34. Dal Norgare AR: Nosocomial pneumonia in the medical and surgical patient, *Med Clin North Am* 78:1081, 1994.
35. Timby BK: Pneumocystosis in patients with acquired immunodeficiency syndrome, *Crit Care Nurs* 12(5):64, 1992.
36. Thompson R: Prevention of nosocomial pneumonia, *Med Clin North Am* 78:1185, 1994.
37. Pürlä P: Changes in crackle characteristics during the clinical course of pneumonia, *Chest* 102:176, 1992.
38. Elpern EH, Jacobs ER, Bone RC: Incidence of aspiration in tracheally intubated adults, *Heart Lung* 16:527, 1987.
39. Methany NA, Eisenberg P, Spies M: Aspiration pneumonia in patients fed through nasoenteral tubes, *Heart Lung* 15:256, 1986.
40. DePaso WJ: Aspiration pneumonia, *Clin Chest Med* 12:269, 1991.
41. Saleh KL: Practical points in understanding aspiration, *J Post Anesth Nurs* 6:347, 1991.
42. Tietjen PA, Kaner RJ, Quinn CE: Aspiration emergencies, *Clin Chest Med* 15:117, 1994.
43. West JW: Pulmonary embolism, *Med Clin North Am* 70:877, 1986.
44. Counselman FL: Best tests for pulmonary embolism, *Emerg Med* 22(21):66, 1990.
45. Davis LA, O'Rouke NC: Pulmonary embolism: early recognition and management in the postanesthesia care unit, *J Post Anesth Nurs* 8:338, 1993.
46. Roberts SL: Pulmonary tissue perfusion: altered: emboli, *Heart Lung,* 16:128, 1987.
47. Sherman S: Pulmonary embolism update, *Postgrad Med* 89:195, 1991.
48. Schiff MJ: Finding and fighting pulmonary embolism, *Emerg Med* 21(7):47, 1989.
49. Goldhaber SZ and others: Recombinant tissue-type plasminogen activator versus a novel dosing regimen of urokinase in acute pulmonary embolism: a randomized controlled multicenter trial, *J Am Coll Cardiol* 20:24, 1992.
50. Janz MA, Pierson DJ: Pneumothorax and barotrauma, *Clin Chest Med* 15:75, 1994.
51. Committee on Trauma of the American College of Surgeons: *Advanced trauma life support,* Chicago, 1984, American College of Surgeons.
52. Kirby TJ, Ginsberg RJ: Management of the pneumothorax and barotrauma, *Clin Chest Med* 13:97, 1992.
53. Samelson SL, Goldberg EM, Ferguson MK: The thoracic vent: clinical experience with a new device for treating simple pneumothorax, *Chest* 100:880, 1991.
54. Litwack K: Practical points in the care of the thoracic surgery patient, *Post Anesth Nurs* 5:276, 1990.
55. Simonson G: *Cancer of the lung.* In Sexton DL, editor: *Nursing care of the respiratory patient,* Norwalk, Conn, 1990, Appleton & Lange.
56. Cottrell JJ, Ferson PF: Preoperative assessment of the thoracic surgical patient, *Chest* 13:47, 1992.
57. O'Byrne C: Postoperative care and complications in the thoracotomy patients, *Crit Care Q* 7(4):53, 1985.
58. Finkelmeier B: Difficult problems in postoperative management, *Crit Care Q* 9(3):59, 1986.
59. Forshag MS, Cooper AD: Postoperative care of the thoracotomy patient, *Clin Chest Med* 13:33, 1992.
60. Daitch JS: *Post anesthesia care after thoracic surgery.* In Frost EAM, editor: *Post anesthesia care unit current practices,* ed 2, St Louis, 1990, Mosby.
61. Whitman G, Weber MM: Postoperative care after thoracic surgery, *Curr Rev PACU* 14:137, 1992.

13

Pulmonary Therapeutic Management

KATHLEEN M. STACY

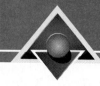

Management of patients with pulmonary dysfunction employs a wide variety of therapeutic interventions. This chapter focuses on the priority interventions that are used to manage pulmonary disorders in the critical care environment.

Oxygen Therapy

Normal cellular function depends on a supply of oxygen adequate to meet metabolic needs. The goal of oxygen-administration is to provide a sufficient concentration of inspired oxygen to permit full use of the oxygen-carrying capacity of the arterial blood, thus ensuring adequate tissue oxygenation if the cardiac output (CO) is adequate and the hemoglobin (Hgb) concentration and structure are normal.[1,2]

Oxygen Delivery

Oxygen therapy devices come in many different forms (Table 13-1).[2,3] Oxygen is generally ordered in liters per minute (L/min), as a concentration of oxygen expressed as a percent (such as 40%), or as a fraction (such as 0.4)[3] of inspired oxygen (FIO_2).[3] The amount of oxygen administered depends on the pathophysiologic mechanisms affecting patients' oxygenation status. In most cases the amount required should provide an arterial partial pressure of oxygen (PaO_2) of 60 to 90 mm Hg, so a Hgb saturation of greater than 90% is achieved. The concentration of oxygen given to individual patients is a clinical judgment based on the many factors that influence oxygen transport, such as Hgb concentration, CO, and the arterial oxygen tension.[2]

Complications

Oxygen, like most drugs, has adverse effects and complications resulting from its use. The lungs are designed to handle a concentration of 21% oxygen, with some adaptability to higher concentrations, but adverse effects can result if a high concentration is administered for too long.

Hypoventilation

The first adverse effect of oxygen administration is hypoventilation. In patients with severe chronic obstructive pulmonary disease (COPD) and certain types of drug overdoses, the normal stimulus to breathe (increasing carbon dioxide levels) is muted. In these patients decreasing oxygen levels stimulate breathing. When oxygen is administered and hypoxemia corrected, the stimulus to breathe is abolished and hypoventilation develops, resulting in a further increase in the arterial partial pressure of carbon dioxide ($PaCO_2$). Eventually, patients become somnolent and even obtunded because of carbon dioxide narcosis. Because of the risk of hypoventilation and carbon dioxide accumulation, all chronically hypercapnic patients require careful low-flow oxygen administration.[2,3]

Absorption atelectasis

Another adverse effect of high concentrations of oxygen is absorption atelectasis. Administering high concentrations of oxygen washes out the nitrogen that normally fills the alveoli and helps hold them open (residual volume). As oxygen replaces the nitrogen in the alveoli, the alveoli start to shrink and collapse because oxygen is absorbed into the blood stream faster than it can be replaced in the alveoli, particularly in areas of the lungs that are minimally ventilated.[1]

Oxygen toxicity

The most detrimental effect of breathing a high concentration of oxygen is the development of oxygen toxicity, which can occur in patients breathing oxygen concentrations of greater than 50% for more than 24 hours. Patients most likely to develop oxygen toxicity are those who require intubation, mechanical ventilation, and high oxygen concentrations for extended periods. Hyperoxia, or the administration of higher-than-normal oxygen concentrations, produces an overabundance of oxygen-free radicals. These radicals are responsible for the initial damage to the alveolar-capillary membrane. Oxygen-free radicals are toxic metabolites of oxygen metabolism. Normally, enzymes neutralize the radicals, which prevents any damage from occurring. During the administration of high levels of oxygen, the large number of oxygen-free radicals produced exhausts the supply of neutralizing enzymes, damaging the lung parenchyma and vasculature.[4]

CLINICAL MANIFESTATIONS. A number of clinical manifestations are associated with oxygen toxicity. The first symptom is substernal chest pain exacerbated by deep breathing. A dry cough and tracheal irritation follow. Eventually, definite pleuritic pain occurs on inhalation, followed by dyspnea. Upper airway changes may include a sensation of nasal stuffiness, sore throat, and eye and ear discomfort. Chest radiographs and pulmonary function tests show no abnormalities until symptoms are severe. Complete, rapid reversal of these symptoms occurs as soon as normal oxygen concentrations return.[4] These abnormalities are reversible several days after normal oxygen concentrations return. If high oxygen concentrations are still needed, permanent damage may occur.[3]

Nursing Management

Nursing priorities for patients receiving oxygen include assuring the oxygen is being administered as ordered and observing patients for complications of the therapy. Confirming that the oxygen therapy device is properly positioned and replacing it after removal is important. During meals an oxygen mask should be changed to a nasal cannula if patients can tolerate one. Patients on oxygen therapy should also be transported with the oxygen. In addition, the oxygen saturation should be periodically monitored using a pulse oximeter.[5]

Artificial Airways

Oropharyngeal and Nasopharyngeal Airways

Pharyngeal airways are made of rubber or plastic and are used to maintain airway patency by keeping the tongue from obstructing the upper airway. An oral airway is inserted upside down and rotated 180 degrees as it is passed

TABLE 13-1
OXYGEN ADMINISTRATION DEVICES

EQUIPMENT	OBJECTIVES	L/MIN	Fio₂ (%)	ADVANTAGES/DISADVANTAGES
LOW FLOW SYSTEMS				
Nasal cannula	Provides oxygen through a low flow oxygen delivery system.	1 2 3 4 5 6	24 28 32 36 40 44	Can be used with mouth breathers Convenient Comfortable Good low flow Allows for talking and eating Fio₂ not really accurate because it depends on patients' respiratory pattern May cause sinus pain >2 L/min requires added humidity Easily displaced Nasal passages must be patent
Simple face mask*	Provides oxygen through a mask and low flow oxygen delivery system.	5 6 8	40 50 60	Simple set-up; good for emergency situations Can get uncomfortable Poor patient tolerance Fio₂ not really accurate because it depends on patients' respiratory pattern Cannot provide enough humidity for prolonged use Must be removed at meals Tight fitting mask can cause pressure sores Aspiration of vomitus is a potential problem
Partial rebreathing mask	Provides a high oxygen concentration through a low flow delivery system.	6 8 10-15	35 45-50 In excess of 60 depending on patient's ventilatory pattern	Simple set-up; good in emergency situations Can be uncomfortable Does not provide adequate humidity for long-term use
Nonrebreathing mask	Provides high oxygen concentration.	6 8 10-15	55-60 60-80 80-90	Delivers the highest possible oxygen concentration (55%-90%) possible from a low flow system Good for short-term therapy and transport Has three one-way valves Requires a tight seal May irritate skin
HUMIDIFYING SYSTEMS				
Aerosol mask (high humidity face mask)	Delivers a specific Fio₂ through an aerosol device.		28-100 (variable)	High humidity Accurate Fio₂ Does not dry mucous membranes Can be uncomfortable May need extra equipment for higher Fio₂ Moisture build-up in tube
Face tent	Delivers high humidity.		21-55	Used for patients with facial trauma Does not dry mucous membranes Can function as high flow system when attached to Venturi system Interferes with eating and talking Impractical for long-term use Possible to rebreathe CO_2

From Flynn JBM, Bruce NP: *Introduction to Critical Care Skills,* St Louis, 1993, Mosby.
*A minimum flow rate of 5 L/min to flush expired carbon dioxide from the mask is needed.

TABLE 13-1—cont'd

OXYGEN ADMINISTRATION DEVICES

EQUIPMENT	OBJECTIVES	L/MIN	FIO$_2$ (%)	ADVANTAGES/DISADVANTAGES
HUMIDIFYING SYSTEMS—cont'd				
Trach mask T-tube	Delivers a specific FIO$_2$ through an aerosol system.		28-100 (variable)	High humidity Accurate FIO$_2$ Can control oxygen Does not need vent May need extra equipment for higher FIO$_2$
HIGH FLOW SYSTEMS				
Venturi mask†	Provides high flow oxygen with a precise FIO$_2$ in a selected range.	Blue-4 Yellow-4 White-6 Green-8 Pink-8	24 28 31 35 40	Can provide humidity Accurate oxygen levels Simple set-up; good for emergency situations Well tolerated Can only have FIO$_2$ in selected range Hot and confining Must fit snugly
CONTINUOUS POSITIVE AIRWAY PRESSURE (CPAP)				
CPAP mask	Provides continual positive airway pressure through a mask without the use of a ventilator.		30-100	Do not need ventilator Do not need to be intubated Can get gastric distension Mask is uncomfortable Not useful if patient becomes apneic

From Flynn JBM, Bruce NP: *Introduction to Critical Care Skills*, St Louis, 1993, Mosby.
†Jet adapters on Venturi masks are color coded.

into the mouth. It should be used only in unconscious patients who have absent or diminished gag reflexes. A nasal airway is placed by lubricating the tube and inserting it midline along the floor of the naris into the posterior pharynx. Respirations should be assessed after placement of either airway to ensure proper position. Complications of these airways include trauma to the oral or nasal cavity, obstruction of the airway, laryngospasm, and gagging and vomiting.[6-8]

Endotracheal Tubes

An **endotracheal tube** (ETT) is the most commonly used artificial means for short-term airway management. Indications for endotracheal intubation include airway maintenance, secretion control, oxygenation, and ventilation.[8] An endotracheal tube may be placed through the orotracheal or nasotracheal route. In most situations involving emergency placement, the orotracheal route is used because the approach is simpler and affords use of a larger diameter endotracheal tube. A larger diameter tube facilitates secretion removal, decreases the work of breathing, and allows for fiberoptic bronchoscopy, if necessary. The orotracheal route also avoids nasal and sinus complications. Nasotracheal intubation provides greater

patient comfort over time and is preferred when patients have a jaw fracture. In addition, the nasotracheal route facilitates oral hygiene and tube stability.[7,9,10]

ETTs are available in a variety of sizes, according to the internal diameter of the tube, and have a radiopaque marker that runs the length of the tube. On one end of the tube is a cuff that is inflated using the pilot balloon. Because of the high incidence of cuff-related problems, low-pressure, high-volume cuffs (soft cuffs) are preferred. On the other end of the tube is a 15 mm adaptor that facilitates the connection of the tube to a manual resuscitation bag (MRB), T-tube, or ventilator (Fig. 13-1).[11]

Intubation

Equipment that should be readily available to facilitate the insertion of an ETT includes a suction system with catheters and tonsil suction, an MRB with a mask connected to 100% oxygen, a laryngoscope handle with assorted blades, a variety of sizes of ETTs, and a stylet. Before the procedure is initiated, all equipment should be inspected to ensure its effectiveness. The procedure should be explained to the patient, if possible. The patient should have a patent intravenous catheter and be monitored with a pulse oximeter. The patient should be sedated before the procedure and a topical anesthetic ap-

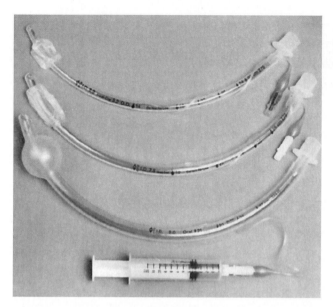

FIG. 13-1 Endotracheal tubes. (From Perry AG, Potter PA: *Clinical nursing skills and techniques,* ed 3, St Louis, 1994, Mosby.)

plied to facilitate placement of the tube. In some cases a paralytic agent may be necessary if the patient is extremely agitated.[7-9]

The procedure is initiated by positioning patients with their neck flexed and head slightly extended in the "sniff" position. The oral cavity and pharynx should be suctioned and any dental devices removed. Patients should be preoxygenated and ventilated using the MRB and mask with 100% oxygen.[7-9] Cricoid pressure should be applied to decrease the risk of aspiration.[6,9] Each intubation attempt should be limited to 30 seconds. Once the ETT is inserted, patients should be assessed for bilateral breath sounds and bilateral chest movement. The tube should then be secured and a chest radiograph obtained to confirm placement.[7,8,12] The tip of the endotracheal tube should be at least 2 cm above the carina but with the cuff below the cricoid cartilage.[13] Once final adjustment of the position is complete, the level of insertion (marked in centimeters on side of tube) should be noted.[8]

COMPLICATIONS. Intubation presents a number of complications, including gastric intubation; right mainstem bronchus intubation; vomiting with aspiration; trauma to the mouth, nose, pharynx, trachea, esophagus, eyes, or facial tissue; laryngospasm; hypoxemia; and hypercapnia. Hypoxemia and hypercapnia can cause bradycardia, tachycardia, dysrhythmias, hypertension, and hypotension.[8,9,13]

Complications

A number of factors predispose patients to the development of complications during intubation (Box 13-1). Complications include tube obstruction and displacement, sinusitis, nasal injury, and tracheoesophageal fistu-

---

BOX 13-1

FACTORS THAT PREDISPOSE DAMAGE TO THE AIRWAYS BY ARTIFICIAL TUBES

GENERAL FACTORS

Prolonged intubation
Prolonged mechanical ventilation
Inadequate patient sedation
Repeated flexion and extension of the neck
Decerebrate or decorticate movements
Patient out of phase with controlled mechanical ventilation ("bucking" the ventilator)
Traction on the tube during turning, suctioning, and ventilator connection and disconnection
Previous prolonged intubation
Chronic airway or lung disease (especially sputum-producing disease) requiring frequent suctioning procedures
Airway infection
Hypotension

SITE-SPECIFIC FACTORS
Laryngeal

Multiple orotracheal or nasotracheal intubations
Inexperienced laryngoscopist, an emergency intubation, or self-extubation
Too large a translaryngeal tube

Tracheal

Cuff overinflation
Combination of high positive end-expiratory pressure (PEEP) and low lung compliance
Too small or large a cuff in relation to the tracheal size
Noncircular cross-sectional tracheal shape

---

las (Table 13-2). A number of complications can occur days to weeks after the ETT is removed. These include mucosal lesions, laryngeal and/or tracheal stenosis, and cricoid abscess (Table 13-2). Delayed complications usually require some form of surgical intervention to correct.[9,10,13]

Tracheostomy Tubes

A **tracheostomy tube** is the preferred method of airway maintenance in patients requiring intubation for more than 21 days and is also indicated in several other situations. These include upper airway obstruction or malformation, failed intubation, repeated intubations, presence of complications of endotracheal intubation, glottic incompetence, sleep apnea, and chronic inability to clear secretions.[7] A tracheostomy tube provides the best route for long-term airway maintenance and avoids the oral, nasal, pharyngeal, and laryngeal complications of endotracheal intubation. The tube is shorter, of wider diam-

TABLE 13-2
ENDOTRACHEAL TUBES: COMPLICATIONS, CAUSES, AND TREATMENT

COMPLICATIONS	CAUSES	PREVENTION/TREATMENT
Tube obstruction	Patient biting tube Tube kinking during repositioning Cuff herniation Dried secretions, blood, or lubricant Tissue from tumor Trauma Foreign body	*Prevention:* Place bite block. Sedate patient PRN. Suction PRN. Humidify inspired gases. *Treatment:* Replace tube.
Tube displacement	Movement of patient's head Movement of tube by patient's tongue Traction on tube from ventilator tubing Self-extubation	*Prevention:* Secure tube to upper lip. Restrain patients' hands. Sedate patient PRN. Ensure that only 2 inches of tube extend beyond lip. Support ventilator tubing. *Treatment:* Replace tube.
Sinusitis and nasal injury	Obstruction of the paranasal sinus drainage Pressure necrosis of nares	*Prevention:* Avoid nasal intubations. Cushion nares from tube and tape/ties. *Treatment:* Remove all tubes from nasal passages. Administer antibiotics.
Tracheoesophageal fistula	Pressure necrosis of posterior tracheal wall resulting from overinflated cuff and rigid nasogastric tube	*Prevention:* Inflate cuff with minimal amount of air necessary. Monitor cuff pressures every 8 hours. *Treatment:* Position cuff of tube distal to fistula. Place gastrostomy tube for enteral feedings. Place esophageal tube for secretion clearance proximal to fistula.
Mucosal lesions	Pressure at tube and mucosal interface	*Prevention:* Inflate cuff with minimal amount of air necessary. Monitor cuff pressures every 8 hours. Use appropriate size tube. *Treatment:* May resolve spontaneously. Perform surgical intervention.
Laryngeal or tracheal stenosis	Injury to area from end of tube or cuff, resulting in scar tissue formation and narrowing of airway	*Prevention:* Inflate cuff with minimal amount of air necessary. Monitor cuff pressures every 8 hours. Suction area above cuff frequently. *Treatment:* Perform tracheostomy. Place laryngeal stint. Perform surgical repair.
Cricoid abscess	Mucosal injury with bacterial invasion	*Prevention:* Inflate cuff with minimal amount of air necessary. Monitor cuff pressures every 8 hours. Suction area above cuff frequently. *Treatment:* Perform incision and drainage of area. Administer antibiotics.

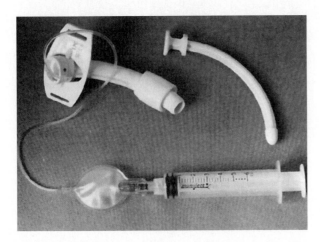

FIG. 13-2 Tracheostomy tubes. (From Perry AG, Potter PA: *Clinical nursing skills and techniques,* ed 3, St Louis, 1994, Mosby.)

eter, and less curved than the endotracheal tube; thus the resistance to air flow is less, and breathing is easier. The tracheostomy has other advantages over endotracheal intubation, including easier secretion removal, increased patient acceptance and comfort, the possibility of patients' eating and talking, and the facilitation of ventilator weaning because a tracheostomy tube is easier to breathe through when patients are off the ventilator.[7,10,14]

Tracheostomy tubes are made of plastic or metal and may be single-lumen or double-lumen tubes. Single-lumen tubes consist of two parts: (1) the tube and a built-in cuff, which is connected to a pilot balloon for inflation purposes and (2) an obturator, which is used during tube insertion. The double-lumen tubes consist of the tube with the attached cuff, the obturator, and an inner cannula that can be removed for cleaning and reinserted or, if disposable, replaced by a new sterile inner cannula. The inner cannula can quickly be removed if it becomes obstructed, making the system safer for patients with significant secretion problems. Single-lumen tubes provide a larger inside diameter for air flow than do double-lumen tubes, thus reducing air-flow resistance and allowing patients to ventilate through the tube with greater ease. Plastic tracheostomy tubes also have a 15 mm adaptor on the end (Fig. 13-2).[15]

Complications

Tracheostomy tubes are inserted via a tracheostomy procedure. Inoperative complications of a tracheotomy include hemorrhage, pneumothorax, pneumomediastinum, tracheoesophageal fistula, laryngeal nerve injury, and cardiopulmonary arrest. Immediate postoperative complications include hemorrhage, wound infection, subcutaneous emphysema, tube obstruction, and displacement of the tube (Table 13-3).[9,16] Later complications of a tracheotomy include tracheal stenosis, tracheoesophageal

fistula, tracheoinnominate artery fistula, and tracheocutaneous fistula (Table 13-3).[9,17]

Nursing Management

Patients with an endotracheal or tracheostomy tube require some additional measures to address the effects associated with tube placement on the respiratory and other body systems. **Nursing priorities in the management of patients with an artificial airway include humidification, cuff management, suctioning, and communication.** Because the tube bypasses the upper airway system, warming and humidifying of air must be performed by external means. Because the cuff of the tube can cause damage to the walls of the trachea, proper cuff management is imperative. In addition, the normal defense mechanisms are impaired and secretions may accumulate; thus suctioning may be necessary to promote secretion clearance. Because the tube does not allow air flow over the vocal cords, developing a method of communication is also very important.

Lastly, observing patients to ensure proper placement of the tube and patency of the airway is essential. **In the event of unintentional extubation or decannulation, patients' airways should be opened with the head-tilt/chin lift maneuver and maintained with an oropharyneal or nasopharyngeal airway. If patients are not breathing, they should be manually ventilated with an MRB and face mask with 100% oxygen. In the case of a tracheostomy, the stoma should be covered to prevent air from escaping through it.**

Humidification

Humidification of air is normally performed by the mucosal layer of the upper respiratory tract. When this area is bypassed, such as in endotracheal intubation and tracheostomy or use of supplemental oxygen, humidification by external means is necessary. Various humidification devices add water to inhaled gas to prevent drying and irritation of the respiratory tract, prevent undue loss of body water, and facilitate secretion removal.[18]

Bubble diffusion humidifiers are commonly used to provide moisture to inhaled gas. They may be warm or cold humidifiers. With a cold humidifier, the gas diffuses out of a stem submerged in water, breaks into small bubbles, and vaporizes. At room temperature the gas provides only approximately 50% of the humidification needed by the body. This method of humidification can therefore lead to drying and irritation of mucous membranes when used for a significant time. Diffusion humidifiers cannot humidify gas adequately at higher rates of flow, making them more suitable for low-flow oxygen delivery over short time spans. Relatively simple and reliable devices, cold humidifiers are available as disposable units, thus decreasing maintenance time and eliminating the potential for infection associated with reusable equipment. Warm humidifiers provide better humidification than cold humidifiers because they supply both heat and

TABLE 13-3
TRACHEOTOMY: COMPLICATIONS, CAUSES, AND TREATMENT

COMPLICATIONS	CAUSES	PREVENTION/TREATMENT

Hemorrhage	Vessels' opening after surgery
	Vessel erosion caused by tube
		Prevention:
		  Use appropriate size tube.
		  Treat local infection.
		  Suction gently.
		  Humidify inspired gases.
		  Position tracheal window not lower than third tracheal
		    ring.
		Treatment:
		  Pack lightly.
		  Perform surgical intervention.

Wound infection	Colonization of stoma with hospital flora	*Prevention:*
		  Perform routine stoma care.
		Treatment:
		  Remove tube, if necessary.
		  Perform aggressive wound care and debridement.
		  Administer antibiotics.

Subcutaneous emphysema	Positive pressure ventilation
	Coughing against a tight, occlusive dressing or sutured or packed wound
		Prevention:
		  Avoid suturing or packing wound closed around tube.
		Treatment:
		  Remove any sutures or packing if present.

Tube obstruction	Dried blood or secretions
	False passage into soft tissues
	Opening of cannula positioned against tracheal wall
	Foreign body
	Tissue from tumor
		Prevention:
		  Suction PRN.
		  Humidify inspired gases.
		  Use double-lumen tube.
		  Position tube so that opening does not press against tracheal wall.
		Treatment:
		  Remove/replace inner cannula.
		  Replace tube.

Displacement of tube	Patient movement
	Coughing
	Traction on ventilatory tubing
		Prevention:
		  Tie tapes to allow only one finger width between the tape and neck.
		  Suture tube in place.
		  Use tubes with adjustable neck plates for patients with short necks.
		  Support ventilator tubing.
		  Sedate patients PRN.
		  Restrain patients PRN.
		Treatment:
		  Cover stoma and manually ventilate patients via mouth
		  Replace tube

Tracheal stenosis	Injury to area from end of tube or cuff, resulting in scar tissue formation and narrowing of airway	*Prevention:*
		  Inflate cuff with minimal amount of air necessary.
		  Monitor cuff pressures every 8 hours.
		Treatment:
		  Perform surgical repair.

Tracheoesophageal fistula	Pressure necrosis of posterior tracheal wall resulting from overinflated cuff and rigid nasogastric tube	*Prevention:*
		  Inflate cuff with minimal amount of air necessary.
		  Monitor cuff pressures every 8 hours.
		Treatment:
		  Perform surgical repair.

Continued.

	T A B L E 1 3 - 3 — c o n t ' d	
	TRACHEOTOMY: COMPLICATIONS, CAUSES, AND TREATMENT	
COMPLICATIONS	**CAUSES**	**PREVENTION/TREATMENT**
Tracheoinnominate artery fistula	Direct pressure from the elbow of the cannula against the innominate artery Placement of tracheal stoma below fourth tracheal ring Downward migration of the tracheal stoma resulting from traction on tube High-lying innominate artery	*Prevention:* Position tracheal window no lower than third tracheal ring. *Treatment:* Hyperinflate cuff to control bleeding. Remove tube and replace with endotracheal tube and apply digital pressure through stoma against the sternum. Perform surgical repair.
Tracheocutaneous fistula	Failure of stoma to close after removal of tube	*Treatment:* Perform surgical repair.

moisture and break gas into smaller particles at higher flow rates. Heated cascade humidifiers are preferred for use with intubated patients because 100% humidification of inhaled gas can be ensured.[18]

Cuff management

Because the cuff of the endotracheal or tracheostomy tube is a major source of the complications associated with artificial airways, proper **cuff management** is essential. To prevent the complications associated with cuff design, only low-pressure, high-volume cuffed tubes should be used in clinical practice. Even with these tubes, cuff pressures can be high enough to cause tracheal ischemia and injury. Both cuff-inflation techniques and cuff-pressure monitoring are critical components in the care of patients with an artificial airway.[7,10]

CUFF-INFLATION TECHNIQUES. Two different cuff-inflation techniques are currently being used—the minimal leak (ML) technique and the minimal occlusion volume (MOV) technique. The ML technique consists of injecting air into the cuff until no leak is heard and then withdrawing the air until a small leak is heard on inspiration.[15] Problems with this technique include difficulty maintaining positive end-expiratory pressure (PEEP),[7] aspiration around the cuff,[7,19] and increased movement of the tube in the trachea.[19] The MOV technique consists of injecting air into the cuff until no leak is heard, withdrawing the air until a small leak is heard on inspiration, and then adding more air until no leak is heard on inspiration.[19] The problem with this technique is that it generates higher cuff pressures than the ML technique.[20] The selection of technique should be based on the needs of individual patients. If patients need a seal to provide adequate ventilation or are at high risk for aspiration, the MOV technique should be used. Otherwise, the ML technique should be used.[20]

CUFF PRESSURE MONITORING. Cuff pressures should be monitored at least every 8 hours with a mercury or an-

eroid manometer.[7,19,20] Cuff pressures should be maintained at 18 to 22 mm Hg (25 to 30 cm H_2O) because greater pressures decrease blood flow to the capillaries in the tracheal wall and lesser pressures increase the risk of aspiration. Pressures in excess of 22 mm Hg (30 cm H_2O) should be reported to physicians. In addition, cuffs should not be routinely deflated because this increases the risk of aspiration.[20] One cuff on the market, made of foam, is self-inflating and often used with tracheostomy tubes. It is deflated during tube insertion, after which the air line is opened to room air and the cuff self-inflates. It maintains a constant pressure of 20 mm Hg. Removal can be complicated if the plastic sheath covering the foam is perforated. When perforation occurs, the foam may not be deflated because the air cannot be completely aspirated.

Suctioning

Suctioning is often required to maintain a patent airway in patients with an endotracheal or tracheostomy tube. Suctioning is a sterile procedure that should be performed only when patients need it. A number of complications are associated with suctioning, including hypoxemia, atelectasis, bronchospasms, cardiac dysrhythmias, hemodynamic alterations, increased intracranial pressure,[21] and airway trauma.[7]

COMPLICATIONS. Hypoxemia can result from disconnecting the oxygen source from patients and/or removing the oxygen from patients' airways when suction is applied. Atelectasis is thought to occur when the suction catheter is larger than one half of the diameter of the ETT. Excessive negative pressure occurs when suction is applied, promoting collapse of the distal airways. Bronchospasms result when the suction catheter stimulates the airways.[21] Cardiac dysrhythmias, particularly bradycardias, are attributed to vagal stimulation.[22] Some hemodynamic alterations—such as increases in mean arterial pressure, CO, and pulmonary artery pressure—result

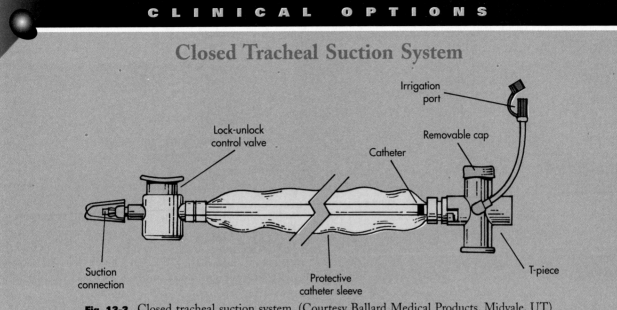

Closed Tracheal Suction System

Irrigation port

Lock-unlock control valve

Removable cap

Catheter

Suction connection

Protective catheter sleeve

T-piece

Fig. 13-3 Closed tracheal suction system. (Courtesy Ballard Medical Products, Midvale, UT)

One of the newer devices to facilitate suctioning patients on the ventilator is the closed tracheal suction system (CTSS). This device consists of a suction catheter in a plastic sleeve that attaches directly to the ventilator tubing, allowing patients to be suctioned while remaining on the ventilator. Advantages of the CTSS include the maintenance of oxygenation and PEEP during suctioning, reduction of hypoxemia-related complications, and protection of staff members from patients' secretions. The CTSS is convenient to use, requiring only one person to perform the procedure. Concerns related to the CTSS include autocontamination, inadequate removal of secretions, and increased risk of unintentional extubation resulting from the extra weight of the system on the ventilator tubing. Autocontamination is not an issue if the catheter is cleaned properly after every use and changed every 24 hours. Inadequate removal of secretions may not be a problem; further investigation is required to settle this issue.[29]

from lung hyperinflation during the procedure.[23] Airway trauma occurs with impaction of the catheter in the airways and excessive negative pressure applied to the catheter.[21]

PROTOCOL FOR LIMITING COMPLICATIONS. A number of protocols regarding suctioning have been developed. Several different practices have been found helpful in limiting the complications of suctioning. Hypoxemia can be minimized by giving patients three hyperoxygenation-hyperinflation breaths (breaths at 100% FIO_2 and 150% tidal volume) with either the ventilator or MRB before the procedure and after each pass of the suction catheter.[21,24] An alternative to this recommendation is to use hyperoxygenation alone before and after each suction pass and only add hyperinflation if patients exhibit signs of desaturation.[25] Atelectasis can be avoided by using a suction catheter with an external diameter less than one half of the internal diameter of the ETT. Using 100 mm Hg of suction or a flow rate of 15 to 20 L/min decreases the chances of hypoxemia and airway trauma.[21] Limiting the duration of each suction pass to 10 seconds and the number of passes to only those necessary also helps

minimize hypoxemia, airway trauma, cardiac dysrhythmias, and hemodynamic alterations.[21,24] The process of applying intermittent rather than continuous suction has been shown to be of no benefit.[26] In addition, the instillation of normal saline to help remove secretions has not proved beneficial and may actually contribute to lower airway colonization and development of nosocomial pneumonia.[27,28]

Communication

One of the major stressors for patients with an artificial airway is impaired **communication**. This is related to the inability to speak, insufficient explanations from staff members, inadequate understanding, fear of being unable to communicate, and difficulty with communication methods. A number of interventions can facilitate communication in patients with an endotracheal or tracheostomy tube. These include performing a complete assessment of patients' ability to communicate, teaching patients a variety of ways to communicate, and facilitating their ability to communicate by providing them with their eye glasses and hearing aids.[30]

COMMUNICATION METHODS. A number of methods are available to facilitate communication, including the use of verbal and nonverbal language and a variety of devices that assist patients undergoing long-term and short-term ventilation therapy. Nonverbal communication may include the use of sign language, hand signals, lip reading, pointing, facial expressions, or eye blinking. Simple devices available include pencil and paper; magic slates; magnetic boards with plastic letters; picture, alphabet, or symbol boards; and flash cards. More sophisticated devices include typewriters, computers, talking tracheostomy and endotracheal tubes, and external hand-held vibrators. Regardless of the method selected, patients must be taught how to use the device.[30] Patients with ETTs should be encouraged to communicate in writing because attempts at speech cause tube movement and increase tracheal injury.[7]

Extubation

An ETT is removed when no longer needed. Extubation is a simple procedure that can be accomplished at the bedside. Before removal of the tube, the airway, mouth, and pharynx are suctioned. Next, all the air in the cuff of the tube is removed, as well as any tape or ties securing the tube. Patients are then given several breaths using an MRB, and the tube is removed quickly after peak inflation.[7] A tracheostomy tube is removed in a similar fashion, except patients do not usually require any manual inflations during the procedure. Once the tube is removed, the stoma is covered with a dry dressing. The stoma should close within several days.[31] Complications of extubation include glottic edema, laryngeal dysfunction, sore throat and hoarseness, and vocal cord paralysis.[10]

Mechanical Ventilation

Indications

Mechanical ventilation is indicated in a variety of situations, including ventilatory failure, respiratory failure,[32,33] some operative procedures, and during impending collapse of other body systems.[33] Clinical indicators of mechanical ventilation include a respiratory rate of greater than 35, maximal inspiratory pressure of less than 20 mm Hg, vital capacity of less than 10 ml/kg, minute ventilation of less than 3 or greater than 20 L/min, $Paco_2$ levels of greater than 50 mm Hg with a pH of less than 7.25, or Pao_2 levels (with supplemental oxygen) of less than 55 mm Hg.[33]

Types of Ventilators

The two main types of ventilators currently available are **positive-pressure ventilators** and negative-pressure ventilators. Rarely used in the critical care environment, negative-pressure ventilators are applied externally and decrease the atmospheric pressure surrounding the tho-

rax to initiate a breath.[34] Positive-pressure ventilators use positive pressure to deliver oxygen to patients' lungs through an endotracheal or tracheostomy tube.[35] This process reduces the work of breathing and promotes gas exchange. There are three categories of positive pressure ventilators: volume-cycled, pressure-cycled, and time-cycled.[32]

Volume-cycled ventilators

Volume-cycled ventilators are designed to deliver a preset volume of gas to patients. The machine can deliver the volume of gas despite changes in pressure within patients' lungs. The major disadvantage of this type of ventilation is increased risk of barotrauma. To avoid this complication, pressure limits are programmed into the ventilator. When the pressure limit is exceeded, the ventilator will "spill" the remaining volume of gas out of the system. Volume-cycled ventilators are the most commonly used type of ventilator in critical care.[32] Fig. 13-4 depicts three volume-cycled ventilators commonly used in critical care.

Pressure-cycled ventilators

Pressure-cycled ventilators deliver gas until a preset pressure is reached. The disadvantage of this type of ventilation is that the volume of gas varies with the pressure in patients' lungs. This type of ventilation can be useful in short-term ventilation situations.

Time-cycled ventilators

Time-cycled ventilators deliver gas over a preset time interval. The advantage of this type of ventilator is that the inspiratory phase can be held constant. The disadvantage is that pressure and volume change with each breath. Rarely used for adults, this type of ventilation is employed more frequently for neonates and children.[32]

Modes of Ventilation

The term *ventilator mode* refers to the means by which the machine ventilates patients. In other words, selection of a particular mode of ventilation determines the extent to which patients participate in their own ventilatory pattern. The choice depends on patients' situations and the goals of treatment.[33] A large variety of modes are available (Table 13-4); and many of these modes may be used in conjunction with each other. Because brands of ventilators vary in their ability to perform certain functions, not all modes are available on all ventilators.

Ventilator Settings

A variety of settings on the ventilator allow the ventilator parameters to be individualized to patients' needs and the mode of ventilation selected (Box 13-2 on p. 260). In addition, each ventilator has a patient-monitoring system that allows all aspects of patients' ventilatory pat-

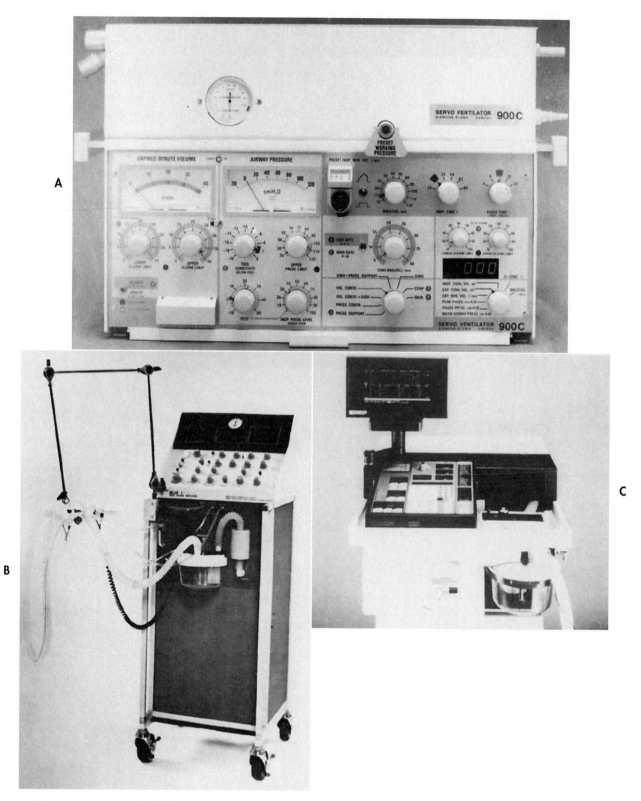

FIG. 13-4 Three types of volume-cycled ventilators. **A,** Servo 900C ventilator. **B,** Bear 1 adult volume ventilator. **C,** Puritan-Bennett 7200 microprocessor ventilator. (From Dupuis YG: *Ventilators: theory and clinical application,* ed 2, St Louis, 1992, Mosby.)

TABLE 13-4
MODES OF MECHANICAL VENTILATION

MODE OF VENTILATION	CLINICAL APPLICATION	NURSING IMPLICATIONS
Controlled ventilation (CV)—delivers gas at preset rate and tidal volume, regardless of patients' inspiratory efforts[32,35,36]	CV is used as the primary ventilatory mode in patients who are apneic.[32,36]	CV is used in patients unable to initiate a breath.[32] Spontaneously breathing patients must be sedated and/or paralyzed.[35]
Assist-Control ventilation (A/C)—delivers gas at preset tidal volume in response to patients' inspiratory efforts and will initiate breath if patient fails to do so within preset time[32,35,36]	A/C is used as primary mode of ventilation in spontaneously breathing patients with weak respiratory muscles.[32]	Hyperventilation can occur in patients with increased respiratory rates.[32,35] Sedation may be necessary to limit the number of spontaneous breaths.[32]
Synchronous intermittent mandatory ventilation (SIMV)—delivers gas at preset tidal volume and rate while allowing patients to breathe spontaneously; ventilator breaths are synchronized to patients' respiratory effort[32,35,36]	SIMV is used both as primary mode of ventilation in a wide variety of clinical situations and as a weaning mode.[32,36]	SIMV may increase the work of breathing and promote respiratory muscle fatigue.[32,35]
Positive end-expiratory pressure (PEEP)—positive pressure applied during ventilator breaths Constant positive airway pressure (CPAP)—positive pressure applied during spontaneous breaths[36]	PEEP and CPAP are used in patients with hypoxemia refractory to oxygen therapy; they increase functional residual capacity and improve oxygenation by opening collapsed alveoli and preventing them from collapsing at end expiration.[36] PEEP is used with CV, A/C, or SIMV. CPAP is used as primary mode of ventilation.	Side effects include decreased cardiac output (CO), barotrauma, and increased intracranial pressure.[33,36]
Pressure support ventilation (PSV)—preset positive pressure used to augment patients' inspiratory efforts; patient controls rate, inspiratory flow, and tidal volume[36-39]	PSV is used as the primary mode of ventilation in patients with stable respiratory drive, with SIMV to support spontaneous breaths, and as a weaning mode in patients who are difficult to wean.[36-39]	Advantages include increased patient comfort, decreased work of breathing and respiratory muscle fatigue, and promotion of respiratory muscle conditioning.[36-39]
Independent lung ventilation (ILV)—ventilation of each lung separately[36,40]	ILV is used in patients with unilateral lung disease, bronchopleural fistulas, and bilateral asymmetric lung disease.[40]	ILV requires double-lumen endotracheal tube, two ventilators,[35,40] sedation, and/or pharmacologic paralysis.[35]
High-Frequency ventilation (HFV)—delivers a small volume of gas at a rapid rate Three different types: High-Frequency positive-pressure ventilation (HFPPV)—delivers 60-100 breaths/min High-Frequency jet ventilation (HFJV)—delivers 100-600 cycles/min High-Frequency oscillation (HFO)—delivers 900-3000 cycles/min[39]	HFV is used in situations in which conventional mechanical ventilation compromises hemodynamic stability, with bronchopleural fistulas, during short-term procedures, and with diseases that create a risk of barotrauma.[39]	Patients may need to be sedated. Inadequate humidification can compromise airway patency. Assessment of breath sounds is difficult.[38,39]
Mandatory minute volume (MMV)—allows patients to breathe spontaneously while ensuring delivery of constant minute volume if patients' minute volume falls below preset level[36]	MMV is used as a weaning mode and with PSV as a backup in patients with unstable respiratory drives.[36]	MMV does not evaluate respiratory pattern. MMV may be achieved with rapid, shallow breathing.[36]

TABLE 1 3 - 4 — c o n t ' d

MODES OF MECHANICAL VENTILATION

MODE OF VENTILATION	CLINICAL APPLICATION	NURSING IMPLICATIONS
Inverse ratio ventilation (IRV)—ventilation in which the proportion of inspiratory time to expiratory time is ≥1:1; can be initiated using pressure-controlled breaths (PC-IRV) or volume-controlled breaths (VC– IVR)[36,41]	IRV is used in patients with hypoxemia refractory to PEEP; the longer inspiratory time increases functional residual capacity and improves oxygenation by opening collapsed alveoli, and the shorter expiratory time induces intrinsic PEEP (auto-PEEP) that prevents alveoli from recollapsing.[36,41]	IRV requires sedation and/or pharmacologic paralysis because of discomfort. Increased intrathoracic pressure can result in excessive air trapping and decreased cardiac output (CO).[31,36]
Nasal positive-pressure ventilation (NPPV)—positive pressure delivered via a nasal mask with a volume ventilator[39,42]	NNPPV is used at night for patients with respiratory muscle weakness or nighttime hypoventilation.[39,42]	Mask should fit well and have soft padding. Equipment should be positioned to facilitate sleep.[39,42]

tern to be assessed, monitored, and displayed. These monitoring capabilities include exhaled minute volume, exhaled tidal volume, total respiratory rate, peak pressure, plateau pressure, PEEP, mean airway pressure, spontaneous minute volume, spontaneous respiratory rate, circuit temperature, FIo_2, inspired tidal volume, pressure waveform, flow waveform, auto-PEEP, and respiratory mechanics. Monitoring capabilities vary slightly from one brand of ventilator to another.[43]

Complications

Mechanical ventilation often saves lives, but similar to other interventions, it is not without complications. Some complications are preventable, whereas others can be minimized but not eradicated. Physiologic complications associated with mechanical ventilation include decreased CO, unintentional acute respiratory alkalosis, increased intracranial pressure, gastric distention, and barotrauma.[44]

Decreased CO

Positive-pressure ventilation increases intrathoracic pressure, which decreases venous return to the right side of the heart. Impaired venous return decreases preload, which results in a decrease in CO. Decreased CO is thought to further impair hepatic and renal function.[44]

Unintentional respiratory alkalosis

Unintentional respiratory alkalosis may occur secondary to alveolar hyperventilation as a result of pain, anxiety, dyspnea, agitation, or inappropriate ventilator settings. Respiratory alkalosis can impair cerebral perfusion and predispose patients to the development of cardiac dysrhythmias.[44]

Increased intracranial pressure

Positive-pressure ventilation impairs cerebral venous return. Thus in patients with impaired autoregulation, positive-pressure ventilation can result in increased intracranial pressure.[44]

Gastric distention

Gastric distention occurs when air leaks around the endotracheal or tracheostomy tube cuff and overcomes the resistance of the lower esophageal sphincter. This problem can be prevented by inserting a nasogastric tube and ensuring appropriate cuff inflation.[44]

Barotrauma

Barotrauma occurs in mechanically ventilated patients as a result of alveolar overdistention. Usually occurring with any ventilatory mode using high tidal volumes and/or high pressures, barotrauma causes alveolar rupture and leakage of the air, fluid, and protein into the pulmonary interstitial space. Once in the space, the air travels out through the hilum and into the mediastinum, pleural space, subcutaneous tissues, pericardium, peritoneum, and retroperitoneum. This occurrence can result in a number of disorders, the most lethal of which is a pneumothorax. The fluid and protein contribute to the development of pulmonary edema.[45]

Weaning

Weaning should begin only after the original process requiring ventilator support has been corrected and patient stability achieved. Other factors to consider when weaning are length of time on ventilator, sleep deprivation, nutritional status, and psychologic readiness. Three areas that should be reviewed to determine readiness to wean are patients' level of oxygenation, CO_2 elimination, and

BOX 13-2

VENTILATOR SETTINGS

RESPIRATORY RATE (F)

Number of breaths the ventilator will deliver per minute.

TIDAL VOLUME (V_T)

Volume delivered to patients during a normal ventilator breath. Usual volume selected is 10 to 15 ml/kg.

OXYGEN CONCENTRATION (FIO_2)

Selects delivery of oxygen between 21% and 100%.

I:E RATIO

Ratio of inspiratory time to expiratory time. Determined by adjusting the inspiratory flow rate. Usually 1:2, unless inverse ratio ventilation is in use.

INSPIRATORY FLOW RATE (PEAK FLOW)

Flow of tidal volume delivery.

SENSITIVITY

Control that adjusts the ventilatory response to patients' respiratory effort. It determines the amount of effort patients must generate to initiate a breath.

SIGHS

Allows periodic selection of a larger-than-normal tidal volume. Usual volume is $1\frac{1}{2}$ to 2 times tidal volume, and usual rate is 4 to 5 times an hour.

PRESSURE LIMITS

Adjustable setting to regulate the maximal pressure the machine can generate to deliver the tidal volume. Once the pressure limit is reached, the ventilator will spill the undelivered volume into the atmosphere to protect patients from barotrauma. The limit is usually set at 10 to 20 cm H_2O above the normal peak pressure.

BOX 13-3

WEANING CRITERIA

FIO_2 of <50%
PEEP of <5 cm H_2O
Respiratory rate <30 breaths/min
Minute ventilation <10 L/min
Static compliance >25-30 cm H_2O
Maximal inspiratory pressure < −20 cm H_2O
Vital capacity >10-15 ml/kg
Spontaneous tidal volume >4-5 ml/kg
Maximal voluntary ventilation > twice minute ventilation
PaO_2 >60 mm Hg on an FIO_2 of <50%
Shunt <15%-20%
Alveolar-arterial oxygen tension difference <350 torr on an FIO_2 of 100%
$PaCO_2$ within normal range

BOX 13-4

WEANING INTOLERANCE INDICATORS

Dysrhythmias
Increase or decrease in heart rate of >20 beats/min
Increase or decrease in blood pressure of >20 mm Hg
Increase in respiratory rate of >10 above baseline
Tidal volumes of <250 ml
Increase in minute ventilation of >5 L/min
Diaphoresis
Dyspnea
Shortness of breath
Restlessness
Decrease in level of consciousness
SpO_2 <90%
PaO_2 <60 mm Hg
Increase in $PaCO_2$ with a decrease in pH of <7.35

mechanical efficiency (Box 13-3).[45,46] Once readiness to wean has been established, patients should be prepared for the process. Patients should be positioned upright to facilitate breathing and suctioned to ensure airway patency. In addition, nurses should explain the process and offer reassurance. During the weaning process, patients should be continuously monitored for signs of weaning intolerance (Box 13-4).[45]

Methods

A number of methods can be used to wean patients from the ventilator. The method selected depends on patients' condition, their pulmonary status, and the length of time they have been on the ventilator. The four main methods for weaning are T-tube, constant positive airway pressure (CPAP), intermittent mandatory ventilation (IMV), and pressure support ventilation (PSV).[45]

T-TUBE. T-tube weaning consists of removing patients from the ventilator and having them breathe spontaneously on a T-tube (T-piece). After a predetermined time, patients are placed back on the ventilator, the goal being to progressively increase the time spent off the ventilator. During the weaning process patients should be closely observed for respiratory muscle fatigue.[45,46] Extubation is considered once patients are able to maintain adequate spontaneous respirations for at least 2 hours.[46]

CPAP. CPAP weaning is very similar to T-tube weaning, except patients are placed on the CPAP mode instead of a T-tube.[45]

IMV. IMV weaning consists of placing the ventilator in the SIMV mode and slowly decreasing the rate until

TABLE 13-5
TROUBLESHOOTING THE VENTILATOR

ALARM	CAUSES	NURSING IMPLICATIONS
Low exhaled volume	Cuff leak	Evaluate patency of cuff. Reinflate if necessary. If the cuff is ruptured, the tube will need to be replaced.
	Disruption in ventilatory tubing	Evaluate ventilator tubing and tighten or replace as necessary.
High pressure	Patients disconnected from ventilator	Reconnect to ventilator.
	Secretions in airway	Suction patients.
	Patients biting tube	Insert bite block.
	Tube kinked in airway	Reposition patients' head and neck.
	Cuff herniation	Deflate and reinflate cuff.
	Increased airway resistance/decreased lung compliance (e.g., caused by bronchospasm, pneumothorax, pulmonary edema)	Auscultate breath sounds. Notify physician if problem suspected. Evaluate static and dynamic compliance. Evaluate placement of tube on chest x-ray film (it may be touching the carina). Stabilize tube to prevent movement in airway.
	Patients coughing and/or fighting the machine	Explain all procedures to patients in calm, reassuring manner. Sedate patients as necessary.
Inoperative ventilator	Ventilator malfunction	Remove patients from ventilator, and ventilate manually with MRB. Call respiratory therapy.
Low oxygen pressure	Oxygen malfunction	Remove patients from ventilator, and ventilate manually with MRB. Call respiratory therapy.

zero (or close) is reached. The rate is usually decreased one to three breaths at a time, and an ABG analysis is usually obtained 30 minutes afterward. This method allows patients gradually to increase their spontaneous rate until they no longer need support.[45,46]

PSV. PSV weaning consists of placing patients on the pressure support mode and setting the pressure support at a level that facilitates a spontaneous tidal volume of 10 to 12 ml/kg. PSV augments patients' spontaneous breaths with a positive-pressure "boost" during inspiration. During the weaning process the level of pressure support is gradually decreased in increments of 3 to 6 cm H_2O until a level of 5 cm H_2O is achieved. If patients are able to maintain adequate spontaneous respirations at this level, extubation is considered.[45,46] PSV can also be used with CPAP and IMV weaning to help overcome the resistance in the ventilator system.[37]

Nursing Management

Nursing priorities for patients on a ventilator include regular monitoring for both patient-related and ventilator-related complications. Interventions should include a routine total assessment, with particular em-phasis on the pulmonary system, placement of the endotracheal tube, and observation for subcutaneous emphysema and synchrony with the ventilator. Assessment of the ventilator should include a review of all the ventilator settings and alarms.

Bedside evaluation of vital capacity, minute ventilation, arterial blood gas values, and other pulmonary function tests may be warranted, according to patients' condition. The use of pulse oximetry can facilitate continuous, noninvasive assessment of oxygenation.[47] Static and dynamic compliance should also be monitored to assess for changes in lung compliance (see Appendix B).

Some additional measures are required to maintain a trouble-free ventilator system. These include maintaining a functional MRB connected to oxygen at the bedside, ensuring that the ventilator tubing is free of water, positioning the ventilator tubing to avoid kinking, maintaining the patency of ventilator tubing and connections, changing ventilator tubing according to hospital policy, and monitoring the temperature of the inspired air. In addition, a clear understanding of alarms and their related problems is important (Table 13-5).[48] **If the ventilator malfunctions, patients should be removed from the ventilator and ventilated manually with an MRB.**

MEDICATION	DOSAGE	ACTIONS	SPECIAL CONSIDERATIONS
NEUROMUSCULAR BLOCKING AGENTS (NMBA)		Used to paralyze patients to decrease oxygen demand and avoid ventilator asynchrony.	• Administer sedative and analgesic agents concurrently because NMBAs have no sedative or analgesic properties.
Atracurium (Tracrium)	Loading dose of 0.4-0.5 mg/kg IV followed by 5.0-9.0 µg/kg/min IV infusion		
Vecuronium (Norcuron)	Loading dose of 0.08-0.1 mg/kg IV followed by 1.0 µg/kg/min IV infusion		• Evaluate the level of paralysis q4h using a peripheral nerve stimulator.
Pancuronium (Pavulon)	Loading dose of 0.06-0.1 mg/kg IV followed by 1.0 µg/kg/min IV infusion		• Monitor patients for the immobility complications. • Protect patients from the environment because they are unable to do so. • Prolonged muscle paralysis may occur following discontinuation of the paralysis.
BRONCHODILATORS			
Beta-agonists		Used to relax bronchial smooth muscle and dilate airways and prevent bronchospasms.	• May cause nervousness, tremors, insomnia, tachycardia, dysrhythmias, hypertension, and angina.
Albuterol (Proventil)	Nebulizer: 0.5 ml q4-6h Metered-dose inhaler (MDI): 2 puffs q4-6h		• Treatment is usually considered effective when breath sounds improve and dyspnea is lessened.
Bitolterol (Tornalate)	MDI: 2-3 puffs q6h		
Isoetharine (1%) (Bronkosol)	Nebulizer: 0.25-1 ml q3-6h		• Efficiency of administration is significantly decreased when administered through an endotracheal tube.
Metaproterenol (5%) (Alupent)	Nebulizer: 0.2-0.3 ml q3-6h MDI: 2-3 puffs q3-6h		
Terbutaline (Brethine)	MDI: 1-2 puffs q4-6h		• Racemic epinephrine is the drug of choice in the treatment of acute bronchospasm or laryngospasm.
Racemic epinephrine	Nebulizer: 0.3-1 ml q2-4h		
Vagal blockers		Used to block the constriction of the bronchial smooth muscles and reduce mucus production.	• Relatively few adverse effects because systemic absorption is poor.
Ipratropium (0.025%) (Atrovert)	Nebulizer: 1-2 ml q4-6h MDI: 2-4 puffs q4-6h		
Xanthines		Used to dilate bronchial smooth muscles.	• Administer loading dose over 30 minutes.
Theophylline	Loading dose of 5 mg/kg followed by 0.5-0.7 mg/kg/h IV infusion		• Monitor serum blood levels; therapeutic level is 10-20 µg/dl.
Aminophylline	Loading dose of 6 mg/kg followed by 0.5-0.7 mg/kg/h IV infusion		• Should be administered with caution in patients with cardiac, renal, or hepatic disease. • Sign of toxicity include CNS excitation, seizures, confusion, irritability, hyperglycemia, headache, nausea, hypotension, and dysrhythmias.

Pulse Oximetry

Pulse oximetry is a noninvasive method for monitoring oxygen saturation (SpO_2) and is indicated whenever patients' oxygenation status requires continuous observation. It consists of a microprocessor and a probe that attaches to patients (finger, ear, toe, or nose). The probe consists of two light-emitting diodes and a photodetector. The diodes transmit red and infrared light wavelengths through the pulsating vascular bed to the photodetector on the other side. The photodetector converts the light signals into an electric signal, which is then sent to a microprocessor that converts it to a digital reading. The pulse oximeter is considered very accurate ($+/-4\%$ to 5% at a saturation greater than 70%).[49]

Nursing Management

Nursing priorities are directed toward minimizing the physiologic and technical factors that can limit the monitoring system.

Physiologic limitations

Physiologic limitations include elevated levels of abnormal hemoglobins, presence of vascular dyes, and poor tissue perfusion. The pulse oximeter cannot differentiate between normal and abnormal hemoglobin. Elevated levels of abnormal hemoglobin falsely elevate the SpO_2. Vascular dyes, such as methylene blue, indigo carmine, indocyanine green, and fluorescein also interfere with pulse oximetry and can lead to falsely low readings. Poor tissue perfusion to the area with the probe leads to loss of pulsatile flow and signal failure.[49]

Technical limitations

Technical limitations include bright lights, excessive motion, and incorrect placement of the probe. Bright lights may interfere with the photodetector and cause inaccurate results. The probe should be covered to limit optical interference. Excessive motion can mimic arterial pulsations and lead to false readings. Incorrect placement of the probe can lead to inaccurate results because part of the light can reach the photodetector without having passed through blood (optical shunting). Interventions to limit these problems include using the proper probe in the appropriate spot (e.g., not using a finger probe on the ear), applying the probe according to the directions, and ensuring that the area being monitored has adequate perfusion.[49]

Pharmacology

There are a number of pharmacologic agents used in the care of patients with pulmonary disorders. Table 13-6 reviews the various agents used and any special considerations necessary for administering them.[50-52]

References

1. Shapiro BA, Peruzzi WT, Kozelowski-Templin R: *Clinical application of blood gases*, St Louis, ed 5, 1994, Mosby.
2. Levitzky MG, Cairo JM, Hall SM: *Introduction to respiratory care*, Philadelphia, 1990, WB Saunders.
3. Thalken FR: *Medical gas therapy*. In Scanlon CL, Spearman CB, Sheldon RL, editors: *Egan's fundamentals of respiratory care*, ed 6, St Louis, 1994, Mosby.
4. Brown LH: Pulmonary oxygen toxicity, *Focus Crit Care* 17(1):68, 1990.
5. Nelson DM: Interventions related to respiratory care, *Nurs Clin North Am* 27:301, 1992.
6. Albarran-Solelo R and others: *Textbook of advanced cardiac life support*, ed 3, Dallas, 1994, American Heart Association.
7. Stauffer JL: Medical management of the airway, *Clin Chest Med* 12:449, 1991.
8. Victor LD: *Endotracheal intubation*. In Victor LD, editor: *Manual of critical care procedures*, Rockville, Md, 1989, Aspen.
9. Einarsson O, Rochester CL, Rosenbaum S: Airway management in respiratory emergencies, *Clin Chest Med* 15:13, 1994.
10. Stone DJ, Bogdonoff DL: Airway considerations in the management of patients requiring long-term endotracheal intubation, *Anesth Anal* 74:276, 1992.
11. Colice GL: Technical standards for tracheal tubes, *Clin Chest Med* 12:433, 1991.
12. Zarshenas Z, Sparschu RA: Catheter placement and misplacement, *Crit Care Clin* 10:417, 1994.
13. McCulloch TM, Bishop MJ: Complications of translaryngeal intubation, *Clin Chest Med* 12:507, 1991.
14. Wenig BL, Applebaum EL: Indications for and techniques of tracheotomy, *Clin Chest Med* 12:545, 1991.
15. Weilitz PB, Dettenmeier PA: Back to basics: test your knowledge of tracheostomy tubes, *Am J Nurs* 94:46, 1994.
16. Myers EN, Carrau RL: Early complications of tracheotomy: incidence and management, *Clin Chest Med* 12:589, 1991.
17. Wood DE, Mathisen DJ: Late complications of tracheotomy, *Clin Chest Med* 12:597, 1991.
18. Scanlan CL: *Humidity and aerosol therapy*. In Scanlan CL, Spearman CB, Sheldon RL, editors: *Egan's fundamentals of respiratory care*, ed 6, St Louis, 1994, Mosby.
19. Goodnough SKC: Reducing tracheal injury and aspiration, *Dimens Crit Care Nurs* 7:324, 1988.
20. Tyler DO, Clark AP, Ogburn-Russell L: Developing a standard for endotracheal tube cuff care, *Dimens Crit Care Nurs* 10:54, 1991.
21. Stone KS: Endotracheal suctioning in the critically ill, *Crit Care Nurs Curr* 7:5, 1989.
22. Gunderson LP, Stone KS, Hamlin RL: Endotracheal-suctioning-induced heart rate alterations, *Nurs Res* 40:139, 1991.
23. Stone KS and others: The effect of lung hyperinflation and endotracheal suctioning on cardiopulmonary hemodynamics, *Nurs Res* 40:76, 1991.
24. Stone KS: Ventilator versus manual resuscitation bag as the method of delivering hyperoxygenation before endotracheal suctioning, *AACN Clin Iss Crit Care Nurs* 1:289, 1990.
25. Maninelli-Van Atta J, Beck SL: Preventing hypoxemia and hemodynamic compromise related to endotracheal suctioning, *Am J Crit Care* 1:62, 1992.
26. Czarnik RE and others: Deferential effects of continuous versus intermittent suction on tracheal tissue, *Heart Lung* 20:144, 1991.
27. Gray JE, MacIntyre NR, Kronenberger WG: The effects of bolus normal saline instillation in conjunction with endotracheal suctioning, *Respir Care* 25:785, 1990.

28. Hagler DA, Traver GA: Endotracheal saline and suction catheters: sources of lower airway contamination, *Am J Crit Care* 3:444, 1994.

29. Johnson KL and others: Closed versus open endotracheal suctioning: costs and physiologic consequences, *Crit Care Med* 22:658, 1994.

30. Williams ML: An algorithm for selecting a communication technique with intubated patients, *Dimens Crit Care Nurs* 11:222, 1992.

31. Godwin JE, Heffner JE: Special critical care considerations in tracheostomy management, *Clin Chest Med* 12:573, 1991.

32. Vasbinder-Dillon D: Understanding mechanical ventilation, *Crit Care Nurs* 8(7):42, 1988.

33. Grum CM, Morganroth ML: Initiating mechanical ventilation, *Intensive Care Med* 3:6, 1988.

34. Levine S, Levy S, Henson D: Negative-pressure ventilation, *Crit Care Clin* 6:505, 1990.

35. Luce JM: What to consider when choosing a positive-pressure ventilation mode, *J Crit Ill* 6:339, 1991.

36. Sassoon CSH, Mahutte K, and Light RW: Ventilatory modes: old and new, *Crit Care Clin* 6:605, 1990.

37. Pierce JD and others: Pressure support ventilation: reducing the work of breathing during weaning, *Dimens Crit Care Nurs,* 12:283, 1993.

38. St John RE, Lefrak SS: Alternate modes of mechanical ventilation, *AACN Clin Iss Crit Care Nurs* 1:248, 1990.

39. Burns SM: Advances in ventilatory therapy, *Focus Crit Care* 17:227, 1990.

40. Simons B, Borg U: Independent lung ventilation, *Crit Care Rep* 1:398, 1990.

41. Marcy TW, Marini JJ: Inverse ratio ventilation in ARDS: rationale and implementation, *Chest* 100:494, 1991.

42. Spessert CK, Weilitz PB, Goodenberger DM: A protocol for initiation of nasal positive pressure ventilation, *Am J Crit Care* 2:54, 1993.

43. Kacmarek RM, Meklaus GJ: The new generation of mechanical ventilators, *Crit Care Clin* 6:551, 1990.

44. Pierson DJ: Complications associated with mechanical ventilation, *Crit Care Clin* 6:711, 1990.

45. Geisman LK: Advances in weaning from mechanical ventilation, *Crit Care Clin North Am* 1:697, 1989.

46. Tobin MJ, Yang K: Weaning from mechanical ventilation, *Crit Care Clin* 6:725, 1990.

47. Hess D: Noninvasive respiratory monitoring during ventilatory support, *Crit Care Clin North Am* 3:565, 1991.

48. Grossbach I: Troubleshooting ventilator- and patient-related problems/Part 1, *Crit Care Nurs* 6:58, 1986.

49. Rueden KT: Noninvasive assessment of gas exchange in the critically ill patient, *AACN Clin Iss Crit Care Nurs* 1:239, 1990.

50. Susla GM: Neuromuscular blocking agents in critical care, *Crit Care Nurs Clin North Am* 5:297, 1993.

51. Dettenmeier PA: *Pulmonary nursing care,* St Louis, 1992, Mosby.

52. Reading PM, St. John RE: Aerosolized therapy for ventilator-assisted patients, *Crit Care Nurs Clin North Am* 5:271, 1993.

Neurologic Alterations

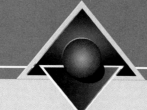

14

Neurologic Assessment and Diagnostic Procedures

KATHLEEN A. MENDEZ

Assessment of patients with neurologic dysfunction is the beginning point in the nursing process and forms the basis for nursing diagnosis. The following chapter focuses on priority clinical assessments and diagnostic procedures currently used in the critical care setting.

History

All neurologic assessments require a comprehensive history of events preceding hospitalization. An adequate neurologic history includes information about clinical manifestations, associated complaints, precipitating factors, progression, and familial occurrences. If patients are incapable of providing this information, family members or significant others should be contacted as soon as possible. When patients are not the source of the history, someone who was in daily contact with them should be selected. Frequently, the neurologic history provides valuable information that directs caregivers to focus on certain aspects of patients' clinical assessment.

Physical Examination

Five major components make up the neurologic examination of critically ill patients. **These assessment priorities are evaluation of level of consciousness, motor function, pupils and eyes, respiratory patterns, and vital signs.** Until all five components have been assessed, the neurologic examination is incomplete.

Level of Consciousness

Assessment of the level of consciousness is the most important aspect of the neurologic examination. In most situations, patients' level of consciousness deteriorates before any other neurologic changes are noted. These deteriorations are often subtle and must be monitored carefully. The following categories are often used to describe patients' level of consciousness:[1]

- Alert—Patients respond immediately to minimal external stimuli.
- Lethargic—State of drowsiness or inaction in which patients need an increased stimulus to be awakened.
- Obtunded—A duller indifference to external stimuli exists, and response is minimally maintained.
- Stuporous—Patients can be aroused only by vigorous and continuous external stimuli.
- Comatose—Vigorous stimulation fails to produce any voluntary neural response.

Assessment of level of consciousness should focus on two priorities: (1) evaluation of arousal or alertness and (2) appraisal of content of consciousness or awareness.[2]

Arousal

Evaluation of **arousal** is an assessment of the reticular activating system and its connection with the thalamus and cerebral cortex. Arousal is the lowest level of consciousness, and observation centers on patients' ability to respond to verbal or noxious stimuli in an appropriate manner.[1] To stimulate patients, nurses should begin with verbal stimuli in a normal tone. If patients do not respond, nurses should increase stimulation by shouting at patients. If patients still do not respond, nurses should increase the stimulation again by shaking patients. Noxious stimuli should follow if previous attempts to arouse the patient were unsuccessful.

NOXIOUS STIMULI. There are two types of noxious stimuli—central and peripheral. Central stimulation stimulates the brain and is used to assess arousal. Peripheral stimulation is used to assess motor function and will be discussed later. Acceptable methods of central stimulation are as follows:[2]

1. Trapezius pinch—performed by squeezing the trapezius muscle between the thumb and first two fingers.
2. Sternal rub—performed be applying firm pressure to the sternum with the knuckles, using a rubbing motion. If this technique is used repeatedly, the sternum can become bruised.
3. Supraorbital pressure—performed by pressing the notch in the orbital rim with the fingertips. Patients with head injuries, frontal craniotomies, or facial surgery should not be evaluated with this method because of the possibility of an underlying fractured or unstable cranium.

Awareness

Appraisal of content of consciousness or **awareness** is a higher-level function concerned with patients' orientation to person, place, and time. Assessment of content of consciousness requires patients to give appropriate answers to a variety of questions. Changes in patients' answers that indicate increasing degrees of confusion and disorientation may be the first sign of neurologic deterioration.[3]

GLASGOW COMA SCALE. The most widely recognized tool for assessing level of consciousness is the **Glasgow Coma Scale** (GCS). This scored scale is based on evaluation of three categories: eye opening, verbal response, and best motor response (Table 14-1). The best possible score on the GCS is 15, and the lowest score is 3. Generally a score of 7 or less on the GCS indicates coma. Several points should be kept in mind when the GCS is used for serial assessment. It provides data about level of consciousness only and should never be considered a complete neurologic assessment. It is not a sensitive tool for evaluation of an altered sensorium, nor does it account for possible aphasia. The GCS is also a poor indicator of lateralization (decreasing motor response on one side or changes in pupillary reaction) of neurologic

Motor Function

Assessment of motor function should focus on three priorities: (1) observation of involuntary motor movements, (2) evaluation of muscle tone, and (3) estimation of muscle strength. Nurses should assess each extremity individually and then compare one side to another. Lateralizing signs are neurologic findings that occur only on one side of the body, such as unilateral deterioration in **motor movements.**[5]

Involuntary motor movement

Initially the muscles should be inspected for size and shape and presence of atrophy. During this inspection the muscles should also be observed for the presence of involuntary movements indicating neurologic dysfunction.[3,5] Table 14-2 lists a variety of abnormal motor movements and their causes.

Muscle tone

Muscle tone is assessed by evaluating the opposition to passive movement. Patients are instructed to relax the extremity while nurses perform a passive range of motion test and evaluate the degree of resistance. Muscle tone is appraised for signs of hypotonia, flaccidity, hypertonia, spasticity, or rigidity.[5]

Muscle strength

Muscle strength is assessed by having patients perform a number of movements against resistance. The strength of the movement is then graded using a six point scale:

- ◆ 0—no muscular contraction
- ◆ 1—trace of contraction
- ◆ 2—active movement with gravity eliminated
- ◆ 3—active movement against gravity
- ◆ 4—active movement with some resistance
- ◆ 5—active movement with full resistance

The upper extremities may be tested by asking patients to grasp, squeeze, and release nurses' index and middle fingers. If weakness or asymmetry is suspected, patients may be instructed to extend both arms with the palms turned upward and hold that position with their eyes closed. If patients have a weaker arm, it will drift downward and pronate. The lower extremities may be tested by asking patients to push and pull their feet against resistance.[5]

NOXIOUS STIMULI. If patients are incapable of comprehending and following a simple command, noxious stimuli is required to determine motor responses. The stimuli is applied to each extremity to allow evaluation of the individual extremity function. Peripheral stimulation is used to assess motor function. Acceptable methods of peripheral stimulation are as follows:[2]

1. Nailbed pressure—performed by applying firm pressure, using an object such as a pen, to the nailbed. Patients' movement must not be inter-

---

TABLE 14-1
GLASGOW COMA SCALE

CATEGORY	SCORE	RESPONSE
Eye opening	4	Spontaneous—eyes open spontaneously without stimulation
	3	To speech—eyes open with verbal stimulation but not necessarily to command
	2	To pain—eyes open with noxious stimuli
	1	None—no eye opening regardless of stimulation
Verbal response	5	Oriented—accurate information about person, place, time, reason for hospitalization, and personal data
	4	Confused—answers not appropriate to question, but use of language is correct
	3	Inappropriate words—disorganized, random speech, no sustained conversation
	2	Incomprehensible sounds—moans, groans, and incomprehensible mumbles
	1	None—no verbalization despite stimulation
Best motor response	6	Obeys commands—performs simple tasks on command; able to repeat performance
	5	Localizes to pain—organized attempt to localize and remove painful stimuli
	4	Withdraws from pain—withdraws extremity from source of painful stimuli
	3	Abnormal flexion—decorticate posturing spontaneously or in response to noxious stimuli
	2	Extension—decerebrate posturing spontaneously or in response to noxious stimuli
	1	None—no response to noxious stimuli; flaccid

deterioration.[4] Whatever assessment tool is chosen to measure level of consciousness, the goal is to identify subtle changes in consciousness responses. Communication of small signs of deteriorating consciousness may allow early intervention and thus prevent neurologic disaster.

	T A B L E 1 4 - 2	
	TYPES OF HYPERKINESIAS AND DYSKINESIAS	
TYPE	**CHARACTERISTICS**	**CAUSE**
Fasciculations	Rapid muscle contractions involving several motor units; may involve hands and feet, tongue, or entire body	Most cases are evidence of damage to either anterior horn cells or the motor axon as it travels to the motor unit
	Occasionally related to a rare familial muscle disorder called *benign fasciculations*	
Clonus	Repetitive, sustained stretch reflex from over-excitement of the muscle	Usually occurs in a severely spastic limb but may occur in any muscle
Myoclonus	Series of shock-like contractions that cause throwing movements of a limb	Associated with an irritable nervous system and spontaneous electrical discharge of neurons
	Usually reappear at random but frequently triggered by sudden startling.	Structures associated with myoclonus include the cerebral cortex, cerebellum, reticular formation, and spinal cord
	Does not appear during sleep	
Chorea	Brief, irregular, symmetric movements present at rest but accentuated by movement	Associated with excess concentration of or a supersensitivity to dopamine within the synapses of the basal ganglia
	Tend to flow from one muscle to another in various parts of the body	
Ballism	Gross form of chorea consisting of continuous, irregular contraction of muscles; complex movement with violent flinging of extremities	Results from injury to subthalamus nucleus (one of the nuclei that make up the basal ganglia)
	Movements are augmented by physical effort or excitement and diminished by rest	Thought to be due to reduced inhibitory influence in the nucleus
	Ballism is seen most commonly on one side of the body, a condition termed *hemiballism*	Hemiballism results from injury to the contralateral subthalamic nucleus
	Decreased dopamine concentration may reduce or eliminate ballism	
Athetosis	Slower, more fluid-like movements than chorea	Occurs most commonly as a result of injury to the basal ganglia in infancy that allows the release of primitive reflex movements
	Typically consists of flexion and extension of fingers, wrist, and elbows, abduction and adduction of the arm	Exact pathophysiologic mechanism is not known
Choreathetosis	Involves both chorea and athetosis	Precise pathophysiologic mechanism is not known
Tics	Rapid, occasionally sustained movements that appear in a sequential pattern; the pattern is repeated at the next occurrence of the tic	Associated with excess dopamine, but structures involved are not conclusively known
	Movements may be simple or complex	
	Typically preceded by a compulsive urge to carry out the pattern	
Spasm	A strong muscle contraction	Originates locally from muscle or from some level of the nervous system
Hiccup	A spasm	Produced by irritation of the sensory nerves in the stomach or diaphragm or by injuries causing pressure on the myelencephalon

From McCance KL, Huether SE: *Pathophysiology: the biological basis for disease in adults and children,* ed 2, St Louis, 1984, Mosby.

rupted while nurses are applying the nailbed pressure.

2. Pinching of the inner aspect of the arm or leg—performed by firmly pinching a small portion of patients' tissue on the sensitive inner aspect of the arm or leg. Although this form of noxious stimuli is the most apt to cause bruising, it is also the most sensitive for eliciting a movement response.

ABNORMAL MOTOR RESPONSES. Motor responses elicited by noxious stimuli are interpreted differently than those elicited by voluntary demonstration. These responses may be classified in four categories:[3]

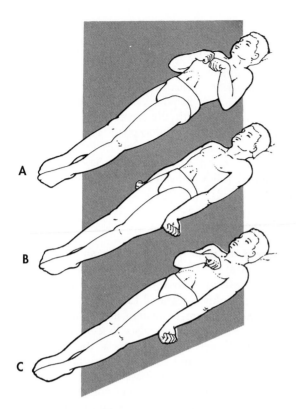

FIG. 14-1 Abnormal motor responses. **A,** Decorticate posturing. **B,** Decerebrate posturing. **C,** Decorticate posturing on right side and decerebrate posturing on left side.

1. Spontaneous—occurs without regard to external stimuli and may not occur by request.
2. Withdrawal—occurs when the extremity receiving the painful stimulus flexes normally in an attempt to avoid the noxious stimulus.
3. Localization—occurs when the extremity opposite to the extremity receiving pain crosses the midline of the body in an attempt to remove the noxious stimulus from the affected limb.
4. Abnormal (Fig. 14-1):
   a. Decortication—an abnormal flexion response that can occur spontaneously or in response to painful stimuli.
   b. Decerebration—an abnormal extension response that may also occur spontaneously or in response to painful stimuli.
   c. Flaccid—no response to painful stimuli.

Pupils and Eyes

Assessment of pupils and eyes should focus on two priorities: (1) appraisal of pupillary function and (2) evaluation of eye movements.[5] In unconscious patients or patients receiving neuromuscular blocking agents and sedation, pupillary response is one of the few neurologic signs that can be assessed.

Pupillary function

Pupillary function is an extension of the autonomic nervous system. Parasympathetic control of pupillary reaction occurs through innervation of the oculomotor nerve (cranial nerve [CN] III), which exits from the brainstem in the midbrain area. When the parasympathetic fibers are stimulated, the pupil constricts. Sympathetic control of the pupil originates in the hypothalamus and travels down the entire length of the brainstem. When the sympathetic fibers are stimulated, the pupil dilates. Evaluation of pupillary response includes assessment of size, shape (round, irregular, or oval), and degree of reactivity to light. The two pupils should be compared for equality. Any of these components of the pupil assessment could change in response to increasing pressure on the oculomotor nerve at the tentorium.[5]

Pupil size. Pupil size should be documented in millimeters with the use of a pupil gauge to reduce the subjectivity of description. Although most people have pupils of equal size, a discrepancy of up to 1 mm between the two pupils is normal. Inequality of pupils is known as *anisocoria,* which occurs in 15% to 17% of the human population.[6] Change or inequality in pupil size, especially in patients who previously have not shown this discrepancy, is a significant neurologic sign that should be reported immediately because it may indicate impending danger of herniation. With the location of the oculomotor nerve (CN III) at the notch of the tentorium, pupil size and reactivity play a key role in the physical assessment of intracranial pressure changes and herniation syndromes. In addition to CN III compression, changes in pupil size occur for other reasons. Large pupils can result from the instillation of cycloplegic agents such as atropine or scopolamine or can indicate extreme stress. Extremely small pupils can indicate narcotic overdose, lower brainstem compression, or bilateral damage to the pons.[2]

Pupil shape. Pupil shape is also noted in the assessment of pupils. Although the pupil is normally round, an irregularly shaped or oval pupil may be noted in patients with elevated intracranial pressure. An oval pupil can indicate the initial stages of CN III compression. An oval pupil is almost always associated with an intracranial pressure (ICP) between 18 and 35 mm Hg. The oval pupil appears to represent a transitional pupil that will return to normal size if ICP can be controlled but will progress to dilation and unreactivity if ICP is not treated or cannot be controlled.[7]

Reactivity to light. Evaluating direct pupillary response to light involves use of a narrow-beamed, bright light shone into the pupil from the outer canthus of the eye. If the light is shone directly onto the pupil, glare or reflection of the light may prevent proper visualization. Consensual pupillary response is the constriction of the pupil in response to a light shone into the opposite eye.[6-] Pupillary reactivity is affected by medications, particularly sympathetic and parasympa-

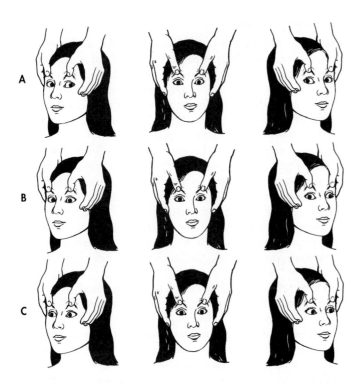

FIG. 14-2 Oculocephalic reflex (doll's eyes). **A,** Normal. **B,** Abnormal. **C,** Absent.

thetic agents, direct trauma, and eye surgery. Pupillary reactivity is also relatively resistant to metabolic dysfunction and can be used to differentiate between metabolic and structural causes of decreased levels of consciousness.[5]

Eye movements

Control of **eye movements** occurs with interaction of three cranial nerves: oculomotor (CN III), trochlear (CN IV), and abducens (CN VI).[3] The pathways for these cranial nerves provide integrated function through the internuclear pathway of the medial longitudinal fasciculus (MLF) located in the brainstem. The MLF provides coordination of eye movements with the vestibular and reticular formation.[5]

CONSCIOUS PATIENTS. In conscious patients the function of the three cranial nerves of the eye and their MLF innervation can be assessed by asking patients to follow nurses' finger through the full range of eye motions. If the eyes move together into all six fields, extraocular movements are intact.[5]

UNCONSCIOUS PATIENT. In unconscious patients assessment of ocular function and the innervation of the MLF is performed by eliciting the oculocephalic (doll's eyes) reflex. If patients are unconscious as a result of trauma, nurses should ascertain the absence of cervical injury before performing this examination. To assess the oculocephalic reflex, nurses should hold patients' eyelids open and briskly turn the head to one side while observing

eye movements, then briskly turn the head to the other side and observe. If the oculocephalic reflex is intact, the doll's eyes reflex occurs. The eyes deviate in a direction opposite to the movement of the head. If the oculocephalic reflex is not intact, the reflex is absent. This lack of response, wherein the eyes remain midline and move with the head, indicates significant brainstem injury. If the oculocephalic reflex is abnormal, the doll's eyes reflex is abnormal. In this situation the eyes rove or move in opposite directions. Abnormal oculocephalic reflex indicates some degree of brainstem injury (Fig. 14-2).[3]

Respiratory Function

Assessment of respiratory function should focus on two priorities: (1) observation of respiratory pattern and (2) evaluation of airway status.[5] The activity of respiration is a highly integrated function that receives input from the cerebrum, brainstem, and metabolic mechanisms. A close correlation exists in clinical assessment among altered levels of consciousness, the level of brain or brainstem injury, and the respiratory pattern noted.[2] Under the influence of the cerebral cortex and the diencephalon, three brainstem centers control respirations. The lowest center, the medullary respiratory center, sends impulses through the vagus nerve to innervate muscles of inspiration and expiration. The apneustic and pneumotaxic centers of the pons are responsible for the length of inspiration and expiration and underlying respiratory rate.[3]

Respiratory pattern

Changes in **respiratory patterns** assist in identifying the level of brainstem dysfunction or injury (Table 14-3). Evaluation of respiratory pattern should also include evaluation of the effectiveness of gas exchange in maintaining adequate oxygen and carbon dioxide levels. Hypoventilation is not uncommon in patients with an altered level of consciousness. Alterations in oxygenation or carbon dioxide levels can result in further neurologic dysfunction. ICP increases with hypoxemia or hypercapnia.[1]

Airway

Finally, assessment of the respiratory function in patients with neurologic deficit should include assessment of airway maintenance and secretion control. Cough, gag, and swallow reflexes responsible for protection of the airway may be absent or diminished.[5]

Vital Signs

The final portion of the neurologic examination is the evaluation of vital signs. **Assessment of vital signs should focus on two priorities: (1) monitoring blood pressure and (2) observing heart rate and rhythm.**[5] As a result of the brain and brainstem influences on cardiac,

TABLE 14-3
RESPIRATORY PATTERNS

PATTERN OF RESPIRATION	DESCRIPTION OF PATTERN	SIGNIFICANCE
Cheyne-Stokes	Rhythmic crescendo and decrescendo of rate and depth of respiration; includes brief periods of apnea	Usually seen with bilateral deep cerebral lesions or some cerebellar lesions
Central neurogenic hyperventilation	Very deep, very rapid respirations with no apneic periods	Usually seen with lesions of the midbrain and upper pons
Apneustic	Prolonged inspiratory and/or expiratory pause of 2-3 sec	Usually seen in lesions of the mid to lower pons
Cluster breathing	Clusters of irregular, gasping respirations separated by long periods of apnea	Usually seen in lesions of the lower pons or upper medulla
Ataxic respirations	Irregular, random pattern of deep and shallow respirations with irregular apneic periods	Usually seen in lesions of the medulla

respiratory, and body temperature functions, changes in vital signs can indicate deterioration in neurologic status.

Blood pressure

A common manifestation of the intracranial injury is systemic hypertension. Cerebral autoregulation, responsible for the control of cerebral blood flow, is frequently lost with any type of intracranial injury. After cerebral injury the body is often in a hyperdynamic state (increased heart rate, blood pressure, and cardiac output) as part of a compensatory response. With the loss of autoregulation and an increase in blood pressure, cerebral blood flow and cerebral blood volume increase, causing an increase in ICP. Control of systemic hypertension is necessary to stop this cycle.[5]

Heart rate and rhythm

The medulla and the vagus nerve provide parasympathetic control to the heart. When stimulated, this lower brainstem system produces bradycardia. Increasing ICP frequently causes bradycardia. Abrupt ICP changes can also produce dysrhythmias such as premature ventricular contractions, atrioventricular block, or ventricular fibrillation.[5]

Cushing's triad

Cushing's triad is a set of three clinical manifestations (bradycardia, systolic hypertension, and bradypnea) related to pressure on the medullary area of the brainstem. These signs often occur in response to intracranial hypertension or herniation syndrome. The appearance of Cushing's triad is a late finding that may be absent in neurologic deterioration.[1]

Diagnostic Procedures

Skull and Spine Films

Skull and spine radiographs assist in the determination of the size and shape of cranial and spinal bones.[8]

Procedure

The procedure for obtaining skull and spine radiographs is relatively painless. A wide variety of views are available, depending on the area to be studied. Lateral and posteroanterior skull films are probably the most commonly ordered radiographs.[9] A C1-2 view is obtained by taking the x-ray through the open mouth of patients (Water's view). For C6-7 views, adequate visualization often requires nurses or technicians to pull down firmly on patients' arms while the film is being taken.[5]

Significance

Skull and spinal films are helpful in identifying fractures, cranial and spinal abnormalities, vascular abnormalities, and degenerative changes.[9] Whenever traumatic injury, especially head injury, is the reason for admission to the critical care unit, cervical spine films should be obtained to rule out cervical spine injuries.[5]

Computed Tomography

The purpose of the **computed tomography (CT) scan** is to obtain rapid, noninvasive visualization of structures.[8,9]

Procedure

CT scanning provides clinicians with a mathematically reconstructed view of multiple sections of the head and body and is accomplished by passing intersecting x-ray beams through the examined area and measuring the density of substances through which the x-ray beam passes. The denser the substance through which the x-ray beam passes, the whiter it will appear on the finished film. The less dense a substance, the blacker it will appear. Therefore with normal findings in a CT scan of the head, bone appears white, blood appears off-white, brain tissue appears shaded gray, cerebrospinal fluid (CSF) appears off-black, and air appears black.[9]

There are two types of CT scans—contrast and noncontrast scans. The noncontrast scan is noninvasive, requires no premedication of the patient, and is good for analysis and location of normal brain structures and in diagnosis of hydrocephalus. The contrast CT scan involves the use of an intravenously injected contrast medium. The use of contrast enhances the vascular areas and allows for detection of vascular lesions or further definition of lesions noted on a noncontrast scan. If patients are to receive a contrast CT scan, their possible sensitivity to iodine-based dye should be determined beforehand, if at all possible. During the infusion of the dye and for 10 to 30 minutes afterwards, patients should be observed closely for anaphylactic reaction.[5,9]

Significance

CT scanning is indicated in the diagnostic work-up of severe headache, head trauma with associated loss of consciousness, seizures, hydrocephalus, suspicion of space-occupying lesions, hemorrhage, or vascular lesions and edema.[9,10]

Magnetic Resonance Imaging

Magnetic resonance imaging (MRI) evaluates structural and biochemical abnormalities, detects necrotic or ischemic tissue, and distinguishes white matter changes.[9]

Procedure

The procedure is performed by placing patients in a large magnetic field. The nuclei of the atoms of the body are stimulated and momentarily absorb some of the energy generated by the magnetic field. Different tissue densities absorb and subsequently release differing amounts of energy. The release of the energy (resonance frequency) is then measured and plotted.[10,11]

The procedure is lengthy and requires patients to lie motionless in a tight, enclosed space. Many patients experience anxiety, panic, and an acute sense of claustrophobia. Mild sedation or a blindfold or both may be necessary. Neurologically impaired patients may not be able to comprehend the instructions, and sedation will be required. Removal of all metal from patients' bodies and clothing is essential because the basis of MRI is a magnetic field. Any questions about specific devices or metals should be directed to the neuroradiologist before testing.[10]

Significance

MRI is useful in identifying a wide variety of neurologic alterations, including edema, ischemia, tumors, infection, hemorrhage and other vascular malformations, and congenital and degenerative disorders.[5]

Cerebral Angiogram

The purpose of **cerebral angiography** is to evaluate the cerebral circulation.[5]

Procedure

Cerebral angiography involves injecting radiopaque contrast medium into the intracranial or extracranial vasculature. With the use of serial radiologic filming, an angiogram traces the flow of blood from the arterial circulation through the capillary bed to the venous circulation. The procedure involves placing a catheter in the femoral artery and threading it up the aorta and into the origin of the cerebral circulation. Other injection sites include a direct carotid or vertebral artery puncture or placement of a catheter in the brachial, axillary, or subclavian artery. Once the catheter is appropriately placed, the contrast medium is injected. Then a rapid succession of radiographs is taken as the contrast medium progresses through the cerebral circulation. Separate contrast medium injections are administered for each vessel being studied.[10]

Before and after the procedure, adequate hydration is necessary to assist the kidneys in clearing the heavy dye load. Inadequate hydration may lead to an acute tubular necrosis and renal shutdown. If patients are unable to tolerate oral fluids, an intravenous line should be placed before the procedure begins.[10] Postprocedure assessment involves vital sign measurement, neurologic evaluation, observation of the injection site, and assessment of neurovascular integrity distal to the injection site every 15 minutes for the first 1 to 2 hours. Any abnormalities must be reported immediately.[5,10]

COMPLICATIONS. Complications associated with cerebral angiography include cerebral embolus caused by the catheter dislodging a segment of atherosclerotic plaque in the vessel, hemorrhage or clot formation at the insertion site, vasospasm of a vessel caused by the irritation of catheter placement, thrombosis of the extremity distal to the injection site, and allergic reaction to the contrast medium.[5]

Significance

Cerebral angiography allows the lumen of vessels to be visualized, providing information about patency, size (narrowing or dilation), irregularities, and occlusion. Angiography is necessary in the diagnosis of cerebral aneurysm, arteriovenous malformation, carotid artery disease, and some vascular tumors.[9,10]

Myelography

The purpose of myelography is to evaluate the spinal canal, the subarachnoid space around the spinal cord, and the spinal nerve roots.[5]

Procedure

The procedure involves a lumbar or cisternal puncture followed by an injection of contrast medium. It is performed fluoroscopically; the infusion of the dye is observed, and radiographic films are taken. Two basic types of contrast medium are used—an oil-based preparation (isothendylate) and a water-based preparation (metrizamide).[9]

OIL-BASED CONTRAST. Use of an oil-based preparation, which is heavier than the CSF, allows the radiologist to place patients in a variety of positions while observing the flow of dye through the spinal subarachnoid space. Disadvantages of the oil-based preparation include the lack of absorption of the dye from the subarachnoid space. Isothendylate (Pantopaque) must be removed at the end of the procedure. Use of an oil-based preparation is associated with a higher incidence of severe postprocedure headache as a result of CSF loss. Postprocedure care of patients who have undergone oil-based contrast myelogram involves ensuring that they lie flat in bed for 4 to 6 hours to prevent headache and CSF leak from the puncture site. To ensure clearance of dye through the urine, adequate hydration is necessary for patients who undergo a metrizamide myelogram.[5]

WATER-BASED CONTRAST. Use of the water-based preparation, which is lighter than CSF, allows for better visualization of nerve roots and projections off the spinal cord. Metrizamide (Amipaque) is absorbed by the arachnoid system and therefore does not require removal after the procedure. The disadvantages of a water-based preparation include rapid dissolution of the dye into the subarachnoid space. Patients cannot be rolled into different positions to reveal dye flow. Because water-based preparations may be toxic to the cerebral tissue, care must be taken to ensure that a large dye load does not reach the surface of the brain. This is accomplished by keeping patients' heads elevated 30 to 45 degrees after the procedure. Toxicity is evidenced by grand mal seizures.[5]

COMPLICATIONS. Possible risks of myelography include injection of the dye outside the subarachnoid space; arachnoiditis as a result of irritation of the arachnoid membranes from a foreign material; and allergic reactions to the dye that may cause confusion, disorientation, anaphylactic reaction, headache, or grand mal seizure.[12]

Significance

Myelography is useful in identifying a wide variety of spinal abnormalities, including spinal canal blockage caused by herniated intervertebral disks, spinal cord tumors, bony fragments or growths, and congenital anomalies.[9]

Cerebral Blood Flow Studies

Cerebral blood flow studies measure the amount of blood flow to the different regions of the brain.[10]

Procedure

Methods of determining cerebral blood flow range from intracarotid or intravenous injection of radioisotopes to inhalation of isotopes or nitrous oxide. The most clinically acceptable method of cerebral blood flow analysis

involves inhalation of xenon-133 for 3 to 5 minutes. Clearance of this isotope from brain tissue is then monitored by means of 16 to 32 probes that are placed externally around the head. Information from the probes is passed to a computer that calculates regional cerebral blood flow.[10]

Significance

Uses of cerebral blood flow studies include evaluation of cerebral vasospasm after subarachnoid hemorrhage and measurement of cerebral blood flow during operative procedures that require extreme hypotension, such as aneurysm clipping. It is also beneficial in monitoring changes in cerebral blood flow after cerebral vascular surgery, such as carotid endarterectomy, cerebral revascularization (superficial temporal artery-middle cerebral artery bypass), or arteriovenous malformation excision.[5]

Ultrasound Studies

A noninvasive technique, ultrasound studies provide information about the flow velocity of blood through cerebral vessels.[13]

Procedure

A Doppler probe is placed externally over the vessel where ultrasonic waves are generated and blood flow velocities are calculated. As the diameter of the vessel changes, the velocity of the flow of blood through the vessel changes. The higher the flow velocity, the narrower the vessel. This narrowing can be the result of vasospasm or vessel plaque.[13]

Significance

Extracranial Doppler studies are used as a routine screening procedure for intraluminal narrowing of the common and internal carotid arteries as a result of arteriosclerotic plaques or atheromata. When changes in flow velocities are noted that may indicate significant occlusion of the vessel, a cerebral angiogram is often required to verify the degree of severity of the narrowed vessel.[7]

Transcranial Doppler studies monitor cerebral blood flow velocity through cranial "windows" or thinned areas of the skull. Depending on the angle of the Doppler probe, flow velocities can be measured in the anterior, middle, or posterior cerebral arteries. Current use of transcranial Doppler studies is mainly for postintracranial aneurysm rupture when concern about vasospasm development is a factor. Use of serial transcranial Doppler studies for the detection of cerebral vasospasm greatly reduces the need for cerebral angiograms to verify and follow postsubarachnoid hemorrhage vasospasm.[13]

Electroencephalography

The purpose of an electroencephalography (EEG) is to record the brain's electrical impulses, commonly called *brain waves* (Table 14-4).[5]

TABLE 14-4

TYPES OF ELECTRICAL BRAIN WAVES

WAVE	DURATION	DESCRIPTION
Delta	1 to 4 cycles/second	Normal, seen in stages 3 and 4 of sleep
Alpha	8 to 13 cycles/second	Normal, relaxed state with eyes closed, seen often in occipital leads
Theta	4 to 7 cycles/second	Less common in adults than in children, characteristic of coma in brain injury
Beta	12 to 40 cycles/second	Fast waves indicating mental or physical activity
Sleep spindles	12 to 14 cycles/second	Seen in stage 2 sleep, not REM
Spike and slow wave	Variable	Seen in irritable brain tissue (such as seizure)

Procedure

Noninvasive electrodes are placed on the head, and electrical impulses detected are transferred to a central recording device that records the information as a wave form.[1] In preparing patients for an EEG, nurses should stress the noninvasive aspects of this procedure. Conscious patients may be asked to perform certain simple tasks during the procedure, such as blinking, closing the eye, or swallowing. Occasionally, testing needs to be performed during sleep or after a period of sleep deprivation.[5]

Significance

EEG detects and localizes abnormal electrical activity. This abnormal activity is manifested as slowing, which occurs in areas of injury or infarct, or as spikes and waves, which are seen in irritated tissue. Indications for the use of EEG include seizure focus identification, infarct, metabolic disorders, confirmation of brain death (electrocerebral silence), and some head injuries.[9]

Evoked Potentials/Responses

Evoked potentials/responses record the electrical impulses generated by a sensory stimulus as it travels through the brainstem and into the cerebral cortex.[9]

Procedure

The three types of evoked potential tests are visual evoked potentials (VEP), brainstem auditory evoked responses (BAER), and somatosensory evoked potentials (SSEP). VEP involves monitoring the visual pathways through the brainstem and cortex in response to patients' viewing a shifting geometric pattern on a screen or placing a mask that sends a flashing light stimulus over the eye. BAER involves monitoring the auditory pathway through the brainstem and cortex in response to a rhythmic clicking sound sent through earphones placed over patients' ears. SSEP involves monitoring sensory pathways from the extremities ascending the spinal cord through the brainstem and into the cortex by administering a small electrical shock to a nerve root in the periphery, such as the ulnar or radial nerve.[10]

Significance

Evoked potentials/responses are used to detect lesions in cerebral cortex, ascending pathways of the spinal cord, brainstem, and thalamus.[9,10] They can also be used during therapeutically induced comas (these sensory pathways are unaffected by the depressive activity of these drugs) to assess patients' neurologic status and determine brainstem or spinal cord injury in traumatically injured patients.[10]

Lumbar Puncture

The purpose of a **lumbar puncture** (LP) is to obtain a CSF sample or measure CSF pressure (Table 14-5).[10]

Procedure

An LP involves the introduction of an 18- to 22-gauge hollow needle into the subarachnoid space at L4-5 below the end of the spinal cord, which is usually at L1-2. Patients are placed either in the lateral recumbent position, with the knees and head tightly tucked, or in the sitting position, leaning over a bedside table or some other support. After the procedure patients should remain flat for 1 to 6 hours to prevent a spinal headache.[10]

COMPLICATIONS. Risks associated with an LP include possible brainstem herniation if intracranial pressure is elevated and respiratory arrest associated with neurologic deterioration. During the procedure nurses must monitor patients' neurologic and respiratory status.[9]

Significance

CSF samples assist in the diagnosis of subarachnoid hemorrhage, meningitis, and multiple sclerosis. CSF pressures facilitate the evaluation of hydrocephalus and space-occupying lesions.[10]

Nursing Management

Nursing management of patients undergoing a diagnostic procedure involves a variety of interventions. **Priorities are directed toward preparing patients psychologically and physically for the procedure, monitoring pa-**

TABLE 14-5

CEREBROSPINAL FLUID ANALYSIS

PARAMETERS	NORMAL	ABNORMAL	POSSIBLE CAUSE
Pressure (initial readings)	75-180 mm H_2O (5-15 mm Hg)	<60 mm	Faulty needle placement Dehydration Spinal block along subarachnoid space Block of foramen magnum
		>200 mm	Muscle tension Abdominal compression Brain tumor Subdural hematoma Brain abscess Brain cyst Cerebral edema (any cause) Hydrocephalus
Color	Clear, colorless	Cloudy	Increased cell count Increased microorganisms
		Yellow	Xanthochromic (RBC pigments) High protein content
		Smoky	Presence of RBCs
Red blood cells	None	Blood-tinged	Traumatic tap
		Grossly bloody	Traumatic tap Subarachnoid hemorrhage

White blood cells	0-6 mm^3	>10 mm^3 (Cell counts range from below 100 to many thousands depending on causative factor; all are abnormal findings)	Occurs in many conditions:
			  Bacterial infections of meninges
			  Viral infections of meninges
			  Neurosyphilis
			  Tuberculous meningitis
			  Metastatic neoplastic lesions
			  Parasitic infections
			  Acute demyelinating diseases
			  Following introduction of air or blood into subarachnoid space

Protein*	15-45 mg/100 ml (1% of serum protein)	<10 mg/100 ml	Little clinical significance

		>60 mg/100 ml	Occurs in many conditions:
			  Complete spinal block
			  Guillain-Barré syndrome
			  Carcinomatosis of meninges
			  Tumors close to pial or ependymal surfaces, or in cerebello-positive angle
			  Acute and chronic meningitis
			  Meningeal hemorrhage
			  Demyelinating disorders
			  Degenerative diseases

Glucose	50-75 mg/100 ml (approximately 60% of blood glucose level)	<40 mg/100 ml	Acute bacterial meningitis Tuberculous meningitis Meningeal carcinomatosis
		>100 mg/100 ml	Diabetes
Chloride	700-750 mg/100 ml; 125 mM	<625 mg/100 ml	Hypochloremia Tuberculous meningitis
		>800 mg/100 ml	Not of neurologic significance; correlated with blood levels of chloride

*NOTE: If CSF contains blood, this will raise the protein level.

From Rudy E: *Advanced neurological and neurosurgical nursing,* ed 4, St. Louis, 1984, Mosby.

tients' responses to the procedure, and assessing patients after the procedure. Preparing patients includes teaching them about the procedure, answering their questions, and positioning them for the procedure. Monitoring patients' responses to the procedure includes observing patients for signs of pain, anxiety, or change in level of consciousness and monitoring vital signs. Assessing patients after the procedure includes observing them for complications related to the procedure and medicating them for any postprocedure discomfort. **Nurses should immediately report any evidence of increasing intracranial pressure to physicians and initiate emergency measures to decrease the pressure.**

References

1. Ackerman LL: Alteration in level of responsiveness: a proposed nursing diagnosis, *Nurs Clin North Am* 28:729, 1993.
2. Lower J: Rapid neuro assessment, *Am J Nurs* 92(6):38, 1992.
3. Sullivan J: Neurologic assessment, *Nurs Clin North Am* 25:795, 1990.
4. Segatore M, Way C: The Glascow Coma Scale: time for change, *Heart Lung* 21:548, 1992.
5. Barker E: *Neuroscience nursing,* St Louis, 1994, Mosby.
6. Bishop BS: Pathologic pupillary signs: self-learning module, part 1, *Crit Care Nurs* 11(6):59, 1991.
7. Marshall SB and others: *Neuroscience critical care: pathophysiology and patient management,* Philadelphia, 1990, WB Saunders.
8. Sullivan TE and others: Closed head injury assessment and research methodology, *J Neurosci Nurs* 26:24, 1994.
9. Shpritz DW: *Neurodiagnostic studies.* In Cammermeyer M, Appledorn C: *Core curriculum for neuroscience nursing,* Chicago, 1990, American Association of Neuroscience Nurses.
10. Mason PJB: Neurodiagnostic testing in critically injured adults, *Crit Care Nurs* 12(6):64, 1992.
11. Lee BCP: Magnetic resonance imaging of the central nervous system, *Hosp Med* 29(2):130, 1993.
12. Jones AG: Side effects following metrizamide myelography and lumbar laminectomy, *J Neurosci Nurs* 1:90, 1987.
13. Marsh K: Transcranial Doppler sonography: non-invasive monitoring of intracranial vasculature, *J Neurosci Nurs* 22:113, 1990.

15

Neurologic Disorders

KATHLEEN A. MENDEZ

CHAPTER OBJECTIVES

- Describe the etiology and pathophysiology of various neurologic disorders.
- Identify the clinical manifestations of various neurologic disorders.
- Explain the treatment of various neurologic disorders.
- Discuss the nursing management of patients with various neurologic disorders.

KEY TERMS

An understanding of the pathology of a disease, the areas of assessment on which to focus, and the usual medical management allows critical care nurses more accurately to anticipate and plan nursing interventions. Although a wide array of neurologic disorders exists, only a few routinely require care in the critical care environment. This chapter focuses on priority neurologic disorders that nurses commonly encounter in the critical care environment.

Hemorrhagic Cerebrovascular Accident

Cerebrovascular accident, commonly known as *stroke,* is a descriptive term for the onset of neurologic symptoms caused by interruption of blood flow to the brain. Stroke is the third leading cause of death in the United States, preceded only by heart disease and cancer. Two basic types of stroke exist: ischemic and hemorrhagic. Ischemic stroke produces symptoms resulting from occlusion of a blood vessel. (This type of stroke is not presented in this book because it does not generally require admission to the critical care unit.) Hemorrhage stroke produces symptoms resulting from rupture of a blood vessel. Hemorrhagic strokes are classified as intracerebral hemorrhage and subarachnoid hemorrhage (SAH). Intracerebral hemorrhage is usually caused by hypertensive rupture of a cerebral vessel. SAH can be caused by aneurysm rupture or arteriovenous malformation rupture.[1]

Cerebral Aneurysm

Description and etiology

An aneurysm is an outpouching of the wall of a blood vessel caused by weakening of the vessel wall. Aneurysms can occur in vessels in other parts of the body, but this section focuses on **cerebral aneurysms.** Most cerebral aneurysms are saccular or berrylike, with a stem and neck. Aneurysms are usually small (2 to 6 mm in diameter) but may be as large as 6 cm. An aneurysm that ruptures or becomes large enough to exert pressure on surrounding structures is cause for clinical concern.[2]

Etiologies of aneurysms include congenital formation, traumatic injury that stretches and tears the muscular middle layer of the arterial vessel, infectious material that lodges against a vessel wall and erodes the muscular layer (most often infectious vegetation on valves of the left side of the heart after bacterial endocarditis), and atherosclerosis.[3] Multiple aneurysms occur in 20% to 25% of the cases and are often bilateral, occurring in the same location on both sides of the head.[2] Aneurysms frequently

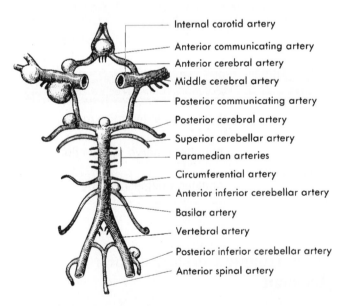

Internal carotid artery

Anterior communicating artery

Anterior cerebral artery

Middle cerebral artery

Posterior communicating artery

Posterior cerebral artery

Superior cerebellar artery

Paramedian arteries

Circumferential artery

Anterior inferior cerebellar artery

Basilar artery

Vertebral artery

Posterior inferior cerebellar artery

Anterior spinal artery

FIG. 15-1 The common sites of berry aneurysms. The size of the aneurysm in the drawing is proportional to the frequency of occurrence at the various sites. (From Wyngaarden JB, Smith LH, editors: *Cecil's textbook of medicine,* ed 16, Philadelphia, 1982, WB Saunders.)

occur at the base of the brain on the circle of Willis. Distribution is as follows: anterior communicating artery, 30%; posterior communicating artery, 25%; branching of the middle cerebral artery, 13%; and all other locations, 32% (Fig. 15-1). Most cerebral aneurysms, especially those that are congenital, occur at the bifurcation of blood vessels.

Pathophysiology

The cause of the defect in vessel development that occurs in the congenital aneurysm is unknown. A small portion of the inner muscular or elastic layer of the vessel is poorly developed, leaving a thin vessel wall. As individuals mature, blood pressure rises and puts more stress on this thin vessel wall. The vessel balloons out, creating a berrylike appearance. The aneurysm becomes clinically significant when the vessel wall becomes so thin that it ruptures, sending arterial blood at a high pressure into the subarachnoid space. An unruptured aneurysm may be equally problematic because it places pressure on surrounding structures. This is particularly true of the posterior communicating artery aneurysm that puts pressure on the oculomotor nerve (CN III), causing ipsilateral pupil dilation and ptosis.[2,3]

Assessment and diagnosis

Patients with an aneurysm are usually seen after the SAH. SAH becomes the working diagnosis until the cause of the hemorrhage is determined. Clinical manifestations of SAH range from the sudden onset of an excruciating headache to coma or death. Vomiting, nuchal rigidity (stiff neck), photophobia, seizure, hemiplegia, and other focal neurologic deficits are common.[2,3]

Diagnosis of SAH is based on clinical presentation, computed tomography (CT) scan, and lumbar puncture. When SAH is suspected, a CT scan is performed to identify subarachnoid blood. In 75% of the cases blood is present in the basal cisterns if the CT scan is performed within 48 hours of the hemorrhage. On the basis of the appearance and location of the SAH, diagnosis of cause, such as aneurysm or AVM, may be made from the CT scan.[4] If results of the CT scan are unequivocal, a lumbar puncture is performed to obtain cerebrospinal fluid (CSF) for analysis. After the SAH, CSF may appear red or xanthochromic (dark amber) because blood products have broken down.[2] Once the SAH has been documented, a cerebral angiogram is necessary to identify its exact cause. If a cerebral aneurysm rupture is the cause, angiogram is also essential to define the exact location of the aneurysm in preparation for surgery.[3] Once the aneurysm has been located, it is graded using a classification scale based on the severity of the neurologic deficits associated with the bleed (Box 15-1).

Medical management

Medical management of patients with SAH is complex. It involves monitoring for and treating complications

HUNT AND HESS CLASSIFICATION OF SUBARACHNOID HEMORRHAGE

Grade I   Asymptomatic, minimal headache, slight nuchal rigidity

Grade II   Moderate to severe headache, nuchal rigidity, minimal neurologic deficit

Grade III Drowsiness, confusion, mild focal neurologic deficit

Grade IV Stupor, moderate to severe hemiparesis, early decerebrate posturing

Grade V   Comatose, decorticate or decerebrate posturing, moribund appearance

that can occur and deciding when surgical intervention should take place. The three major complications after SAH from aneurysm rupture are rebleeding, vasospasm, and hydrocephalus. Preserving an adequate cerebral blood flow is essential for a positive outcome after SAH.[3]

REBLEEDING. *Rebleeding* refers to the occurrence of a second SAH at any time in an unsecured aneurysm. The incidence of rebleeding is highest during the first 3 weeks, with the highest incidence in the first 24 hours after the hemorrhage. Mortality rates for rebleeding have been reported to be as high as 70%.[4]

TREATMENT. Definitive treatment for prevention of rebleeding is surgical clipping of the aneurysm.[5] While awaiting surgery, patients should have blood pressure high enough to maintain adequate cerebral blood flow but low enough to prevent rebleeding. The exact level for patients will vary depending on their level of consciousness. Wide fluctuations in blood pressure should also be avoided. Patients should be placed in a quiet, nonstressful environment to prevent increases in blood pressure.[3]

VASOSPASM. Another complication of SAH is **cerebral vasospasm.** Vasospasm, or the narrowing of the lumen of the vessel, is believed to be sustained arterial contraction as a response to subarachnoid blood clots coating the outer surface of the blood vessels. It is a critical issue because of its location in the cerebral vasculature.[6] Inasmuch as aneurysms occur at the circle of Willis, the major vessels responsible for feeding cerebral circulation are affected by vasospasm. Depending on the arterial vessels involved in the vasospasm reaction, arterial flow decreases in large areas of the cerebral hemispheres, causing ischemic stroke. The peak period for vasospasm is 4 to 12 days after rupture. Vasospasm, which occurs in 40% to 60% of patients with SAH,[3] begins around the third day after rupture and can last for 3 to 4 weeks.

TREATMENT. A variety of therapies designed to reverse or overcome vasospasm have been evaluated. Two treatments that seem to have potential benefit are hypervolemic hyperperfusion with or without induced hyperten-

sion and the administration of calcium channel blockers.[7]

Designed to maximize cardiac performance and improve cerebral blood flow, hypervolemic hyperperfusion therapy involves the use of crystalloids and volume expanders. The goal is to increase the central venous pressure 10 to 12 mm Hg or bring pulmonary artery wedge pressure to 18 to 20 mm Hg.[10] Induced hypertension is usually used as an adjunct therapy when vasospasm is present. Induced hypertension involves the use of vasoactive agents to raise systolic blood pressure to the point at which the neurologic dysfunction improves or returns to baseline. In an unsecured aneurysm the systolic pressure should be maintained no higher than 160 mm Hg. In a secured aneurysm the systolic pressure may be elevated as high as 240 mm Hg. This increase in pressure forces blood at higher pressures through the vasospastic area. Complications associated with this therapy include cardiac failure, pulmonary edema, and increased intracranial pressure (ICP). Careful monitoring of patients' pulmonary artery wedge pressure, cardiac output, oxygenation status, chest x-ray, and ICP is important.[8]

The exact mechanism behind calcium channel blockers, which constitute the second regimen for the prevention and treatment of vasospasm, is unknown. Calcium channel blockers are believed to affect the influx of calcium that occurs in an injured cell. Some calcium channel blockers (particularly nimodipine) have a selective cerebral vasodilator effect.[7,8] Growing evidence supports the effectiveness of these agents if treatment begins immediately after the initial hemorrhage. Results of ongoing clinical trials indicate that treatment with calcium channel blockers is beneficial, both in reducing ischemic deficit attributable to vasospasm and promoting positive clinical outcomes, if given prophylactically. No apparent therapeutic benefit is evident once a neurologic deficit has developed.[9]

HYDROCEPHALUS. Hydrocephalus is a late complication that frequently occurs after SAH. Blood that has circulated in the subarachnoid space and been absorbed by the arachnoid villi may obstruct these villi and reduce the rate of CSF absorption. Over time, increasing volumes of CSF in the intracranial space produce communicating hydrocephalus.[3]

TREATMENT. Treatment consists of placing a drain to remove CSF. This can be a temporary measure, with a catheter inserted in the lateral ventricle and attached to an external drainage bag, or permanent, with the placement of a ventriculoperitoneal shunt.[3]

SURGICAL INTERVENTION. A key issue in medical management is timing of surgery. It provokes much discussion focused on the difference in patient outcome when surgery is performed within 3 days of the bleed versus when it is postponed 10 to 14 days after the bleed. The International Cooperative Study on the Timing of Aneurysm Surgery found no difference in patient outcome between early and late surgery. The risk of rebleeding and vasospasm in patients who waited for surgery was found to equal the risk of postoperative complications in those who had early surgery.[10]

Aneurysm clipping is the surgical procedure for repair of the aneurysm. This procedure involves a **craniotomy** to expose the area of aneurysm. The aneurysm is isolated, and a clip is placed over the neck of the aneurysm to eliminate the area of weakness. Aneurysms that cannot be isolated for clipping are wrapped with plastic coating or other materials.[2]

Arteriovenous Malformation

Description and etiology

Arteriovenous malformation (AVM) is a tangled mass of arterial and venous blood vessels that shunt blood directly from the arterial side into the venous side, bypassing the capillary system. AVMs may be small, focal lesions or large lesions that occupy almost an entire hemisphere. The cause of an AVM is always congenital. The exact embryonic reason for the development of this malformation is unknown.[11]

Pathophysiology

The pathophysiologic features of the AVM are related to the size and location of the malformation. The AVM can be fed by one or more cerebral arteries. Known as *feeders,* these arteries tend to enlarge over time and increase the volume of blood shunted through the malformation, as well as increase the overall mass effect. Large, dilated, tortuous draining veins also develop as a result of the increasing flow of blood. Blood flows into the venous side of the AVM at a higher than normal pressure. In a normal vascular flow, mean arterial pressure is 70 to 80 mm Hg, mean arteriole pressure is 35 to 45 mm Hg, and mean capillary pressure drops from 35 to 10 mm Hg as it connects with the venous side. Lack of this capillary bridge allows blood with a mean pressure of 35 to 45 mm Hg to flow into the venous system. Because there is no muscular layer in the vein as there is in the artery, veins become extremely engorged. As a result of the shunting of blood through the AVM and away from normal cerebral circulation, poor perfusion occurs in the underlying cerebral tissues. This decreased perfusion produces a chronic ischemic state that results in cerebral atrophy.[11]

Assessment and diagnosis

Initial assessment of patients' condition depends on the presenting symptoms. Although SAH is one of the most common and severe presenting symptoms, other clinical manifestations may also occur before SAH. The onset of seizures is frequently the reason that patients with an AVM seek medical attention. As the mass of the AVM enlarges and the flow of blood increases, the pulsation of the blood vessel against the cerebral tissue surface causes a disturbance of the electrical activity of the area.

Seizures can be focal or generalized. Headaches are another common symptom of patients with an AVM. Headache may occur as a result of the increasing mass effect of the lesion or vascular changes in response to the shunted blood. Headaches are not in themselves cause to suspect AVM because of the wide variety of reasons for them.[11]

Diagnostic evaluation includes CT scan, EEG, and angiogram. CT scanning is performed initially as a noninvasive study to begin the diagnostic process. If an AVM is suspected from the results of the noncontrast scan, a contrast scan is performed. An EEG is obtained in an attempt to localize any seizure focus or define areas of cortical injury caused by cerebral ischemia or atrophy. Finally, for confirmation and definition of the AVM an angiogram is performed. If surgical intervention is planned, an angiogram is required to identify the feeding arteries and draining veins of the AVM.[2]

Medical management

Medical management of an AVM usually involves surgical excision, embolization, or conservative management of symptoms such as seizures and headache.

SURGICAL INTERVENTION. Whether surgical excision is performed depends on the location and size of the AVM. Some malformations are located so deep in cerebral structures (the thalamus or midbrain) that attempts to remove the AVM would cause severe neurologic deficits. The history of previous hemorrhage and the age and general condition of patients are also taken into account in decisions about surgical intervention.[11]

Surgical excision of large AVMs includes the risk of reperfusion bleeding. As feeding arteries of the AVM are clamped off, the arterial blood that usually flows into the AVM is now diverted into the surrounding circulation. In many cases the surrounding tissue has been in a state of chronic ischemia and the arterial vessels feeding these areas are maximally dilated. As arterial blood begins to flow at a higher volume and pressure into these dilated arteries, seeping of blood from the vessels may occur. The evidence of reperfusion bleeding in the operating room indicates that no more arterial blood can be diverted from the AVM without risk of serious intracerebral hemorrhage. In the postoperative phase, low blood pressure is maintained to prevent further reperfusion bleeding. In large AVMs, two to four stages of surgery might be required over a 6- to 12-month period.[11]

EMBOLIZATION. Embolization is another method to reduce the size of an AVM. It may also be used on surgically inaccessible AVMs. Embolization is an interventional radiologic technique in which a catheter is placed in the groin or other site in a manner similar to that for an angiogram. Under fluoroscopy, the catheter is threaded up to the internal carotid artery. Small Silastic beads or a variety of other materials, such as glue, are then slowly introduced through the catheter. The increased flow to the AVM usually carries the blocking material into the AVM. This procedure is designed to block the feeding arterial portion of the AVM and therefore eliminate it. Frequently, embolization and surgery are combined. Patients undergo one to three sessions of embolization to reduce the size of the lesion and then receive a craniotomy for total excision. Lodging of the substance in a vessel that feeds normal tissue is one of the risks associated with the procedure. This occurrence creates an embolic stroke with the immediate onset of neurologic symptoms.[11]

Intracerebral Hemorrhage

Description and etiology

Intracerebral hemorrhage is the escape of blood into cerebral tissue, resulting in cerebral tissue destruction, cerebral edema, and ICP. Causes of intracerebral hemorrhage include aneurysm or AVM rupture, trauma, blood dyscrasia (leukemia, hemophilia, sickle cell disease), anticoagulation therapy, brain tumors, and systemic hypertension.[12]

Pathophysiology

The pathophysiology of intracerebral hemorrhage is caused by continued elevated blood pressure exerting force against smaller arterial vessels that have become damaged from arteriosclerotic changes. Eventually this artery breaks, and blood bursts from the vessel into the cerebral tissue, creating a hematoma. ICP rises precipitously in response to the increased overall intracranial volume.[12]

Assessment and diagnosis

Initial assessment usually reveals unconscious, critically ill patients with deep, labored respirations. Patients often have many of the presenting symptoms of increased ICP.[2]

Medical management

An antihypertensive medication is usually administered immediately to reduce the blood pressure to a relatively normal reading. If the hemorrhage is significant enough to cause increased ICP, the blood pressure should not be allowed to drop too low or too rapidly. If blood pressure drops below 140 mm Hg systolic and ICP remains high, cerebral perfusion may be compromised.[2]

Definitive management of a hypertensive hemorrhage is similar to that of a traumatic hemorrhage. Surgical removal of the clot depends on the size and location of the clot, patients' ICP, and other neurologic symptoms. If the hematoma is large and causes a shift in structures or ICP is elevated despite routine methods to lower it, a craniotomy is performed to remove the hematoma. Nonsurgical management includes measures to maintain the ICP within normal limits and support all other vital functions until patients regain consciousness.[12]

BOX 15-2

NURSING DIAGNOSIS PRIORITIES

HEMORRHAGIC CEREBROVASCULAR ACCIDENT

Altered Cerebral Tissue Perfusion related to increased intracranial pressure, p. 492

Altered Cerebral Tissue Perfusion related to vasospasm, p. 491

Unilateral Neglect related to perceptual disruption, p. 495

Impaired Verbal Communication related to speech center injury, p. 497

Anxiety related to threat to biologic, psychologic, and/or social integrity, p. 464

Knowledge Deficit related to lack of previous exposure to information, p. 455

Nursing Management

Nursing management of patients with a hemorrhagic cerebrovascular accident incorporates a variety of nursing diagnoses (Box 15-2). **Nursing priorities are directed toward administering medications to maintain patients' blood pressure within the prescribed range, monitoring for complications, and educating patients and families.**

Administering medications to maintain patients' blood pressure within the prescribed limit

Adequate blood pressure is necessary to continue to supply the brain with the appropriate amount of oxygen and nutrients. However, when damage or disease of the cerebrovascular system is the cause of hospitalization, the actual level of blood pressure most appropriate for patients depends on the underlying condition. After spontaneous intracerebral hemorrhage or initial subarachnoid hemorrhage, for example, keeping the blood pressure relatively low is important. In vasospasm after subarachnoid hemorrhage, relatively high blood pressures are required for adequate perfusion. Nurses must monitor blood pressure constantly, administer medications as necessary, and observe patients' activities and interactions in response to blood pressure.[2]

Monitoring for complications

Patients should be monitored for signs of rebleeding, vasospasm, hydrocephalus, and increased intracranial pressure. Two other complications commonly found in patients with a hemorrhagic CVA are unilateral neglect and impaired communication.

INCREASED INTRACRANIAL PRESSURE. The numerous signs and symptoms of **increased intracranial pressure** include decreased level of consciousness, Cushing's triad (bradycardia, systolic hypertension, and bradypnea), diminished brainstem reflexes, papilledema, decerebrate posturing (abnormal extension), decorticate posturing (abnormal flexion), unequal pupil size, projectile vomiting, decreased pupillary reaction to light, altered breathing patterns, and headache.[13]

SENSORY PERCEPTUAL DISTURBANCES. Damage to the temporoparietal area can create a variety of disturbances that affect patients' ability to interpret sensory information.[14] Damage to the dominant hemisphere (usually left) produces problems with speech and language and abstract and analytical skills. Damage to the nondominant hemisphere (usually right) produces problems with spatial relationships.[15] The resulting deficits include agnosias, apraxias, and visual field defects.[2] Perceptual defects are not as readily noticeable as motor deficits but may be more debilitating, leading to the inability to perform skilled or purposeful tasks.[15]

AGNOSIAS. An agnosia is a disturbance in the perception of familiar sensory (verbal, tactile, visual) information. **Unilateral neglect** is a form of agnosia characterized by an unawareness or denial of the affected half of the body. This denial may range from inattention to an actual refusal to acknowledge paralysis by neglecting the involved side or denying ownership of the side, attributing the paralyzed arm or leg to someone else. This neglect may also extend to extrapersonal space. This defect usually results from right hemispheric brain damage that causes left hemiplegia.[15,16]

A variety of other agnosias exist in addition to unilateral neglect. Some people are unable to recognize objects visually (visual object agnosia), whereas others cannot recognize faces (prosopagnosia) and may have to rely on the voice or characteristic mannerisms when identifying a person. Tactile agnosia is a perceptual disorder in which patients are unable to recognize by touch alone an object that has been placed in their hands. This may occur even when sense of touch is intact. If allowed to see or hear the object, patients usually recognize it.[14,15]

Spatial orientation is also affected, resulting in interference with patients' ability to judge position, distance, movement, form, and the relationship of their body parts to surrounding objects. Patients may confuse such concepts as *up* and *down* and *forward* and *backward.* They may have difficulty following a route from one place to another and get lost even in areas that were once familiar. Stroke patients may also experience reading and writing problems related to visual perception and visuospatial deficits. One type of spatial dyslexia is related to unilateral spatial neglect. Patients may not look at the beginning of a line of written material that appears on the left. Instead patients fix their attention on a point to the right of the beginning of the line and read to the end of the line. If asked to draw a design, they complete only half of it.[16]

VISUAL FIELD DEFECTS. Visual field defects may accompany the agnosia, although they do not cause it. A hemispheric lesion can interrupt the visual pathways, with the resulting visual defect dependent on the location and extent of the lesion. At the optic chiasm, nerve fibers coming from the nasal half of each retina cross to the opposite side, whereas fibers coming from the temporal half of each retina do not cross. This partial crossing allows binocular vision. In the optic chiasm, fibers from the nasal half of each retina join the uncrossed fibers from the temporal half of the retina to form the optic tract. Impulses conducted to the right hemisphere by the right optic tract represent the left field of vision, and those conducted to the left hemisphere by the left optic tract represent the right field of vision. Optic radiations extend back to the occipital lobes. Visual defects restricted to a single field (right or left) are termed *homonymous hemianopsia.*[17]

Nurses may be the first to detect this defect in patients. Patients with hemianopsia may neglect all sensory input from the affected side and appear unresponsive when approached from the affected side; however, if nurses approach patients from the healthy side, patients appear quite alert. Nurses may also observe that patients eat food from only one half of the tray.[15] Hemianopsia may recede gradually with time. Many patients can learn to scan their environment visually to compensate for the defect, although in the acute stage of stroke, patients may be too lethargic to learn methods of visual scanning. This visual defect can lead to fear and confusion and jeopardize patients' safety.[17]

APRAXIA. Lesions in the parietal lobe, as well as in other cortical structures, can result in apraxia, an inability to perform a learned movement voluntarily. Even though patients may understand the task and have intact motor ability, they are unable to perform the task and often fumble and make mistakes. Patients suffering from dressing apraxia, for example, may be unable to orient clothing in space, becoming tangled in their clothes when attempting to dress.[14,15]

IMPAIRED COMMUNICATION. **Impaired communication** is a condition that makes expressing and exchanging thoughts, ideas, or desires difficult. The posterior temporoparietal area contains the receptive speech center known as *Wernicke's area.* The center for the perception of written language lies anterior to the visuoreceptive areas. Located at the base of the frontal lobe's motor strip and slightly anterior to it is Broca's area, also known as the *motor speech center.* These sensory and motor areas are connected by a large bundle of nerve fibers. Receptive and motor language functions do not occur entirely within discrete areas; language is believed to be an integrated sensorimotor process, roughly located in these areas in the dominant cerebral hemisphere. The elaborately complex functions of speech and language are also believed to depend on other associative areas of the cerebrum and their thalamic connections. Consequently the degree of communication impairment among patients with lesions located in the same area of the brain varies.[18]

Aphasia is a loss of language abilities caused by brain injury, usually to the dominant hemisphere.[24] Language abilities involve more than just comprehension and expression. *Language* is a broad term, referring to the content individuals attempt to interpret or convey through listening, speaking, reading, writing, and gesturing. The severity of aphasia depends on the area and extent of cerebral damage.[18]

RECEPTIVE APHASIA. Receptive aphasia, also referred to as *sensory, Wernicke's,* or *fluent aphasia,* occurs when the connection between the primary auditory cortex in the temporal lobe and the angular gyrus in the parietal lobe is destroyed. Comprehension of speech is impaired, but patients can still talk if the motor area for speech, Broca's area, is intact. Patients may in fact talk excessively, making many errors in word usage. They are able to hear examiners but can neither comprehend their words nor repeat them. Such patients may speak nonsensically, rambling and giving little information. Patients with receptive aphasia are also unable to read words, although they can see them.[18]

EXPRESSIVE APHASIA. Expressive aphasia, also known as *motor, Broca's,* or *nonfluent aphasia,* is primarily a deficit in language output or speech production. Depending on the lesion's size and exact location, a wide variation in the motor deficit can result. Expressive aphasia can range from a mild dysarthria (imperfect articulation as a result of weakness or lack of coordination of speech musculature) to incorrect tonation and phrasing and, in its most severe form, to complete loss of all ability to communicate through verbal and written means. With this severe form of aphasia, people also lose the ability to communicate through conventional gestures such as nodding or shaking the head for *yes* or *no.* In most cases of expressive aphasia, the muscles of articulation are intact. If speech is possible at all, occasionally the words *yes* or *no* are uttered, sometimes appropriately. Some people may sing the words of well-known songs. Others may utter expletives when excited or angered. Some people with expressive aphasia hesitate in trying to express words. They struggle to form words while using motor musculature (verbal apraxia), an articulatory disorder associated with some expressive aphasias. All these difficulties may cause patients to experience exasperation and despair. Most patients with nonfluent aphasia also have severely impaired writing ability. Even though their penmanship may be adequate, they are unable to express themselves through writing—a deficit termed *agraphia.* If the right hand is paralyzed, as is often the case, patients cannot write or print with the left hand.[18] In the recovery phase of severe expressive aphasia, patients regain the ability to speak aloud, albeit slowly and laboriously. Many patients learn to communicate ideas to some extent.

GLOBAL APHASIA. Global aphasia results when a massive lesion affects both the motor and sensory speech areas. Patients are unable to transform sounds into words and comprehend speech. All language modalities are affected, and impairment may be so severe that patients are unable to communicate on any level. These patients generally have severe hemiplegia and homonymous hemianopsia. These patients rarely regain a significant degree of language function, unless the lesion is caused by a transient disorder such as cerebral edema or metabolic derangement.[18]

Educating patients and families

Educating patients and families includes teaching them about stroke and its management, answering their questions, and preparing them for discharge or rehabilitation. Discharge teaching should include methods to compensate for residual deficits. Nurses should also encourage participation in rehabilitation and support groups and stress the importance of taking prescribed medications.[19]

Cerebral Tumors

Description and Etiology

The overall incidence of central nervous system (CNS) tumors in the United States is 36,000 cases annually, with 80% involving the brain and 20% involving the spinal cord.[20] The incidence of tumors peaks in two age groups: childhood (ages 3 to 12) and in later years (ages 50 to 70).

In the CNS, most primary neoplastic growths result from irregular mitosis of the support cells, the neuroglia. Neurons themselves have little ability to regenerate and little to no mitotic capability. Primary CNS tumors are classified as *benign* or *malignant,* but the definition of these terms varies from the tumor classification system used for the rest of the body. Benign CNS tumors are those growths lying in accessible areas of the CNS, with slow growth and lack of invasiveness. They can be completely removed without significant neurologic deficit. Malignant tumors are neoplasms (such as glioblastoma multiforme) that have multiple, fingerlike projections into normal tissue. Attempts to completely remove all of the tumor would cause unacceptable neurologic damage. Another type of CNS malignancy is the presence of a usually benign growth that lies deep in vital structures of the CNS where attempt at removal would cause severe neurologic deficit. It is malignant by location, not by histologic classification.[2] Generally CNS tumors do not metastasize outside the CNS, but metastatic cells from the body can reproduce in the CNS. Primary lesions of the lung, breast, and prostate contribute most significantly to metastatic lesions in the brain.[20]

Pathophysiology

The accurate identification of the cell of origin and assessment of the aggressiveness of the cells of the tumor is essential to understand the pathophysiology associated with any tumor of the brain or spinal cord. A variety of classification systems have been developed over the years to categorize CNS tumor cells. For the purposes of this

TABLE 15-1
CEREBRAL TUMORS

TYPE	INCIDENCE	ETIOLOGY	PATHOPHYSIOLOGY
MENINGIOMA	10%-15% of all intracranial tumors	Arise from the meninges and their derivatives; generally benign, malignant form rare	Highly vascular tumor that receives its blood supply from the meninges; slow-growing; firm, rubbery consistency that is easy to differentiate from normal tissue; most frequent location is the parasagittal region; may erode into bone of skull
GLIOMA Astrocytoma (grades I-IV)	30%-40% of intracranial tumors; 30% of tumors in children	Derived from astrocytes, which are the support framework for neurons and capillaries in the CNS	More rapid growing than meningiomas and not well-differentiated from edematous or necrotic brain; rarely metastasizes outside the CNS. Classified in ascending grades of malignancy; grade IV also known as *glioblastoma multiforme*
Oligodendroglioma	4%-5% of intracranial tumors	Arise from oligodendroglial cells, which are normally responsible for the myelin sheath in the CNS	May be slow-growing or a rapidly growing, highly malignant form. Well-defined, globular or cystic; can be soft, gelatinous, or mucinous. Located in the cerebral hemispheres, primarily frontal lobe, and occasionally in the ventricles
Ependymoma	5%-6% of intracranial tumors; most often seen in children and young adults	Arise from ependymal cells, which are responsible for the lining of the ventricular system and the choroid plexus	Slow-growing and usually benign histology but difficult to remove because of location in ventricles; fourth ventricle most common site. Causes obstruction of CSF outflow or erosion into the surrounding structures.
CRANIOPHARYN-GIOMA	Small percentage of intracranial tumors (2%-4%); most common in 30-40 year age group; may be seen in children	Arise from squamous cell nests	Benign, congenital, slow-growing tumor; largely cystic, solid; well-defined and firmly attached to surrounding brain tissue. Location usually midline at the base of the brain near the pituitary stalk; often causes depressed anterior pituitary function. Could fill third ventricle, causing obstruction; could place pressure on optic chiasm or invade sella turcica, basal ganglia, or brainstem. Tends to recur because of embryonic remnants
PINEAL TUMOR	More common in men than in women between 20-30 years of age; may be called *teratoma*	Arise from primitive germ cells that migrate during fetal development	Most often located near the pineal gland; well-defined white-yellow or dark-brown cystic areas that contain remnants of bone, cartilage, teeth, or hair. Pinealoma also contains melatonin, which inhibits sexual development. Can extend and recur; can obstruct the cerebral aqueduct and third ventricle
PITUITARY TUMOR	8%-12% of all intracranial tumors	Arise from selected cells of the anterior pituitary gland	Causes endocrine system dysfunction resulting from dysfunction of pituitary hormone secretion through hypersecretion (eosinophilic or basophilic), hyposecretion, or disruption of function because of mass effect (chromophobic adenoma). Also can cause pressure on the optic chiasm, hypothalamic dysfunction, or erosion through sella turcica into nasal sinuses

TABLE 15-1—cont'd
CEREBRAL TUMORS

TYPE	INCIDENCE	ETIOLOGY	PATHOPHYSIOLOGY
VASCULAR TUMOR	Small percentage of intracranial tumors; more common in females	Called *hemangiomas* or *hemangioblastoma;* arise from abnormally developed blood vessels	Most located near skull or vertebral column; dura often involved; slow-growing mass, cavernous type; has a honeycomb appearance with irregular margins. Potential danger from this tumor type includes hemorrhage
METASTATIC TUMOR	10% of intracranial tumors	Arise from cells that have metastasized from primary site, particularly lung, breast, kidney, or melanoma	Metastasis that could appear anywhere in the intracranial space; single or multiple sites in brain. Usually well-defined, circumscribed, and solid; easy to distinguish from brain tissue. Can be area of initial symptoms before primary site is discovered.

TABLE 15-2
BRAIN TUMORS AND RELATED SYMPTOMS

TUMOR LOCATION	SYMPTOMS
Frontal lobe	Disturbed mental state, apathy, inappropriate behavior, dementia, depression, emotional lability, inattentiveness, inability to concentrate, indifference, loss of self-restraint and social behavior, impaired recent memory, difficulty with abstraction, quiet but flat affect, speech disturbance, impaired sphincter control with bowel and bladder incontinence, motor disorders, gait disturbances, paralysis, "frontal release signs," seizures
Temporal lobe	Aphasia, generalized psychomotor seizures, visual field changes, personality changes, ataxia, headache, signs and symptoms of increased ICP, tinnitus, memory impairment
Parietal lobe	Sensory deficits, motor and sensory focal seizures, agnosias, dominant hemisphere speech deficits/receptive aphasia, hypesthesias, paresthesias, dyslexia, visual field cut, diminished appreciation of the side opposite the tumor, headache, apraxia, tactile inattention, right and left disorientation
Occipital lobe	Headache, signs and symptoms of increased ICP, visual impairment (homonymous hemianopsia), visual agnosia, cortical blindness, hallucinations, seizures
Cerebellar	Unsteady gait, falling, ataxia, incoordination, tremors, head tilt, nystagmus, CSF obstruction/hydrocephalus, lower cranial dysfunction of CN VIII-XII, truncal ataxia if vermis is tumor site
Brainstem	Vertigo, dizziness, vomiting, CN IV-XII palsies/dysfunction, nystagmus, decreased corneal reflex, headache, vomiting, gait disturbance, motor and sensory deficits, deafness, intranuclear ophthalmoplegia, sudden death from cardiac and respiratory failure
Pituitary and hypothalamus	Visual deficits, headache, hormonal dysfunction, sleep disturbances, water imbalance, temperature fluctuations, imbalance in fat and carbohydrate metabolism, Cushing's syndrome
Ventricular	Obstruction of CSF circulation, hydrocephalus, rapid rise in ICP, postural headache

From Barker E: *Neuroscience nursing,* St Louis, 1994, Mosby.

discussion, tumors are grouped by the cell of origin and order of frequency (Table 15-1).[21]

Assessment and Diagnosis

Assessment of a suspected CNS tumor focuses on patients' specific neurologic abnormalities. Possible neurologic dysfunctions are as varied as the different portions of the CNS (Table 15-2). Patients may initially have focal neurologic deficit, history of increasing headaches that are worse in the morning than in the evening, seizure activity, hormonal changes, and personality changes.[2]

Physical examination serves to define further the focal neurologic deficit. If the tumor is large enough to create a mass effect, the classic triad of papilledema, vomiting, and headache may be found.[22] Depending on the suspected abnormality, diagnostic workup may include a CT scan, magnetic resonance imaging, electroencephalogram, neuroendocrine tests, cerebral angiogram, chest x-ray examination, and bone scan. After a specific lesion has been identified, a biopsy specimen is frequently obtained for histologic examination.[2] Once the type of tumor has been diagnosed, medical management can be planned.

Medical Management

Medical management of a CNS tumor centers on surgery, radiation, and chemotherapy. Depending on the type and location of the tumor, any or all of these treatment modalities may be employed. If cerebral edema is a major factor associated with the identified tumor, steroid therapy is often the beginning point of medical management. Steroids, particularly dexamethasone (Decadron), can produce a significant but temporary reversal of neurologic symptoms. Steroids, believed to reduce cerebral edema by strengthening the cell membrane, decrease neurologic deficit by reducing ICP.[2]

Surgical intervention

Removal of the entire lesion is the goal but not always the outcome of surgery. In benign, well-defined lesions, surgical removal may be the only treatment necessary. In invasive, poorly defined lesions, surgery is the beginning point of treatment. Even though a craniotomy will not remove 100% of an invasive tumor, "debulking" of the tumor mass reduces pressure on surrounding structures and may slow the growth process.[23]

Radiation

With incompletely excised tumors, radiation is often the next step of medical management. Some tumors that occur in functionally critical areas such as the brainstem, hypothalamus, and thalamus are not surgically accessible without significant neurologic deficit. Radiation may be the primary method for medical management of these tumors. The goal of radiation is to destroy or retard the growth of tumor cells without damaging normal tissue. Histologic diagnosis of the tumor cell is essential in planning the type of radiation to be used. The total dose of radiation varies, depending on the tumor type, location, size of the field, and prior or concurrent chemotherapy.[24]

Chemotherapy

Chemotherapy treatment is another option for patients with malignant brain tumors. Cytotoxic agents are usually used because of their ability to cross the blood-brain barrier. In addition, multiple chemotherapeutic agents are usually used because of their synergistic effects. The agents may be administered intravenously, intraarterially, or through an Ommaya reservoir.[2]

Investigational therapy

A new technique for tumor management under clinical investigation is stereotactic radiosurgery. Radiosurgery is performed by directing a single high dose of ionizing radiation toward a small, well-defined intracranial lesion without significantly affecting surrounding tissue. This technique employs a "gamma knife," or external high-energy photon beams, from a linear accelerator.[25] The fact that radiosurgery is often performed with local anesthesia and without surgical incision makes radiosurgery a primary treatment alternative for older patients and those who are medically infirm or resistant to microsurgical removal.[26]

Nursing Management

The major part of nursing management of patients with a CNS tumor does not occur in the critical care environment. Generally patients are in the critical care unit during the postoperative stage of a craniotomy with a variety of nursing diagnoses (Box 15-3). **Nursing priorities are directed toward observing for signs of increased intracranial pressure and other complications of surgery, offering psychosocial support, and educating patients and families.**

Observing for signs of increased intracranial pressure

With the advent of steroids, the cerebral edema associated with brain tumors and craniotomy has virtually been eliminated, although patients should still be observed for signs of increased intracranial pressure. Generally patients with an uncomplicated craniotomy for removal of a brain tumor remain in the critical care unit overnight. Patients who have had a cervical or high thoracic spinal cord tumor excised remain in the unit postoperatively for close observation of respiratory status and motor/sensory function of the extremities.[2]

Offering psychological support

Nurses should never ignore the psychosocial aspects facing patients with a CNS tumor, even in the immediate postoperative period. Nurses should offer support to family members and significant others, as well as to patients.[2]

Educating patients and families

Educating patients and families includes teaching them about intracranial tumors and their management, answering their questions, and preparing them for discharge or rehabilitation. Discharge teaching should include methods to compensate for residual deficits and manage seizures. Nurses should encourage participation in rehabilitation and support groups and stress the importance of taking prescribed medications.[19]

Guillain-Barré Syndrome

Description and Etiology

Guillain-Barré syndrome (GBS) is an inflammatory peripheral polyneuritis characterized by a rapidly progressive, ascending **peripheral nerve dysfunction** leading to paralysis. Because of the ventilatory support required for these patients, GBS is one of the few peripheral neurologic diseases requiring a critical care environment. The cause of GBS is unknown, but more than 60% of patients report a viral infection 2 to 4 weeks before the onset of clinical manifestations. The result is an autoimmune response of the peripheral nervous system.[27,28]

Pathophysiology

This disease affects the motor and sensory pathways of the peripheral nervous system, as well as the autonomic nervous system functions of the cranial nerves. The major finding in GBS is a segmental demyelination process of the peripheral nerves. GBS is believed to be an autoimmune response to antibodies formed against a recent viral illness, usually upper respiratory or gastrointestinal. T-cells migrate to the peripheral nerves, resulting in edema and inflammation. Macrophages then invade the area and break down the myelin.[29] Inflammation around this demyelinated area causes further dysfunction.[28]

The myelin sheath of the peripheral nerves is generated by Schwann's cells and acts as an insulator for the peripheral nerve. Myelin promotes rapid conduction of nerve impulses by allowing the impulses to jump along the nerve via the nodes of Ranvier. Disruption of the myelin fiber slows and may eventually stop the conduction of impulses along the peripheral nerves. In GBS the more thickly myelinated fibers of motor pathways and cranial nerves are more severely affected than the thinly myelinated sensory fibers of cutaneous pain, touch, and temperature.[29]

Once the temporary inflammatory reaction stops, myelin-producing cells begin to reinsulate the demyelinated portions of the peripheral nervous system. When remyelination occurs, normal neurologic function should return. In some instances the axon may be damaged during the inflammatory process. The degree of axonal damage is responsible for the degree of neurologic dysfunction that persists after recovery.[28]

Assessment and Diagnosis

Symptoms of GBS include motor weakness, paresthesias and other sensory changes, cranial nerve dysfunction (especially oculomotor, facial, glossopharyngeal, vagal, spinal accessory, and hypoglossal), and some autonomic nervous system dysfunction.[2] The usual course of GBS begins with an abrupt onset of lower extremity weakness that progresses to flaccidity and ascends over a period of hours to days. Motor loss is usually symmetric, bilateral, and ascending. In the most severe cases complete flaccidity of all peripheral nerves, including spinal and cranial nerves, occurs.[27,29]

Admission to the hospital occurs when lower extremity weakness prevents mobility. Admission to the critical care unit occurs when progression of the weakness threatens respiratory muscles. As patients' weakness progresses, close observation is essential. Frequent assessment of the respiratory system, including ventilatory parameters such as inspiratory force and tidal volume, is necessary. The most common cause of death in patients with GBS is respiratory arrest. As the disease progresses and respiratory effort weakens, intubation and mechanical ventilation are necessary. Continued, frequent assessment of neurologic deterioration is required until patients reach the peak of the disease and plateau occurs.[2,28]

The diagnosis of GBS is based on clinical findings, CSF analysis, and nerve conduction studies. CSF analysis demonstrates a protein that appears normal initially but elevates in the fourth to sixth week. No other changes in the CSF occur. Nerve conduction studies that test the velocity at which nerve impulses are conducted show significant reduction, as the demyelinating process of the disease suggests.[28]

Medical Management

With no curative treatment available, the medical management of GBS is limited. It must simply run its course, which is characterized by ascending paralysis that advances over 1 to 3 weeks and then remains at a plateau for several weeks. The plateau stage is followed by descending paralysis and return to normal or near-normal function. The main focus of medical management is the support of bodily functions and the prevention of complications.[28]

Plasmapheresis

Often used in the treatment of GBS, plasmapheresis involves plasma exchanges or washes that remove the antibodies causing GBS.[27] A recently published study of

NURSING DIAGNOSIS PRIORITIES

GUILLAIN-BARRÉ

Ineffective Breathing Pattern related to musculoskeletal or neuromuscular impairment, p. 486

Acute *Pain* related to transmission and perception of cutaneous, visceral, muscular, or ischemic impulses, p. 499

Anxiety related to threat to biologic, psychologic, and/or social integrity, p. 464

Powerlessness related to health care environment and illness-related regimen, p. 460

Knowledge Deficit related to lack of previous exposure to information, p. 455

220 patients in a multicenter clinical trial demonstrated that 71% of the plasmapheresis treatment group (versus 52% of the control group) had full muscular strength recovery at 1 year.[30]

Nursing Management

Nursing management of patients with GBS incorporates a variety of nursing diagnoses (Box 15-4). The goal of nursing management is to support all normal body functions until patients can do so on their own. Patients with GBS may be immobile for months. Although the condition is reversible, recovery from GBS is a long process. **Nursing priorities are directed toward providing ventilatory support and pulmonary toilet, facilitating nutritional support, providing comfort and emotional support, and educating patients and families.**

Providing ventilatory support and pulmonary toilet

Total ventilatory support and pulmonary toilet are required at the peak level of the illness. As patients' symptoms recede, weaning from the ventilator and initiation of coughing and deep breathing exercises are important ways to prevent pulmonary complications.[27]

Facilitating nutritional support

Nutritional support should be implemented early in the course of the disease. Because GBS recovery is a long process, adequate nutritional support over an extended period of time presents problems. Nutritional support is usually accomplished through enteral feeding, which is preferable to total parenteral nutrition because it is less invasive and reduces the risk of infection in patients who are highly vulnerable.

Providing comfort and emotional support

Pain control is another important component in the care of patients with GBS. Although patients have minimal to no motor function, most sensory functions remain, causing them considerable muscle ache and pain. Because of the length of this illness, nurses must work closely with physicians and patients to identify a safe, effective, long-term solution to pain management. These patients require extensive emotional support. Although the illness is almost 100% reversible, the total helplessness of patients, their constant pain or discomfort, and the length of the disease create difficulties in coping with this condition. Nurses should remember that GBS does not affect the level of consciousness or cerebral function. Interaction and communication are necessary elements of the nursing management plan.

Educating patients and families

Educating patients and families includes teaching them about Guillain-Barré and its management, answering their questions, and preparing them for discharge or rehabilitation. Discharge teaching should include methods to compensate for any residual deficits and techniques for pain management. Nurses should encourage participation in rehabilitation and stress the importance of taking prescribed medications.[19]

References

1. Mitiguy J: Spontaneous intracranial hemorrhage: the brain under attack, *Headlines* 2(3):2, 1991.
2. Barker E: *Neuroscience nursing*, St Louis, 1994, Mosby.
3. Cook H: Aneurysmal subarachnoid hemorrhage: neurosurgical frontiers and nursing challenges, *AACN Clin Iss Crit Care Nurs* 2:665, 1991.
4. Welty TE, Horner TG: Pathophysiology and treatment of subarachnoid hemorrhage, *Clin Pharm* 9:35, 1990.
5. Manifold SL: Aneurysmal SAH: cerebral vasospasm and early repair, *Crit Care Nurs* 10(8):62, 1990.
6. Findlay JM, Macdonald RL, Weir BK: Current concepts of pathophysiology and management of cerebral vasospasm following aneurysmal subarachnoid hemorrhage, *Cerebrovasc Brain Metab Rev* 3(4):336, 1991.
7. Armstrong SL: Cerebral vasospasm: early detection and intervention, *Crit Care Nurs* 14(4):33, 1994.
8. Sikes PJ, Nolan S: Pharmacologic management of cerebral vasospasm, *Crit Care Nurs Q* 15(4):79, 1993.
9. Robinson MJ, Teasdale GM: Calcium antagonists in the management of subarachnoid hemorrhage, *Cerebrovasc Brain Metab Rev* 2(3):205, 1990.
10. Kassell NF and others: The International Cooperative Study on the Timing of Aneurysm Surgery, *Neurosurg* 73:37, 1990.
11. McNair N: Arteriovenous malformation, *Crit Care Nurs* 8(4):35, 1988.
12. Davis A: *Intracerebral hemorrhage.* In Commermeyer M, Appledorn C: *Core curriculum for neuroscience nursing,* ed 3, Chicago, 1990, American Association of Neuroscience Nurses.
13. Wall BM, Philips JP, Howard JC: Validation of increased intracranial pressure and high risk for increased intracranial pressure, *Nurs Diagnosis* 5:74, 1994.
14. Olson E: Perceptual deficits affecting the stroke patient, *Rehabil Nurs* 16(4):213, 1991.
15. Baggerly J: Sensory perceptual problems following stroke: the "invisible" deficits, *Nurs Clin North Am* 26:997, 1991.

16. Kalbach LR: Unilateral neglect: mechanisms and nursing care, *J Neurosci Nurs* 23(2):125, 1991.
17. Phipps MA: Assessment of neurologic deficits in stroke: acute and rehabilitation implications, *Nurs Clin North Am* 26:957, 1991.
18. Boss BJ: Managing communication disorders in stroke, *Nurs Clin North Am* 26:985, 1991.
19. Chipps EM, Clanin NJ, Campbell VG: *Neurologic disorders*, St Louis, 1992, Mosby.
20. American Cancer Society: *Facts on cancer of the brain*, Atlanta, 1988, American Cancer Society.
21. Zulch DJ: Principles of the new World Health Organization (WHO) classification of brain tumors, *Neuroradiology* 19:59, 1980.
22. Barker E: Brain tumor: frightening diagnosis, nursing challenge, *RN* 53(9):46, 1990.
23. Cammermeyer M: *Cerebral tumors.* In Commermeyer M, Appeldorn C: *Core curriculum for neuroscience nursing*, ed 3, Chicago, 1990, American Association of Neuroscience Nurses.
24. Association for Brain Tumor Research: *Radiation therapy of brain tumors*, Chicago, 1990, Association for Brain Tumor Research.
25. Mughmaw SB: An overview of methods in stereotactic surgery, *Radiol Tech* 63:402, 1992.
26. Stephanian E and others: Gamma knife surgery for sellar and suprasellar tumors, *Neurosurg Clin North Am* 3:207, 1992.
27. Mascarella JJ, Hudson DC: Dysimmune neurologic disorders, *AACN Clin Iss Crit Care Nurs* 26:985, 1991.
28. Hund EF and others: Intensive management and treatment of severe Guillain-Barré syndrome, *Crit Care Med* 21:433, 1993.
29. Ross AP: Nursing interventions for persons receiving immunosuppressive therapies for demyelinating pathology, *Nurs Clin North Am* 28:829, 1993.
30. French Cooperative Group on Plasma Exchange: Plasma exchange in Guillain-Barré syndrome one year follow-up, *Ann Neurol* 32:94, 1992.

16

Neurologic Therapeutic Management

KATHLEEN A. MENDEZ

CHAPTER OBJECTIVES

- Discuss the concept of cerebral autoregulation.
- Calculate cerebral perfusion pressure.
- Describe the therapies commonly used to treat intracranial hypertension.

- Identify the different types of intracranial pressure monitoring devices.
- List the four supratentorial herniation syndromes.

KEY TERMS

TABLE 16-1
MECHANISMS OF ICP ELEVATION

PATHOPHYSIOLOGY	EXAMPLE	TREATMENT
Disorders of CSF space		
Overproduction of CSF	Choroid plexus papilloma	Diuretics, surgical removal
Communicating hydrocephalus from obstructed arachnoid	Old subarachnoid hemorrhage	Surgical drainage from lumbar intrathecal site
Noncommunicative hydrocephalus	Posterior fossa tumor obstructing aqueduct	Surgical drainage by ventricular drainage
Interstitial edema	Any of above	Surgical drainage of CSF
Disorders of intracranial blood		
Intracranial hemorrhage causing increased ICP	Epidural hematoma	Surgical drainage
Vasospasm	Subarachnoid hemorrhage	Hypervolemia and hypertensive therapy Calcium channel antagonists
Vasodilation	Elevated $Paco_2$	Hyperventilation and adequate oxygenation
Increasing cerebral blood volume and ICP	Hypoxia	
Disorders of brain substance		
Expanding mass lesion with local vasogenic edema causing increased ICP	Brain tumor	Steroids Surgical removal
Ischemic brain injury with cytotoxic edema increasing ICP	Anoxic brain injury from cardiac or respiratory arrest	Resistant to therapy
Increased cerebral metabolic rate increasing cerebral blood flow and ICP	Seizures, hyperthermia	Anticonvulsant medications, especially barbiturates, control fever

From: Helfaer MA, Kirsch JR: Intracranial vault pathophysiology, *Crit Care Rep* 1:12, 1989.

Despite the diversity of neurologic abnormalities, one aspect of the critical care management of patients with neurologic disorders is common to a wide variety of these pathologic conditions. This chapter focuses on the priority interventions used to manage increased intracranial pressure in the critical care environment.

Assessment of Intracranial Pressure

Monro-Kellie Hypothesis

The intracranial space comprises brain substance (80%), cerebrospinal fluid (CSF) (10%), and blood (10%).[1] Under normal physiologic conditions ICP is maintained below 15 mm Hg mean pressure. Essential for understanding the pathophysiology of ICP, the Monro-Kellie hypothesis proposes that an increase in volume of one intracranial component must be compensated by a decrease in one or more of the other components, so total volume remains fixed. This compensation, although limited, includes displacing CSF from the intracranial vault to the lumbar cistern, increasing CSF absorption, and compressing the low-pressure venous system.[2] Pathophysiologic alterations that can elevate ICP are outlined in Table 16-1.

Volume-Pressure Curve

When capable of compliance, the brain can tolerate significant increases in intracranial volume without much increase in ICP. The amount of intracranial compliance, however, is limited. Once this limit has been reached, a state of decompensation with increased ICP results. As ICP rises, the relationship between volume and pressure changes, and small increases in volume may cause major elevations in ICP (Fig. 16-1). The exact configuration of the volume-pressure curve and point at which the steep rise in pressure occurs vary among patients. The configuration of this curve is also influenced by the cause and rate of volume increases within the intracranial vault; for example, neurologic deterioration occurs more rapidly in patients with an acute epidural hematoma than in patients with a meningioma of the same size.[2,3]

Cerebral Blood Flow and Autoregulation

Cerebral blood flow (CBF) corresponds to the metabolic demands of the brain. Although the brain makes up only 2% of body weight, it requires 15% to 20% of the resting cardiac output and 15% of the body's oxygen demands. The normal brain has a complex capacity to maintain a constant CBF despite wide ranges in arterial

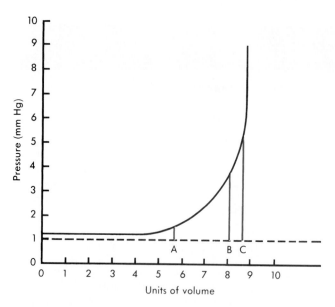

FIG. 16-1 Intracranial volume-pressure curve. **A,** Pressure is normal, and increases in intracranial volume are tolerated without increase in intracranial pressure. **B,** Increases in volume may cause increases in pressure. **C,** Small increases in volume may cause large increases in pressure.

pressure—an effect known as *autoregulation.* Mean arterial pressure (MAP) of 50 to 150 mm Hg does not alter CBF when autoregulation is present. Outside the limits of this autoregulation, CBF becomes passively dependent on the perfusion pressure.[2]

Factors other than arterial blood pressure affecting CBF are conditions that result in acidosis, alkalosis, and changes in metabolic rate. Conditions causing acidosis (hypoxia, hypercapnia, and ischemia) result in cerebral vascular dilation. Conditions causing alkalosis (e.g., hypocapnia) result in cerebral vascular constriction. Normally, a reduction in metabolic rate (e.g., from hypothermia or barbiturates) decreases CBF, and increases in metabolic rate (e.g., from hyperthermia) increase CBF.[4]

Arterial blood gases exert a profound effect on CBF. Carbon dioxide, which affects the pH of the blood, is a potent vasoactive substance. Carbon dioxide retention (hypercapnia) leads to cerebral vasodilation, and increased cerebral blood volume, whereas hypocapnia leads to cerebral vasoconstriction and reduced cerebral blood volume.[2] Prolonged hypocapnia, however, especially at an arterial partial pressure of carbon dioxide ($Paco_2$) less than 20 mm Hg, can produce cerebral ischemia.[5] Low arterial partial pressure of oxygen (Pao_2), especially below 40 mm Hg, leads to cerebral vasodilation, which increases the intracranial blood volume and can contribute to increased ICP. The brain is thus exposed to ischemia directly through arterial hypoxemia, as well as through increased ICP. High Pao_2 levels have not been shown to affect CBF in either direction.[2]

Metabolic activity in the brain significantly influences CBF. Normally, when cerebral metabolic activity in-

creases, CBF also increases to meet the demand. Any pathologic process that decreases CBF could lead to a mismatch between metabolic demand and blood supply, resulting in cerebral ischemia.[2,5]

Cerebral Perfusion Pressure

Measuring CBF in the clinical setting is difficult. **Cerebral perfusion pressure** (CPP), an estimated pressure, is the blood pressure gradient across the brain and is calculated as the difference between the incoming MAP and the opposing ICP on the arteries (CPP = MAP − ICP). The CPP in the average adult is approximately 80 to 100 mm Hg, with a range of 60 to 150 mm Hg. The CPP should be maintained near 80 mm Hg to provide adequate blood supply to the brain. If the CPP drops below this point, ischemia may develop. A sustained CPP of 30 mm Hg or less will usually result in neuronal hypoxia and cell death. When the mean systemic arterial pressure equals the ICP, CBF may cease.[6]

Assessment Techniques

Signs and symptoms

The numerous signs and symptoms of increased ICP include decreased level of consciousness, Cushing's triad (bradycardia, systolic hypertension, and bradypnea), diminished brainstem reflexes, papilledema, decerebrate posturing (abnormal extension), decorticate posturing (abnormal flexion), unequal pupil size, projectile vomiting, decreased pupillary reaction to light, altered breathing patterns, and headache.[7] Patients may exhibit one or all of these symptoms, depending on the underlying cause of the elevation in ICP. **One of the earliest and most important signs of increased ICP is a decrease in the level of consciousness. This change should be reported immediately to physicians.**

Monitoring techniques

The common sites for monitoring ICP are the intraventricular, subarachnoid, and epidural spaces and the parenchyma. Each system has advantages and disadvantages for monitoring ICP (Table 16-2).[1,8] The type of monitor chosen depends on both the suspected pathologic condition and physicians' preferences.

VENTRICULOSTOMY. The type of monitor placed in the ventricular system is usually a small catheter known as a *ventriculostomy catheter.* Inserted through a burr hole while patients are under local anesthesia, it is usually placed in the anterior horn of the lateral ventricle. If at all possible, the ventriculostomy catheter is placed in the nondominant hemisphere (Fig. 16-2, *A*).[1,8,9]

SUBARACHNOID BOLT. The second type of monitor frequently used is the subarachnoid bolt or screw. This small, hollow device is inserted through a burr hole, with the distal end lying in the subarachnoid or subdural space, while patients are under local anesthesia. Inserting this device (Fig. 16-2, *B*) is easier than inserting the ventriculostomy catheter.[1,8]

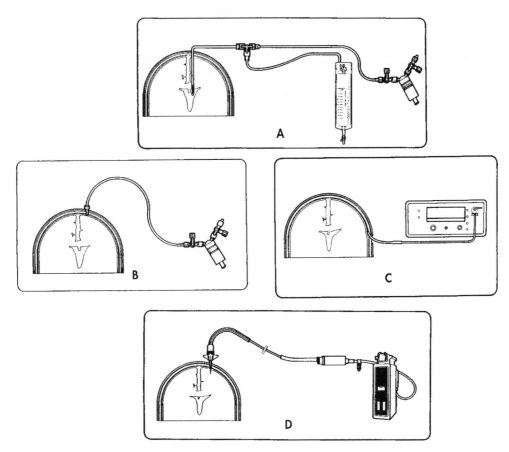

FIG. 16-2 A, Ventricular pressure monitoring system. **B,** Subarachnoid pressure monitoring system. **C,** Epidural pressure monitoring system. **D,** Intraparenchymal pressure monitoring system. (Courtesy Camino Laboratories, San Diego, CA.)

EPIDURAL MONITOR. Another type of device commonly used is the epidural monitor, also placed through a burr hole while patients are under local anesthesia. Physicians strip the dura away from the inner table of the skull before inserting the epidural monitor. The most common type of epidural monitor is the fiberoptic or pneumatic sensor, although other implantable epidural transducers are often used for long-term monitoring (Fig. 16-2, *C*).[1,8]

FIBEROPTIC CATHETER. The fourth type of ICP monitoring system is the fiberoptic transducer-tipped catheter (Fig. 16-2, *D*). This small (4F) catheter can be placed intraventricularly, intraparenchymally, in the subarachnoid space, or in the subdural space.[1,8]

Intracranial pressure waves

Since the beginning of ICP monitoring, clinicians have been interested in the waveforms associated with intracranial dynamics. As with arterial and pulmonary artery waves, the normal **ICP wave** has a distinct waveform (Fig. 16-3). Three different abnormal waveforms have also been identified. These are known as A, B, and C waves (Fig. 16-4). These waves reflect spontaneous alterations in ICP associated with respiration, systemic blood pressure, and deteriorating neurologic status.[8]

NORMAL ICP WAVEFORM. Intracranial pressure waveforms have three distinct peaks known as P_1, P_2, and P_3. P_1, also called the *percussion wave*, is the first peak and is associated with arterial pulsations. P_2, also known as

the *tidal wave*, and P_3, also known as the *dicrotic wave*, are associated with venous pulsations. With increased intracranial pressure, the amplitude of P_2 becomes greater than that of the other two waves.[8]

A WAVES. A waves, also called *plateau waves* because of their distinctive shape, are the most clinically significant of the three types. A waves usually occur in an already elevated baseline ICP (greater than 20 mm Hg) and are characterized by sharp increases in ICP of 30 to 69 mm Hg, which remain at a plateau for 2 to 20 minutes and then return to baseline. The actual cause of A waves is unknown, but they may result from vasodilation and increased CBF, decreased venous outflow (and therefore increased cerebral blood volume), fluctuations in $Paco_2$ (and therefore changes in cerebral blood volume), or decreased CSF absorption. B waves frequently precede A waves. Plateau waves are considered significant because of the reduced cerebral perfusion pressure associated with ICP in the 50 to 100 mm Hg range. Transient signs of intracranial hypertension such as a decreased level of consciousness, bradycardia, pupillary changes, and respiratory changes may accompany these waves. Some research suggests that prolonged increases in ICP associated with plateau waves could result in transient as well as permanent cell damage from ischemia. Management of A waves is directed at the reduction of the high pressure and prevention of other plateau waves.[1,8]

B WAVES. B waves are sharp, rhythmic oscillations with a sawtooth appearance that occur every 30 seconds to 2 minutes and can raise the ICP from 5 to 70 mm Hg. B waves are a normal physiologic phenomenon that occur in everyone but are amplified in states of low intracranial compliance. B waves appear to reflect fluctuations in cerebral blood volume. Decompensation of normal intracranial volume compensatory capacity is indicated by B waves with a high amplitude (greater than 15 mm Hg pressure change from peak to trough of wave).[1,8]

C WAVES. C waves, smaller rhythmic waves that occur every 4 to 8 minutes, occur at normal levels of ICP. C waves are related to normal fluctuations in respirations and systemic arterial pressure.[1,8]

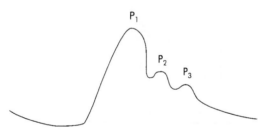

FIG. 16-3 Components of a normal intracranial pressure waveform. (From Barker E: *Neuroscience nursing*, St Louis, 1994, Mosby.)

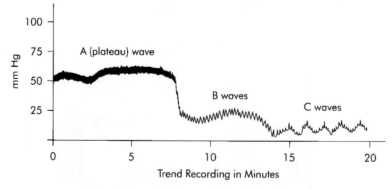

FIG. 16-4 Abnormal intracranial pressure waveforms. (From Barker E: *Neuroscience Nursing,* St Louis, 1994, Mosby.)

Management of Intracranial Hypertension

Once intracranial hypertension is documented, therapy must be prompt to prevent secondary insults. Although the exact pressure level denoting intracranial hypertension remains uncertain, most current evidence suggests ICP should generally be treated when it exceeds 20 mm Hg.[4] All therapies are directed toward reducing the volume of one or more of the components (blood, brain, CSF) that lie within the intracranial vault. A major goal of therapy is to determine the cause of the elevated pressure and, if possible, remove the cause.[10] In the absence of a surgically treatable mass lesion, intracranial hypertension is treated medically. Nurses play an important role in rapid assessment and implementation of appropriate therapies for reducing ICP. **Nursing priorities for the management of intracranial hypertension include keeping patients' heads elevated 30-45° and in a neutral plane; maintaining normothermia and controlled ventilation to ensure a $Paco_2$ level of 25-30 mm Hg and Pao_2 level greater than 70 mm Hg; administering diuretic agents, anticonvulsants, and medications to ensure systolic blood pressure between 140-160 mm Hg; and performing ventricular drainage (if ventriculostomy catheter is present).**

Patient Positioning

Positioning of patients is a significant factor in the prevention and treatment of elevated ICP. Positions that keep the head and neck elevated 30 to 45 degrees and in a neutral position at all times allow proper venous return. In these positions, gravity enhances venous drainage from the brain and head.[11,12] Positions that impede venous return from the brain cause elevations in ICP. Obstruction of jugular veins or an increase in intrathoracic or intraabdominal pressure is communicated as increased pressure throughout the open venous system, thereby impeding drainage from the brain and increasing ICP. Positions that decrease venous return from the head (i.e., Trendelenburg, prone, extreme flexion of the hips, and angulation of the neck) should be avoided if possible. If changes to positions such as Trendelenburg are necessary to provide adequate pulmonary care, critical care nurses must closely monitor ICP and vital signs. Mechanisms to reduce ICP (e.g., sedation, ventricular drainage) may also be employed while patients are in Trendelenburg's position.[13] Other impediments to cerebral venous drainage are positive end-expiratory pressure (PEEP) greater than 5 to 10 cm H_2O pressure, coughing, suctioning, tight tracheostomy tube ties, and Valsalva's maneuver.[3]

Hyperventilation

Controlled **hyperventilation** is an important adjunct of therapy for patients with increased ICP. If the carbon dioxide pressure ($Paco_2$) can be reduced from its normal level of 35 to 40 mm Hg to a range of 25 to 30 mm Hg in patients with intracranial hypertension, vasoconstriction of cerebral arteries, reduction of cerebral blood flow, and increased venous return will result. Reducing the intracranial blood volume results in a general reduction in ICP.[4] The use of controlled hyperventilation is currently under investigation. Research indicates that in certain situations of increased ICP, vasoconstriction of the cerebral vessels has already occurred. In these cases further application of controlled hyperventilation could cause vasoconstriction to such an extent that cerebral ischemia occurs.[14] Documentation shows that high levels of $Paco_2$ cause cerebral vasodilation and contribute to elevated ICP. For this reason $Paco_2$ levels greater than 40 mm Hg are considered dangerous.[2]

Although hypoxemia should obviously be avoided, excessively high levels of oxygen offer no benefits.[3] In fact, increasing inspired oxygen concentrations (FIO_2) above 60% may lead to toxic changes in lung tissue. The increasing use of devices for monitoring oxygen saturation (e.g., pulse oximeter) has led to a greater awareness of circumstances such as suctioning and restlessness that can cause oxygen desaturation and therefore elevate ICP.

Sedation and Neuromuscular Blocking Agents

Any treatment modality that increases the incidence of noxious stimulation can increase ICP. Such noxious stimuli include pain as a result of injuries sustained with the initial trauma, presence of an endotracheal tube, coughing, suctioning, repositioning, bathing, and many routine nursing care procedures. To ensure adequate ventilation ($Paco_2$ level of 25 to 30 and Pao_2 level greater than 70) and in anticipation of the deleterious effects of noxious stimuli on ICP, nurses may use sedatives alone or in combination with nondepolarizing neuromuscular blocking agents. Use of these medications is recommended only in patients who have an ICP monitor in place because sedatives and neuromuscular blocking agents in particular affect the reliability of neurologic assessment. Although sedation of unconscious patients can obscure portions of the neurologic examination, its benefit may outweigh the risks.[15]

Temperature Control

Directly proportional to body temperature, cerebral metabolic rate increases 5% to 7% per degree centigrade of increase in body temperature.[5] This fact is significant because as the cerebral metabolic rate increases, blood flow to the brain must increase to meet tissue demands. To avoid the increase in blood volume associated with increased cerebral metabolic rate, nurses must prevent hyperthermia in patients with a brain injury. Antipyretics and cooling devices should be used when appropriate while the source of the fever is being determined.[15]

Blood Pressure Control

Sustained systolic arterial hypertension (greater than 160 mm Hg) in conjunction with elevated ICP requires vigorous treatment. Control of systemic arterial hypertension may require nothing more than the administration of a sedative agent. Small, frequent doses may be sufficient to blunt noxious stimuli and prevent them from triggering rises in blood pressure. When sedation proves inadequate in controlling systemic arterial hypertension, primary antihypertensive agents are used. Care must be taken in choosing these agents because many of the peripheral vasodilators are also cerebral vasodilators (e.g., nitroprusside and nitroglycerin). However, all antihypertensives are believed to cause some degree of cerebral vasodilation. To reduce this vasodilating effect, cotreatment with beta blockers (e.g., propranolol and labetalol) may be beneficial.[15]

Seizure Control

The incidence of posttraumatic seizures in people with head injuries has been estimated at 5%. Because of the risk of a secondary ischemic insult associated with seizures, many physicians prescribe anticonvulsant medications prophylactically. Seizures cause metabolic requirements to increase, which results in elevation of cerebral blood flow, cerebral blood volume, and ICP—even in paralyzed patients. If blood flow cannot match demand, ischemia develops, cerebral energy stores are depleted, and irreversible neuronal destruction occurs. The usual anticonvulsant regimen for seizure control includes phenytoin or phenobarbital, or both, in therapeutic doses.[15]

Lidocaine

Various forms of sensory stimulation (including tracheal intubation, laryngoscopy, and endotracheal suctioning) may provoke marked increases in ICP and MAP. One therapy used to prevent cerebral ischemia and acute intracranial hypertension has been the administration of lidocaine through an endotracheal tube or intravenous infusion before nasotracheal suctioning.[4] Lidocaine is believed to be effective in blunting ICP spikes secondary to tracheal stimulation. Studies have found that peak lidocaine concentrations are linearly related to the administered dose and that the rate of absorption depends on the vascularity of the site of administration.[4] It has also been documented that lidocaine is initially distributed to the lungs, then to the heart and kidneys, and then to muscle and adipose tissue.[16]

Prophylactic administration of lidocaine before endotracheal suctioning is widely practiced. In most cases 50 to 100 mg is administered intravenously approximately 2 minutes before suctioning is performed. If the endotracheal route is chosen, 2 ml of 4% lidocaine is the preferred dose, and suctioning must be completed within 5 minutes of administering the drug. Adherence to this procedure is believed to protect patients from the associated increases in ICP that occur with suctioning. A number of studies in progress are investigating the usefulness of lidocaine in this area.[16]

Cerebrospinal Fluid Drainage

Cerebrospinal fluid drainage for intracranial hypertension may be used along with other treatment modalities. CSF drainage is accomplished by the insertion of a pliable catheter into the anterior horn of the lateral ventricle (ventriculostomy), preferably on the nondominant side. Such drainage can help support patients through periods of cerebral edema by controlling spikes in ICP. One of the major advantages of the ventriculostomy is its dual role as a monitoring device and treatment modality. Because CSF provides a favorable medium for infection, flawless aseptic technique must be followed during insertion and maintenance of the system. The ventricular system is connected to a drainage bag and then maintained as a closed system for the period of time the ventriculostomy catheter remains in place—usually 3 to 5 days (see Clinical Options box).[8]

Diuretics

Osmotic agents

Clinicians have known for decades that osmotic agents effectively reduce ICP. The mechanism by which these **diuretics** reduce ICP continues to be a subject of investigational interest. One theory is that these agents act by remaining relatively impermeable to the blood-brain barrier, thereby drawing water from normal brain tissue to plasma. The direction of flow is from the hypoconcentrated tissue to the hyperconcentrated cerebral vasculature. If the situation becomes reversed and the tissue becomes hyperconcentrated in relation to the cerebral vasculature, a rebound phenomenon could occur. These agents have little direct effect on edematous cerebral tissue situated in an area of defective blood-brain barrier; instead, they require an intact blood-brain barrier for osmosis to occur.[15]

The most widely used osmotic diuretic is mannitol, a large molecule that is retained almost entirely in the extracellular compartment and has little to none of the rebound effect noted with other osmotic diuretics. Mannitol may improve perfusion to ischemic areas of the brain, producing cerebral vasoconstriction and resulting in reduced ICP.[15]

Perhaps the most common difficulty associated with the use of osmotic agents is the production of electrolyte disturbances. Careful attention should be paid to body weight and fluid and electrolyte stability. Serum osmolality should be kept between 300 and 320 mOsm/L. Hypernatremia and hypokalemia are frequently associated with repeated administration of osmotic agents. Central venous pressure readings should be monitored to prevent hypovolemia.[15] Smaller doses of mannitol simplify fluid

CLINICAL OPTIONS

Intermittent vs. Continuous CSF Drainage

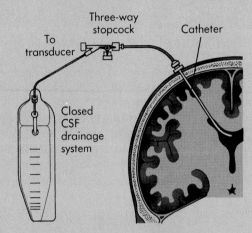

INTRAVENTRICULAR CATHETER

Fig. 16-5 Intermittent drainage system. (From Barker E: *Neuroscience nursing*, St Louis, 1994, Mosby.)

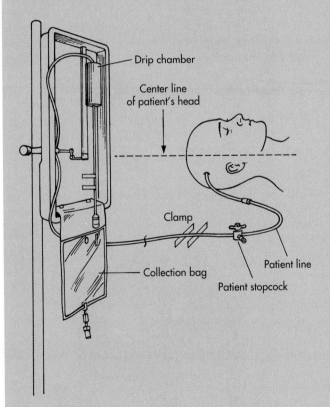

Fig. 16-6 Continuous drainage system. (Courtesy Codman & Shurtleff, Randolf, Mass.)

INTERMITTENT DRAINAGE SYSTEM

Intermittent drainage involves draining CSF via a ventriculostomy when ICP exceeds the upper pressure parameter set by physicians. Intermittent drainage involves opening the three way stopcock to allow CSF to flow into the drainage bag for brief periods (30 to 120 seconds) until the pressure is below the upper pressure parameter.

CONTINUOUS DRAINAGE SYSTEM

Continuous drainage involves placing the drip chamber of the drainage system at a specified level above the foramen of Monroe (usually 15 cm). The system is left open to allow continuous drainage of CSF into the chamber (which drains into a collection bag) against a pressure gradient that prevents excessive drainage and ventricular collapse.

and electrolyte management, and their use is encouraged whenever possible.[4]

Nonosmotic agents

Loop diuretics have also been used to decrease ICP. Furosemide, one such nonosmotic diuretic, may act differently from osmotic agents by pulling sodium and water from edematous areas and, perhaps, decreasing CSF production. One advantage of furosemide over osmotic diuretics is that its effect is not generally associated with increases in serum osmolality. Therefore electrolyte imbalances may not be as severe with the use of nonosmotic diuretics.[15]

High-Dose Barbiturate Therapy

Barbiturate therapy is a treatment protocol developed for the management of uncontrolled intracranial hypertension that does not respond to the conventional treatments previously described. *Uncontrolled ICP* is defined as an ICP greater than 20 mm Hg lasting 30 minutes or more that does not respond to aggressive use of conventional therapies, as an ICP greater than 40 mm Hg lasting 15 minutes or more, or CPP lower than 50 mm Hg.[5]

Although the specific action of barbiturates in the reduction of ICP is unclear, several theories explain their effect on the central nervous system and the subsequent cerebral protection they provide. Barbiturates increase cerebral vascular resistance in the undamaged portions of the brain, resulting in a decrease in cerebral blood flow and shunting of blood to the damaged portions of the brain. Barbiturates also slow cerebral metabolism by reducing the functional electrical generation of the neurons. This decreased cerebral metabolism thus lessens the glucose and oxygen demands of the brain. Barbiturates are also effective anticonvulsants and may suppress subclinical seizure activities (Table 16-3). Finally, some researchers postulate that barbiturates are scavengers of free radicals and thereby prevent cell membrane damage and destruction.[15]

The two most commonly used drugs in high-dose barbiturate therapy are pentobarbital and thiopental. The goal of either of these drugs is a reduction of ICP to 15 to 20 mm Hg while a MAP of 70 to 80 mm Hg is maintained. Patients are maintained on high-dose barbiturate therapy until ICP has been controlled within the normal range for 24 hours. Barbiturates should never be stopped abruptly but should be tapered slowly over approximately 4 days.[5]

Complications of high-dose barbiturate therapy can be disastrous without a specific and organized approach. The most frequent complications are hypotension and myocardial depression. If any complications occur and are allowed to persist unchecked, they may cause secondary insults to an already damaged brain. Hypotension, the most common complication, results from peripheral vasodilation and can be compounded in already dehydrated patients who have received large doses of an osmotic diuretic in an attempt to control ICP. Careful monitoring of fluid status by central venous pressure or a pulmonary artery catheter can help prevent this complication. Myocardial depression results from cardiac muscle suppression and can be avoided by frequent monitoring of fluid status, cardiac output, and serum drug levels. If an adequate cardiac output cannot be maintained in the presence of normothermia, barbiturates must be reduced, regardless of serum levels.[15]

The major unresolved issue in the use of high-dose barbiturates is their effect on outcome after head injury. Several laboratory and clinical trials have been undertaken to address this issue. A multicenter randomized trial of barbiturates demonstrated that most elevations of ICP could be controlled with aggressive use of standard therapies of ICP management. For the small subset of patients in whom standard therapy fails to achieve ICP control, judicious, carefully monitored and administered high-dose barbiturate therapy is beneficial.[17]

Herniation Syndromes

The goal of neurologic evaluation, ICP monitoring, and treatment of increased ICP is to prevent **herniation.** Herniation of intracerebral contents results in the shifting of tissue from one compartment of the brain to another and places pressure on cerebral vessels and vital function centers of the brain. If unchecked, herniation rapidly causes death from the cessation of cerebral blood flow and respirations.

Supratentorial Herniation

There are four types of supratentorial herniation syndromes: central or transtentorial, uncal, cingulate, and transcalvarial (Fig. 16-7).

Uncal herniation

Uncal herniation is the most frequently noted herniation syndrome. In uncal herniation a unilateral, expanding

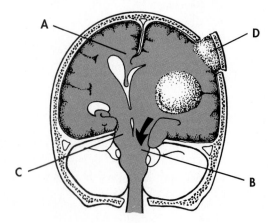

FIG. 16-7 Supratentorial herniation. **A,** Cingulate. **B,** Uncal. **C,** Central. **D,** Transcalvarial.

mass lesion, usually of the temporal lobe, increases ICP, causing lateral displacement of the tip of the temporal lobe (uncus). Lateral displacement pushes the uncus over the edge of the tentorium, puts pressure on the oculomotor nerve (cranial nerve III) and posterior cerebral artery ipsilateral to the lesion, and flattens the midbrain against the opposite side.[3,18]

Clinical manifestations of uncal herniation include ipsilateral pupil dilation, decreased level of consciousness, respiratory pattern changes leading to respiratory arrest, and contralateral hemiplegia leading to decorticate or decerebrate posturing. If no intervention occurs, uncal herniation results in fixed and dilated pupils, flaccidity, and respiratory arrest.[3,18]

Central or transtentorial herniation

In central herniation an expanding mass lesion of the midline, frontal, parietal, or occipital lobes results in downward displacement of the hemispheres, basal ganglia, and diencephalon through the tentorial notch. Central herniation is often preceded by uncal and cingulate herniation.[3,18]

TABLE 16-3

Pharmacologic Agents Used in the Management of Neurologic Disorders

MEDICATION	DOSAGE	ACTIONS	SPECIAL CONSIDERATIONS
ANTICONVULSANTS Phenytoin (Dilantin)	Loading dose of 18 mg/kg IV followed by 3-5 mg/kg q12h IV	Used to prevent the influx of sodium at the cell membrane and inhibit cell depolarization; blocks the spread of a seizure rather than preventing initial neuronal discharge	• Infuse no faster than 50 mg/min to prevent hypotension and bradycardia • Administer with normal saline only as it precipitates with other solutions • Monitor serum level closely, therapeutic level is 10-20 µg/ml.
BARBITURATES Phenobarbital	Loading dose of 6-8 mg/kg IV followed by a maintenance dose q12-24h IV	Used to produce CNS depression and reduce the spread of an epileptic focus	• Administer at a rate of 60 mg/minute • Monitor serum level closely, therapeutic level is 15-40 µg/ml • May depress cardiac and respiratory function
OSMOTIC DIURETICS Mannitol	0.5-2.0 g/kg IV	Used to treat cerebral edema by pulling fluid from the extravascular space into the intravascular space; requires intact blood-brain barrier	• Side effects include hypovolemia and increased serum osmolality • Monitor serum osmolality and notify physician if >310 mOsm/liter • Warm and shake before administering to ensure crystals are dissolved.
LOOP DIURETICS Furosemide (Lasix)	0.1-2.0 mg/kg IV	Used to decrease sodium transport within the brain and thereby reduce cerebral edema; may inhibit CSF production	• Side effects include hypovolemia and hypokalemia
CALCIUM CHANNEL BLOCKERS Nimodipine (Nimotop)	60 mg q4h NG or PO	Used to decrease cerebral vasospasm	• Side effects include hypotension, palpitations, headache, and dizziness • Monitor blood pressure frequently when implementing therapy

Clinical manifestations of central or transtentorial herniation include loss of consciousness; small, reactive pupils progressing to fixed, dilated pupils; respiratory changes leading to respiratory arrest; and decorticate posturing progressing to flaccidity. In the late stages, uncal and central herniation syndromes affect the brainstem similarly.[3,18]

Cingulate herniation

Cingulate herniation occurs when an expanding lesion of one hemisphere shifts laterally and forces the cingulate gyrus under the falx cerebri. Cingulate herniation occurs frequently. Whenever a lateral shift is noted on a CT scan, cingulate herniation has occurred. Little is known about the effects of cingulate herniation, and there are no clinical manifestations that assist in its diagnosis. Cingulate herniation is not in itself life threatening, but if the expanding mass lesion that caused cingulate herniation is not controlled, uncal or central herniation follows.[3,18]

Transcalvarial herniation

Transcalvarial herniation is the extrusion of cerebral tissue through the cranium. In the presence of severe cerebral edema, transcalvarial herniation occurs through an opening from a skull fracture or craniotomy site.[3]

Infratentorial Herniation

There are two infratentorial herniation syndromes: upward transtentorial herniation and downward cerebellar herniation.

Upward transtentorial herniation

Upward transtentorial herniation occurs when an expanding mass lesion of the cerebellum causes protrusion of the vermis (central area) of the cerebellum and the midbrain upward through the tentorial notch. Compression of the third cranial nerve and diencephalon occurs. Blockage of the central aqueduct and distortion of the third ventricle obstructs CSF flow. Deterioration progresses rapidly.[3,18]

Downward cerebellar herniation

Downward cerebellar herniation occurs when an expanding lesion of the cerebellum exerts pressure downward, sending the cerebellar tonsils through the foramen magnum. Compression and displacement of the medulla oblongata occur, rapidly resulting in respiratory and cardiac arrest.[3,18]

Pharmacologic Agents

A number of pharmacologic agents are used in the care of patients with neurologic disorders. Table 16-3 reviews the various agents used and any special considerations necessary for administering them.[19]

References

1. Richmond TS: Intracranial pressure monitoring, *AACN Clin Iss Crit Care Nurs* 4:148, 1993.
2. Helfaer MA, Kirsch JR: Intracranial vault pathophysiology, *Crit Care Rep* 1:12, 1989.
3. Barker E: *Neuroscience nursing*, St Louis, 1994, Mosby.
4. Chesnut RM, Marshall LF: Management of head injury: treatment of abnormal intracranial pressure, *Neurosurg Clin North Am* 2:267, 1991.
5. Marshall SB and others: *Neuroscience critical care: pathophysiology and patient management*, Philadelphia, 1990, WB Saunders.
6. Vos HR: Making headway with intracranial hypertension, *Am J Nurs* 93(2):28, 1993.
7. Wall BM, Philips JP, Howard JC: Validation of increased intracranial pressure and high risk for increased intracranial pressure, *Nurs Diagnosis* 5:74, 1994.
8. Cummings R: Understanding ventricular drainage, *J Neurosci Nurs* 24:84, 1992.
9. McQuillan KA: Intracranial pressure monitoring: technical imperatives, *AACN Clin Iss Crit Care* 2:623, 1991.
10. Wrobel CJ, Marshall LF: *Closed head injury management dilemmas*. In Long DM, editor: *Current therapy in neurological surgery*, ed 3, St Louis, 1992, Mosby.
11. Mitchell PH: Intracranial hypertension: influence of nursing care activities, *Nurs Clin North Am* 21:563, 1986.
12. Feldman Z and others: Effect of head elevation on intracranial pressure, cerebral perfusion pressure, and cerebral blood flow in head-injured patients, *J Neurosurg* 76:207, 1992.
13. Fontaine DK, McQuillan K: Positioning as a nursing therapy in trauma care, *Crit Care Nurs Clin North Am* 1:105, 1990.
14. Muizelaar JP and others: Adverse effects of prolonged hyperventilation in patients with severe head injury: a randomized clinical trial, *J Neurosurg* 75:731, 1991.
15. Frank JI: Management of intracranial hypertension, *Med Clin North Am* 77:61, 1993.
16. Brucia JJ, Owen DC, Rudy EB: The effects of lidocaine on intracranial hypertension, *J Neurosci Nurs* 24:205, 1992.
17. Eisenberg HM and others: High-dose barbiturate control of elevated intracranial pressure in patients with severe head injury, *J Neurosurg* 69:15, 1988.
18. Morrison CAM: Brain herniation syndromes, *Crit Care Nurs* 7(5):34, 1987.
19. Rose BA: Neurologic therapies in critical care, *Crit Care Nurs Clin North Am* 5:237, 1993.

UNIT SIX

Renal Alterations

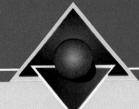

17

Renal Assessment and Diagnostic Procedures

LOIS CATTS

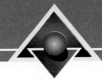

History

A renal history begins with patients' descriptions of the chief symptom. These descriptions include onset, location, duration, and factors that lessen or aggravate the problem.[1,2] Descriptions of any current treatment, medi-cations taken to alleviate symptoms, and procedures performed to ameliorate the condition are helpful in delin-eating the extent of the current complaint. A complete renal and fluid history should always include patients' medical history. Similar symptoms, problems, and treat-ment for past complaints may offer important clues for current treatment or aid in establishing the cause of the problem. Patients and their families or significant others are asked to provide as much detail as possible about the history.

Physical Examination

Inspection

Inspection of patients is focused on five priorities: observation of neck veins, evaluation of hand veins, assessment of skin turgor, identification of skin changes in renal failure, and estimation of peripheral edema.

Observation of neck veins

Renal assessment begins with an inspection of the neck veins. The supine position facilitates normal venous distention. The absence of distention may indicate hypovolemia. Assessment continues with the head of the bed elevated to 45 to 90 degrees. If the veins remain distended more than 2 cm above the sternal notch when the bed is at 45 degrees, fluid overload may be suspected.[3] (Chapter 8 provides a detailed description of neck vein assessment on pages 91 to 93.)

Evaluation of hand veins

Examiners observe hand veins when the hand is in a dependent position. Venous filling that takes longer than 5 seconds suggests hypovolemia. When the hand is elevated, distention should disappear within 5 seconds. If it does not, fluid overload is suspected.

Assessment of skin turgor

Assessment of skin turgor provides additional data for identifying fluid-related problems. As examiners pick up and release the skin over the forearm, they note the speed with which it returns to a normal position. If elasticity and fluid status are normal, the skin returns to its usual shape almost immediately. In hypovolemia the skin remains raised and does not return to its normal position for several seconds. Because people lose skin elasticity as they age, the test on the arm is not considered accurate in older persons. However, skin turgor can still be assessed in the shoulder area, which retains its elasticity.

Evaluation of skin changes in renal failure

Changes in skin texture and overall appearance reveal much about fluid status. For example, patients with end-stage renal failure have rough, dry skin covered with deposits of urate crystals called *uremic frost*. These patients frequently have scratch marks because of the pruritus (itching) associated with renal failure.

Estimation of peripheral edema

Edema is defined as the presence of excess fluid in the interstitial space. Presence of peripheral edema is assessed by applying fingertip pressure on the skin over a bony prominence such as the ankles, pretibial areas (shins), or sacrum. If the indentation made by the fingertip does not disappear within 30 seconds, "pitting" edema is present. **Pitting edema** indicates increased interstitial volume and is not evident until a weight gain of approximately 10% has occurred.[3] It is gauged on a subjective scale of 1 to 4, with +1 indicating only minimum pitting and +4 indicating severe pitting. Edema may appear in any dependent area. In ambulatory patients it is most likely in the legs and feet. In patients on bed rest the sacrum and back are more likely to reveal edema. The presence of edema, however, does not always indicate true fluid overload; a loss of albumin from the vascular space can also cause peripheral edema, yet hypovolemia may be present as described later, in the section on serum albumin.

Auscultation

Auscultation of patients is focused on four priorities: evaluation of heart sounds, assessment of lung sounds, measurement of blood pressure, and identification of orthostatic hypotension.

The purpose of auscultation is to provide additional information about extracellular fluid status. Listening for specific sounds in the heart and lungs provides information about the presence or absence of increased fluid in the interstitium or vascular space.

Evaluation of heart sounds

Auscultation of the heart requires listening for extra sounds indicative of fluid overload, such as third and fourth heart sounds. Increased heart rate alone does not offer much data about fluid volume, but combined with a low blood pressure, it may indicate hypovolemia. Patients in renal failure often have hypertension accompanied by a third or fourth heart sound. Caution should be exercised, however, in making assumptions about fluid status on the basis of a murmur because murmurs may also be present in other cardiac disorders.[1]

Assessment of lung sounds

Lung assessment is extremely important in gauging fluid status. Crackles indicate fluid volume excess. Dyspnea with any mild exertion or dyspnea at night that prevents sleeping in a supine position may indicate fluid overload. Shallow, gasping breaths punctuated by periods of apnea may reflect severe acid-base imbalances. Because the lungs are among the primary controllers of acid-base balance, identifying the types of respiratory changes associated with each condition is important.

Measurement of blood pressure

Hypertension, which may indicate fluid overload, can also be caused by atherosclerotic or arteriosclerotic vessel changes. Blood pressure readings are taken at rest with patients lying, sitting, and standing. A comparison of the three readings helps establish a baseline from which to compare subsequent readings.

Identification of orthostatic hypotension

A drastic drop in pressure from lying to sitting or from sitting to standing is known as **orthostatic hypotension.** A drop of 20 mm Hg in pressure, which can indicate a fluid volume deficit, occurs when the volume of venous circulation is so depleted that a sufficient preload is not immediately available after the position change. Orthostatic hypotension produces feelings of weakness or faintness. Causes of orthostatic hypotension include peripheral vascular disease, which often damages the venous circulation of the lower extremities, and some medications used in the treatment of hypertension.

Palpation

Palpation of patients is focused on one priority: determining the size and shape of the kidney.

Determining the size and shape of the kidney

Palpation of the kidneys is not a routine part of the critical care nursing assessment. Used to determine organ size and shape, kidney palpation employs the bimanual capturing approach. Examiners place one hand posteriorly under the flank of supine patients, with fingers pointing to the midline while positioning the opposite hand just below the rib cage anteriorly. Patients are asked to inhale deeply while pressure is used to bring the hands together. As patients exhale, examiners feel each kidney between their hands, comparing the organs' size and shape. Each kidney should be firm and smooth and of equal size.[3,4] Palpation is a useful technique, although not always practical for critically ill adults.

Percussion

Percussion of patients is focused on three priorities: detecting kidney pain, assessing the abdomen, and identifying ascites.

Detecting kidney pain

Kidney percussion is used to detect pain in the renal area. Percussion of the kidney is performed while patients are lying on their sides or sitting. Examiners place one of their hands over the costovertebral angle (lower border of the rib cage on the flank) and strike the back of the hand with the opposite fist. A dull thud is considered normal. Pain may indicate infection.

Assessing the abdomen

Using the same procedure as for the kidneys but with patients supine, nurses percuss the abdomen to assess fluid status. A dull sound indicates solid bowel contents or fluid, and a hollow sound denotes a gaseous bowel.[1]

Identifying ascites

An important symptom of fluid imbalance, **ascites** is defined as severe fluid distention of the abdominal cavity. Ascites may be differentiated from distention caused by solid bowel contents by producing what is called the *fluid wave.* Nurses elicit the fluid wave by exerting pressure to the abdominal midline while one hand is placed on the right or left flank. Tapping the opposite flank produces a wave in the accumulated fluid that can be felt under the hands. Other signs of ascites are a protuberant, rounded abdomen and abdominal striae. Ascites may represent fluid volume excess. In people with renal failure, ascites is caused by volume overload, which forces fluid into the abdomen because of increased capillary hydrostatic pressures. In liver failure the ascites occurs because increased hepatic vascular pressure forces fluid and plasma proteins from the vascular space into the interstitial space and abdominal cavity. (The section on serum albumin in this chapter provides more information on liver failure and ascites.)

Fluid Balance Assessment

Fluid balance assessment in patients with renal failure is focused on three priorities: monitoring weight, comparing intake and output, and identifying electrolyte imbalances.

Monitoring weight

The most important factor in the assessment of fluid status is patients' weight. Significant fluctuations in body weight (over 2 kg) over a 1- to 2-day period indicate fluid gains and losses. Patients are weighed on admission to the critical care unit. Thereafter, their daily weight is used for comparison with the previous day's weight. Fluctuations in weight are of critical importance to nurses caring for patients with renal failure. As a method of comparison, 1 L of fluid equals 1 kg, or approximately 2.2 pounds. Differences in daily weight are often used for determining diuretic drug dosages and calculating the amount of fluid to remove during a dialysis treatment.

Comparing intake and output

Patients' intake and output of fluids can be compared with their weight to evaluate the gain or loss of fluid. Urinary output and insensible fluid losses (perspiration and water vapor from the lungs) can range widely from 750 to 2400 ml daily. When intake exceeds output, a positive fluid balance exists. If renal failure perpetuates the positive fluid gain, fluid overload results. Conversely, if output exceeds intake (e.g., from fever, increased respiration, profuse sweating, vomiting, diarrhea, gastric suction, wound drainage), a negative fluid balance exists. Abnormal output of body fluids creates not only fluid imbalances but also electrolyte and acid-base disturbances. For example, gastrointestinal suction or loss by diarrhea can result in fluid deficit, sodium and potassium deficits, and metabolic acidosis (from excessive loss of bicarbonate). During a 24-hour period, fever can increase skin and respiratory losses by as much as a

TABLE 17-1
NORMAL ELECTROLYTE VALUES AND FUNCTIONS

ELECTROLYTE	NORMAL SERUM VALUE	FUNCTIONS
Sodium	135-145 mEq/L	Maintains extracellular osmolality Maintains the active transport mechanism in conjunction with potassium Controls body fluids (largely responsible for water movement and retention) Aids in maintaining neuromuscular activity Aids in some enzyme activities (helping to create energy) Influences acid-base balance
Potassium	3.5-5.0 mEq/L	Promotes transmission of nerve impulses Maintains intracellular osmolality Activates several enzymatic reactions Aids in regulation of acid-base balance Promotes myocardial, skeletal, and smooth muscle contractility
Chloride	98-108 mEq/L	Maintains body osmolality (in conjunction with sodium) Aids in body water balance (in conjunction with sodium) Competes with bicarbonate for recombination with sodium to maintain acid-base balance Maintains acidity of body fluids (gastric juice)
Calcium	8.5-10.5 mg/dl or 4.5-5.8 mEq/L	Maintains hardness of bone and teeth (crystalline in nature) Contracts skeletal muscle Coagulates blood Maintains cellular permeability Contracts heart muscle
Phosphorus	2.7-4.5 mg/dl	Aids in structure of cellular membrane Helps deliver oxygen to the tissues Is integral part of intracellular energy production (ATP) Helps maintain bone hardness Aids in enzyme regulation (ATPase)
Magnesium	1.5-2.5 mEq/L	Aids in neuromuscular transmission Aids in contraction of heart muscle Activates enzymes for cellular metabolism of carbohydrates and proteins Aids in maintaining the active transport mechanism at the cellular level Aids in transmission of hereditary information to offspring
Bicarbonate	24-28 mEq/L	Buffers the acidity of body fluids (controls the hydrogen ion concentration and combines with other body salts to maintain acid-base balance)

75 ml/1 SD F rise. In maintaining daily records of intake and output, nurses must record all gains and losses. A running total fluid balance, positive or negative, over several days may reveal several liters of fluid gain or loss. A standard list of the fluid volume held in various containers (e.g., milk cartons, juice containers) expedites this process. Discussions about the importance of accurate intake and output with patients, families, and friends are necessary and can improve the accuracy of record keeping.

Identifying electrolyte imbalances

Often accompanied by clinical manifestations such as changes in level of consciousness, disturbances in fluid and electrolyte levels are expected in renal failure. Changes in mental status include disorientation, lethargy, coma, and confusion. These symptoms may result from excesses or deficits of sodium, calcium, and magnesium. Table 17-1 lists the normal values for the major serum electrolytes, and Table 18-2 describes changes in serum electrolyte values with renal failure and other conditions.

Laboratory Assessment

Serum Albumin

Slightly more than 50% of total plasma protein consists of serum albumin, which is manufactured in the liver. Its normal blood levels are 3.5 to 5.5 g/dl. Albumin is primarily responsible for maintaining colloid osmotic pressure, which holds fluid in the vascular space. A decreased albumin level results in a plasma-to-interstitium fluid shift, which creates edema. A decreased albumin level can result from a critical illness that causes a protein-calorie malnutrition. This condition depletes available stores of albumin and causes oncotic pressure to fall and fluid to move from the vascular space to the interstitial space. Generalized edema results. Liver disease can also cause albumin levels to fall because the diseased liver fails to synthesize sufficient albumin. Severe portal hypertension can force albumin and other plasma proteins into the abdominal cavity, creating ascites. Increased albumin levels are rare. The body uses a fixed amount of protein for energy and body cell replacement and converts excess protein into stored fat. If all plasma proteins are elevated, fluid volume deficit (hemoconcentration) is usually suspected.

Hemoglobin and Hematocrit

Hemoglobin (Hgb) and hematocrit (Hct) levels can indicate increases or decreases in intravascular fluid volume. Both Hgb and Hct values vary according to gender: The Hgb value in males is normally 13.5 to 17.5 g/dl, and in females, 12 to 16 g/dl. Hemoglobin values do not change with changes in fluid volume status. However, Hct levels change according to intravascular fluid volume. The Hct value expresses the percentage of red blood cells (RBCs) in a volume of whole blood. The Hct value ranges from 40% to 54% in males and 37% to 47% in females. An increase in the Hct value, with a stable Hgb value, may indicate hemoconcentration. Conversely a decreased Hct level without a change in Hgb level indicates hemodilution. Anemia is frequently associated with renal failure because of (1) a shortened RBC lifespan and (2) the kidney's inability to produce erythropoietin, which stimulates the bone marrow to produce RBCs.[5,6]

Blood Urea Nitrogen and Creatinine

Blood urea nitrogen (BUN) and creatinine are both by-products of protein metabolism. The normal value for BUN is 9 to 20 mg/dl, and the normal value for creatinine is 0.7 to 1.5 mg/dl.

Creatinine

Creatinine is a by-product of normal cell metabolism and appears in serum in amounts proportional to the body muscle mass. Creatinine is easily excreted by the renal tubules. Measuring the amount of creatinine in the excreted urine over 24 hours (creatinine clearance) and the simultaneous creatinine level in the blood (serum creatinine) provides accurate information about kidney function. An excess of creatinine in critically ill patients usually occurs with renal failure, when diminished renal function impairs creatinine excretion.

Blood urea nitrogen

Blood urea nitrogen (BUN) levels do not indicate renal failure as accurately as the creatinine level. BUN levels fluctuate greatly with protein intake, whereas creatinine levels are relatively unaffected by protein intake. Increased levels of BUN, often called *urea,* also occur with fluid volume deficit (hemoconcentration), infection, medications, excessive protein intake, and renal failure.

Significance

Both BUN and creatinine levels become elevated when renal function deteriorates.

Serum electrolytes

Serum electrolyte values are often abnormal as a result of renal insufficiency or failure. Normal electrolyte values are shown in Table 17-1. Electrolyte abnormalities seen in renal failure are described in Table 18-2.

Anion Gap

The anion gap is the difference between the number of measurable cations (sodium and potassium) and the number of measurable anions (chloride and bicarbonate) in the serum. The value represents the remaining unmeasurable anions present in the extracellular fluid. These include phosphates, sulfates, ketones, pyruvate, and lactate. The following formula is generally used in the calculation of the anion gap:

$$Na^+ - (Cl^- + HCO_3^-)$$

The normal value is 10 to 12 mEq/L and should not exceed 14 mEq/L.

Significance

An increased anion gap level reflects overproduction or poor excretion of acid products. Renal failure can increase the anion gap value because of retention of acids and altered bicarbonate reabsorption. Diabetic ketoacidosis also results in ketone production, which elevates the level of the anion gap.

Osmolality

Osmolality can be measured in the urine and serum. The simultaneous measurement of the serum and urinary os-

T A B L E 1 7 - 2	
ESSENTIAL URINALYSIS TESTS FOR DIAGNOSING RENAL DISORDERS	
SUBSTANCE	**NORMAL VALUES**
Specific gravity	1.003-1.030
Urinary osmolality	300-1200 mOsm/L
Urinary pH	4.5-8.0
Urinary electrolytes	
Sodium	80-180 mEq/24 hr
Potassium	40-80 mEq/24 hr
Chloride	110-20 mEq/24 hr
Calcium	50-300 mEq/24 hr
Glucose	0
Protein	0

molality levels provides the most accurate assessment of fluid status.

Serum osmolality

The serum osmolality level reflects the concentration or dilution of vascular fluid. The normal serum osmolality level is 275 to 295 mOsm/L.[5] Antidiuretic hormone (ADH) plays an important role in maintaining the serum osmolality level. When the serum osmolality level increases above 295 mOsm/L, the release of ADH from the pituitary gland stimulates increased water reabsorption. This expands the vascular space and brings the serum osmolality level down to the normal range. A more concentrated urine also results. The inverse occurs with a decreased serum osmolality (below 275 mOsm/L), which inhibits the production of ADH and results in increased excretion of water through the kidneys, producing dilute urine.

Urine osmolality

The normal level of urinary osmolality is 300 to 1200 mOsm/kg. Urine osmolality depends on reabsorption or excretion of water in the kidney tubules, increasing if patients are dehydrated because of the retention of fluid by the body and decreasing during hypervolemia. With a fluid volume overload the kidneys excrete more water. In late renal failure the urinary osmolality value is usually low because solutes and fluids are being abnormally retained. Specific urinalysis tests are summarized in Table 17-2.

Urine pH Level

Urine pH level indicates the acidity or alkalinity of the urine. The normal level of urinary pH is 6.0, but it may range from 4.5 to 8.0. As the kidney regulates acid-base balance, far more hydrogen ions are excreted than bicarbonate ions, which accounts for the acidity of the urine. Therefore changes in renal function produce changes in urinary pH value.

Significance

An increase in urinary acidity (decreased level of pH) indicates excretion of acids by the body. Conversely a decrease in urinary acidity (increased pH or higher alkaline level) means the body is excreting bicarbonate.

Urine Specific Gravity

Specific gravity measures the density or weight of urine compared with that of distilled water. The normal urinary specific gravity level is 1.003 to 1.030 as compared with the normal specific gravity level of distilled water at 1.000. Because urine is composed of many solutes and substances suspended in water, its specific gravity level should always be higher than that of water and thereby indicate the ability of the kidney to dilute or concentrate the urine.

Significance

Decreases in specific gravity values reflect the kidneys' inability to excrete the usual solute load into urine (dilute urine with fewer solutes). Increases in specific gravity values (a more concentrated urine) occur with a body fluid volume deficit caused by fever, vomiting, or diarrhea. An increased specific gravity value can also occur with diabetes or glomerular membrane permeability changes, which allow glucose and protein in the urine. These substances increase the urine specific gravity.[5]

Glycosuria

Glucose is normally reabsorbed by the renal tubules; therefore urine should be free of glucose.

Significance

The transient appearance of glucose in the urine may be brought on by ingestion of a heavy carbohydrate load, stress, or renal changes that accompany pregnancy. The consistent appearance of glycosuria signals the onset of diabetes mellitus.

Proteinuria

Like glucose, protein is normally absent from urine because the size of the protein molecule prevents it from passing across the normal glomerular capillary membrane.

Significance

Thus the consistent appearance of protein in urine suggests compromise of the glomerular membrane and possible renal disease. The transient appearance of protein in the urine can result from efferent arteriole constriction caused by stress, medications, vigorous exercise, or extreme cold. Also, proteinuria can accompany the renal changes associated with pregnancy.

Urine Electrolytes

Levels of urinary electrolytes are not measured as frequently as serum electrolytes because urinary findings are less significant. Measuring urinary electrolyte levels requires a 24-hour urine sample.

Significance

Electrolyte levels are highly variable, and the electrolytes depend on the kidneys for adequate excretion. Consequently, changes in urinary electrolyte levels strongly suggest renal failure.[5] Table 17-1 lists the normal values for urinary electrolytes, and Table 18-3 describes the urinalysis findings in acute tubular necrosis.

Urine Sediment

The presence of epithelial cells and casts aids in identifying problems related to the kidneys. Casts are shells or clumps of cellular breakdown or proteinaceous materials that form in the renal tubular system and are washed out in the urinary flow.

Significance

Although small numbers of epithelial cells normally appear in the urine and an occasional cast may be found, their consistent appearance is abnormal.

Diagnostic Procedures

Radiologic Assessment

Although laboratory assessment is the primary method to diagnose renal and urologic problems, radiologic assessment confirms or clarifies causes of particular disorders. Specific tests are described in Box 17-1.

Renal Biopsy

Renal biopsy is the definitive tool for diagnosing disease processes of the kidney.

Procedure

Two methods are used in renal biopsy—closed biopsy and open biopsy. Percutaneous needle biopsy (closed method) involves introducing a cannula into the flank to obtain a specimen of cortical and medullary kidney tissue. Open biopsy involves surgical visualization of the kidney, at which time a tissue sample is obtained. Specimens are then examined in the laboratory.

BOX 17-1

RENAL IMAGING TESTS

KIDNEY-URETER-BLADDER (KUB)

Flat-plate x-ray film of abdomen determines position, size, and structure of kidneys and urinary tract. KUB is usually followed by more sophisticated tests.

INTRAVENOUS PYELOGRAPHY (IVP)

Intravenous injection of contrast media plus x-ray film allows visualization of internal kidney (parenchyma, calyces, pelves, ureters, bladder). Timing of stages can delineate size and shape. Obstructions and tumors can be found. Drawback can be hypersensitivity to contrast medium.

RETROGRADE PYELOGRAPHY

Injection of iodine-based contrast medium through ureteral catheter into collection system (calyces, pelves, and ureters) allows visualization of clots, stones, and strictures. It may be useful when allergy to IVP dye exists (less chance of hypersensitivity in this test).

RENAL ANGIOGRAPHY

Injection of contrast medium into arterial blood perfusing the kidney allows x-ray visualization of renal vessels. Stenoses, cysts, clots, and tumors may be visualized, as may infarctions, traumas, and torn kidneys.

RENAL COMPUTED TOMOGRAPHIC (CT) SCAN

After administration of a radioisotope, which is absorbed by the kidneys, scintillation photography is performed in several planes. Density of the image helps determine tumor, cysts, hemorrhage, calcification, adrenal tumors, or necrosis. It may be used before or instead of renal biopsy.

RENAL ULTRASONOGRAPHY (ECHO)

High-frequency sound waves are transmitted to the kidneys and urinary tract and viewed on an oscilloscope. This type of test is usually used to search for fluid accumulation or obstruction.

MAGNETIC RESONANCE IMAGING (MRI)

A scanner produces three-dimensional images in response to the application of high-energy radiofrequency waves to the tissues. MRI produces clear images; the density of the image may indicate lesions; malformation of tissue, vessels, or tubules; and necrosis. MRI is more specific than renal ultrasonography or CT scan. It is helpful in the detection of renal masses, particularly in distinguishing simple cysts from those complicated by hemorrhage. MRI is noninvasive and painless, does not expose patients to any known risks, and has no known complications.

Significance

Renal biopsy can identify the presence of diseases such as glomerulonephritis, amyloidosis, and lupus erythematosus.

References

1. Bates B: *A guide to physical examination,* ed 5, Philadelphia, 1991, JB Lippincott.
2. Baer CL, Lancaster LE: Acute renal failure, *Crit Care Nurs Q* 14(4):1, 1992.
3. Grimes J, Burns E: *Health assessment in nursing practice,* ed 3, Boston, 1992, Jones & Bartlett.
4. Malasanos L, Barkauskas V, Stoltenberg-Allen K: *Health assessment,* ed 4, St Louis, 1990, Mosby.
5. Fischbach F: *A manual of laboratory diagnostic tests,* ed 4, Philadelphia, 1992, JB Lippincott.
6. Binkley LS, Whittaker A: Erythropoietin use in the critical care setting, *AACN Clin Issues Crit Care Nurs* 3(3):640, 1992.

18

Renal Disorders and Therapeutic Management

LOIS CATTS

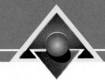

Acute Renal Failure

Description and Etiology

Acute renal failure (ARF) can be defined as any rapid decline in glomerular filtration rate (GFR) with subsequent retention of metabolic waste products (azotemia). Usually accompanied by oliguria or anuria, ARF is a short-term condition that lasts 10 to 25 days or longer. If the appropriate treatment is not initiated or patients do not respond to treatment, the acute condition may lead to chronic renal failure. ARF is a serious complication in critically ill patients, and mortality rates remain

BOX 18-1

ETIOLOGY OF ACUTE RENAL FAILURE

PRERENAL

Hemorrhage
Severe GI losses
Burns
Shock
Cirrhosis
Renal trauma
Volume depletion (actual loss or "third-spacing")
Heart failure
Renal losses (diuretics, diabetes insipidus, osmotic diuresis)

INTRARENAL

Thrombus
Stenosis
Hypertensive sclerosis
Glomerulonephritis
Pyelonephritis
Acute tubular necrosis
Diabetic sclerosis
Toxic damage

POSTRENAL

Obstructions (stenosis, calculi)
Prostatic disease
Tumors

BOX 18-2

ETIOLOGY OF ACUTE TUBULAR NECROSIS

ISCHEMIC

Hemorrhage
Excessive diuretic use
Burns
Peritonitis
Sepsis
Heart failure
Myocardial ischemia
Pulmonary emboli
Transfusion reactions
Obstetric complications (severe toxemia, abruptio placentae, placenta previa, uterine rupture)

TOXIC

Rhabdomyolysis
Hypercalcemia
Gram-negative sepsis
Nephrotoxic medications (aminoglycosides, cephalosporins, antimicrobials, antineoplastic agents, analgesics containing phenacetin)
Heavy metals
Radiocontrast media
Insecticides
Carbon tetrachloride
Methanol
Street drugs such as phencyclidine (PCP)

---

high, ranging from 35% to 86% even with advanced critical care and hemodialysis techniques. Gastrointestinal (GI) bleeding, sepsis, and neurologic changes are often implicated in deaths related to acute renal failure. Causes of ARF are categorized in three areas: prerenal, intrarenal, and postrenal (Box 18-1).

Prerenal

Causes of prerenal failure are associated with any insult that reduces vascular perfusion to the kidney. The GFR is decreased, leading to oliguria. The nephrons are not damaged, and return to normal renal function is possible with prompt treatment of the underlying cause of the prerenal condition.

Postrenal

Causes of postrenal failure are usually obstructive disorders occurring beyond the kidney in the remainder of the urinary tract. As with prerenal conditions, prompt treatment restores normal kidney function and prevents permanent kidney damage.

Intrarenal

Causes of intrarenal failure, also known as *intrinsic, primary,* or *parenchymal damage,* are insults to the kidney tissue from infections, insults to the nephron such as glo-

merulonephritis, and scleroses from hypertension and diabetes mellitus. Damage from intrarenal conditions primarily affects the tubular component of the nephron. The most common intrarenal condition is acute tubular necrosis.

Acute Tubular Necrosis

Description and Etiology

Acute tubular necrosis (ATN) refers to damage occurring within the epithelium of the tubular portions of the nephron. Although *ATN* and *ARF* are sometimes used interchangeably, ATN is actually a cause of ARF; of all ARF patients, 75% to 90% of cases are caused by ATN. Damage to the cellular structures in this area prevents normal concentration of urine, filtration of wastes, and regulation of acid-base, electrolyte, and water balances. A number of disorders can result in ATN, and several contributing factors may work together to bring about tubular damage. Causes are divided into two categories—ischemic and toxic (Box 18-2). Ischemic damage occurs irregularly along the tubular membranes, causing areas of tubular cell damage and cast formation. Toxic damage results from nephrotoxins, usually drugs, chemical agents, or bacterial endotoxins, which cause uniform, widespread damage. The renal tubular cells are constantly at risk for damage because of their normally high blood flows, high oxygen requirements, and constant reabsorption and secretion of metabolites.

Pathophysiology

Several theories have been proposed to explain the pathophysiology underlying ATN:

1. The back-leak theory suggests that tubular injury, whether ischemic or toxic, causes return of metabolites such as creatinine to the peritubular circulation. This causes decreased urinary production.[1]
2. The tubular obstruction theory suggests that interstitial edema or an accumulation of casts and sloughing tissue creates a tubular obstruction. Filtration ceases when tubular hydrostatic pressure reaches that of glomerular filtration. This decreases the formation of urine.[1]
3. The vascular theory suggests that damage to the tubules is mediated by obstruction in the renal capillary beds. Prolonged ischemia results in afferent arteriolar constriction and a reduction of GFR, which decreases the available filtrate. The exchange between tubules and capillaries is obliterated, and tubular cells fail to receive the necessary blood flow and oxygen to sustain them.[1]
4. The decreased glomerular membrane permeability theory suggests that restrictive filtration occurs at the cellular level independent of blood flow.
5. The vasoconstriction theory suggests that reduced renal perfusion and reduced capillary flow in the cortical region of the kidney (site of most of the glomeruli) result in ATN.[1]

Phases of ATN

Onset phase

The onset phase is the period from the occurrence of the insult to cell injury. The phase can last from hours to days depending on the causative factor, with toxic factors lasting longer. Treatment during this time may prevent irreversible damage.

Oliguric/anuric phase

The second phase of ATN lasts 1 to 2 weeks. Urine output is less than 400 ml/24 hours. Oliguria is encountered more commonly in ischemic damage, whereas nonoliguria is usually seen after a toxic insult to the kidneys[2,3] (Box 18-3). The mortality rate is 25% in patients with nonoliguric ATN, but it climbs to 66% if oliguria is present. Anuria occurs more commonly in postrenal obstruction. During this phase the GFR is significantly decreased, which leads to increased levels of abnormalities (e.g., hyperkalemia, hyperphosphatemia, hypocalcemia) and metabolic acidosis[2] (Table 18-1).

BOX 18-3

DEFINITION OF URINE VOLUME IN RENAL FAILURE

Anuria: Urine volume of less than 100 ml/24 hr
Oliguria: Urine volume of 100 to 400 ml/24 hr
Polyuria: Urine volume greater than 400 ml/24 hr in patients with renal failure; urine volume possibly as high as 1.5 L/24 hr but without clearance of solutes and waste products from the body

---

TABLE 18-1

EXPECTED LABORATORY FINDINGS WITH ACUTE TUBULAR NECROSIS

INDICATOR	VALUE	RATIONALE
BLOOD		
Blood urea nitrogen	Elevated	Damaged tubules allow urea to be reabsorbed
SERUM		
Serum creatinine	Elevated	Damaged tubules cannot rid the blood of creatinine
Serum potassium	Elevated	Damaged tubules cannot excrete potassium to clear the blood
Serum pH	Usually lower	Damaged tubules cannot excrete hydrogen ions and save bicarbonate ions
URINE		
Creatinine clearance	Decreased	Damaged tubules cannot excrete creatinine

Modified from Norris MK: *DCCN* (8)1:16, 1989.

Diuretic phase

Lasting from 7 to 14 days, the diuretic phase is characterized by increases in GFR and urine output to as much as 2 to 4 L/24 hours. During this phase, tubular function returns slowly, and tubular reabsorption may not be able to increase as quickly as GFR. The result of this inequality is sodium and water loss in the urine, which leads to volume depletion.

Recovery phase

During this stage renal function slowly returns to normal or near normal, with GFR 70% to 80% of normal within 1 to 2 years. If significant renal parenchymal damage has occurred, blood urea nitrogen (BUN) and creatinine levels may never return to normal.

Assessment and Diagnosis

Laboratory assessment

Laboratory assessment usually includes both serum and urinary values. This information has been compiled into several tables for easy reference:

1. Table 17-1 summarizes normal serum electrolyte values.
2. Table 18-1 summarizes serum and urinary findings in ATN.
3. Table 18-2 summarizes abnormal serum electrolyte values.
4. Table 17-2 summarizes normal urinalysis values.
5. Table 18-3 on p. 320 summarizes urinalysis findings in ATN.

BUN and creatinine levels

Although it reflects cellular damage, BUN is not the most reliable indicator of renal damage because it can also indicate protein intake, blood in the GI tract, and cell catabolism. Creatinine, on the other hand, is an accurate reflection of renal damage because it is almost totally excreted by the renal tubules. Elevated levels of creatinine can reflect damage to as many as 50% of the nephrons. The creatinine level does not rise as rapidly as the BUN level because creatinine is independent of urinary flow. (See p. 309 for more information on BUN and creatinine laboratory assessment values.)

Electrolyte levels

Most of the electrolytes in the extracellular fluid become increasingly elevated depending on the cause of damage and length of time the damage has been present. As urinary output decreases, serum electrolyte levels increase. Typically, elevation of potassium and phosphorus levels and depression of sodium and calcium levels occur. The retention of large amounts of fluids depresses sodium levels and produces a dilutional effect.

Radiologic assessment

Radiologic tests used in diagnosing renal disorders have become increasingly sophisticated and valuable. Sonography, tomography, and angiography can help pinpoint the causal mechanism and even help differentiate between ARF and chronic renal failure (see Table 17-3). Radiologic contrast media have been implicated in the development and worsening of renal disorders.

Medical Management

The goals of treatment in ARF are to (1) correct the cause, (2) promote regeneration of any remaining functional renal capacity, and (3) prevent complications. Management strategies are based on the three causes of ARF. In critical care the most common ARF etiologies are prerenal and intrarenal. Postrenal failure is infrequent as an admission diagnosis to the critical care unit.

Prerenal failure

Patients in prerenal failure require two management approaches: fluid replacement and stimulation of urine output with diuretics. Also, correction of the problem causing the initial poor renal perfusion is necessary.

Intrarenal failure

Patients with intrarenal failure may have had increased amounts of water, solutes, and potential toxins introduced into the circulation; thus prompt measures are needed to decrease their levels. Hemodialysis is the usual treatment of choice, particularly if volume overload creates pulmonary and cardiac compromise. Severe hyperkalemia almost always necessitates hemodialysis because of the life-threatening cardiac dysrhythmias resulting from high serum potassium.

Fluid restriction

Fluids are restricted to prevent the circulatory overload and interstitial edema associated with ARF. The amount of fluid restriction required depends on daily urinary volumes, insensible losses, daily weights, and intake and output records. Patients are usually restricted to 1 L of fluid if urinary output is 500 ml or less and insensible losses range from 500 to 750 ml/day. In the absence of oliguria, however, fluid intake may be matched to daily fluid output.

Management of electrolyte imbalances

Serum electrolyte levels require frequent observation, especially in the initial critical phases of acute renal failure.[4-6]

HYPERKALEMIA. Potassium may quickly reach levels of 6.0 mEq/L and above, and patients can develop life-threatening dysrhythmias. Three strategies are used to treat hyperkalemia:

1. Stop all potassium supplements.
2. Temporarily control symptoms by IV infusion of insulin and glucose. An infusion of 100 ml of 50% dextrose accompanied by 20 units of regular insulin forces potassium back into the cells. Sodium bicarbonate (40 to 160 mEq) may be infused to promote higher excretion of potassium in the urine.
3. Eliminate potassium from the body by use of cation-exchange resins such as sodium polystyrene sulfonate (Kayexalate), which is mixed in water and sorbitol and given orally, rectally, or through a nasogastric tube.[6] The resin captures potassium in the bowel, and it is eliminated in the feces. Dialysis is another mechanism for permanent removal of potassium from the body.

HYPONATREMIA. Sodium levels may be low due to the dilutional effect of fluid volume overload.[7] This condition is treated by fluid restriction.

HYPERPHOSPHATEMIA AND HYPOCALCEMIA. Aluminum hydroxide preparations are administered to bind phos-

TABLE 18-2

...ES IN ACUTE RENAL FAILURE AND OTHER CONDITIONS

		CAUSES	FINDINGS
...L		Metabolic alkalosis	Muscular weakness
		Decreased potassium intake	Cardiac irregularities
		Use of diuretics without potassium supplementation	Abdominal distention and flatulence
		Loss of gastrointestinal (GI) fluids (suction, nausea and vomiting, diarrhea)	Paresthesia
			Decreased reflexes
			Anorexia
		Hyperaldosteronism (primary and secondary Cushing's syndrome)	Dizziness
			Confusion
			Increased sensitivity to digitalis
			ECG changes
...I/L		Acute or chronic renal failure	Irritability and restlessness
		Excess intake of potassium	Anxiety
		Excess intake through infusions	Nausea and vomiting
		Burns	Abdominal cramps
		Crushing injuries	Weakness
		Potassium-sparing diuretics	Numbness and tingling (fingertips and circumoral)
		Metabolic acidosis	
		Transfusions of old blood	Cardiac irregularities (first tachycardia, then bradycardia)
			ECG changes
SODIUM			
Hyponatremia			
Water intoxication	Possibly less than 125 mEq/L (very mild to severe); serum sodium value of 110-115 mEq/L known to occur	Excess D₅W solution intravenously	Disorientation
		Excess plain water intake	Muscle twitching
		Renal failure	Nausea and vomiting
			Abdominal cramps
			Headaches
			Seizures
True hyponatremia	Less than 135 mEq/L	Gastric suction	Apprehension
		Vomiting	Dizziness
		Burns	Postural hypotension
		Use of potent diuretics	Cold, clammy skin
		Heat exhaustion (excessive sweating)	Decreased skin turgor
			Tachycardia
		Loss from wounds and drainage	Oliguria
		Use of tap-water enemas	
		Diarrhea	
		Adrenal insufficiency	
Syndrome of inappropriate release of ADH (SIADH)	Less than 120 mEq/L	Central nervous system (CNS) disorders	Anorexia
		Major trauma (stress)	Nausea and vomiting
		Malignancies (lung, pancreas, thymus)	Abdominal cramps
			Lethargy and withdrawal
		Certain drugs (oral hypoglycemics, antineoplastics, diuretics, analgesics, bronchodilators)	Convulsions
			Coma
			Urinary osmolality greater than plasma

ECG, Electrocardiogram; *ADH,* antidiuretic hormone.

Continued.

TABLE 18-2			
ELECTROLYTE DISTURBANCES IN ACUTE RENAL FAILURE AND OTHER CONDITIONS— cont'd			
DISTURBANCE	**SERUM VALUE**	**CAUSES**	**FINDINGS**
SODIUM—cont'd			
Hypernatremia	Greater than 145 mEq/L	Inability to respond to thirst (decreased fluid intake) Heatstroke Diarrhea (excess fluid loss) Severe insensible loss (ventilation, sweating) Diabetes insipidus Excessive administration of sodium solutions (e.g., hypertonic saline, sodium bicarbonate) Hypertonic tube feedings without water supplement NOTE: Hypernatremia is usually the result of dehydration of the ECF and subsequent hyperconcentration of the sodium.	Extreme thirst Fever Dry, sticky mucous membranes Altered mentation Seizures (later stages)
CALCIUM			
Hypocalcemia	Less than 8.5 mg/dl or 4.5 mEq/L	Protein malnutrition (decreased albumin causes decreased calcium) Decreased calcium intake Burns or infection Decreased parathyroid function (PTH controls serum calcium availability) Decreased GI absorption of calcium (diarrhea) Excessive antacid use (prevents absorption) Renal failure (decreased vitamin D available to stimulate absorption) alkalosis	Irritability Muscular tetany Muscle cramps Decreased cardiac output (decreased contractions) Bleeding (decreased ability to coagulate) ECG changes Positive Chvostek's sign Positive Trousseau's sign
Hypercalcemia	Greater than 10.5 mg/dl or 5.8 mEq/L	Increased parathyroid activity (increased bone resorption of calcium) Multiple fractures Prolonged immobilization Bone tumors Other malignancies Decreased phosphorus (inverse relationship between calcium and phosphate) acidosis	Deep bone pain Excessive thirst Anorexia Lethargy Weakened muscles
MAGNESIUM			
Hypomagnesemia	Less than 1.4 mEq/L	Malnutrition Chronic alcoholism (malnutrition) Diuretics (prolonged use) Severe diarrhea Severe dehydration	Choroid and athetoid muscle activity Facial tics Spasticity Cardiac dysrhythmias

ECF, Extracellular fluid; *PTH,* parathyroid hormone.

TABLE 18-2
ELECTROLYTE DISTURBANCES IN ACUTE RENAL FAILURE AND OTHER CONDITIONS—cont'd

DISTURBANCE	SERUM VALUE	CAUSES	FINDINGS
MAGNESIUM—cont'd			
Hypermagnesemia	Greater than 2.5 mEq/L	Excessive intake of magnesium products (antacids and laxatives) Renal failure Severe dehydration if oliguria present	CNS depression (especially respiratory) Lethargy Coma Bradycardia ECG changes
PHOSPHATE			
Hypophosphatemia	Less than 3.0 mg/dl	Diabetic ketoacidosis (renal wasting) Malabsorption disorders Renal wasting of phosphorus Prolonged use of IV dextrose infusions Low-phosphate diets in patients with renal failure Phosphate-poor total parenteral nutrition solutions	Hemolytic anemias Depressed white cell function Bleeding (decreased platelet aggregation) Nausea, vomiting, and anorexia
Hyperphosphatemia	Greater than 4.5 mg/dl	Renal failure Lactic acidosis Catabolic stress Chemotherapy for certain malignancies	Tachycardia Nausea Diarrhea Abdominal cramps Muscle weakness Flaccid paralysis Increased reflexes
CHLORIDE			
Hypochloremia	Less than 98 mEq/L	Loss of gastric contents (vomiting, suction) Diarrhea (prolonged) Excessive diuretic use Excessive sweating Prolonged use of IV dextrose Metabolic alkalosis	Hyperirritability Tetany or muscular excitability Slow respirations Decreased blood pressure (with fluid loss)
Hyperchloremia	Greater than 108 mEq/L	Severe diarrhea Urinary diversions Renal failure Metabolic acidosis Excessive parenteral administration of isotonic saline solution	Weakness Lethargy Deep, rapid breathing Possible unconsciousness (later stages)
ALBUMIN			
Hypoalbuminemia	Less than 3.8 g/dl	Protein-deficient diet Burns Starvation Surgeries (major, with prolonged recovery phase) Digestive diseases	Muscle wasting Peripheral edema (fluid shift) Decreased resistance to infection Poorly healing wounds

Continued.

TABLE 18-2
ELECTROLYTE DISTURBANCES IN ACUTE RENAL FAILURE AND OTHER CONDITIONS—cont'd

DISTURBANCE	SERUM VALUE	CAUSES	FINDINGS
ACIDOSIS/ALKALOSIS			
Metabolic acidosis	Bicarbonate level less than 22 mEq/L Partial pressure of carbon dioxide (P_{CO_2}) normal or less than 35 mm Hg to compensate for the low bicarbonate level pH below 7.35	Diabetic ketoacidosis Lactic acidosis Uremia Ingestion of acids (e.g., salicylates, alcohol, boric acid) Starvation Diarrhea Some diuretics	Weakness Dizziness Rapid respirations Coma (later stages)
Metabolic alkalosis	Bicarbonate level greater than 26 mEq/L P_{CO_2} level normal or greater than 45 mm Hg to compensate for the elevated bicarbonate level pH level greater than 7.45	Vomiting (with loss of chloride) Excessive intake of alkalies Primary aldosteronism (because of loss of potassium) Diuretic use in patient with heart failure	Hyperexcitability of muscles Bradycardia Bradypnea Numbness and tingling

TABLE 18-3
URINALYSIS FINDINGS WITH ACUTE TUBULAR NECROSIS

INDICATOR	VALUE	RATIONALE	INDICATOR	VALUE	RATIONALE
Volume	Decreased	Damaged tubules cannot excrete	Urine osmolality	250-350 mOsm/L regardless of hydration	Damaged tubules cannot concentrate or dilute urine
Creatinine	60 mg/dl	Damaged tubules cannot excrete urea properly	Casts	Present (epithelial)	Results from direct damage to the epithelium of the tubules
Urea	300 mg/dl	Damaged tubules cannot excrete urea properly and urea may be reabsorbed	Red blood cells	Present	Results from glomerular and/or tubular damage
Potassium	21 mEq/24 hr	Decreased urine output and tubular dysfunction prevent K^+ from being secreted	Cellular debris	Present	From tubular damage, actual sloughing of tubular walls possibly occurring
Specific gravity	1.012 regardless of hydration	Damaged tubules cannot concentrate or dilute urine			

Modified from Norris MK: *DCCN* (8)1:16, 1989.

phorus in the bowel and thereby lower its level.[8] High phosphorous levels inhibit calcium. The reverse is also true. Calcium may be increased by use of calcium supplements, vitamin D preparations, and synthetic calcitriol (Rocaltrol).

Nutrition

The nutritional aspect of nursing management in renal failure involves both replacement and restriction. If patients are anorexic and malnourished, TPN can be provided in a renal formula. The diet prescription for pa-

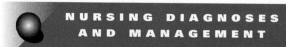

BOX 18-4

NURSING DIAGNOSES AND MANAGEMENT

ACUTE RENAL FAILURE

- *Risk for Fluid Volume Excess* risk factor: renal failure, p. 503
- *Risk for Infection* risk factors: protein-calorie malnourishment, invasive monitoring devices, p. 482
- *Body Image Disturbance* related to functional dependence on hemodialysis life-sustaining technology, p. 459
- *Knowledge Deficit: Fluid Restriction, Reportable Symptoms,* and *Medications* related to lack of previous exposure to information, p. 455

tients in renal failure is restrictive. Protein, potassium, sodium, and phosphorus are usually limited. Protein is restricted to limit azotemia.[9] Carbohydrates are encouraged to provide energy for healing. (see Chapter 6).

Nursing Management

Nursing management of patients with ARF incorporates a variety of nursing diagnoses (Box 18-4). **Nursing priorities are directed toward preventing infectious complications, optimizing fluid balance, preventing electrolyte imbalance, and educating patients and families.**

Preventing infectious complications

Nursing management for patients with ARF focuses on prevention and control of complications secondary to the disease process. In preventing infection, nurses not only monitor for signs of infection but maintain patients' pulmonary hygiene, skin integrity, and nutrition. Nurses also provide strict asepsis when changing dressings and performing urinary catheterizations and other invasive procedures. If patients are immobile, frequent turning and observation of potential sites for skin breakdown decrease the risk of infection. If significant anasarca (severe generalized edema) has developed, the use of a circulating air or air-fluid mattress may help prevent skin breakdown.

Optimizing fluid balance

Maintenance of optimal fluid balance for patients with ARF involves monitoring the urine output in response to diuretics, accurately maintaining intake and output records, tracking fluid losses, assessing for compartmental fluid shifts with development of interstitial edema, and if patients are critically ill, evaluating cardiovascular function using pulmonary artery pressure measurements and cardiac outputs. Daily patient weights are correlated with fluid intake and output to determine fluid balance. Because hypovolemia usually precedes ischemic tubular damage, careful assessment of fluid intake and losses

from all sources is important. Hypervolemia is often seen when patients move from impaired renal function into complete renal failure. Cardiac output can also decrease with a severe initial insult such as hemorrhage. Measures to prevent blood loss in patients with renal failure include minimizing unnecessary blood draws for laboratory analysis, observing for signs of bleeding, and testing all stools, nasogastric drainage, and emesis for occult blood.

Correcting electrolyte imbalance

Hyperkalemia, hypocalcemia, hyponatremia, and hyperphosphatemia may all occur during ARF.[4-8] Knowledge of the clinical manifestations of these electrolyte imbalances enables nurses to prevent or control their associated side effects. The most potentially hazardous imbalances are hyperkalemia and hypocalcemia, which can result in life-threatening cardiac dysrhythmias. Hyperphosphatemia may result in severe pruritus. Thus nursing care is directed at soothing the itching by lubricating skin with emollients, discouraging scratching, and administering phosphate-binding medications.

Educating patients and families

Nurses provide uncomplicated information about ARF to patients and families. Topics include prognosis, treatment, and possible complications. Nurses explain that sleep-rest disorders and emotional upset can occur as complications of ARF and encourage patients and families to voice concerns, frustrations, and fears. Providing ways for patients to control some aspects of the acute care environment and treatment is helpful.

Dialysis

A wide range of dialysis options is available for the treatment of ARF: hemodialysis, peritoneal dialysis, and continuous renal replacement therapy.[10,11]

Hemodialysis

Hemodialysis roughly translates as "separating from the blood."[12] It has two parts: the dialysis part that removes excess electrolytes, fluids, and toxins from the blood and the ultrafiltration part that removes fluid. Many therapeutic medications are also removed from the body during hemodialysis (Table 18-4).

Hemodialyzer

Hemodialysis works by circulating blood outside the body through synthetic tubing to a dialyzer, which consists of several membrane pockets or tubes (Fig. 18-1). While the blood flows through the semipermeable membranes, a fluid (dialysate bath) bathes the membranes and, through osmosis and diffusion, performs exchanges of fluid, electrolytes, and toxins from the blood to the bath[13] (Box 18-5). The blood and bath are shunted in opposite directions through the dialyzer to maintain the highest osmotic and chemical gradients.

Text continued on p. 326.

TABLE 18-4

IMPACT OF RENAL FAILURE AND HEMODIALYSIS ON SELECTED DRUGS USED IN CRITICAL CARE

DRUG	NORMAL DRUG METABOLISM AND EXCRETION	% OF NORMAL DOSE ADJUSTMENT IN RENAL FAILURE DUE TO DECREASED CREATININE CLEARANCE (ML/MIN)*	EFFECT OF HEMODIALYSIS
ANTIINFECTIVES			
Antibiotics			
Amikacin†	94%-99% renal excretion	—	Dialyzed
Ampicillin	73%-92% renal excretion 12%-24% hepatic metabolism	Creatinine clearance 10-50: 100% of normal dose every 6-12 hours Creatinine clearance < 10: 50%-100% of normal dose every 12 hours	Moderately dialyzed
Clindamycin	10% renal excretion 85% hepatic metabolism (some active metabolites)	No change	Not dialyzed
Cefazolin	>95% renal excretion	Creatinine clearance 10-50: 50%-100% of normal dose every 12 hours Creatinine clearance < 10: 50% of normal dose every 24 hours	Moderately dialyzed
Cefotaxime	40%-65% renal excretion 40%-60% hepatic metabolism (active metabolite has 25% activity of parent)	Creatinine clearance 10-50: 50%-100% of normal dose every 8-12 hours Creatinine clearance < 10: 50% of normal dose every 8-12 hours	Moderately dialyzed
Ceftriaxone	40%-67% renal excretion 40% hepatic metabolism	Creatinine clearance 10-50: No change Creatinine clearance < 10: Decrease dose only with hepatic failure	Questionably dialyzed
Cefoxitin	78%-99% renal excretion	Creatinine clearance 10-50: 50%-100% of normal dose every 12-24 hours Creatinine clearance < 10: 25% of normal dose every 24 hours	Moderately dialyzed
Ceftazidime	>85% renal excretion	Creatinine clearance 10-50: 50% of normal dose every 6-8 hours Creatinine clearance < 10: 25% of normal dose every 12-24 hours	Dialyzed
Ciprofloxacin	62% renal excretion 38% hepatic metabolism	Creatinine clearance 10-50: 75% of normal dose every 12 hours Creatinine clearance < 10: 50%-75% of normal dose every 24 hours	Slightly dialyzed

Modified from Bubp JL, Rodondi LC, Gamberloglio JG: *Renal dialysis.* In Koda-Kimble MA, Young LY: *Applied therapeutics: the clinical use of drugs,* ed 5, Vancouver, Wash., 1992, Applied Therapeutics; and Aweeka FT: *Drug dosing in renal failure.* In Koda-Kimble MA, Young LY: Applied therapeutics: the clinical use of drugs, ed 5, Vancouver, Wash., 1992, Applied Therapeutics.
*The degree of renal failure is assessed by the creatinine clearance. Normal creatinine clearance is 120 ml/min; it decreases in renal failure. In renal failure, drug dosages are reduced either by decreasing the amount of drug administered each dose, lengthening the time between doses, or both.
†Aminoglycosides (Amikacin, Gentamycin, and Tobramycin): These drugs have a narrow therapeutic window, which means that the range between the therapeutic level and the toxic level is small, and they require close monitoring. In addition, drug clearance is affected by multiple factors. Refer to a pharmacist or pharmacokinetic text for recommendations.

T A B L E   1 8 - 4 — c o n t ' d

IMPACT OF RENAL FAILURE AND HEMODIALYSIS ON SELECTED DRUGS USED IN CRITICAL CARE

DRUG	NORMAL DRUG METABOLISM AND EXCRETION	% OF NORMAL DOSE ADJUSTMENT IN RENAL FAILURE DUE TO DECREASED CREATININE CLEARANCE (ML/MIN)*	EFFECT OF HEMODIALYSIS
ANTIINFECTIVES—cont'd			
Antibiotics—cont'd			
Cefotetan	50%-89% renal excretion 12% hepatic metabolism	Creatinine clearance 10-50: 50%-100% of normal dose every 12-24 hours Creatinine clearance < 10: 25%-50% of normal dose every 24 hours	Moderately dialyzed
Erythromycin	5%-15% renal excretion 85%-95% hepatic metabolism	No change	Slightly dialyzed
Gentamicin†	90%-97% renal excretion	—	Dialyzed
Imipenem	60%-75% renal excretion 22% hepatic metabolism	Creatinine clearance 10-50: 50%-75% of normal dose every 8-12 hours Creatinine clearance < 10: 25%-50% of normal dose every 12 hours	Moderately dialyzed
Mezlocillin	45%-65% renal excretion 35%-55% hepatic metabolism	Creatinine clearance 10-50: 100% of normal dose every 6-8 hours Creatinine clearance < 10: 50% of normal dose every 8 hours	Slightly dialyzed
Nafcillin	25%-30% renal excretion Up to 70% hepatic metabolism	No change	Not dialyzed
Penicillin‡	50% renal excretion 19% hepatic metabolism	—	Moderately dialyzed
Piperacillin	50%-60% renal excretion Up to 30%-40% hepatic metabolism	Creatinine clearance 10-50: 100% of normal dose every 6-8 hours Creatinine clearance < 10: 50%-75% of normal dose every 8 hours	Moderately dialyzed
Sulfamethoxazole	10% renal excretion 65%-80% hepatic metabolism	Creatinine clearance 10-50: 100% of normal dose every 12-24 hours Creatinine clearance < 10: 100% of normal dose every 24 hour	Slightly dialyzed
Tobramycin†	90%-97% renal excretion	—	Dialyzed
Trimethoprim	20%-35% renal excretion 53%-80% hepatic metabolism	Creatinine clearance 10-50: 100% of normal dose every 12-24 hours Creatinine clearance <10: 100% of normal dose every 24 hours	Slightly dialyzed
Vancomycin	80%-90% renal excretion 10%-20% hepatic metabolism	Requires individualized dosing regimens	Not dialyzed

*The degree of renal failure is assessed by the creatinine clearance. Normal creatinine clearance is 120 ml/min; it decreases in renal failure. In renal failure, drug dosages are reduced either by decreasing the amount of drug administered each dose, lengthening the time between doses, or both.
†Aminoglycosides (Amikacin, Gentamycin, and Tobramycin): These drugs have a narrow therapeutic window, which means that the range between the therapeutic level and the toxic level is small, and they require close monitoring. In addition, drug clearance is affected by multiple factors. Refer to a pharmacist or pharmacokinetic text for recommendations.
‡Penicillin G: Methods have been developed to calculate dosage based on changes in creatinine clearance. However, none of these methods have been subjected to careful clinical trials. Other factors can also affect patients' responses to therapy. Refer to a pharmacist or pharmacokinetic text for recommendations.

Continued.

TABLE 18-4—cont'd
IMPACT OF RENAL FAILURE AND HEMODIALYSIS ON SELECTED DRUGS USED IN CRITICAL CARE

DRUG	NORMAL DRUG METABOLISM AND EXCRETION	% OF NORMAL DOSE ADJUSTMENT IN RENAL FAILURE DUE TO DECREASED CREATININE CLEARANCE (ML/MIN)*	EFFECT OF HEMODIALYSIS
ANTIINFECTIVES—cont'd			
Antifungal			
Amphotericin B	3%-5% renal excretion 95%-97% hepatic metabolism	Creatinine clearance 10-50: 100% of normal dose every 24 hours Creatinine clearance < 10: 100% of normal dose every 24-48 hours	Not dialyzed
Fluconazole	70% renal excretion Some hepatic metabolism	Creatinine clearance 10-50: 50% of normal dose every 24 hours Creatinine clearance < 10: 25% of normal dose every 24 hours	Moderately dialyzed
Ketoconazole	3% renal excretion 51% hepatic metabolism	No change	Not dialyzed
Antiviral			
Acyclovir	70-80% renal excretion 14% hepatic metabolism	Creatinine clearance 10-50: 100% of normal dose every 12-24 hours Creatinine clearance < 10: 50% of normal dose every 24 hours	Dialyzed
Gancyclovir	>90% renal excretion	Creatinine clearance 10-50: 1.25-2.5 mg/Kg every 24 hours Creatinine clearance < 10: 1.25 mg/Kg every 24 hours	Dialyzed
CARDIOVASCULAR DRUGS			
Beta blockers			
Atenolol	75% renal excretion 10% hepatic metabolism	Creatinine clearance <50: 50% dose reduction and titrate as needed	Moderately dialyzed
Labetalol	5% renal excretion 95% hepatic excretion	No change	Not dialyzed
Metoprolol	10% renal excretion 90% hepatic metabolism	No change	Metabolites dialyzed
Nadolol	75% renal excretion 25% hepatic metabolism	Creatinine clearance <50: 50% dose reduction and titrate as needed	Moderately dialyzed
Propranolol	<1% renal excretion Primarily hepatic metabolism	No change	Not dialyzed

Modified from Bubp JL, Rodondi LC, Gamberloglio JG: *Renal dialysis.* In Koda-Kimble MA, Young LY: *Applied therapeutics: the clinical use of drugs,* ed 5, Vancouver, Wash., 1992, Applied Therapeutics; and Aweeka FT: *Drug dosing in renal failure.* In Koda-Kimble MA, Young LY: Applied therapeutics: the clinical use of drugs, ed 5, Vancouver, Wash., 1992, Applied Therapeutics.

*The degree of renal failure is assessed by the creatinine clearance. Normal creatinine clearance is 120 ml/min; it decreases in renal failure. In renal failure, drug dosages are reduced either by decreasing the amount of drug administered each dose, lengthening the time between doses, or both.

TABLE 18-4—cont'd
IMPACT OF RENAL FAILURE AND HEMODIALYSIS ON SELECTED DRUGS USED IN CRITICAL CARE

DRUG	NORMAL DRUG METABOLISM AND EXCRETION	% OF NORMAL DOSE ADJUSTMENT IN RENAL FAILURE DUE TO DECREASED CREATININE CLEARANCE (ML/MIN)*	EFFECT OF HEMODIALYSIS
CARDIOVASCULAR DRUGS—cont'd			
ACE inhibitors			
Captopril	36%-42% renal excretion 50% hepatic metabolism	Creatinine clearance 10-50: No change Creatinine clearance < 10: 25% dose reduction and titrate as needed	Moderately dialyzed
Enalapril	61% renal excretion 33% hepatic metabolism	Creatinine clearance <50: 50% dose reduction and titrate as needed	Moderately dialyzed
Calcium channel blockers			
Nifedipine	100% hepatic metabolism	No change	Not known
Verapamil	100% hepatic metabolism	No change	Not dialyzed
Antidysrhythmics			
Digoxin	70% renal excretion	Creatinine clearance 10-50: 50% dose reduction and titrate as needed Creatinine clearance < 10: 75% dose reduction and titrate as needed	Not dialyzed
Lidocaine	100% hepatic metabolism	No change	Not dialyzed
Procainamide	50%-60% renal excretion Hepatic metabolism to active NAPA metabolite	Creatinine clearance 10-50: 100% of normal dose every 6-12 hours Creatinine clearance < 10: 100% of normal dose every 12-24 hours	Moderately dialyzed
ANALGESICS			
Codeine	Hepatic metabolism	Creatinine clearance 10-50: 25% of normal dose and titrate as needed Creatinine clearance < 10: 50% of normal dose and titrate as needed	Not known
Ibuprofen	45%-60% excreted unchanged and as metabolites	No change	Not dialyzed
Meperidine	10% renal excretion Hepatic metabolism	Creatinine clearance 10-50: 75%-100% of normal dose every 6 hours Creatinine clearance < 10: 50% of normal dose every 6-8 hours and use with caution	Not known

*The degree of renal failure is assessed by the creatinine clearance. Normal creatinine clearance is 120 ml/min; it decreases in renal failure. In renal failure, drug dosages are reduced either by decreasing the amount of drug administered each dose, lengthening the time between doses, or both.

Continued.

TABLE 18-4 — cont'd

IMPACT OF RENAL FAILURE AND HEMODIALYSIS ON SELECTED DRUGS USED IN CRITICAL CARE

DRUG	NORMAL DRUG METABOLISM AND EXCRETION	% OF NORMAL DOSE ADJUSTMENT IN RENAL FAILURE DUE TO DECREASED CREATININE CLEARANCE (ML/MIN)*	EFFECT OF HEMODIALYSIS
ANTICONVULSANTS/SEDATIVES			
Anticonvulsants			
Phenobarbital	10%-40% renal excretion Hepatic metabolism	Creatinine clearance 10-50: No change Creatinine clearance < 10: Slight dosage decrease	Moderately dialyzed
Phenytoin	Hepatic metabolism	No change	Not dialyzed
Sedatives			
Diazepam	Renal excretion of active metabolites Hepatic metabolism	Reduction of dose and titration as needed	Not dialyzed
Midazolam	Not known	Not known	Not dialyzed
H₂ BLOCKERS			
Cimetidine	40%-80% renal excretion	Creatinine clearance 10-50: 25% dose reduction Creatinine clearance < 10: 50% dose reduction	Slightly dialyzed
Famotidine	Significant renal excretion Small hepatic metabolism	Creatinine clearance < 10: 100% of normal dose every 24-48 hours	
Ranitidine	70% renal excretion	Creatinine clearance 10-50: 25% dose reduction	Slightly dialyzed

Modified from Bubp JL, Rodondi LC, Gamberloglio JG: *Renal dialysis.* In Koda-Kimble MA, Young LY: *Applied therapeutics: the clinical use of drugs,* ed 5, Vancouver, Wash., 1992, Applied Therapeutics; and Aweeka FT: *Drug dosing in renal failure.* In Koda-Kimble MA, Young LY: Applied therapeutics: the clinical use of drugs, ed 5, Vancouver, Wash., 1992, Applied Therapeutics.

*The degree of renal failure is assessed by the creatinine clearance. Normal creatinine clearance is 120 ml/min; it decreases in renal failure. In renal failure, drug dosages are reduced either by decreasing the amount of drug administered each dose, lengthening the time between doses, or both.

BOX 18-5

COMPOSITION OF HEMODIALYSATE BATH

Purified water (reverse osmosis process)
Sodium chloride
Potassium chloride
Sodium bicarbonate (used frequently, although sodium acetate may be used as a substitute)
Calcium chloride
Magnesium chloride
Lactic acid

Ultrafiltration

A positive hydrostatic pressure is applied to the blood, and a negative hydrostatic pressure is applied to the dialysate bath for fluid removal. The two forces together, called *transmembrane pressure,* pull and squeeze the excess fluid from the blood. The difference between the two values (expressed in millimeters of mercury [mm Hg]) represents the transmembrane pressure and results in fluid extraction, known as *ultrafiltration,* from the vascular space.[9] The anticoagulant heparin is added to the system just before the blood enters the dialyzer. Without heparin the blood would clot because its presence outside the body and its passage through synthetic tubing initiate the clotting mechanism. Heparin can be administered by bolus injection or intermittent infusion. The components of a hemodialysis system are shown in Fig. 18-2.

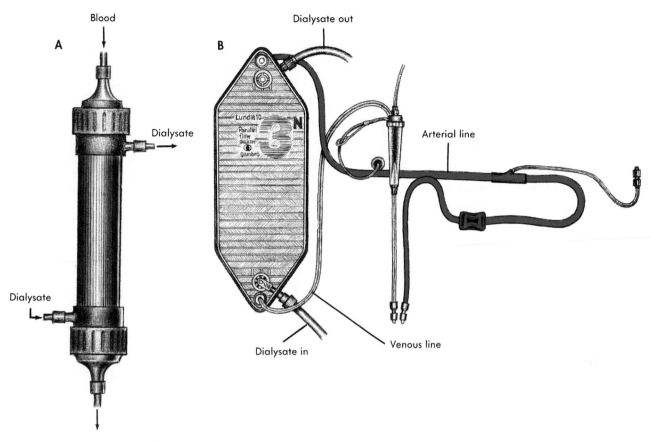

FIG. 18-1 Types of dialyzers. **A,** Hollow fiber. **B,** Flat plate. (From Thompson JM and others: *Mosby's clinical nursing,* ed 3, St Louis, 1993, Mosby.)

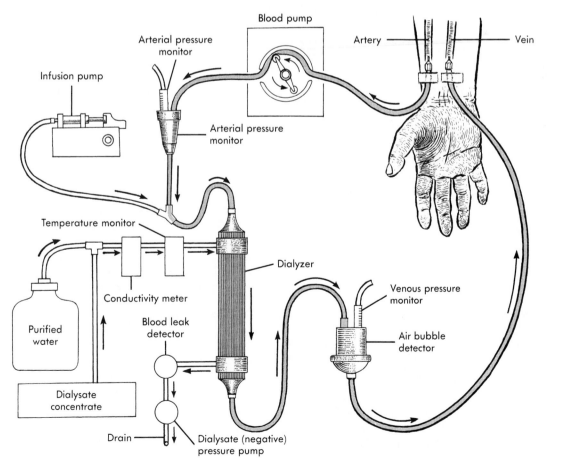

FIG. 18-2 Components of a hemodialysis system.

Vascular Access for Hemodialysis

Hemodialysis requires access to the bloodstream. Over many years various types of permanent arteriovenous (A-V) accesses have been created. The common denominator is access to the arterial circulation and return to the venous circulation. Femoral and subclavian catheters (used most often in critical care patients) permit access to the venous circulation only.

Subclavian and femoral vein catheters

Subclavian and femoral vein catheters are used in the critical care unit for patients in ARF who require short-term hemodialysis. Both subclavian and femoral catheters can be inserted at the bedside. A dual-lumen catheter is the type most frequently used to obtain vascular access in acute hemodialysis.[13] It has a central partition running the length of the catheter. The outflow catheter pulls the blood through openings that are proximal to the inflow openings to avoid dialyzing the blood just returned to the area (i.e., recirculation), which would severely reduce the procedure's effectiveness. In addition, some catheters incorporate a Dacron cuff that decreases the incidence of catheter-related infections.[13] After the insertion of any new subclavian

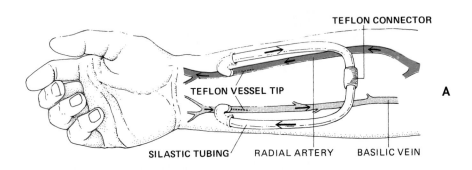

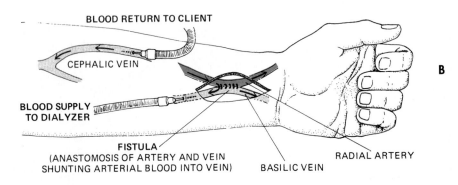

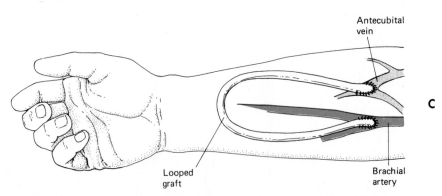

FIG. 18-3 Methods of vascular access for hemodialysis. **A,** External cannula or shunt. **B,** Internal A-V fistula. **C,** Looped graft in forearm. (From Kaga L: *Renal disease: a manual of patient care,* New York, 1979, McGraw-Hill.)

access, a chest x-ray is performed to rule out the possibility of pneumothorax or hemothorax resulting from the catheter insertion. Femoral catheter sites are monitored carefully for any signs of hematoma or bleeding.

A-V shunt

A-V shunts are used infrequently. The shunt consists of Teflon vessel tips, Silastic tubing, and a connection joint for creating the circuit between the arterial and venous circulation. (Fig. 18-3, *A*). The shunt requires a peripheral artery, usually radial or ulnar, and a peripheral vein such as the cephalic or basilic. A surgical cutdown is performed on each vessel. Tubing extends from each vessel tip (outside the body) and is connected, when not being used for dialysis, by a straight connector or a heparin-T device. Blood flows in a U-shaped fashion from artery to vein. Shunts may also be inserted in the thigh or ankle. Complications common to A-V shunts are thrombosis, infection, and skin erosion. (Nursing management considerations for A-V shunts are listed in Table 18-5.)

A-V fistula

The A-V fistula is created surgically. A peripheral artery and vein are connected under the skin. The anastomoses may be side to side, end to side, or end to end. The high arterial flow creates swelling of the vein, or a pseudoaneurysm, that on healing permits the insertion of large-bore needles for inflow and outflow vascular access (Fig. 18-3, *B*). If patients' vessels are adequate, A-V fistulas are the preferred mode of access because of the relatively few complications. However, complications such as decreased perfusion to the affected extremity, thrombosis, infection, and venous hypertension can occur. (The care of the fistula and nursing considerations are listed in Table 18-5.)

A-V grafts

Currently, A-V grafts are the most frequently used long-term access for treating chronic renal failure. Synthetic materials (such as Goretex) and biologic materials (such as human umbilical veins) provide a wide range of lumen sizes and graft lengths. The graft is a tube made from the desired material (usually Goretex) and surgically implanted between the selected artery and vein un-

---

TABLE 18-5

COMPLICATIONS AND NURSING MANAGEMENT OF A-V SHUNT, A-V FISTULA, AND A-V GRAFTS

TYPE	COMPLICATIONS	NURSING MANAGEMENT
A-V shunt	Clotting Dislodgment Skin erosion Infection Bleeding	Monitor for clinical manifestations of infection. Monitor for clinical manifestations of thrombosis (darkening of blood, separation of serum or cellular compartment blood in tubing, decreased temperature of tubing). Assess insertion site daily for erosion around insertion sites. Use strict aseptic technique during dressing changes at insertion sites. Teach patients to avoid sleeping on or prolonged bending of accessed limbs. Keep two shunt clamps attached to patients' clothing or access dressing at all times.
A-V fistula	Thrombosis Infection Pseudoaneurysm Vascular steal syndrome Venous hypertension Carpal tunnel syndrome Inadequate blood flow	Teach patients to avoid wearing constrictive clothing on limbs containing access. Teach patients to avoid sleeping on or prolonged bending of accessed limb. Use aseptic technique when cannulating access. Avoid repetitious cannulation of one segment of access. Offer comfort measures, such as warm compresses and ordered analgesics, to lessen pain of vascular steal. Teach patients to develop blood flow in the fistulas through exercises (squeezing a rubber ball) while applying mild impedance to flow just distal to the access (at least once per day for 10 to 15 minutes).
A-V graft	Bleeding Thrombosis False aneurysm formation Infection Arterial or venous stenosis Vascular steal syndrome	Avoid too early cannulation of new access. Teach patients to avoid wearing constrictive clothing on accessed limbs. Avoid repeated cannulation of one segment of access. Use aseptic technique when cannulating access. Monitor for changes in arterial or venous pressure while patients are on dialysis. Provide comfort measures to reduce pain of vascular steal (e.g., warm compresses, analgesics as ordered).

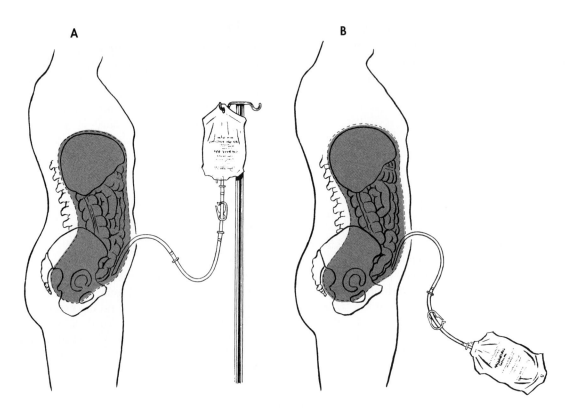

FIG. 18-4 Peritoneal dialysis. **A,** Inflow. **B,** Outflow (drains by gravity). (From Thompson JM and others: *Mosby's clinical nursing,* ed 3, St Louis, 1993, Mosby.)

der the skin. The graft creates a raised area that looks like a large vein, just under the skin (Fig. 18-3, *C*). Two large-bore needles are used for outflow and inflow to the graft. For both grafts and fistulas, firm pressure must be applied to stop bleeding after needle removal at the end of the hemodialysis treatment. (Nursing management and complications of the A-V graft are listed in Table 18-5.)

Peritoneal Dialysis

Peritoneal dialysis (PD) involves the introduction of sterile dialyzing fluid through an implanted catheter into the abdominal cavity. The dialysate bathes the peritoneal membrane, which covers the abdominal organs and overlies the capillary beds that support the organs. By the processes of osmosis, diffusion, and active transport, excess fluid and solutes travel from the peritoneal capillary fluid through the capillary walls, through the peritoneal membrane, and into the dialyzing fluid. After a selected time (dwell time), the fluid is drained out of the abdomen by gravity (Fig. 18-4). The process is then repeated. (Indications and contraindications for PD[10,11] are summarized in Box 18-6.) The volume of dialysate instilled into the abdomen affects clearance. During acute PD, 3.5 L/hr provides a urea clearance of 26 ml/min. During chronic, continuous PD, 2-L exchanges every 4 hours provide a clearance of 7 ml/min. The dialysate is instilled at normal body temperature for comfort, vasodilatation,

---

BOX 18-6

Indications and Contraindications for Peritoneal Dialysis

INDICATIONS

Uremia
Volume overload
Electrolyte imbalances
Hemodynamic instability
Lack of access to circulation
Removal of high-molecular-weight toxins
Patients with nonrenal critical illness who are receiving
 PD for chronic renal failure
Severe cardiovascular disease
Inability to anticoagulate
Contraindication to hemodialysis

CONTRAINDICATIONS

Recent abdominal surgery
History of abdominal surgeries with adhesions and
 scarring
Significant pulmonary disease
Need for rapid fluid removal
Peritonitis

T A B L E 1 8 - 6		
DIALYSATE CONCENTRATIONS FOR PERITONEAL DIALYSIS (PD)		
PD-1 SOLUTION	**PD-2 SOLUTION**	**LOW CALCIUM SOLUTION**
Na, 132 mmol/L	Na, 132 mmol/L	Na, 132 mmol/L
Ca, 3.5 mmol/L	Ca, 3.5 mmol/L	Ca, 2.5 mmol/L
Mg, 1.5 mmol/L	Mg, 0.5 mmol/L	Mg, 0.5 mmol/L
Cl, 102 mmol/L	Cl, 96 mmol/L	Cl, 95 mmol/L
Lactate, 35 mmol/L	Lactate, 40 mmol/L	Lactate, 40 mmol/L
Dextrose, 1.5%, 2.5%, 4.25%	Dextrose, 1.5%, 2.5%, 3.5%, 4.25%	Dextrose, 1.5%, 2.5%, 3.5%, 4.25%

Modified from Smith LJ: *AACN Clin Issues* 3(3):558, 1992.

and increased solute transport in the peritoneum. The various glucose concentrations of the dialysate allow different rates of fluid removal. (Dialysate concentrations are summarized in Table 18-6.) PD is not routinely used as an emergency treatment in renal failure. However, the use of PD is growing annually, and when patients on PD are admitted to the critical care unit for reasons other than renal failure, the PD is continued (Table 18-7).

PD catheters

Two types of catheters are used for PD: the rigid stylet and silicone catheters. The single-use rigid stylet catheter can be inserted at the bedside for immediate initiation of dialysis. Patient mobility is limited when the rigid stylet catheter is in place because of the possibility of perforation.[14] The silicone catheter is usually inserted surgically, although it can be inserted at the bedside. This catheter is extremely flexible, allowing patients to move freely with minimal discomfort.[14] Most catheters have a tunnel segment that passes through subcutaneous tissue and muscle and a cuff for stabilization at the peritoneal membrane. Disposable external Y-tubing is used for delivery and drainage of dialysate (Fig. 18-4).

PD complications

The numerous complications of PD, which range from annoying to severe, require careful observation and intervention to control or prevent further problems.[15] The most serious complication is peritonitis. (Complications and nursing management related to PD are listed in Table 18-4.)

Continuous Renal Replacement Therapy

Continuous renal replacement therapy (CCRT) is a newer mode of dialysis used in critically ill patients with ARF. CRRT is a continuous therapy lasting 12 hours or longer in which blood is circulated from an artery to a vein through a highly porous hemofilter.[10,16,17] The system allows for slow volume removal (5 to 15 ml/min), plus removal of urea, creatinine, and electrolytes.[16,17] The hydrostatic pressure exerted by

B O X   1 8 - 7
INDICATIONS AND CONTRAINDICATIONS FOR CONTINUOUS RENAL REPLACEMENT THERAPY

INDICATIONS

Need for large fluid volume removal in hemodynamically unstable patients
Hypervolemic or edematous patients unresponsive to diuretic therapy
Patients with multiple organ dysfunction syndrome
Ease of fluid management in patients requiring large daily fluid volume, such as replacement for oliguria, TPN administration
Contraindications to hemodialysis and peritoneal dialysis
Inability to anticoagulate

CONTRAINDICATIONS

Hematocrit >45%
Lack of arterial access
TPN, total parenteral nutrition.

patients' mean arterial pressure (MAP) forms the "push" for continuous flow of blood through the hemofilter. A MAP of greater than 70 mm Hg is necessary to maintain this flow. The ultrafiltrate can be drained by gravity flow or by a suction-assisted collection system.[16] (Indications and contraindications for CRRT[10,11,16-21] are summarized in Box 18-7.) Because controlled removal and replacement of fluid are possible with CRRT, hemodynamic stability is maintained. This makes CRRT highly advantageous for use in patients with myocardial failure, shock, and multiple organ dysfunction syndrome.[11,18,20] The three common forms of CRRT are slow continuous ultrafiltration (SCUF), continuous arteriovenous hemofiltration (CAVH), and continuous arteriovenous hemodialysis (CAVHD). (A comparison of CRRT methods is found in Table 18-8.)

TABLE 18-7
COMPLICATIONS AND NURSING MANAGEMENT OF PERITONEAL DIALYSIS

COMPLICATIONS	NURSING MANAGEMENT
Peritonitis	Assess for signs and symptoms: cloudy effluent, abdominal pain, rebound tenderness, nausea and vomiting, and fever. Obtain effluent sample for culture. Administer antibiotics as ordered. Teach patients and families signs and symptoms and their prevention.
Exit site infection	Monitor site daily for signs and symptoms of infection: enduration, erythema, purulence, and hyperthermia. Increase daily cleaning of site. Apply topical antibiotics as ordered (controversial). Teach patients and families to avoid agents such as creams and lotions around exit site.
Catheter-tunnel infection	Assess for signs and symptoms of infection: pain along tunnel, enduration for several centimeters away from catheter, erythema leading away from the exit site, and drainage at exit site or as tunnel is "milked" toward exit site. Teach patients and families signs and symptoms of infection. Teach patients and families to avoid pulls or tugs on the catheter or trauma to the exit site. Emphasize the need to maintain cleansing regimen at exit site.
Fluid obstruction	Change position of patients (i.e., standing, lying, side lying, knee chest). Relieve patients' constipation. Irrigate the catheter. Ensure that sufficient fluid is in abdomen (sometimes requires a residual reservoir of approximately 50 ml).
Rectal pain	Ensure a sufficient reservoir of fluid. Use slow infusion rate.
Shoulder pain	Ensure that all air is primed from infusion tubing. Attempt draining the effluent with patients in knee-chest position. Administer mild analgesics as ordered.
Hernias	Monitor for increase in size of or pain in area of hernia. Decrease volume of exchanges as ordered. Dialyze with patients in the supine position. Use abdominal binder or support for patients (as long as not binding on catheter exit site). Avoid initiation of PD until exit site healing has taken place (approximately 1 to 2 weeks) if possible.
Fluid overload	Increase use of hypertonic solutions. Decrease by mouth (PO) fluid intake. Shorten dwell times. Weigh patients frequently. Monitor lung sounds and peripheral edema.
Dehydration	Assess patients for decreased skin turgor, muscle cramps, hypotension, tachycardia, and dizziness. Discontinue hypertonic solutions. Increase PO fluid intake. Lengthen dwell times.
Blood-tinged effluent	Monitor for change in effluent color (clear yellow to pink or rusty). Administer heparin, as ordered, to avoid fibrin formation. Obtain patient history about catheter trauma and patient activity before appearance of complication.

Slow continuous ultrafiltration (SCUF)

SCUF, as the name implies, slowly removes fluid, 100 to 300 ml/hr, through a process of convection.[10,17,18,20] This process consists of an exchange of solutes and solvents across a semipermeable membrane.[18] Because fluid is removed slowly, it is used for patients who have acute heart failure with mild renal compromise.[16] (The SCUF system setup is illustrated in Fig. 18-5, *A*.)

Continuous arteriovenous hemofiltration (CAVH)

CAVH is a process in which both fluid and solute are removed through convection in volumes of 500 to 800 ml/hr. In addition, fluid replacement with appropriate and sufficient electrolytes is administered to patients.[16,18] Replacement solutions may consist of standard solutions of bicarbonate or acetate and also include dextrose and electrolytes such as potassium, magnesium, sodium, and

TYPE	ULTRAFILTRATION RATE	FLUID REPLACEMENT	INDICATION
SCUF	100 to 300 ml/hr	None	Fluid removal
CAVH	500 to 800 ml/hr	Predilution or postdilution, calculating an hourly net loss	Fluid removal, moderate solute removal
CAVHD	500 to 800 ml/hr	Predilution or postdilution, subtracting the dialysate and then calculating an hourly net loss	Fluid removal, maximum solute removal

SCUF, Slow continuous ultrafiltration; *CAVH,* continuous arteriovenous hemofiltration; *CAVHD,* continuous arteriovenous hemodialysis.
Modified from Price CA: *AACN Clin Issues* 3(3):597, 1992.

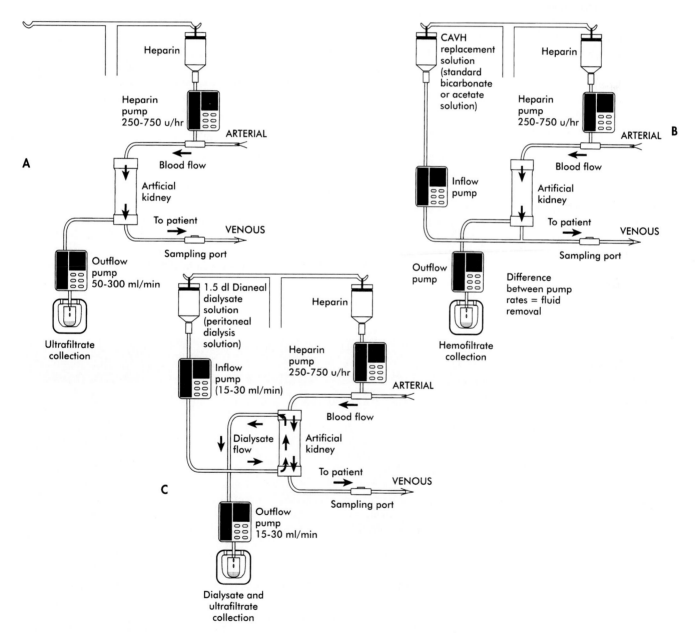

FIG. 18-5   **A,** SCUF system setup. **B,** CAVH system setup. **C,** CAVHD system setup.
(Modified from Bosworth C: SCUF/CAVH/CAVHD: critical differences, *Crit Care Nurs Q* 14(4):45, 1992.)

calcium.[18] CAVH is indicated when patients' clinical conditions warrant moderate removal of fluid and solutes. Because large volumes are removed, fluid may be replaced hourly with a continuous infusion. Fluid volume monitoring is of particular importance to patients with hemodynamic compromise.[16,20]

HEMOFILTERS. Hemofilters are designed to clear solutes and unbound molecules of up to 50,000 daltons. Typical hemodialysis clears only particles of up to 10,000 daltons. The hemofilter clears many drugs that dialysis cannot remove. Hemofilters can remove fluid at the rate of 35 to 45 ml/min. Significant fluid removal (ultrafiltration) alone can be accomplished by simply allowing the blood pressure to push the blood continuously through the circuit.

FLUID REPLACEMENT. Fluid replacement is based on fluid losses and electrolyte values, with consideration given to achieving the desired reduction in the extracellular fluid volume. The following fluid replacement calculation is performed every hour: Total output per hour minus IV/oral intake per hour minus desired hourly output (loss) equals amount of IV replacement fluid to be infused the next hour.[20] Replacement fluids may range from potassium-free lactated Ringer's solution to normal saline solution.

ANTICOAGULATION. Anticoagulation is important because blood is traveling through an extracorporeal circuit. Commonly, a 2000-U bolus of heparin is given before initiation of CRRT. Thereafter, 5 to 10 U/kg/hr is infused throughout the treatment. Clotting times are frequently calculated to monitor anticoagulation. The CAVH system setup is illustrated in Fig. 18-5, *B*. The system is identical to the SCUF system, with the addition of a replacement solution.[18,20]

Continuous arteriovenous hemodialysis (CAVHD)

The CAVHD method accomplishes both fluid removal and maximal removal of solutes. In addition, the process of conduction allows the passive diffusion of solutes across the semipermeable membrane so that solute removal is enhanced. This form of CRRT is similar to traditional hemodialysis.[18] A peritoneal or custom dialysate solution is infused into the hemofilter to remove fluids. Instead of a replacement fluid, the dialysate solution is added, infused through the hemofilter, and removed with the ultrafiltrate.[18] CAVHD is indicated in patients who require large-volume removal for severe uremia or severe acid-base imbalances. Although it is rather expensive, CAVHD is the most efficient form of CRRT.[16,20] (The system setup for CAVHD is illustrated in Fig. 18-5, *C*.)

Vascular access for CRRT

Single-lumen, large-bore catheters are placed into an artery and vein. Usually the femoral site is selected because of its large size and accessibility. Additional access sites for CRRT include the subclavian vein and an A-V shunt.[18]

Complications of CRRT

Although CRRT is a successful treatment for ARF, potential complications are numerous (Table 18-9). Patients with ARF undergoing CRRT present special challenges to critical care nurses. Nurses have a crucial role in the early detection and treatment of any complications that result from CRRT therapy.[16,17,19-21] Table 18-10 describes problems, etiologies, and clinical manifestations related to CRRT, as well as nursing management priorities.

TABLE 18-9
POTENTIAL COMPLICATIONS RELATED TO CRRT

CLINICAL FINDING	POTENTIAL RATIONALES
Dehydration, hypotension	Incorrect intake/output calculations, inadequate prescription for fluid replacement
Electrolytes, acid-base abnormalities	Incorrect replacement fluids, incorrect dialysate, lactate intolerance
Hypothermia	Extracorporeal system, cool replacement fluids, cool dialysate
Hyperglycemia	High dextrose in dialysate
Decreased ultrafiltrate	Clotted hemofilter, poor blood flow through the hemofilter, need for predilution replacement fluid, hemoconcentration with hematocrit level above 35%, hypotension
Inadequate blood flow through the hemofilter	Clotted hemofilter, hypotension, kinked or positional catheters or tubing, too-small arterial and/or venous catheter
Clotted hemofilter	Improper heparinization, prolonged hypotension, poor blood flow rate, secondary to vascular accesses
Blood leak with blood in ultrafiltrate	Defective hemofilter, break in membrane integrity secondary to blunt trauma or high vacuum suction
Disconnection at catheter or hemofilter	Non–Luer-locked syringe connections, connections not secured with tape, patients out of bed

Modified from Price CA: *AACN Clin Issues* 3(3):597, 1992.

TABLE 18-10

PROBLEMS, ETIOLOGIES, CLINICAL MANIFESTATIONS, AND NURSING INTERVENTIONS RELATED TO CRRT

PROBLEM	ETIOLOGY	CLINICAL MANIFESTATIONS	NURSING MANAGEMENT
Decreased ultrafiltration rate	Hypotension Dehydration Kinked lines Bending of catheters Clotting of filter	Ultrafiltration rate decreased Minimal flow through blood lines	Observe filter and arteriovenous system. Control blood flow. Control coagulation time. Position patients on back. Lower height of collection container.
Filter clotting	Obstruction Insufficient heparinization As above	Ultrafiltration rate decreased, despite height of collection container being lower	Control heparinization. Maintain continuous heparinization. Call physicians. Remove system. Prime catheters with heparin. Prime a new system and connect it. Start predilution with 1000 ml saline 0.9% solution per hour. Do not use three-way stopcocks.
Hypotension	Increased ultrafiltration rate Blood leak Disconnection of one of lines	Bleeding	Control amount of ultrafiltration. Control access sites. Clamp lines. Call physician.
Fluid and electrolyte changes	Too much/little removal of fluid Inappropriate replacement of electrolytes Inappropriate dialysate	Changes in mentation ↑ or ↓ CVP, PAWP ECG change ↑ or ↓ BP and heart rate Abnormal electrolyte levels	Observe for changes in central venous pressure or pulmonary capillary wedge pressure. Observe for changes in vital signs. Observe electrocardiogram for changes as result of electrolyte abnormalities. Monitor output values every hour. Control ultrafiltration.
Bleeding	System disconnection ↑ Heparin dose	Oozing from catheter insertion site or connection	Monitor activated clotting time (ACT) no less than once every hour. Adjust heparin dose within specifications to maintain ACT. Observe dressing on vascular access for blood loss. Observe for blood in filtrate (filter leak).
Access dislodgment or infection	Catheter/connections not secured Break in sterile technique Excessive patient movement	Bleeding from catheter site or connections Inappropriate flow/infusion Fever Drainage at catheter site	Observe access site at least once every 2 hr. Ensure that clamps are available within easy reach at all times. Observe strict sterile technique when dressing vascular access.

Modified from Lievaart A, Voerman HJ: *Heart Lung* 20(2):152, 1991.

Fluid Volume Replacement

Intravenous Volume Replacement

Hypovolemia is a risk factor for prerenal failure. If IV volume replacement is administered, one of the IV solutions listed in Table 18-11 may be used. Intravascular solutions are generally classified as crystalloid, colloid, or blood products. An understanding of the differences among the various types of intravenous fluids is essential for safe critical care nursing practice.

Crystalloid solutions

These IV solutions consist of electrolytes in water or dextrose in water in a variety of combinations (Table 18-11). They are described as isotonic, hypotonic, or hypertonic compared with the normal serum osmolality (tonicity) of 275 to 295 mOsm/L. (See Figure 18-6 for further explanation of the effects of the different solution concentrations on the cells within the body.)

ISOTONIC SOLUTIONS. These solutions have the same osmolality, or concentration of particles, as the extracellular and intracellular fluids. The most commonly used isotonic solutions are normal saline (0.9% NaCl) and lactated Ringer's.[22,23]

HYPOTONIC SOLUTIONS. These solutions are more dilute than body fluids. The hypotonic fluid is pulled into the cells, causing them to swell and sometimes burst if sufficient volume is given. The most commonly used hypotonic solution is D_5W. Water is also a hypotonic solution.

HYPERTONIC SOLUTIONS. These solutions contain greater than 285 to 295 mOsm/L. Hypertonic solutions pull water out of the cells so the cells shrink (Fig. 18-6); 3% saline is an example of a hypertonic solution.

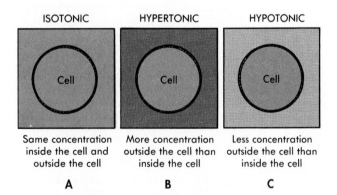

FIG. 18-6 **A,** *Isotonic solution:* The extracellular solution concentration is the same as the intracellular concentration, with no movement of water into or out of the cell. **B,** *Hypertonic solution:* The extracellular solution concentration is greater than the intracellular concentration. Water moves from the cell into the extracellular compartment. **C,** *Hypotonic solution:* The extracellular solution concentration is less than the intracellular concentration. Water moves from the extracellular compartment into the cell.

Colloids

Colloids contain large molecules that contribute to the plasma colloid osmotic pressure within the intravascular space and help keep fluid within the blood vessels. Used for rapid volume expansion, colloid solutions work by pulling fluids from the interstitium into the bloodstream to expand the circulating volume. Albumin is the major natural colloid in the blood plasma. A 10-ml infusion of albumin (25%) can pull as much as 350 ml into the vascular system. Synthetic volume expanders such as Dextran and Hetastarch are also available. The effects from volume expanders can last as long as 24 hours, with corresponding rises in pulmonary artery wedge pressure, MAP, and cardiac index. (Specific colloid solutions are described in more detail in Table 18-11.)

Blood products

Blood products are derived from human blood donors. Whole blood is not usually administered, but rather the specific product required to treat the clinical deficit.

Medications

Diuretics

Used to increase water excretion via the kidneys, **diuretics** are frequently prescribed in the critical care setting. Several classes of diuretics are available (Table 18-12).[24,25] In critically ill patients, diuretics are usually administered by IV bolus, although some recent studies suggest that continuous diuretic infusion may be as or more effective in selected patient populations.[26,27]

Impact of Renal Failure on Medications

In general, medications are either eliminated from the body unchanged by renal excretion or metabolized by the liver. The amount of unchanged drug normally excreted by the kidney is a major factor in determining whether renal failure will affect drug clearance from the body. Drugs that are excreted primarily by the liver are not significantly affected by changes in renal function, unless drug metabolites produce a pharmacologic action or the metabolites are excreted by the kidney. If a drug is normally excreted via the kidney, either the dose must be reduced, the interval between doses lengthened, or a combination of both actions taken to avoid accumulation of the drug. (See Table 18-4 for more information on changes in medications recommended with low creatinine clearance.)

Impact of Hemodialysis on Medications

If hemodialysis is required, drugs that are primarily eliminated by the kidney are dialyzed and a posthemodialysis dose may be prescribed. Three factors affect the degree to which a drug will be removed by hemodialysis. First, drugs with low molecular weight and high water

TABLE 18-11		
MOST FREQUENTLY USED INTRAVENOUS SOLUTIONS		
NAME	**ELECTROLYTES**	**INDICATIONS**
CRYSTALLOIDS*		
Dextrose in water (D_5W)—isotonic	None	To maintain volume To replace mild loss To provide minimal calories
Normal saline (0.9% NaCl)	Sodium 154 mEq/L Chloride 154 mEq/L Osmolality 308 mEq/L	To maintain volume To replace mild loss To correct mild hyponatremia
Half-strength saline (0.45% NaCl)	Sodium 77 mEq/L Chloride 77 mEq/L	For free water replacement To correct mild hyponatremia For free water and electrolyte replacement (used in fluid and electrolyte-restricted conditions)
Lactated Ringer's	Sodium 130 mEq/L Potassium 4 mEq/L Calcium 2.7 mEq/L Chloride 107 mEq/L Lactate 27 mEq/L pH 6.5	For fluid and electrolyte replacement (contraindicated for patients with renal or liver disease or in lactic acidosis)
COLLOIDS		
5% Albumin (Albumisol)	Albumin 50 g/L Sodium 130 to 160 mEq/L Potassium 300 mOsm/L Osmolality Osmotic pressure 20 mm Hg pH 6.4 to 7.4	For volume expansion For moderate protein replacement For achievement of hemodynamic stability in shock states
25% Albumin (salt-poor)	Albumin 240 g/L Globulins 10 g/L Sodium 130 to 160 mEq/L Osmolality 1500 mOsm/L pH 6.4 to 7.4	Concentrated form of albumin sometimes used with diuretics to move fluid from tissues into the vascular space for diuresis
Hetastarch	Sodium 154 mEq/L Chloride 154 mEq/L Osmolality 310 mOsm/L Colloid osmotic pressure 30-35 mm Hg	Synthetic polymer (6% solution) used for volume expansion For hemodynamic volume replacement after cardiac surgery, burns, sepsis)
Low-molecular-weight dextran (LMWD)	Glucose polysaccharide molecules with an average molecular weight of 40,000, no electrolytes	For volume expansion and support (contraindicated for patients with bleeding disorders)
High-molecular-weight dextran (HMWD)	Glucose polysaccharide molecules with an average molecular weight of 70,000, no electrolytes	Used prophylactically in some cases to prevent platelet aggregation, available in either saline or glucose solutions

*For the crystalloid solutions that contain electrolytes, specific concentrations of electrolytes and pH will vary according to manufacturers.

TABLE 18-12
DIURETIC EFFECTS ON ELECTROLYTES

AGENTS	MODE OF ACTION	ELECTROLYTE EFFECTS	COMPLICATIONS
LOOP DIURETICS			
Ethacrynic acid, furosemide, bumetanide	Inhibits reabsorption of electrolytes in the ascending loop of Henle	Potassium decreases, uric acid increases, calcium decreases, magnesium decreases, sodium decreases, chloride decreases, bicarbonate decreases	Metabolic alkalosis, hypokalemia, hyponatremia, hypochloremia
THIAZIDE DIURETICS			
Chlorothiazide, hydrochlorothiazide	Acts directly on the nephron to increase sodium chloride excretion with a large volume of water in the distal tubule	Sodium decreases slightly, chloride decreases slightly, potassium decreases, uric acid increases, calcium increases	Most sodium reabsorbed, hypokalemia, hypercalcemia, hypophosphatemia, hyperparathyroidism
OSMOTICS			
Mannitol	Increases urine output because of increased plasma osmolality, increasing flow of water from tissues	Potassium increases, sodium increases	Hypernatremia preceding hyponatremia, acidosis, dehydration
METHYLXANTHINES			
Caffeine, aminophylline	Acts similarly to the thiazide diuretics but on proximal tubule	Sodium decreases, chloride decreases, potassium decreases, calcium increases	Hyponatremia, hypokalemia, hypercalcemia

From Mendyka BE: Fluid and electrolyte disorders caused by diuretic therapy, *AACN Clin Issues Crit Care Nurs* 3(3):674, 1992.

solubility are more easily removed by dialysis. Second, drugs that are protein bound are not significantly removed by hemodialysis because only unbound drugs can cross the hemodialysis membrane. Third, high-flux and peritoneal dialysis can remove larger molecules than hemodialysis. (Table 18-4 summarizes the impact of renal failure and hemodialysis on selected drugs used in critical care.)

References

1. Douglas S: Acute tubular necrosis: diagnosis, treatment, and nursing implications, *AACN Clin Issues Crit Care Nurs* 3(3):688, 1992.
2. Baer CM, Lancaster LE: Acute renal failure, *Crit Care Nurs Q* 14(4):1, 1992.
3. Stark JL: Acute tubular necrosis: differences between oliguria and nonoliguria, *Crit Care Nurs Q* 14(4):22, 1992.
4. Innerarity SA: Electrolyte emergencies in the critically ill renal patient, *Crit Care Nurs Clin North Am* 2(1):89, 1990.
5. DeAngelis R, Lessig ML: Hyperkalemia, *Crit Care Nurs Q* 12(3):55, 1992.
6. Innerarity SA: Hyperkalemic emergencies, *Crit Care Nurs Q* 14(4):32, 1992.
7. Cluitmans FH, Meinders AE: Management of severe hyponatremia: rapid or slow correction, *Am J Med* 88:161, 1990.
8. Workman ML: Magnesium and phosphorus: the neglected electrolytes, *AACN Clin Issues Crit Care Nurs* 3(3):655, 1992.
9. Lancaster LE: Renal response to shock, *Crit Care Nurs Clin North Am* 2(2):221, 1990.
10. Stark J: Dialysis options in the critically ill: hemodialysis, peritoneal dialysis, and continuous renal replacement therapy, *Crit Care Nurse Q* 14(4):40, 1992.
11. Baer CL, Lancaster LE: Acute renal failure, *Crit Care Nurs Q* 14(4):1, 1992.
12. Gutch CF, Stoner MH, Corea AL: *Review of hemodialysis for nurses and dialysis personnel,* ed 5, St Louis, 1993, Mosby.
13. Pechman P: Acute hemodialysis: issues in the critically ill, *AACN Clin Issues Crit Care Nurs* 3(3):545, 1992.
14. Smith LJ: Peritoneal dialysis in the critically ill patient, *AACN Clin Issues Crit Care Nurs* 3(3):558, 1992.
15. Graham-Macaluso MM: Complications of peritoneal dialysis: nursing care plans to document teaching, *ANNA J* 18(5):479, 1991.
16. Price CA: Continuous renal replacement therapy: the treatment of choice for acute renal failure, *ANNA J* 18(3):239, 1992.
17. Price CA: An update on continuous renal replacement therapies, *AACN Clin Issues Crit Care Nurs* 3(3):597, 1992.
18. Bosworth C: SCUF/CAVH/CAVHD: critical differences, *Crit Care Nurs Q* 14(4):45, 1992.
19. Coloski D and others: Continuous arteriovenous hemofiltration patient: nursing care plan, *DCCN* 9(3):130, 1990.

20. Lievaart A, Voerman HJ: Nursing management of continuous arteriovenous hemodialysis, *Heart Lung* 20(2):152, 1991.
21. Pinson JM: Preventing complications in the CAVH patient, *DCCN* 11(5):242, 1992.
22. Metheny NM: Why worry about IV fluids? *Am J Nurs* 90(6):50, 1990.
23. Kuhn MM: Colloids vs crystalloids, *Crit Care Nurs* 11(5):37, 1991.
24. Mendyka BE: Fluid and electrolyte disorders caused by diuretic therapy, *AACN Clin Issues Crit Care Nurs* 3(3):672, 1992.
25. Kellick KA: Diuretics, *AACN Clin Issues Crit Care Nurs* 3(2):472, 1992.
26. Rudy DW and others: Loop diuretics for chronic renal insufficiency: a continuous infusion is more efficacious than bolus therapy, *Ann Intern Med* 115(5):360-366, 1991.
27. Martin S, Danziger LH: Continuous infusion of loop diuretics in the critically ill: a review of the literature, *Crit Care Med* 22(8):1323-1329, 1994.

UNIT SEVEN

Gastrointestinal Alterations

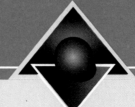

19

Gastrointestinal Assessment and Diagnostic Procedures

WENDY BODWELL

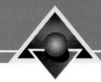

CHAPTER OBJECTIVES

- Identify areas of the health history that should be reviewed in patients with gastrointestinal dysfunction.
- Describe the components of a thorough gastrointestinal assessment.

- Discuss the clinical significance of various laboratory tests used in the assessment of gastrointestinal disorders.
- Outline important diagnostic procedures for detection of various gastrointestinal disorders.

KEY TERMS

Assessment of critically ill patients with gastrointestinal dysfunction includes a review of patients' health history, thorough physical examination, and analysis of patients' laboratory data. Numerous invasive and noninvasive diagnostic procedures may also be performed to help identify the disorder. This chapter focuses on priority clinical assessments, laboratory studies, and diagnostic procedures currently used in the critical care setting.

Clinical Assessment

History

The health history of patients with suspected or confirmed gastrointestinal (GI) disorders should be reviewed for the following:[1]

1. Past health history, including any surgery, diseases, and hospitalizations
2. Potential nonspecific problems that may affect the GI system—changes in weight, appetite, and activity level
3. Location and description of symptoms, including the site, pain characteristics, and temporal relationship to events (e.g., food intake, time of day)
4. Intake and output (food elimination)—diet (food patterns), nutritional status, bowel characteristics (stool descriptions), use of medication and alcohol, and dependence on laxatives or enemas

To help ascertain patients' nutritional status, nurses should review their histories, focusing on weight loss, edema, anorexia, vomiting, diarrhea, decreased or unusual food intake, and chronic illness.

Physical Examination

The clinical assessment helps establish baseline data about the physical dimensions of patients' situations. The assessment should proceed when patients are as comfortable as possible and in a supine position; their position may need readjustment if it causes pain. To prevent stimulation of GI activity, nurses should perform stages of the assessment in the following order: inspection, auscultation, percussion, and palpation. Although assessment of the GI system typically begins with inspection of the abdomen, the oral cavity must also be inspected to determine any unusual findings.[1]

Priorities for clinical assessment, along with normal and abnormal findings and additional related information, are outlined in Box 19-1. **Inspection** and **auscultation** elicit information about the function of the GI tract, and percussion and palpation elicit information about deep organs such as the liver, spleen, and pancreas. Because percussion often helps relax tense muscles, it is performed before palpation. Percussion, in the absence of any disease, is most helpful in delineating the position and size of the liver and spleen. Fluid, gaseous distention, and masses in the abdominal region can also be detected. Palpation is most useful in detecting abdominal pathologic conditions such as masses and areas of tenderness.[1]

Laboratory Studies

The value of various **laboratory studies** used to diagnose and treat diseases of the GI system has often been emphasized. No single procedure, however, provides an overall picture of the various organs' functional states. Also, no single value is predictive by itself. More than 100 laboratory tests have been proposed for the study of the liver and biliary tract alone. Common laboratory tests used in the assessment of GI disorders are found in Table 19-1.[2]

Diagnostic Procedures

Endoscopy

Available in several forms, **endoscopy** is a diagnostic and therapeutic procedure for the direct visualization and evaluation of the GI tract. The main difference between the different forms is the length of anatomic area that can be examined. An esophagogastroduodenoscopy allows viewing of the esophagus, stomach, and upper duodenum. A colonoscopy permits viewing of the colon and rectum. A proctosigmoidoscopy is used to examine the sigmoid colon, rectum, and anus.[3] In addition, endoscopy provides therapeutic benefits for a variety of conditions. Specifically, endoscopy is used to achieve hemostasis in patients with upper GI bleeding.[4]

Procedure

For a procedure involving the upper GI tract, patients should be NPO (nothing by mouth) for at least 4 to 6 hours before the procedure or as ordered by the physician. For a procedure involving the lower GI tract, cleansing enemas may be necessary. Immediately before the procedure a sedative or analgesic is usually administered. The endoscope is passed through the mouth or inserted via the anus and advanced until the region to be examined is visualized. After the procedure, patients should remain NPO until their gag reflex returns (usually 2 to 4 hours).[3]

If the endoscopy is performed to control bleeding, several techniques are available to achieve hemostasis. Thermal techniques use laser photocoagulation or electrocoagulation to control bleeding. Topical or injectable techniques involve the use of sclerotherapy to control bleeding. Mechanical methods such as endoscopic stapling and band ligation may also be used to control bleeding.[4]

COMPLICATIONS. Invasive tests present risks for some patients. Although rare, potential complications include perforation, hemorrhage, vasovagal stimulation, and oversedation. Signs of perforation include pain, bleeding, and fever.[3]

BOX 19-1

CLINICAL ASSESSMENT PRIORITIES OF THE ADULT GASTROINTESTINAL SYSTEM

INSPECTION

Procedure

Perform in warm, well-lighted environment with patients in comfortable position with abdomen exposed; view from slightly above and to one side of abdomen

Observe skin (pigmentation, lesions, striae, scars, dehydration, venous pattern), contour, movement (respiratory, symmetry, peristalsis)

Normal findings

Skin: normal considerable variation in pigmentation because of race, ethnic background, occupation exposure; however, abdomen generally lighter in color than other exposed areas

Contour: slightly concave or slightly round appearance

Movement: symmetric; no visible pulsations or peristaltic waves

Abnormal findings

Skin: jaundice, skin lesions, tenseness, glistening, stretch marks, scars (keloids), masses

Contour: distended (asymmetric/generalized)

Related information

Chart findings, using one of two anatomic maps (four quadrants or nine sections)

AUSCULTATION

Procedure

Listen below and to the right of umbilicus for bowel sounds; proceed methodically through all quadrants, lifting and lightly placing diaphragm of stethoscope

Normal findings

Sounds in small intestine are high pitched and gurgling; colonic sounds are low pitched and have a rumbling quality

Bowel sounds occur at a rate of 5 to 35/min

Abnormal findings

Lack of bowel sounds throughout 5-minute period, extremely soft and widely separated sounds, and increased sounds with characteristically high-pitched, loud, rushing sound (peristaltic rush)

Bruits, peritoneal friction rubs, venous hums

Related information

Normal venous hum audible at times but abnormal when heard in periumbilical region and accompanied by a palpable thrill

Decreased bowel sounds not significant without added data (e.g., nausea, vomiting, digestion)

PERCUSSION

Procedure

Proceed systematically to percuss lightly the entire abdomen, including the liver and spleen

Normal findings

Stomach: tympanic when empty

Intestine: tympanic or hyperresonant

Liver and spleen: dull

Abnormal findings

Flatness over stomach

Solid masses and distended bladder: dull sound

Liver and spleen: dull sounds beyond anatomic borders

Related information

Upper liver border is usually found in fourth or fifth intercostal space

PALPATION

Procedure

Perform both light (tender) and deep palpation of each organ and each quadrant of abdomen

Light: assesses depth of skin and fascia (depth approximately 1 cm)

Deep: assesses beneath rectus abdominis muscle; perform bimanually (4 to 5 cm deep)

Examine last any areas in which patients complain of tenderness

Normal findings

No areas of tenderness or pain

No bulges, masses, or hardening

Abnormal findings

Rebound tenderness, rigidity

If enlarged, gallbladder (right upper quadrant) palpable as small mass attached to liver

Spleen palpable only if enlarged

Related information

Liver sometimes cannot be palpated in healthy adults; however, in extremely thin but healthy adult, it may be felt at the costal margin.

TABLE 19-1
COMMON LABORATORY TESTS USED IN THE ASSESSMENT OF GASTROINTESTINAL DISORDERS

TEST	NORMAL LEVELS	CLINICAL SIGNIFICANCE
LIVER FUNCTION		
Serum bilirubin		
Total	0.0-1.0 mg/dl	Elevated in hepatocellular disease
Direct	0.0-0.4 mg/dl	Elevated in biliary disease
Indirect	0.0-0.6 mg/dl	Elevated in hepatocellular disease
Serum alkaline phosphatase		
Female	30-100 U/L	Elevated in biliary obstruction
Male	45-115 U/L	
Amino transferases		
AST		
Female	9-25 U/L	Elevated in hepatocellular disease
Male	10-40 U/L	
ALT		
Female	7-30 U/L	Elevated in hepatocellular disease
Male	10-55 U/L	
GGT	1.0-60.0 U/L	Elevated in acute liver disease, biliary obstruction, acute pancreatitis
LDH	110-210 U/L	Elevated in hepatocellular disease
Serum total protein	6.0-8.0 g/dl	Decreased in hepatocellular disease
Serum albumin	3.1-4.3 g/dl	Decreased in catabolic states, such as cirrhosis
Serum globulin	2.6-4.1 g/dl	Elevated in chronic liver disease
Plasma ammonia	12-55 mmol/L	Elevated in hepatic failure, hepatic encephalopathy, cirrhosis
PANCREATIC EXOCRINE FUNCTION		
Serum amylase	53-123 U/L	Elevated in acute pancreatitis, biliary obstruction
Serum lipase	4-24 U/dl	Elevated in acute pancreatitis, biliary obstruction

AST, Aspartate aminotransferase (formerly SGOT); *ALT*, alanine aminotransferase (formerly SGPT); *GGT*, Gamma-glutamyltransferase; *LDH*, lactic dehydrogenase.

Significance

An esophagogastroduodenoscopy is used to survey esophageal and gastric bleeding and lesions. A colonoscopy is used to diagnose inflammatory bowel disease and polyps. A proctosigmoidoscopy is used to evaluate rectosigmoidal bleeding. Endoscopy is also used to evaluate the status of surgical anastomoses.[3]

Angiography

Angiography is a diagnostic and therapeutic procedure. Diagnostically, it is used to evaluate the status of the GI circulation. Therapeutically, it is used to achieve transcatheter control of GI bleeding.[5,6]

Procedure

The radiologist cannulates the femoral artery with a needle and passes a guide wire through it into the aorta. The needle is removed, and an angiographic catheter is inserted over the guide wire. The catheter is advanced into the vessel supplying the portion of the GI tract be-ing studied. Once the catheter is in place, contrast medium is injected and serial radiographics are taken.[6] If the procedure is undertaken to control bleeding, vasopressin (Pitressin) or embolic material (Gelfoam) is injected after the site of the bleeding is located.[5,6]

COMPLICATIONS. Complications include overt and covert bleeding at the femoral puncture site, neurovascular compromise of the affected leg, and sensitivity to the contrast medium. Before the procedure, patients should be asked about any sensitivities to contrast. Postprocedural assessment involves monitoring vital signs, observing the injection site for bleeding, and assessing neurovascular integrity distal to the injection site every 15 minutes for the first 1 to 2 hours. Patients should remain flat for at least 12 hours. Any evidence of bleeding or neurovascular impairment must be immediately reported to physicians.[3]

Significance

Angiography is used in the diagnosis of upper GI bleeding only when endoscopy fails.[5] It is used to treat those patients (approximately 15%) whose GI bleeding does not stop after medical measures or endoscopic treatment.[6] Angiography is also used to evaluate cirrhosis, portal hypertension, intestinal ischemia, and other vascular abnormalities.[3]

Abdominal Plain Film Radiologic Studies

Numerous **radiologic studies** are available to further investigate large bowel disease. The most noninvasive studies are plain films such as the abdominal x-ray examination. Air in the bowel serves as a contrast medium to aid in visualization of the bowel. Gas patterns (the presence of gas inside or outside the bowel lumen and the distribution of gas in dilated and nondilated bowel) are best revealed by plain films.[7]

Procedure

Plain films can be obtained at the bedside using a portable x-ray machine. An anteroposterior film of the chest or abdomen is usually obtained. A left lateral decubitus view may also be chosen to evaluate free air or fluid. No special preparation is required for plain films.[7]

Significance

An abdominal film is useful in the diagnosis and evaluation of a bowel obstruction, perforated bowel, ruptured esophagus, and ileus. In addition, abdominal films are used to verify nasogastric and feeding tube placement.[7]

Liver Scans

Designed to assess patients' hepatic status, a **liver scan** is useful in detecting various abnormalities of the liver and spleen.[8]

Procedure

The scan involves injecting intravenous radioisotopes, the uptake of which is primarily in the liver. The liver cells take up 80% to 90% of the isotope, which is then secreted into the bile and transported throughout the system, allowing visualization of the biliary system, gallbladder, and duodenum. Patients are usually not sedated but must be able to lie flat for 60 minutes during the scanning.[8]

Significance

A liver scan yields information about the size, vascularity, and blood flow of the organs. Little or no uptake occurs in patients with cirrhosis or splenomegaly secondary to portal hypertension. Uptake results can indicate cirrhosis, hepatitis, tumors, abscesses, and cysts, whereas nonvisualization indicates obstruction.[8]

Ultrasound

Useful in evaluating the status of the gallbladder and biliary system, liver, spleen, and pancreas, **ultrasound** plays a key role in the diagnosis of many acute abdominal conditions because it is sensitive in detecting obstructive lesions and ascites. Ultrasound is easily performed, noninvasive, and well-tolerated by critically ill patients.[9]

Procedure

Sound waves are used to produce echoes that are converted into electrical energy and transferred to a screen for viewing. A transducer that emits and receives sound waves is moved slowly over the area of the abdomen to be studied. Tissues of varying densities produce different echoes that translate into different structures.[9]

Significance

Ultrasound is used to identify gallstones and hepatic abscesses, candidiasis, and hematomas. It is also effective in the diagnosis of acute cholecystitis and biliary obstructions.[9] Intestinal gas, ascites, and extreme obesity can interfere with transmission of the sound waves and thus limit the usefulness of the procedure. Patients should be NPO 8 to 12 hours before the procedure to limit the effects of intestinal gas on the procedure.[3]

Computed Tomography

Computed tomography (CT) scan is a radiographic examination that provides cross-sectional images of internal anatomy.[10] It may be used to evaluate abdominal vasculature and identify focal points found on nuclear scans as solid, cystic, inflammatory, or vascular.[3]

Procedure

The procedure involves taking patients to a CT scanner, placing them on the table, and inserting the area to be studied into the opening of the scanner. Multiple x-ray films are then taken at a variety of angles. A computer synthesizes images of the structures being studied.[11] Intravenous and GI contrast may also be used to facilitate the imaging of the blood vessels and GI tract, respectively.[3]

Significance

CT detects mass lesions more than 2 cm in diameter and allows visualization and evaluation of many different aspects of GI disease.[10] It is particularly useful in identifying pancreatic pseudocysts, abdominal abscesses, biliary obstructions, and a variety of GI neoplastic lesions.[11,12]

Nursing Management

Nursing management of patients undergoing a diagnostic procedure involves a variety of interventions. **Priorities are directed toward preparing patients psychologically and physically for the procedure, monitoring their responses to the procedure, and assessing them after the procedure.** Preparing patients includes teaching them about the procedure, answering any questions, and transporting and positioning them for the procedure. Monitoring their responses to the procedure includes observing them for signs of pain, anxiety, and hemorrhage and monitoring vital signs. Assessing patients after the procedure includes observing for complications and medicating patients for any postprocedure discomfort. **Any evidence of gastrointestinal bleeding should be immediately reported to physicians, and emergency measures to maintain circulation must be initiated.**

References

1. Bates B: *A guide to physical examination*, ed 5, Philadelphia, 1991, JB Lippincott.
2. Normal reference values, *N Engl J Med* 327(10):718, 1992.
3. Doughty DB, Jackson DB: *Gastrointestinal disorders*, St Louis, 1993, Mosby.
4. Kovacs TOG, Jensen DM: *Therapeutic endoscopy for upper gastrointestinal bleeding*. In Taylor MB, editor: *Gastrointestinal emergencies*, Baltimore, 1992, Williams & Wilkins.
5. Porter DH, Kim D: *Angiographic intervention in upper gastrointestinal bleeding*. In Taylor MB, editor: *Gastrointestinal emergencies*, Baltimore, 1992, Williams & Wilkins.
6. Elta GH: *Approach to the patient with gross gastrointestinal bleeding*. In *Textbook of gastroenterology*, vol 1, Philadelphia, 1991, JB Lippincott.
7. Roszler MH: Plain film radiologic examination of the abdomen, *Crit Care Clin* 10:277, 1994.
8. Davis LP, Fink-Bennet D: Nuclear medicine in the acutely ill patient. Part I, *Crit Care Clin* 10:265, 1994.
9. Ramano WM, Platt JF: Ultrasound of the abdomen, *Crit Care Clin* 10:297, 1994.
10. Dobranowski J and others: *Procedures in gastrointestinal radiology*, New York, 1990, Springer-Verlag.
11. Eisenberg RL: *Gastrointestinal radiology*, ed 2, Philadelphia, 1990, JB Lippincott.
12. Zingas AP: Computed tomography of the abdomen in the critically ill, *Crit Care Clin* 10:321, 1994.

20

Gastrointestinal Disorders and Therapeutic Management

WENDY BODWELL

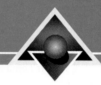

Understanding the pathology of a disease, areas of assessment on which to focus, and usual medical management allows critical care nurses to anticipate and plan accurate nursing interventions. Although a wide array of gastrointestinal disorders exists, only a few routinely require care in the critical care environment. This chapter focuses on priority gastrointestinal disorders and the therapeutic management of critically ill patients with gastrointestinal dysfunction.

Acute Gastrointestinal Bleeding

Description and Etiology

Gastrointestinal (GI) **hemorrhage** is a medical emergency that accounts for nearly $1 billion of current national health care expenditure[1] and results in almost 300,000 hospital admissions yearly.[2] Despite advances in medical knowledge and nursing care, the mortality rate for acute GI bleeding has not changed in more than 50 years;[2,3] it remains approximately 10%. Most cases of GI hemorrhage result from bleeding in the upper GI tract.[3] Bleeding from lower GI tract lesions can be rapid and life threatening, whereas bleeding from colon cancer and hemorrhoids is usually slow and intermittent and does not require hospitalization.[3]

If unrecognized or treated too late, GI hemorrhage can lead to **hypovolemic shock** and ultimately death, but studies have found that the most common cause of death in GI hemorrhage actually results from exacerbation of underlying disease rather than intractable hypovolemic shock.[1,4] Gogel and Tandberg[1] point out that patients with a history of previous upper gastrointestinal (UGI) hemorrhage have a better prognosis than those with no previous bleeding, perhaps because they have proved their ability to tolerate severe blood loss. Acute GI perforation, peritonitis, and sepsis are rare complications of GI hemorrhage.[1]

Pathophysiology

Stress **ulcers,** peptic ulcers, nonspecific erosive gastritis, and esophageal varices are among the leading causes of UGI hemorrhage.

Stress ulcers

The term *stress ulcer* (erosive **gastritis**) covers a spectrum of diseases ranging from superficial mucosal erosions to discrete, mature ulcers. Almost always limited to the stomach, stress ulcers are lesions that produce diffuse mucosal oozing. Such bleeding does not often cause massive GI hemorrhage and is generally attributed to superficial capillaries. Overt bleeding occurs in 2% to 15% of critically ill patients, typically those who have not received stress ulcer prophylaxis.[5-8] Patients at risk include those in high physiologic stress situations such as occur with thermal injury, head trauma, extensive surgery, shock, and acute neurologic disease. Several pathophysi-

---

BOX 20-1

ETIOLOGY OF STRESS ULCERS

PRECIPITATING FACTORS

Increased stress level (alteration in equilibrium)
Increased acid level in lumen of stomach (pH < 3.5)

COFACTORS

Mucosal ischemia
Hydrogen-ion back diffusion (gastric barrier)
Gram-negative septicemia
Drug intake (e.g., steroids and catecholamines in patients with head trauma)

---

ologic mechanisms have been implicated in stress ulcer formation (Box 20-1). The onset can be rapid (2 to 10 days), and hemorrhage can begin without pain. Mortality rates for untreated hemorrhage can exceed 50%. Patients at risk for development of stress ulcers should be assessed for the presence of hematemesis (red blood or coffee-ground emesis), bloody nasogastric aspirate, and melena (black or dark red stools).

Peptic ulcers

Peptic ulcer disease is the leading cause of UGI hemorrhage, accounting for approximately 50% of cases.[2] The term *peptic ulcer* refers to erosions located primarily in the gastric antrum and duodenum. Such erosions are deep, unlike stress ulcers, which tend to be superficial. Peptic ulcer can be represented by the following ulcer equation: acid + pepsin versus mucosal resistance. This equation implies that the proulcer forces (acid and pepsin) are normally held in check by the opposing forces of gastric mucosal resistance. Peptic ulcer results from an interaction between acid and peptic activity concomitant with a breakdown in the gastroduodenal mucosal defense barrier.[9-12] Other mechanisms that influence ulcer formation include cigarette smoking, familial and genetic factors, emotions, stress, and sociocultural factors.[10,13]

Nonspecific erosive gastritis

Of all UGI hemorrhages, 5% to 25% are the result of nonspecific erosive gastritis, which may be caused by a variety of different agents and disorders (Box 20-2). Nonspecific erosive gastritis is characterized by a wide spectrum of histologic appearances, including inflammation and ulceration. Approximately 200,000 hospitalizations for GI bleeding and 10,000 to 20,000 deaths per year may be attributable to nonsteroidal antiinflammatory drug (NSAID)-induced gastroduodenal mucosal damage,[14,15] which falls into the category of gastritis.[2] As the national population ages, so do patients who are hospitalized in the nation's intensive care units. Nurses should therefore be aware that the GI complications of

ETIOLOGY OF NONSPECIFIC EROSIVE GASTRITIS

Stress-related erosive syndrome (SRES)
Drug-induced
    Ethanol
    Nonsteroidal antiinflammatory drugs
    Iron
    Potassium chloride
    Hepatic arterial chemotherapy
    Corrosives
Prolapse gastropathy
Ischemia
Vasculitis
Occlusive disease
Emboli
Postgastrectomy
Varioliform gastritis
Portal hypertension ("congestive gastropathy")
Radiation
Mechanical (instrumentation, nasogastric tube)

From Lichtenstein DR, Berman MD, Wolfe MM: *Approach to the patient with acute upper gastrointestinal hemorrhage.* In Taylor MB, editor: *Gastrointestinal emergencies,* Baltimore, 1992, Williams & Wilkins, p 104.

NSAIDs[2,11,12,14-18] seriously affect millions of older patients with rheumatoid arthritis.

Esophageal varices

Investigators estimate that 19% to 57% of patients with cirrhosis and esophageal varices experience at least one GI hemorrhage. Significantly, this first bleeding episode is fatal in 28% to 66% of patients.[19] Esophageal variceal hemorrhage carries a poor prognosis—only 10% to 20% of these patients are alive 4 years after their first bleeding episode.[20] Engorged and distended esophageal blood vessels are referred to as *esophageal varices.* Bleeding from such varices is a frequent and significant complication of cirrhosis, a disease that damages the liver sinusoid system. Without adequate sinusoid function, hepatic circulation is impaired and liver pressures are altered. This leads to a rise in portal venous pressure, causing collateral circulation to divert portal blood from high-pressure areas to adjacent low-pressure areas. The tiny esophageal vessels that receive this diverted blood lack sturdy mucosal protection, and as they become engorged and form varices, they become vulnerable to damage from gastric secretions, with subsequent rupture and hemorrhage.[21]

Assessment and Diagnosis

Hematemesis (red blood or coffee-ground emesis), bloody nasogastric aspirate, and melena (black or dark red stools) are hallmark manifestations of GI bleeding.

TABLE 20-1 EFFECT OF GASTRIC BLOOD LOSS ON STOOL CHARACTERISTICS	
VOLUME LOST	**STOOL CHARACTERISTICS**
20 ml	Normal appearance, occult positive
100-200 ml	Melena
1000 ml (<4-hr transit)	Bloody
1000 ml (>4-hr transit)	Melena

From Gogel HK, Tandberg D: *Am J Emerg Med* 4(2):153, 1986.

The effect of blood on stool character is shown in Table 20-1. It may be difficult to estimate the amount of blood in emesis or stool; in these cases a description of the sample and patients' clinical profiles can provide the initial sources for a nursing diagnosis.

Laboratory tests can help determine the extent of bleeding, although nurses should realize that hematocrit values are a poor indicator of the severity and rapidity of acute bleeding episodes. In other words, whole blood is lost, and if a hematocrit value is 45% and patients lose a third of their blood volume in 5 minutes, the hematocrit value remains 45%. Studies have shown that the hematocrit value may take as long as 72 hours to equilibrate after an episode of blood loss.[22] Measurement of arterial blood gases can help in detecting metabolic acidosis associated with severe hypovolemia. Electrolytes should also be assessed because severe hypokalemia and hyponatremia can develop in patients with hypovolemia. Measurement of the prothrombin time, partial thromboplastin time, and total platelet count may help guide blood and blood product replacement therapy. Diagnostic procedures such as endoscopy and arteriography can help establish the site of the bleeding, although these procedures carry a higher risk when performed on an emergent basis.[1]

Medical Management

Medical management for patients at risk for UGI hemorrhage includes the administration of pharmacologic agents for gastric acid neutralization and prevention of bleeding. These agents include antacids, histamine-2 antagonists, and sucralfate[23] and are further discussed in the pharmacology section.

The initial treatment goals for patients with acute GI bleeding are control of bleeding and restoration of adequate circulating blood volume,[1] usually by intravenous infusions of crystalloids and packed red blood cells. Gastric lavage is used to decrease gastric mucosal blood flow, evacuate blood and clots from the stomach, and decrease hemorrhage. Gastric lavage may reduce vomiting and

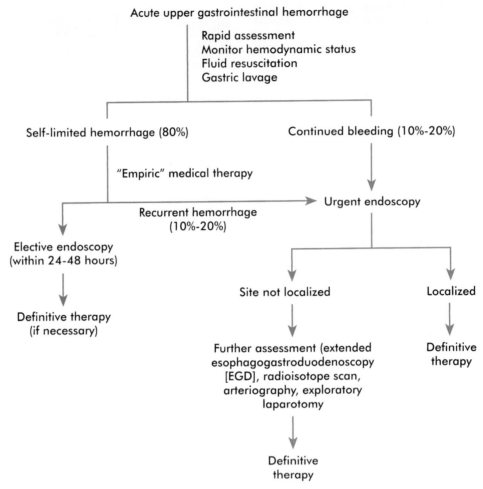

Acute upper gastrointestinal hemorrhage

Rapid assessment
Monitor hemodynamic status
Fluid resuscitation
Gastric lavage

Self-limited hemorrhage (80%)   Continued bleeding (10%-20%)

"Empiric" medical therapy

Recurrent hemorrhage
(10%-20%)   Urgent endoscopy

Elective endoscopy
(within 24-48 hours)

Site not localized   Localized

Definitive therapy
(if necessary)

Further assessment (extended
esophagogastroduodenoscopy
[EGD], radioisotope scan,
arteriography, exploratory
laparotomy

Definitive
therapy

Definitive
therapy

FIG. 20-1 Approach to the patient with acute upper gastrointestinal hemorrhage. (Modified from Lichtenstein DR, Berman MD, Wolfe MM: *Approach to the patient with acute upper gastrointestinal hemorrhage.* In Taylor MB, editor: *Gastrointestinal emergencies,* Baltimore, 1992, Williams & Wilkins.)

lessen the risk of aspiration, and some clinicians find it useful in monitoring the rate of bleeding and preparing patients for endoscopy.[1] Additional treatments include intravenous administration of vasopressin, endoscopic hemostasis, and interventional angiography. Patients who remain hemodynamically unstable despite volume replacement need urgent surgery (Fig. 20-1).[1,24]

In acute variceal hemorrhage, bleeding may be controlled by endoscopic sclerotherapy (the endoscopic injection of a sclerosing agent into the bleeding varix), vasopressin infusion,[1] or balloon tamponade (e.g., the Sengstaken-Blakemore, Linton, Minnesota tubes).[25] Vasopressin reduces portal venous pressure and slows blood flow by constricting the splanchnic arteriolar bed.[26,27] It also causes significant systemic vasoconstriction and can lead to complications such as chest pain or cardiac ischemia, hypertension, congestive heart failure, dysrhythmias, phlebitis, bowel ischemia, and cerebral vascular accident.[28]

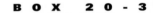

BOX 20 - 3

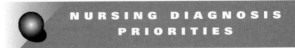

NURSING DIAGNOSIS PRIORITIES

ACUTE GASTROINTESTINAL BLEEDING

- *Fluid Volume Deficit* related to active blood loss, p. 503
- *Decreased Cardiac Output* related to decreased preload, p. 474
- *Anxiety* related to threatened biologic, psychologic, and/or social integrity, p. 464

Nursing Management

Patients with acute GI bleeding may have any number of nursing diagnoses (Box 20-3) depending on the underlying cause of the hemorrhage. **Nursing priorities are direc-**

COMPLICATIONS OF ACUTE PANCREATITIS

RESPIRATORY

Early hypoxemia
Pleural effusion
Atelectasis
Pulmonary infiltration
Adult respiratory distress syndrome
Mediastinal abscess

CARDIOVASCULAR

Hypotension
Pericardial effusion
ST-T changes

RENAL

Acute tubular necrosis
Oliguria
Renal artery or vein thrombosis

HEMATOLOGIC

DIC
Thrombocytosis
Hyperfibrinogenemia

ENDOCRINE

Hypocalcemia
Hypertriglyceridemia
Hyperglycemia

NEUROLOGIC

Fat emboli
Psychosis
Encephalopathy

OPHTHALMIC

Purtscher's retinopathy—sudden blindness

DERMATOLOGIC

Subcutaneous fat necrosis

GASTROINTESTINAL/HEPATIC

Hepatic dysfunction
Obstructive jaundice
Erosive gastritis
Paralytic ileus
Duodenal obstruction
Pancreatic
    Pseudocyst
    Phlegmon
    Abscess
    Ascites
Bowel infarction
Massive intraperitoneal bleed
Perforation
    Stomach
    Duodenum
    Small bowel
    Colon

DIC, Disseminated intravascular coagulation.
From Ranson JHC: *Complications of pancreatitis.* In Taylor MB, editor: *Gastrointestinal emergencies,* Baltimore, 1992, Williams & Wilkins, p 181.

ted toward controlling the bleeding, administering volume replacement, and educating patients and families.

Controlling the bleeding

One measure to control the bleeding is gastric lavage. Historically, iced saline was favored as a lavage irrigant. Research has shown, however, that low-temperature fluids such as iced saline shift the oxyhemoglobin dissociation curve to the left and create adverse effects; these problems can include decreased oxygen delivery to vital organs and prolongation of bleeding time and prothrombin time.[2] Therefore room-temperature water or saline is the currently preferred irrigant for gastric lavage.[1,2]

Administering volume replacement

Measures to facilitate volume replacement include obtaining intravenous access and administering prescribed fluids and blood resuscitation therapy. In addition to monitoring patients' responses to care, nurses should observe patients for complications of acute bleeding. Although a rare complication, gastric perforation constitutes a surgical emergency. Patients report sudden, severe, generalized abdominal pain, with significant rebound tenderness and rigidity. Perforation should be suspected when fever, leukocytosis, and tachycardia persist despite adequate volume replacement.[2]

Educating patients and families

Educating patients and families includes teaching them about GI hemorrhage, answering their questions, and preparing them for discharge. Subjects for discharge teaching include precipitating factors of GI hemorrhage, interventions to reduce further bleeding, and the importance of taking medications.[29]

Acute Pancreatitis

Description and Etiology

Pancreatitis is an inflammation of the pancreas that causes exocrine dysfunction. Infectious complications account for 80% of deaths in patients with acute pancreatitis.[30-34] Other complications of acute pancreatitis affect every organ system and include acute renal failure, myocardial depression, adult respiratory distress syndrome, and disseminated intravascular coagulation (Box 20-4).[31]

From Steer ML: *Acute pancreatitis.* In Taylor MB, editor: *Gastrointestinal emergencies,* Baltimore, 1992, Williams & Wilkins, p 173.

The two most common causes of acute pancreatitis are biliary disease (gallstones) and alcoholism.[31,32] Much less common causes include peptic ulcer disease, surgical trauma, hyperparathyroidism,[35] vascular disease, and use of certain drugs (Box 20-5).[33] In 10% to 25% of patients with acute pancreatitis, no etiologic factor can be determined.[33]

Pathophysiology

In acute pancreatitis the normally inactive digestive enzymes become prematurely activated within the pancreas itself, creating the central pathophysiologic mechanism of acute pancreatitis, which is autodigestion.[30,35] Some authors liken this process to a chemical burn.[30]

The enzyme trypsin initiates the autodigestion process by triggering the secretion of the proteolytic enzymes phospholipase A, elastase, and kallikrein. In the presence of bile, phospholipase A digests the phospholipids of cell membranes, causing severe pancreatic parenchymal and adipose tissue necrosis, with subsequent release of free fatty acids. Elastase activation causes dissolution of the elastic fibers of blood vessels and ducts, leading to hemorrhage. Kallikrein activation causes the release of bradykinin and kallidin, resulting in decreased peripheral vascular resistance, vasodilation, and increased vascular permeability.[35,36]

Together these proteases and phosopholipases cause pancreatic inflammation and swelling. Extravasation of plasma and red blood cells in the area surrounding the pancreas causes fluid to be redistributed from the intravascular space to the retroperitoneum and bowel.[34] With large amounts of plasma volume sequestration, hypovolemia and hypotension occur, causing patients to go into shock.[35]

Assessment and Diagnosis

The clinical manifestations of acute pancreatitis vary from mild to severe and often mimic other disorders. Epigastric to midabdominal pain may vary from mild and tolerable to severe and incapacitating. Patients often report a "boring" or knifelike sensation that radiates to the back. Nausea, vomiting, or both may accompany the pain.[36] Patients may obtain some comfort by leaning forward or lying down with knees drawn up. Other clinical findings seen in acute pancreatitis are abdominal guarding, distention, hypertension, abdominal mass, jaundice, hematemesis, and melena.[31]

The results of GI auscultation vary according to the presence or absence of bowel sounds; abdominal palpation reveals tenderness and guarding. Uncommon inspection findings seen in acute pancreatitis include Grey Turner sign (gray-blue discoloration of the flank) and Cullen's sign (discoloration of the umbilical region).[36] Neuromuscular irritability may result from electrolyte deficiencies, but despite the appearance of muscle weakness and tremors, tetany rarely develops.[35]

Assessment of laboratory data usually demonstrates elevated levels of serum amylase and lipase. Leukocytosis, hypocalcemia, hyperglycemia, hyperbilirubinemia, and hypoalbuminemia may also be present. In addition, patients may experience transient hyperglycemia.[36]

Medical Management

The major goals of therapy are to minimize pancreatic function, ensure adequate circulating volume and oxygenation, correct any metabolic alterations, and manage pain. Immediate treatments include administering intravenous fluids to prevent hypovolemic shock and maintain hemodynamic stability. In severe forms of the disease the use of a pulmonary artery catheter guides fluid management. A nasogastric tube is inserted and gastric suction initiated to minimize pancreatic function. Total parenteral nutrition should begin as soon as possible for patients with severe pancreatitis. Pain relief is another treatment priority, as are recognition and treatment of complications.[36]

Patients should be observed for complications of pancreatitis and treated promptly. Septic complications are

B O X   2 0 - 6

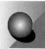

NURSING DIAGNOSIS PRIORITIES

ACUTE PANCREATITIS

- Acute *Pain* related to transmission and perception of cutaneous, visceral, muscular, or ischemic impulses secondary to acute pancreatitis, p. 499
- *Decreased Cardiac Output* related to decreased preload, p. 476
- *Altered Nutrition: Less Than Body Requirements* related to lack of exogenous nutrients and increased metabolic demand, p. 506
- *Anxiety* related to threatened biologic, psychologic, and/or social integrity, p. 464

B O X   2 0 - 7

ETIOLOGY OF INTESTINAL OBSTRUCTIONS

FUNCTIONAL OBSTRUCTION

Prolonged intestinal distention
Hypokalemia
Peritonitis
Narcotic use
Intestinal ischemia
Sepsis

MECHANICAL OBSTRUCTION
Contained within lumen

Intussusception
Large gallstones
Meconium
Bezoars
Neoplasms

Extending into bowel wall

Congenital atresia
Congenital stenosis
Inflammatory bowel disease
Diverticulitis
Radiation
Neoplasms

Outside the bowel

Adhesions
Hernias
Neoplasms
Abscesses
Volvulus
Stomal stenosis

most common; Ranson[33] states that virtually all patients with fever, leukocytosis, or both, after 21 days of continuous treatment, have pancreatic infection. Sepsis without manifestations of leukocytosis or fever can occur and may require the use of antibiotics.[37]

Nursing Management

Patients with acute pancreatitis may have any number of nursing diagnoses (Box 20-6), depending on the severity of the attack. **Nursing priorities are directed toward correcting fluid and electrolyte imbalances, relieving pain, and educating patients and families.**

Correcting fluid and electrolyte imbalances

Assisting with insertion of a pulmonary artery catheter and central venous catheter for fluid replacement therapy is an important nursing function, as are the continuous assessment and monitoring of pressure waveforms once the catheter is in place. Correcting fluid and electrolyte imbalances by administering intravenous infusions is another key nursing task.[36,38]

Relieving pain

Although analgesics should be liberally provided, nurses should keep in mind that high doses of analgesic may impair the ventilatory pattern. Therefore the nursing objective for pain control should be to achieve relief while maintaining ventilation at normal depth and rate. Meperidine (Demerol) is the preferred agent because morphine may produce spasms at Oddi's sphincter.[35] Measures used to rest the pancreas, NPO status, relaxation techniques, and gastric suctioning also help control pain.

Educating patients and families

Educating patients and families includes teaching them about pancreatitis, answering their questions, and preparing them for discharge. Subjects for discharge teaching should include precipitating factors of pancreatitis, interventions to prevent another attack, and the importance of taking prescribed medications.[29]

Acute Intestinal Obstruction

Description and Etiology

Acute intestinal **obstruction** occurs when bowel contents fail to move forward. Functional obstruction, also known as *paralytic ileus*, results from the absence of peristalsis and often occurs with hypokalemia. Mechanical obstruction follows occlusion of the bowel lumen and is usually the result of neoplasms (Box 20-7).[39]

Pathophysiology

The obstructed bowel lumen accumulates fluid and gas proximal to the point of obstruction. Trapped fluids cause bowel distention, which triggers the secretion of fluid and electrolytes into the lumen and perpetuates the distention. Large losses of sodium, potassium, and chloride occur, as well as loss of hydrogen ions from the stomach.[40] As the obstruction persists, the vascular space becomes rapidly depleted, which results in dehydration, hypotension, and hypovolemic shock. If intestinal distention progresses, the bowel wall edema can ultimately impede venous and arterial supply and cause bowel necrosis and perforation. Once the bowel perforates, peritonitis and sepsis ensue.[41]

Assessment and Diagnosis

Sometimes only minimal warning symptoms occur with intestinal obstructions. Typically, patients are first seen in acute distress, with abdominal distention, nausea and vomiting, obstipation, constipation, cramping abdominal pain, and high-pitched bowel sounds.[40] Proximal obstructions are associated with more vomiting and less distention, whereas distal obstructions are associated with more distention and less vomiting. Bowel sounds may be absent or faint and tinkling, depending on the extent of the obstruction.[41]

Diagnosis of intestinal obstruction is aided by radiologic examination. A chest x-ray film and serial abdominal flat-plate films taken with patients standing or sitting and supine reveal dilated loops of gas-filled bowel. Barium or meglumine diatrizoate (Gastrografin) enemas are used to locate the exact site and determine the degree of obstruction.[41]

Medical Management

Medical interventions include replacement of fluids and immediate decompression of the obstruction with nasogastric suction. Use of long GI tubes is contraindicated for colonic obstruction. A sigmoid volvulus can be nonsurgically reduced by inserting a rectal tube during sigmoidoscopy or barium enema and thereby relieving the obstruction. Because the volvulus can recur, elective resection at a later date is desirable.[40]

Surgical intervention is required when the obstruction fails to disappear within 24 hours. When patients are not acutely ill, surgical resection can be a one-stage procedure with reanastomosis of the bowel, which eliminates the need for a temporary colostomy. More often a two- or three-stage procedure is used, and a temporary colostomy created.[40]

Patients should also be observed for complications. Bowel necrosis and perforation are potential complications of colonic obstruction, and both can progress to sepsis. Bowel necrosis occurs as a result of impaired circulation associated with volvulus, closed-loop obstruction, and sustained excessive intraluminal pressure. Bowel perforation often follows overdistention of the bowel lumen and bowel necrosis. These complications carry a high mortality and can be avoided by astute nursing observations followed by prompt surgical intervention.[40]

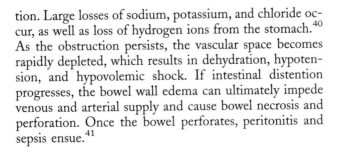

Nursing Management

Patients with an intestinal obstruction may have any number of nursing diagnoses depending on the progression of the illness (Box 20-8). Nursing priorities are directed toward ensuring the patency of the nasogastric tube, monitoring fluid and electrolytes, and educating patients and families.

Ensuring the patency of the nasogastric tube

Placement and patency of the nasogastric tube should be checked as needed to ensure adequate decompression.[29]

Monitoring fluid and electrolytes

Because outputs greater than 1000 ml/8 hr can occur, patients should be monitored for electrolyte imbalance (hyponatremia and hypokalemia) and fluid volume deficit. Accurate intake and output must be maintained. Intravenous fluid and electrolyte solutions should be administered to prevent dehydration and replace lost electrolytes. Administration of antipyretics is necessary for treatment of fever.[42]

Educating patients and families

Educating patients and families includes teaching them about intestinal obstructions, answering their questions, and preparing them for discharge. Subjects for discharge teaching should include precipitating factors of intestinal obstructions and the importance of taking prescribed medications.[29]

Therapeutic Management of Gastrointestinal Intubation

Because **GI intubation** is so commonly used in critical care units, nurses should know the clinical indications and responsibilities inherent in its use. The four categories of GI tubes are based on function: nasogastric suction tubes, long intestinal tubes, balloon tamponade effect tubes, and feeding tubes (see Chapter 6). Indications for GI intubation include gastric or small bowel decompression and control of gastric and esophageal bleeding.[43,44]

Nasogastric Suction Tubes

Nasogastric suction tubes (Levin, Salem sump) remove fluid regurgitated into the stomach, prevent accumulation of swallowed air, partially decompress the bowel in some cases, and reduce the risk of aspiration. These tubes can also be used for collecting specimens and administering tube feedings.[43] The tube is passed through the nose into the nasopharynx and then down through the pharynx into the esophagus and stomach. The length of time the nasogastric tube remains in place depends on its use.

Long Intestinal Tubes

Miller-Abbott, Cantor, Johnston, and Baker tubes are examples of long intestinal tubes that are placed either preoperatively or intraoperatively. Their length allows removal of contents from the intestine that cannot be accomplished by shorter nasogastric tubes. Long intestinal tubes can also decompress the small bowel. In addition, they can splint the small bowel intraoperatively or postoperatively. Because progression of the tubes depends on bowel peristalsis, their use is contraindicated in patients with paralytic ileus and severe mechanical obstruction.[43]

Balloon Tamponade Tubes

Three types of balloon tamponade tubes are currently available: the Sengstaken-Blakemore tube, Linton tube, and Minnesota tube. The Sengstaken-Blakemore tube has three lumens: one for the gastric balloon, esophageal balloon, and gastric suction (Fig. 20-2, *A*). The Linton tube also has three lumens: one for the gastric balloon, gastric suction, and esophageal suction (Fig. 20-2, *B*). The Minnesota tube has four lumens: one for the gastric balloon, esophageal balloon, gastric suction, and esophageal suction (Fig. 20-2, *C*).[44] The Minnesota tube is preferable because it offers both gastric and esophageal balloons and allows suction to be applied above and below the balloons (in the stomach and esophagus).[45]

Physicians insert balloon tamponade tubes. Once the tube is passed into the stomach and placement assessed, the gastric balloon is inflated with 250 to 300 ml of air (or as specified by the tube manufacturer). The tube is then placed under tension so that the gastric balloon can place pressure on the gastroesophageal junction. Tension is usually applied using a helmet with a constant traction spring device. Once in place the esophageal balloon is inflated to a pressure of 25 to 45 mm Hg. Low intermittent suction is applied to the gastric and esophageal ports. When bleeding has stopped for 24 hours, the esophageal balloon is deflated. If no further bleeding occurs in the next 24 hours, the gastric balloon is deflated. If bleeding still does not recur after an additional 24 hours, the tube is discontinued.[44,45]

Nursing Management

Nursing priorities for patients undergoing GI intubation are directed toward preventing the complications associated with the different tubes.

Nasogastric tubes

Nursing care for patients with nasogastric tubes includes interventions to prevent common complications. These include ulceration and necrosis of the nares, esophageal reflux, esophagitis, esophageal erosion and stricture, gastric erosion, and dry mouth and parotitis from mouth breathing; interference with ventilation and coughing; and loss of fluid and electrolytes. Interventions include irrigating the tube every 4 hours with normal saline, ensuring the blue air vent of the Salem sump is patent and maintained above the level of patients' stomachs, and providing frequent care of mouth and nares.[43]

Long intestinal tubes

Interventions used in the care of patients with long intestinal tubes are similar to those used with a nasogastric tube. Patients should also be observed for gaseous distention of the balloon section, which makes removing the tube difficult; rupture of the balloon or spillage of mercury into the intestine; overinflation of the balloon, which can lead to intestinal rupture; and reverse intussusception if the tube is removed rapidly. Intestinal tubes should be removed slowly, usually at the rate of 6 inches per hour.[43]

Balloon tamponade tubes

Nursing management of patients with balloon tamponade tubes includes monitoring them for rebleeding and observing for complications of the tube. The most common complication is pulmonary aspiration. This complication can be limited by first inserting an endotracheal tube for airway management. Additional complications include esophageal erosion and rupture, balloon migration, and nasal necrosis. Balloon migration is potentially life threatening. If the gastric balloon ruptures or is allowed to deflate, the esophageal balloon migrates upward, where it can occlude the airway. **If patients develop respiratory distress, the gastric and esophageal balloon ports should be cut immediately.**[44,45]

Pharmacologic Agents

A number of pharmacologic agents are used in the care of patients with GI disorders. Table 20-2 reviews the various agents and any special considerations necessary for administering them.[23,46]

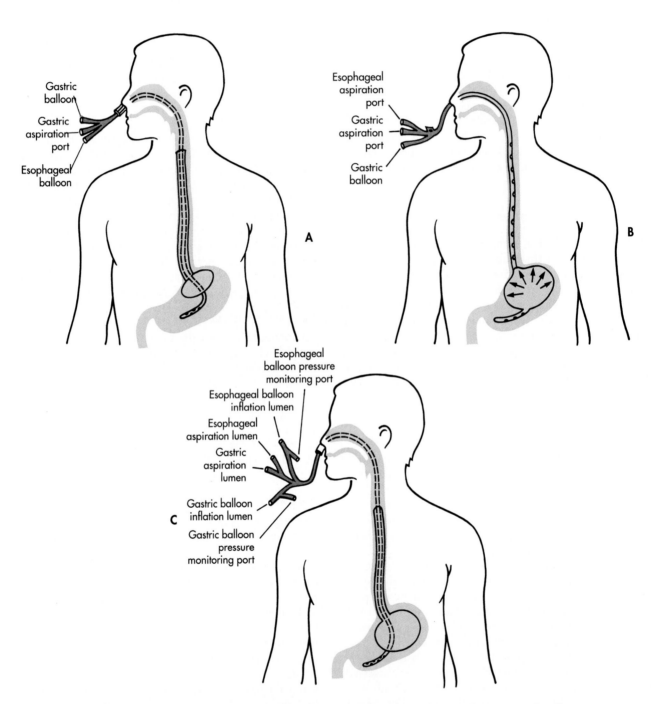

FIG. 20-2 Esophageal tamponade tubes. **A,** Sengstaken-Blakemore tube. **B,** Linton tube. **C,** Minnesota tube. (From Amato EJ: A nursing reference: gastrointestinal tubes and drains. Part II. Esophageal tube, *Crit Care Nurs* 3(1):46, 1983.)

T A B L E   2 0 - 2

Pharmacologic Agents Used in the Management of GI Disorders

MEDICATION	DOSAGE	ACTIONS	SPECIAL CONSIDERATIONS
Antacids	30-90 ml q1-2h PO or NG, possibly titrated to NG pH	Used to buffer stomach acid and raise gastric pH	• Can cause diarrhea or constipation and electrolyte disturbances • Irrigate NG tube with water after administration because antacids can clog tube
Histamine-2 Antagonists • Cimetidine (Tagamet) • Ranitidine (Zantac) • Famotidine (Pepcid)	 300 mg q6h IV or PO 150 mg q12h IV or PO 40 mg qd PO or 20 mg q12h IV	Used to reduce volume and concentration of gastic secretions	• Side effects include CNS toxicity (confusion or delirium) and thrombocytopenia • Separate administration of antacids and histamine blocking agents by 1 hour
Sucralfate (Carafate)	1 g q6h NG or PO	Cytoprotective agent used to increase mucus production, facilitate mucus resistance to back diffusion of hydrogen ions, and bind to erosions	• May cause severe constipation • May cause decreased absorption of certain drugs, separate administration of histamine blocking agents and sucralfate by 2 hours
Vasopressin (Pitressin)	Loading dose of 20 U over 20 min IV followed by 0.2-0.8 U/hr IV infusion	Vasoconstrictor used to lower portal pressure by decreasing blood flow to the splanchnic bed	• Side effects include coronary, mesenteric, and peripheral vasoconstriction • May be administered concurrently with nitroglycerine to minimize side effects

NG, Nasogastric; *CNS*, central nervous system.

References

1. Gogel HK, Tandberg D: Emergency management of upper gastrointestinal hemorrhage, *Am J Emerg Med* 4(2):150, 1986.
2. Lichtenstein DR, Berman MD, Wolfe MM: *Approach to the patient with acute upper gastrointestinal hemorrhage.* In Taylor MB, editor: *Gastrointestinal emergencies,* Baltimore, 1992, Williams & Wilkins.
3. Elta GH: *Approach to the patient with gross gastrointestinal bleeding.* In Yamada T, editor: *Textbook of gastroenterology,* vol 1, Philadelphia, 1991, JB Lippincott.
4. Gogel HK: Personal communication, 1992.
5. Peura DA: Stress-related mucosal damage: an overview, *Am J Med* 83(6A):3, 1987.
6. Peura DA: Prophylactic therapy of stress-related mucosal damage: why, which, who, and so what? *Am J Gastroenterol* 85(8):935, 1990.
7. Konopad E, Noseworthy T: Stress ulceration: a serious complication in critically ill patients, *Heart Lung* 17(4):339, 1988.
8. Zuckerman GR, Shuman R: Therapeutic goals and treatment options for prevention of stress ulcer syndrome, *Am J Med* 83(6A):29, 1987.
9. Mertz HR, Walsh JH: Peptic ulcer pathophysiology, *Med Clin North Am* 75(4):799, 1991.
10. Katz J: The course of peptic ulcer disease, *Med Clin North Am* 75(4):831, 1991.
11. Soll AH: Pathogenesis of peptic ulcer and implications for therapy, *N Engl J Med* 322(13):909, 1990.
12. Ohning G, Soll A: Medical treatment of peptic ulcer disease, *Am Fam Physician* 39(4):257, 1989.
13. Schindler BA, Ramchandani D: Psychologic factors associated with peptic ulcer disease, *Med Clin North Am* 75(4):865, 1991.
14. Agrawal N: Risk factors for gastrointestinal ulcers caused by nonsteroidal anti-inflammatory drugs (NSAIDs), *J Fam Pract* 32(6):619, 1991.
15. Silverstein F: Nonsteroidal antiinflammatory drugs and peptic ulcer disease, *Postgrad Med* 89(7):33, 1991.
16. Peterson WL: Peptic ulcer—an infectious disease? *West J Med* 152(2):167, 1990.
17. Price AH, Fletcher M: Mechanisms of NSAID-induced gastroenteropathy, *Drugs* 40(suppl 5):1, 1990.
18. Holt S, Saleeby G: Gastric mucosal injury induced by nonsteroidal anti-inflammatory drugs, *South Med J* 84(3):355, 1991.
19. Andreani T and others: Preventive therapy of first gastrointestinal bleeding in patients with cirrhosis: results of a controlled trial comparing propranolol, endoscopic sclerotherapy and placebo, *Hepatology* 12(6):1413, 1990.
20. Christensen E and others: Prognosis after the first episode of gastrointestinal bleeding or coma in cirrhosis, *Scand J Gastroenterol* 24:999, 1989.
21. Powell LW, Piper DW: *Fundamentals of gastroenterology,* Sydney, 1991, McGraw-Hill.

22. Laine L: Upper gastrointestinal tract hemorrhage, *West J Med* 155(3):274, 1991.

23. Bezarro ER: Changing perspectives of H₂ antagonists for stress ulcer prophylaxis, *Crit Care Nurs Clin North Am* 2:325, 1993.

24. Sachdeva AK, Zaren HA, Sigel B: Surgical treatment of peptic ulcer disease, *Med Clin North Am* 75(4):999, 1991.

25. Snow ND, Almon M, Baillie J: Minnesota tube placement using a guide wire, *Gastrointest Endosc* 36(4):420, 1990.

26. Ready JB, Robertson AD, Rector WG: Effects of vasopressin on portal pressure during hemorrhage from esophageal varices, *Gastroenterology* 100(5):1411, 1991.

27. Ohnishi K, Sato S: Effects of vasopressin on left gastric venous flow in cirrhotic patients with esophageal varices, *Am J Gastroenterol* 85(3):2933, 1990.

28. Terblance J: *Esophagogastric varices.* In Taylor MB, editor: *Gastrointestinal emergencies,* vol 1, Baltimore, 1992, Williams & Wilkins.

29. Doughty DB, Jackson DB: *Gastrointestinal disorders,* St Louis, 1993, Mosby.

30. Poston GJ, Williamson RCN: Surgical management of acute pancreatitis, *Br J Surg* 77(1):5, 1990.

31. Steer ML: *Acute pancreatitis.* In Taylor MB, editor: *Gastrointestinal emergencies,* Baltimore, 1992, Williams & Wilkins.

32. Singh M, Simsek H: Ethanol and the pancreas, *Gastroenterology* 98(4):1051, 1990.

33. Ranson JHC: *Complications of pancreatitis.* In Taylor MB, editor: *Gastrointestinal emergencies,* Baltimore, 1992, Williams & Wilkins.

34. Smith A: When the pancreas self-destructs, *Am J Nurs* 91(9):38, 1991.

35. Brown A: Acute pancreatitis: pathophysiology, nursing diagnoses, and collaborative problems, *Focus Crit Care* 18(2):121, 1991.

36. Smith SL, Butler RW: *Acute pancreatitis. Part I. An overview,* Aliso Viejo, Calif., 1993, American Association of Critical Care Nurses.

37. Lumsden A, Bradley EL: Secondary pancreatic infections, *Surg Gynecol Obstet* 170(5):459, 1990.

38. Stanten R, Frey CF: Comprehensive management of acute necrotizing pancreatitis and pancreatic abscess, *Arch Surg* 125(10):1269, 1990.

39. Holder WD: Intestinal obstruction, *Gastroenterol Clin North Am* 17(2):317, 1988.

40. Buechter KJ and others: Surgical management of the acutely obstructed colon, *Am J Surg* 156:163, 1988.

41. Steinhagen RM, Aufses AH: Acute abdominal obstruction: when to consider nonoperative therapy, *J Crit Illness* 8:209, 1993.

42. McConnell EA: Meeting the challenge of intestinal obstruction, *Nurs 87* 17(7):34, 1987.

43. Amato EJ: A nursing reference: gastrointestinal tubes and drains. Part I. Intra-abdominal tubes and drains, *Crit Care Nurs* 2(6):50, 1982.

44. Amato EJ: A nursing reference: gastrointestinal tubes and drains. Part II. Esophageal tube, *Crit Care Nurs* 3(1):46, 1983.

45. Pasquale MD, Cerra FB: Sengstaken-Blakemore tube placement, *Crit Care Clin* 8:743, 1992.

46. Kerber K: The adult with bleeding esophageal varices, *Crit Care Nurs Clin North Am* 5:153, 1993.

Endocrine Alterations

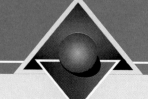

21

Endocrine Assessment and Diagnostic Procedures

JOANN M. CLARK

CHAPTER OBJECTIVES

- Identify two specific assessment differences between diabetic ketoacidosis and hyperglycemic hyperosmolar nonketotic coma.
- Describe two different assessment findings in diabetes insipidus and syndrome of inappropriate antidiuretic hormone.

- Describe the clinical assessment priorities in thyrotoxic crisis.

KEY TERMS

Most of the endocrine glands are deeply encased in the body. This protected position safeguards the glands against injury and trauma but also makes them inaccessible by conventional means of physical examination. Most endocrine glands cannot be assessed by palpation, percussion, or auscultation. Nevertheless the endocrine system may be assessed by clinicians who understand the metabolic actions of the hormones involved. This chapter focuses on the assessment and diagnosis of endocrine disorders of the pancreas, pituitary-hypothalamic system, and thyroid gland that may require admission to a critical care unit.

Clinical Assessment

History

A complete health history includes patients' chief complaints and current health status. Chronic and episodic diseases are discussed. Nurses should question patients about past health history, family history, surgery, medications, recent changes in mental function, and psychosocial history. Patients in the critical care unit may be unable to provide an adequate history because of their altered level of consciousness and need for urgent nursing and medical procedures. In this case, family members or significant others may be questioned, and the previous medical records reviewed. Box 21-1 provides detailed information on the nursing endocrine assessment and history.

The Pancreas

Physical Examination

A major function of the pancreas is to produce insulin, which is responsible for glucose metabolism. Because the pancreas cannot be examined directly, nurses need to be aware of the early clinical effects of hyperglycemia on all body systems. **Nursing physical examination priorities for hyperglycemic patients are focused on the following five areas**[1]: **assessment of neurologic status, evaluation of respirations, identification of cardiac dysfunction, observation of the skin, and measurement of urine output.**

Assessment of neurologic status

Hyperglycemia is associated with fatigue, memory loss, disorientation, and stupor leading to coma.

EVALUATION OF RESPIRATIONS. Hyperglycemic patients often have deep, sighing respirations known as **Kussmaul's respirations.** This is a compensatory hyperventilation that occurs with diabetic ketoacidosis as the body attempts to prevent further decreases in pH, secondary to the ketone-induced metabolic acidosis.

BOX 21-1

IMPORTANT ASPECTS OF ENDOCRINE NURSING HISTORY AND ASSESSMENT

HISTORY

Chief complaint
History of present problem
  Onset
  Duration
  Signs/symptoms
  Treatments
History of pancreatic problems, surgery, diabetes, carbohydrate imbalances, thyroid disease, or kidney problems
Head or neurologic disorders
Recent severe infection or surgical trauma
Past or current treatments using hyperalimentation, peritoneal dialysis, or hemodialysis
Recent, unexplained changes in weight, thirst, hunger, or urination patterns
Changes in mental abilities (i.e., memory loss, momentary disorientation, difficulty concentrating, lethargy)
Recent changes in daily levels of activities, (e.g., decreased endurance level, fatigue, weakness)
Usage of prescription or over-the-counter drugs
Presence of acute stress
Family history of present illness (e.g., carbohydrate imbalance)

ASSESSMENT

Skin turgor
Mucous membranes
Intake and output
Presence of edema
Blood pressure (i.e., hypertension, hypotension, orthostatic hypotension)
Behavioral changes
Decreased muscle strength or muscle coordination
Mental confusion
Weight changes
Presence of thirst

Identification of cardiac dysfunction

Ventricular dysrhythmias are seen secondary to low serum potassium. Orthostatic hypotension occurs secondary to the fluid volume deficit.

Observation of the skin

Hyperglycemia is associated with dry skin. With normal glucose levels, well-hydrated patients have moist and shiny buccal membranes, normal skin turgor, balanced intake and output, absence of thirst, no edema, and stable weight. If hyperglycemia is present, dehydration is ex-

BOX 21-2

HYDRATION ASSESSMENT FOR PATIENTS IN DIABETIC KETOACIDOSIS AND HYPERGLYCEMIC HYPEROSMOLAR NONKETOTIC COMA

Hourly intake
Blood pressure changes
   Orthostatic hypotension
   Pulse pressure
   Pulse rate, character, rhythm
Neck vein filling
Skin turgor
Skin moisture
Body weight
Central venous pressure
Pulmonary arterial wedge pressure
Hourly urine output
Complaints of thirst

pected because of the osmotic diuresis caused by the elevated blood glucose (Box 21-2).

Measurement of urine output

Excessive urination, which frequently leads to dehydration, is expected in hyperglycemia because glucose acts as an osmotic diuretic. The presence of glucose or ketones elevates the urine specific gravity.

Pancreatic Laboratory Assessment

Serum insulin level

The normal **insulin level** is 5 to 20 µU/ml. Blood samples taken from fasting patients are preferred in evaluation of serum insulin levels.

SIGNIFICANCE. Normally the release of insulin depends on the concentration of blood glucose; when glucose levels rise, insulin levels also rise. Conversely, when serum glucose levels are low, insulin secretion is inhibited.

Serum glucose

When patients are fasting, elevated plasma glucose levels range from 70 to 110 mg/dl. The normal fasting **serum glucose** level is measured by laboratory blood test or fingerstick glucometer at the bedside. The normal fasting whole blood value is 60 to 100 mg/dl, and the non-fasting value range is 85 to 125 mg/dl. Fasting glucose levels greater than 140 mg/dl on two occasions represent a positive diagnosis of diabetes mellitus.[2]

SIGNIFICANCE. Consistently elevated glucose levels signal increased glucagon production and an insufficient amount of effective insulin. In healthy individuals a fasting serum glucose level rarely exceeds 110 mg/dl of blood.

Glycosylated hemoglobin

Measuring the **glycosylated hemoglobin** permits a long-term view of glucose levels. During the 120-day life span of red blood cells, the hemoglobin within each cell binds to the available blood glucose through a process known as *glycosylation*. In a blood test, 4% to 7% of hemoglobin is normally glycosylated. Increased levels of circulating glucose cause an increase in glycosylation. Because this process is irreversible, a blood sample provides information about the average amount of blood glucose that has been present over the previous 3 to 4 months.

SIGNIFICANCE. Not routinely performed as a pancreatic screening tool, this test is used most frequently for patients diagnosed with diabetes mellitus. It provides information about the degree of hyperglycemia, including the actual increased values over a specific period. The glycosylated hemoglobin test eliminates many variables that could normally affect the accurate interpretation of a glucose test result. A temporary fasting state, exercise, stress, and medications do not interfere with this test result. Changes in patients' habits initiated the day of the test do not influence test outcome.

Ketones

The normal blood **ketones** level is 2 to 4 mg/dl of blood. Clinically, ketones are detected by a sweet, fruity odor on the exhaled breath. This odor is the result of the body's attempt to keep the pH within the normal range. Sweet-smelling breath occurs when the lungs release carbon dioxide in an attempt to decrease the accumulated acids.

PROCEDURE. Blood and urine specimens can be tested in the laboratory or with reagent strips. Urine samples can also be tested with specially prepared tablets. Both reagent strips and tablets are compared with a color chart. Easily performed, these bedside urine tests provide immediate information regarding ketoacidosis in persons with hyperglycemia.

SIGNIFICANCE. By-products of fat metabolism, ketones are not normally present in the urine. In most cases, when the body uses carbohydrate as its main source of energy, fat metabolism is complete, leaving only a trace of ketones in the blood. In diabetes mellitus, when insulin is not available to move glucose into the body cells for fuel, fats are burned for energy. This lipolysis (fat breakdown) occurs so rapidly that fat metabolism is incomplete and ketone bodies (acetone, beta-hydroxybutyric acid, and acetoacetic acid) collect in the blood (ketonemia) and are excreted in the urine (ketonuria).

Serum osmolality

In blood samples the normal range for **serum osmolality** values is 285 to 295 mOsm/Kg H_2O. Osmolality is a measurement of the number of particles in a solution (concentration of the solution) and not the size or weight of the particles. Used to assess fluid volume status, which can be disrupted in diabetes mellitus, this diagnostic test is not a routine screening tool for pancreatic dysfunction.

SIGNIFICANCE. An accumulation of ketone bodies and ketoacids results from the rapid, incomplete breakdown of fat and protein. The ketone bodies and ketoacids collect in the plasma as metabolic "debris" and, along with the increasing levels of glucose that cannot enter the cell, drastically increase the number of particles that normally circulate in the plasma. This increase in circulating particles, coupled with the fluid loss from hyperglycemic osmotic diuresis, significantly raises the plasma osmolality.

The Hypothalamic-Pituitary System

The hypothalamus and the pituitary glands are not accessible for physical assessment. To identify dysfunction, clinicians must be aware of the systemic effects of a normally functioning hypothalamus and posterior pituitary.

Physical Examination

Nursing physical examination priorities are focused on the following three areas: assessment of fluid balance, evaluation of cardiac function, and evaluation of neurologic status.

Assessment of fluid balance

Released by the posterior pituitary gland, antidiuretic hormone (ADH) controls the amount of fluid lost and retained within the body. Nurses use a **hydration assessment** to determine the effectiveness of ADH function. A hydration assessment includes vital signs, skin integrity, skin turgor, buccal membrane moisture, weight, intake, and output. Daily weight changes coincide with fluid retention and loss. Sudden changes in weight often result from a change in fluid balance. For comparison, 1 L of fluid lost or retained is equal to approximately 1 kg in body weight (2 lb, 2 oz). Physical characteristics of urine such as concentration, color, and specific gravity are significant factors in assessment of fluid balance.

Evaluation of cardiac function

Blood pressure (BP) and pulse rate are carefully evaluated. Decreased BP with an increased pulse is characteristic of hypovolemia, whereas elevated BP and rapid, bounding pulse may indicate hypervolemia. Orthostatic hypotension, which occurs when extracellular fluid volume decreases, is identified by a drop in systolic BP of 20 mm Hg and a drop in diastolic BP of 10 mm Hg when patients change position from supine to upright.

Evaluation of neurologic status

Alterations in serum sodium adversely affect brain tissue and disrupt normal behavioral patterns. Muscle coordination and strength are included in the neurologic assessment.

Pituitary Laboratory Studies

No single diagnostic test identifies a dysfunctional posterior pituitary gland. The diagnosis is usually made by a combination of laboratory tests and patients' clinical profiles. The diagnostic tests measure the amount of ADH released into the bloodstream. The tests include (1) measurement of serum ADH and (2) serum and urine osmolality measurements. Two tests that measure the relationship of serum and urine osmolality are the water deprivation test and the water load test.

Serum antidiuretic hormone

The **serum ADH** test measures the amount of ADH in the bloodstream using a laboratory method called *radioimmunoassay*. This diagnostic procedure provides accurate results and, when available, is the diagnostic test of choice. The normal result of a blood test for serum ADH is 1 to 5 pg/ml (1 picogram = $1 \div 1$ trillion).

PROCEDURE. All medications that can alter the release of ADH are withheld for a minimum of 8 hours before the blood test.

SIGNIFICANCE. The test is read by comparing serum ADH levels with the blood and urine osmolality values. The presence of increased ADH in the bloodstream, compared with a low serum osmolality value and elevated urine osmolality value, confirms the diagnosis of syndrome of inappropriate ADH (SIADH). Reduced serum ADH levels in patients with a high serum osmolality, hypernatremia, and reduced urine concentration signal central diabetes insipidus.

Urine and blood osmolality

Osmolality measurements determine the concentration of dissolved particles in a solution. Normal serum osmolality values range from 285 to 295 mOsm/kg H_2O. **Urine osmolality** values range from 50 to 1200 mOsm/L, with the average within 300 to 800 mOsm/L.

PROCEDURE. The body's ability to maintain a fluid balance is most accurately assessed when urine and blood samples are collected simultaneously.

SIGNIFICANCE. In healthy persons a change in the concentration of solutes triggers a chain of events to maintain normal serum dilution. In well-hydrated persons, the homeostatic mechanism maintains a 1:3 ratio of serum and urine concentrations.

INCREASED SERUM OSMOLALITY. Concentrated plasma stimulates the release of ADH, which reduces the amount of water lost at the renal tubules. Body fluid is then retained to dilute the particle concentration in the blood plasma.

DECREASED SERUM OSMOLALITY. Hypoosmolar plasma inhibits the release of ADH, the kidney tubules increase their permeability, and fluid is eliminated from the body in an attempt to regain normal concentration of particles in the bloodstream.

DECREASED URINE OSMOLALITY. In patients with absent or decreased ADH the urine osmolality is decreased, and serum osmolality is increased.

Water deprivation test

The **water deprivation test** is based on the physiologic premise that ADH is released to conserve urinary water when patients are at risk for dehydration. This procedure requires that all fluid be withheld while laboratory tests are determining the body's response to the pending dehydration. Normal values for this test are urine osmolality levels at greater than 800 mOsm and serum osmolality levels at 285 to 295 mOsm/kg H_2O.

PROCEDURE

1. Clinicians withhold all fluids for 24 hours. Normally, such a deprivation of fluids stimulates the release of ADH to conserve urine and thereby maintain serum osmolality. In healthy persons the serum osmolality remains constant while the urine osmolality increases.
2. BP is taken every 1 to 2 hours to identify decreased blood volume, which could indicate pending vascular collapse.
3. Clinicians weigh patients frequently to detect the amount of fluid lost (for every decrease in weight of 2 lb 2 oz, 1 L of body fluid is lost).
4. Serum sodium levels are monitored for a disproportionate rise in sodium compared with the reduced blood volume.
5. Patients receive subcutaneous injections of aqueous Pitressin (synthetic ADH). This phase of testing helps differentiate the type of diabetes insipidus.
6. Serial urine samples are collected for 2 hours, and the urine volume and osmolality are measured.

COMPLICATIONS. Careful monitoring is important to ensure that patients do not become dehydrated or hypotensive.[3]

SIGNIFICANCE. Patients with reduced levels of ADH are unable to curtail fluid losses through the urine despite increases in blood osmolality. Elevated serum osmolality with urine osmolality equal to or more dilute than the serum concentration indicates continued loss of urinary fluid despite hemoconcentration. Diabetes insipidus is suspected when reduced levels of ADH occur with increased serum osmolality and reduced urine concentration.[3]

Water load test

The **water load test** is based on the physiologic premise that changes in the concentration of particles in the bloodstream affect the release of ADH as the body strives to maintain a homeostatic balance. This test overhydrates patients and then provides a series of blood and urine tests to monitor the sequence of physiologic events leading to normal fluid balance. Normal values of urine osmolality range from 50 to 1200 mOsm/kg H_2O, with a usual range of 300 to 900 mOsm/L.[4] Normal urine specific gravity ranges from 1.005 to 1.030.

PROCEDURE

1. Patients are given nothing by mouth overnight and instructed to refrain from smoking (nicotine can stimulate ADH release) and taking medications that alter ADH levels.
2. Patients are asked to drink 20 ml of water per kilogram of body weight within 15 to 30 minutes. A solution of 5% dextrose in water is administered intravenously over 8 to 10 minutes if oral fluid cannot be tolerated.
3. Serial urine samples are collected for 4 to 5 hours and tested for volume, osmolality, and specific gravity.
4. Information on serum osmolality is obtained at the end of the test and compared with the entire volume of urine collected during the test.

COMPLICATIONS. The water load test may subject patients with cardiac or renal dysfunction to circulatory overload. Frequent assessment for signs of cardiac decompensation such as dyspnea, chest pain, lung crackles, jugular vein distention, and elevated central venous and pulmonary artery pressures is required. In addition, because the serum sodium may be diluted by the excess water, patients are carefully observed for signs of sodium changes such as gastrointestinal cramps, diarrhea, apprehension, and personality changes

SIGNIFICANCE. This hypotonic fluid load test decreases the urine osmolality in healthy subjects. Patients with excessive ADH have decreased serum osmolality while maintaining concentrated urine.

Pituitary Diagnostic Procedures

In addition to laboratory tests, the use of radiographic examination, computerized tomography, and magnetic resonance imaging is helpful in diagnosing pituitary-hypothalamic disease. Although these tests may not lead to a definitive diagnosis of diabetes insipidus or SIADH, they are useful in diagnosing the underlying causes of these diseases. Cranial bone fractures and space-occupying masses (e.g., tumors, blood clots) that interfere with pituitary blood supply are examples of abnormalities identified and studied in diagnostic tests.

Radiologic examination

A basic x-ray examination of the inferior skull reveals the sella turcica and surrounding bone formation. Bone fractures and tissue swelling at the base of the brain, which are apparent on a radiograph, suggest interference with the vascular supply and nerve impulses to the hypothalamic-pituitary system.

Computerized axial tomography

Computerized tomography (CT) of the base of the skull (sella turcica) identifies pituitary tumors, blood clots, cysts, nodules, and other tissue masses. A skull CT scan provides more definitive results than an x-ray examination and, whenever possible, is obtained in addition to a skull radiograph. In a CT scan the x-ray beams pass through the head on a predetermined axis, producing images of layers of brain tissue. As the x-ray beams pass through bone, soft tissue, and body fluid, a portion of the beam is absorbed or scattered, depending on the density of the tissue.

PROCEDURE

1. Patients must lie perfectly still. The 40-minute procedure causes no discomfort.
2. A radiopaque sodium iodine solution may be given intravenously to highlight the hypothalamus, infundibular stalk, and pituitary gland. Because this dye may cause allergic reactions in iodine-sensitive persons, patients are carefully questioned about allergies before the start of the test.
3. Multiple x-ray beams pass through the head from specific angles while detectors record the attenuation (absorption or scattering) of the x-ray beam.
4. A computer calculates the degree of attenuated x-ray beams over very small areas. The resulting data are projected on a viewing screen as an image of the head.

SIGNIFICANCE. The tomogram is interpreted by a radiologist for size and shape of the sella turcica and position of the hypothalamus, infundibular stalk, and pituitary gland. The radiologist notes changes in tissue density and makes a diagnostic impression.

Magnetic resonance imaging

Magnetic resonance imaging (MRI) enables the radiologist to visualize internal organs and examine the cellular characteristics of specific tissue. MRI uses a magnetic field rather than x-rays to produce images of internal structures of the body. The body part under examination is presented in cross-sectional slices as a high-resolution image.

SIGNIFICANCE. Soft fluid tissue in and immediately surrounding the brain makes the brain especially responsive to MRI scanning. Although the MRI is not a definitive diagnostic test for posterior pituitary hormonal imbalance, it identifies anatomic disruption of the gland and the surrounding area that suggests primary causes of diabetes insipidus and SIADH.

The Thyroid

The thyroid gland has an important effect on many systemic functions. Thyrotoxic crisis, also known as *thyroid storm,* is a rare but potentially lethal medical condition that may require admission to a critical care unit. It is the most extreme, severe response to overactive thyroid hormone. Manifestations of thyroid abnormalities are listed in Box 21-3.

Physical Examination

The nursing physical examination priorities focus on the following seven areas: palpation of the thyroid, auscultation of the thyroid, evaluation of neurologic status, monitoring of thermoregulation, detection of cardiac dysrhythmias, and assessment of gastrointestinal motility.

Palpation of the thyroid

The normal thyroid gland is not visible as a bulge in the anterior side of the neck. Palpation may reveal a goiter or enlargement of the thyroid gland.

Auscultation of the thyroid

Auscultation of the thyroid is accomplished by using the bell portion of the stethoscope to identify a bruit, or

---

B O X   2 1 - 3

CLINICAL MANIFESTATIONS OF THYROID ABNORMALITIES

HYPOTHYROIDISM (MYXEDEMA)

Decreased basal metabolic rate
Lethargy
Severe muscle cramps
Chronic anemia
Decreased bowel activity, constipation
Menstrual irregularities
Bradycardia
Bradypnea
Paresthesia
Muscle weakness
Decreased glomerular filtration
Decreased cardiac output

HYPERTHYROIDISM (THYROTOXICOSIS)

Increased basal metabolic rate
Fatigue, exhaustion
Diaphoresis
Intolerance to heat
Goiter
Diarrhea
Ophthalmopathy
Hyperkinesis
Increased cardiac output
Tachydysrhythmias
Frequent urination
Emotional lability
Fine tremors

blowing noise, from the circulation through the thyroid gland. Although the presence of a bruit indicates increased blood flow through the glandular tissue, auscultation does not identify patients in thyroid crisis.

Evaluation of neurologic status

Restlessness, inability to sleep, tremors, fatigue, and emotional lability occur in patients during thyroid crisis.

Monitoring of thermoregulation

Heat intolerance is a frequent finding. Even on the coldest days, patients may complain of profuse sweating and ask caregivers to turn off the room heat, open all windows, and remove bed linens. Nurses should perform a hydration assessment and devise a plan to counter the effects of the hyperthermia and potential fluid losses from vomiting and diarrhea.

Detection of cardiac dysrhythmias

Tachydysrhythmias, premature ventricular contractions, and paroxysmal supraventricular tachycardias result from the increased effect of epinephrine on the myocardium.

Assessment of gastrointestinal motility

Appetite may dramatically increase, but nausea, vomiting, and diarrhea often thwart the body's attempt to increase food intake and replenish fuel for energy expenditure. In addition, hypermotility of the gastrointestinal tract interferes with nutrient absorption, and patients may complain of recent weight loss. Elevated glucose levels may result from insufficient insulin release.

Thyroid Laboratory Studies

Laboratory tests of thyroid function are measured to confirm thyrotoxicosis and distinguish the cause as thyroid or extrathyroid. Clinicians must be aware that specific thyroid blood levels may be altered by medications, as listed in Box 21-4.

T_3 and T_4

Triiodothyronine (T_3) and thyroxine (T_4) are the major thyroid hormones measured by blood test. T_4 makes up 92% of all thyroid hormone. Most T_4 is tightly bound to plasma proteins and not metabolically active. The body metabolizes T_4 to form the more active hormone, T_3. Although T_3 constitutes only 4% of all thyroid hormone, it is more potent than T_4 and is responsible for most thyroid hormonal activity. The normal circulating T_4 level ranges from 4.5 to 11.5 ug/dl. The normal circulating T_3 level ranges from 110 to 230 ng/dl.

PROCEDURE. The laboratory tests to determine T_3 and T_4 levels are not complex and require no special patient preparation. Additional tests commonly performed on a thyroid panel are listed in Table 21-1.

SIGNIFICANCE. Thyrotoxicosis, the precursor of thyrotoxic crisis, is diagnosed in part by elevated T_4 and T_3 serum levels. The T_3 and T_4 levels are often depressed in critically ill patients because of protein malnutrition, renal failure, liver failure, and specific drug interactions.[4]

Thyroid Diagnostic Procedures

Thyroid scanning

Thyroid scanning involves the use of oral radioactive iodine. 123-I is the preferred isotope because of its low-

---

B O X 2 1 - 4

MEDICATIONS THAT INFLUENCE DIAGNOSTIC THYROID LEVELS

TRIIODOTHYRONINE (T_3)

Increase	*Decrease*
Methadone	Anabolic steroid
Estrogens	Androgens
Progestins	Salicylates
Amiodarone	Phenytoin
	Lithium
	Reserpine
	Propranolol
	Sulfonamides
	Propylthiouracil
	Methylthiouracil

THYROXINE (T_4)

Increase	*Decrease*
Oral contraceptives	Phenytoin
Heparin	Steroids
Aspirin	Diphenylhydantoin
Furosemide	Chlorpromazine
Clofibrate	Lithium
Phenylbutazone	Sulfonylurea
Some NSAIDs	Sulfonamides
Propranolol	Reserpine
Corticosteroids	Chlordiazepoxide
Amiodarone	

THYROID-STIMULATING HORMONE (TSH)

Increase TSH	*Decrease TSH and TSH response to TRH*
Metoclopramide	Glucocorticoids
Iodides	Dopamine
Lithium	Heparin
Potassium iodide	Aspirin
Morphine sulfate	Carbamazepine

THYROXINE-BINDING GLOBULIN (TBG)

Increase	*Decrease*
Opiates	Androgen therapy
Oral contraceptives	L-Asparaginase
Estrogens	
Clofibrate	
5-Fluorouracil (5-FU)	
Perphenazine	

TABLE 21-1　TESTS MOST COMMONLY PERFORMED ON A THYROID PANEL

TEST	NORMAL ADULT VALUE	CONDITIONS WITH ABNORMAL VALUES		SPECIAL CONSIDERATION
		DECREASED	INCREASED	
Serum thyroxine (T_4)	T_4, 4.5-11.5 μg/dl T_4RIA, 5-12 μg/dl	Hypothyroidism Protein malnutrition Anterior pituitary hypofunction	Hyperthyroidism Viral hepatitis Acute/chronic illness	Simple peripheral blood withdrawal Identifies amount of hormone in circulation Bound by serum protein, therefore affected by TBG Affected by pregnancy
Free thyroid index (FT_4I)	Free T_4, 0.8-2.3 ng/dl	Hypothyroidism	Hyperthyroidism	Same as above, except this measures amount of free T_4, the unbound portion of which enters the cells T_3 uptake multiplied by T_4 equals FTI
Serum triiodothyronine (T_3) (T_3RIA)	110-230 ng/dl	Hypothyroidism Malnutrition Trauma Critical illness	Thyrotoxicosis Toxic adenoma Thyroiditis	Simple peripheral blood withdrawal Measured directly by RIA Direct measurement of both bound and free T_3 Values increase in pregnancy
T_3 uptake ratio (T_3 UR) T_3 resin uptake	25%-35% uptake 0.8-1.30 ratio of laboratory result to standard control	Hypothyroidism Active hepatitis Thyroiditis	Hyperthyroidism Nephrosis Malignancy Protein malnutrition	Does not measure T_3 as name implies Indirectly measures TBG available to bind T_3 and T_4; increase in thyrotoxicosis related to increase in thyroid hormone binding Affected by pregnancy Affected by diseases that alter these proteins
Serum thyroid-stimulating hormone (TSH) test	2-5.4 mU/L <3 ng/ml	Secondary hypothyroidism Anterior pituitary disorder, very low levels, 0.005 mU/L, indicating hyperthyroidism	Primary hypothyroidism Cirrhosis	Identifies thyroid vs. pituitary-hypothalamus disorder
Serum thyrotropin-releasing hormone (TRH), stimulation test, or thyrotropin-releasing factor (TRF) test	Serum TSH rises approximately twice its normal level 30 min after IV TRH			Confirms presence of thyrotoxicosis by measuring response of the pituitary gland's production of TSH 3-4 wk before test, thyroid medication should be discontinued 500 μg of TRH given IV to mimic the hypothalamus Venous blood samples taken at intervals as stated by processing laboratory; peak response occurs in 20 min and returns to normal within 2 hr

FTI, Free thyroid index; *RIA*, radioimmunoassay; *TBG*, thyroxine-binding globulin.

energy, 13-hour output. This short halflife minimizes patients' exposure to radioactive material.[4]

SIGNIFICANCE. Thyroid scanning is useful in detecting the presence of ectopic thyroid tissue and thyroid carcinomas. Thyroid scans also identify the presence and amount of viable thyroid glandular tissue after irradiation treatment.

References

1. Sauve DE, Kessler CA: Hyperglycemic emergencies, *AACN Clin Issues Crit Care* 3(2):350-360, 1992.
2. American Diabetes Association: Clinical practice recommendations, *Diabetes Care* 18(suppl 1), 1995.
3. Balcheller J: Disorders of antidiuretic hormone secretion, *AACN Clin Issues Crit Care* 3(2):370-378, 1992.
4. Horne M, Easterday Heitz U, Swearingen PL: Fluid, electrolytes and acid-base balance: a case study approach, St Louis, 1991, Mosby.

22

Endocrine Disorders and Therapeutic Management

JOANN M. CLARK

CHAPTER OBJECTIVES

- Summarize the endocrine responses to the physiologic stress of critical illness.
- Explain the pathophysiology of hyperglycemia and describe the priorities of nursing management for patients with diabetic ketoacidosis and those for patients with hyperglycemic hyperosmolar nonketotic coma.

- Discuss the nursing priorities for management of patients with either diabetes insipidus or decreased secretion of antidiuretic hormone.
- Prioritize the essential nursing interventions for patients in thyrotoxic crisis.

KEY TERMS

The endocrine system represents a complex interaction of hormones. Endocrine dysfunction is usually related to excessive hormone production or ineffective to absent hormone function. Not all these conditions require admission to a critical care unit. This chapter describes the normal systemic response to critical illness and identifies specific endocrine pathologies involving the pancreas, pituitary-hypothalamic system, and thyroid gland that may require critical care nursing expertise.

Stress of Critical Illness

The stress of critical illness causes an expected systemic endocrine system response (Table 22-1).[1] The normal

TABLE 22-1
PHYSIOLOGIC RESPONSES BY BODY SYSTEMS TO THE STRESS-INDUCED ENDOCRINE CHANGES ASSOCIATED WITH CRITICAL ILLNESS

BODY SYSTEM	PHYSIOLOGIC RESPONSE	ENDOCRINE CHANGE
Cardiovascular	↓ HR, ↓ SV, ↓ CO	↓ Thyroid
	↑ CO, ↓ SVR	↑ Cortisol
	↑ BP, ↑ CO	↑ Aldosterone
	↑ HR, ↑ CO, ↑ BP, ↑ SVR, ↑ coronary bloodflow	↑ Catecholamine
	↑ BP, ↑ CO, ↑ SVR, ↑ sensitivity of baroreceptor reflexes	↑ Antidiuretic hormone
Pulmonary	↓ Hypoxic and hypercapnic drive → hypoventilation, hypoxia, hypercapnia	↓ Thyroid
	↑ Oxygen consumption	↑ Catecholamine
	Bronchodilation, ↑ RR, ↑ V_T	↑ Catecholamine-epinephrine
Neurologic	Altered behavior and cognitive function	↑ Cortisol, ↑ antidiuretic hormone, ↑ adrenocorticotropic hormone
	Central nervous system stimulant (↑ alertness, attentiveness, anxiety, fear)	↑ Catecholamines
	↑ passive avoidance behavior	↑ Antidiuretic hormone
Renal	↑ Na$^+$ absorption, ↑ water permeability, ↑ K$^+$ excretion	↑ Aldosterone
	Hypercalciuria, ↑ GFR	↑ Cortisol
	↓ GFR, ↓ erythrocyte, ↑ water permeability, ↓ urine, ↑ NaCl reabsorption	↑ Antidiuretic hormone
Gastrointestinal	Ulcerations	↑ Corticosteroid, ↑ glucagon
	↓ Blood flow	↑ Antidiuretic hormone
Hematologic, immunologic	↓ Erythropoietin (from ↓ oxygen consumption)	↓ Thyroid
	↑ Polymorphonuclear leukocytes (PMNs), ↓ lymphocytes, ↓ monocytes, ↓ eosinophils, ↓ migration of inflammatory cells (PMNs, monocytes, lymphocytes) to injury → ↑ susceptibility to infection	↑ Cortisol
	↑ Erythrocyte maturation secondary to ↑ erythropoietin, ↑ immune response	↑ Catecholamines
Musculoskeletal	↓ Bone formation and resorption, ↓ growth in children	↓ Thyroid
	Muscle catabolism, ↓ bone formation, ↑ bone resorption, ↓ growth in children	↑ Cortisol
Metabolic	↑ Cholesterol, ↓ lypolysis, ↓ glucose	↓ Thyroid
	↑ Glucose, ↑ lypolysis → ↑ FFA, ↑ glycerol, negative Ca^{++} balance (↓ absorption, ↑ excretion)	↑ Cortisol, ↑ glucagon
	↑ Metabolic rate, ↑ FFA mobilization, ↑ glucose, ↑ heat production	↑ Catecholamine
Other	Connective tissue impairment (thinning skin, bruising, stria, and poor wound healing)	↑ Cortisol
	↓ Libido, ↓ menstruation, ↓ fertility	↓ Gonadotropins

BP, blood pressure; *CO,* cardiac output; *FFA,* free fatty acid; *GFR,* glomerular filtration rate; *HR,* heart rate; *RR,* respiratory rate; *SV,* stroke volume; *SVR,* systemic vascular resistance; *V_T,* tidal volume.
From Sikes PJ: Endocrine responses to the stress of critical illness, *AACN Clin Issues Crit Care* 3(2):384, 1992.

neuroendocrine stress response is designed to maintain homeostasis during psychologic and physiologic stress. This endocrine response often becomes less effective with prolonged critical illness.[1,2]

Pancreas

Two hyperglycemic emergencies necessitate admission to a critical care unit: diabetic ketoacidosis (DKA) and hyperglycemic hyperosmolar nonketotic coma (HHNC).[3]

Diabetic Ketoacidosis

A serious complication of diabetes mellitus, **diabetic ketoacidosis (DKA)** is life threatening to patients with type I insulin-dependent diabetes, although it rarely affects patients with type II, non–insulin-dependent diabetes. DKA is a significant community health problem with a major financial impact. Approximately 45,000 to 130,000 hospitalizations for DKA occur annually, based on a population of 10 million persons with diabetes. Of DKA episodes, 20% occur in persons with newly diagnosed diabetes and the remaining 80% occur after the diagnosis has been made. The average age of patients with DKA is 43 years, showing that this complication occurs more frequently in older persons with diabetes than in adolescents.[4] Of all deaths attributed to diabetes, 10% result from DKA.[5] However, these deaths are believed to occur not from the ketoacidotic state alone but rather from secondary complications (e.g., pneumonia, myocardial infarction, infection) resulting from DKA.[6] Statistics show that the mortality rate for patients hospitalized for DKA is 9%, with DKA mortality rates for females higher than those for males. The mortality rate in the nonwhite population is 3 times higher than in the white population.[4]

Description and Etiology

External causes

Changes in self-management of diabetes can influence the delicate glucose/insulin balance, as can a decrease in insulin intake, an increase in dietary intake, or a decrease in routine exercise without adequate adjustment in insulin or diet. Major physiologic changes such as growth spurts in the adolescent, surgery, infection, and trauma all require an increase in insulin intake. Emotional stress increases glucose levels by releasing epinephrine, norepinephrine, or both, which triggers increased glucagon secretion. Patients may be continuing a routine insulin dose that is now inadequate for the rate of glucose entry into the bloodstream from gluconeogenesis and glycogenolysis triggered by the stress hormones.

Physiologic response

Ketoacidosis results from an alteration in insulin and counterregulatory hormones glucagon, growth hormone, cortisol, and catecholamines.[4] Ketoacidosis may develop over several hours in people with diabetes. In undiag-

---

BOX 22-1

ETIOLOGY OF DIABETIC KETOACIDOSIS

DECREASED EXOGENOUS INSULIN INTAKE

Lack of knowledge, poor compliance
  Omitting dose
  Insufficient dose to meet glucose requirement
  (e.g., hyperalimentation)
Malfunctioning insulin pump
Pharmacologic drugs
  Phenytoin
  Thiazide/sulfonamide diuretics

INCREASED ENDOGENOUS GLUCOSE

Diabetes management changes
  Decreased exercise without decreased food or increased insulin
  Increased dietary intake
Sympathetic nervous system responses
  Stressful events
    Injury
    Surgery
    Infections
      Respiratory tract
      Urinary tract
      Pancreatitis
    Emotional trauma
Increased glucagon
Increased growth hormone
Pharmacologic drugs
  Steroid therapy
  Epinephrine/norepinephrine

---

nosed diabetic patients, ketoacidosis may take days to develop and signal an abrupt onset of the disease. Box 22-1 lists the possible causes of DKA in terms of decreased insulin availability and increased presence of glucose in the bloodstream.

Pathophysiology

Insulin

Insulin is the metabolic key to the transfer of glucose from the bloodstream into the cell, where it can be used immediately for energy or stored for use at a later time. Without the necessary insulin, glucose remains in the bloodstream and cells are deprived of their energy source. A complex pathophysiologic chain of events follows (Fig. 22-1).

Glucagon

The release of **glucagon** is stimulated when insulin is ineffective in providing the cells with glucose for energy. Glucagon increases the amount of glucose in the bloodstream by breaking down stored glucose (glycogenolysis) and converting noncarbohydrate molecules

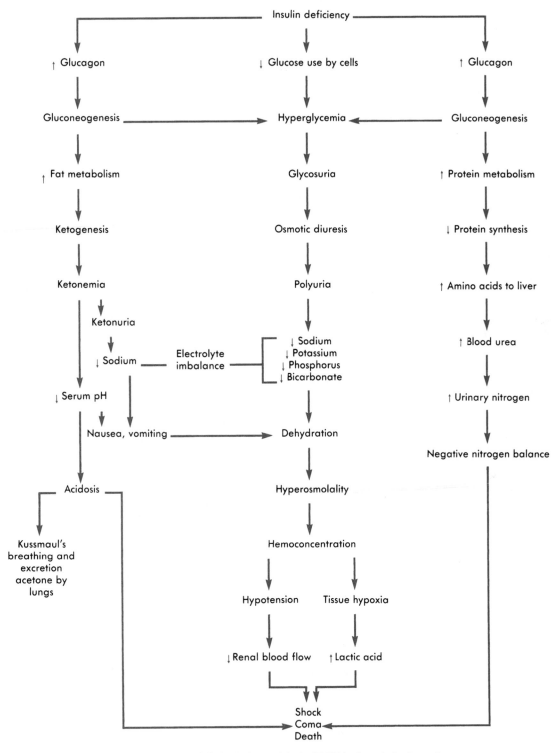

FIG. 22-1 Pathophysiology of diabetic ketoacidosis (DKA). A carbohydrate derangement affects the metabolism of both protein and fat.

into glucose (gluconeogenesis). Blood glucose levels for patients with DKA typically range from 300 to 800 mg/dl of blood. Blood glucose levels alone do not diagnose DKA; ketoacidosis is also a major determining factor.

Hyperglycemia

Hyperglycemia increases plasma osmolality, and blood becomes hyperosmolar. Cellular dehydration occurs as the hyperosmolar extracellular fluid draws the more dilute intracellular and interstitial fluids into the vascular space in an attempt to normalize plasma osmolality. Dehydration stimulates catecholamine production, which stimulates glycogenolysis, lipolysis, gluconeogenesis, and ketogenesis.

Dehydration

Excessive urination and glycosuria occur as a result of the osmotic diuresis. The excess glucose, filtered at the glomeruli, cannot be reabsorbed at the renal tubule and spills into the urine. The unreabsorbed solute exerts its own osmotic pull in the renal tubules, and less water is returned to circulation via the collecting ducts. As a result, large volumes of water, along with sodium, potassium, and phosphorus, are excreted in the urine.

Thirst

Polydipsia occurs as the decrease in the circulating blood volume stimulates the osmoreceptors in the hypothalamus and promotes the release of angiotensin II. This event initiates a strong thirst sensation designed to compensate for the loss of fluids and replenish the circulating blood volume. The fluid volume deficit also stimulates vasoconstriction as a means to preserve blood pressure. Both the vasoconstriction and the extremely elevated levels of glucose impair the delivery of oxygen to the peripheral cells, which impedes the removal of metabolic wastes.

Ketoacidosis

As the insulin/glucose imbalance progresses, gluconeogenesis continues to convert noncarbohydrate molecules into glucose. **Ketoacidosis** occurs as ketoacid end-products accumulate in the blood, and incomplete fatty acid metabolism releases highly acidic substances (acetoacetic acid and β-hydroxybutyric acid) into the bloodstream (ketonemia) and the urine (ketonuria).

Acidosis

Patients with moderate to severe DKA typically have a pH of less than 7.20, whereas in mild DKA the pH may be above 7.20 but less than 7.35.[4] The respiratory rate is increased in an attempt to compensate for the metabolic acid buildup. The deep and rapid breathing pattern that develops is known as **Kussmaul's respirations.** Acetone is exhaled, giving the exhaled breath a characteristic fruity odor.

Gluconeogenesis

Gluconeogenesis stimulates mobilization of protein and increases protein catabolism. Protein is broken down and converted to glucose in the liver. Continuous, uninterrupted gluconeogenesis leaves no reserve protein available for synthesis and repair of vital body tissues.

Urea

Nitrogen accumulates as protein is metabolized. Urea, added to the bloodstream, increases the osmotic diuresis and exacerbates dehydration. Loss of muscle mass and reduced resistance to infection occur with impaired protein use.

Assessment and Diagnosis

DKA is usually preceded by complaints from patients of malaise, headache, polyuria (excessive urination), polydipsia (excessive thirst), and polyphagia (excessive hunger). Nausea, vomiting, extreme fatigue, dehydration, and weight loss follow. Central nervous system depression and changes in the level of consciousness can quickly lead to coma.

Neurologic status

Patients with DKA may be lethargic, stuporous, or unconscious depending on the degree of fluid-balance disturbance.

Fluid balance

Physical examination reveals evidence of dehydration, including flushed, dry skin; dry buccal membranes; and skin turgor that may retain its position for more than 3 seconds. Sunken eyeballs caused by a lack of fluid in the interstitium of the eyeball may be observed. Tachycardia, hypotension, and low central venous pressure (CVP) occur with profound fluid losses. Temperature is normal or subnormal, unless an infection, which may have precipitated the DKA, is present.[4]

Pulmonary

Kussmaul's air hunger is evident. The exhaled breath has the fruity odor of acetone. Arterial blood gas analysis usually reveals metabolic acidosis with partial respiratory compensation.

Laboratory studies

The usual laboratory tests include blood and urine analyses.

BLOOD. The blood test reveals hyperglycemia (blood glucose usually greater than 300 mg/dl), ketonemia, low arterial blood pH, low plasma bicarbonate, increased serum osmolality, elevated hematocrit, marked leukocytosis (regardless of presence of infection), increased blood urea nitrogen (BUN), and imbalances of sodium, potassium, and other electrolytes. If patients do not have diabetes, other causes of metabolic acidosis are ruled out before a course of therapy is begun. Starvation, alcoholism, certain toxic chemicals, lactic acid, and uremia can also produce a ketoacidotic state.[6]

URINE. The urine demonstrates heavy ketonuria, glycosuria, and a high urine specific gravity.

Medical Management

Once diagnosed, DKA requires aggressive management to prevent progressive decompensation. Medical management is focused on the following outcomes:

1. Restore the insulin/glucagon ratio to break the ketotic cycle.
2. Reverse dehydration to treat and prevent circulatory collapse.
3. Replenish electrolytes.

Restore insulin/glucagon ratio to break ketotic cycle

Insulin is given simultaneously with intravenous fluids to reverse ketoacidosis and restore a normal insulin/glucagon ratio.

INSULIN ADMINISTRATION. The traditional use of large bolus doses of insulin has slowly given way to lower, continuous intravenous doses of insulin. A bolus of 0.3 U/kg may be given to saturate the insulin cell receptor sites and compete with any insulin resistance at the cell receptor site. Replacement of low-dose insulin, 0.1 U/kg/hr (approximately 5 to 10 U/hr), is given intravenously until acidosis is reversed. In most patients, serum glucose levels decline 75 to 100 mg/dl/hr.[4]

BREAK KETOTIC CYCLE. The administration of insulin restores the insulin/glucose ratio and inhibits the release of glucagon, so glucose is no longer poured into the bloodstream. This stops production of ketoacids as a by-product of incomplete fat metabolism. Finally, rehydration replenishes the cells and dilutes the serum concentration of ketones, urea, and glucose.

Reverse dehydration to treat and prevent circulatory collapse

Patients with DKA are severely dehydrated, with a possible loss of 5% to 10% of body weight in fluids and a fluid deficit of 3 to 5 L. Initially, normal physiologic saline may be given to reverse the intravascular deficit, hypotension, and extracellular fluid losses. During the first hour, 1 L of normal saline may be infused. The infusion rate varies depending on urinary output, secondary illnesses, and precipitating factors. Infusions of half-strength sodium chloride may follow the initial saline replacement to dilute the serum osmolality. Because the water deficit exceeds the sodium loss, half-strength sodium chloride (0.45 NaCl) can be given at a rate of 300 to 500 ml/hr until serum osmolality returns to normal and blood glucose levels decrease. Once the serum glucose level is 250 to 300 mg/dl, a 5% dextrose (D_5W) solution is infused. Intravenous glucose is necessary to replenish glucose stores and prevent cerebral damage because muscle and liver glycogen reserves may have been depleted during gluconeogenesis. Preventing a further rapid drop in glucose that would mimic hypoglycemia is also necessary. Intravenous glucose is maintained until patients are taking adequate liquids by mouth.

Replenish electrolytes

Hyperkalemia occurs with acidosis. In DKA, this is treated with insulin, which drives the potassium back into the cells. **Hypokalemia** may occur as insulin promotes the return of potassium into the cell, and acidosis is reduced. Potassium replacement is guided by the serum potassium level until the potassium shift stabilizes. Hypokalemia can occur within the first 4 hours of the rehydration-insulin treatment.

Nursing Management

Nursing management of patients with DKA demands astute assessments, critical thinking, and quick decision making. It incorporates a variety of nursing diagnoses (Box 22-2). **Nursing priorities are directed toward normalizing blood glucose, optimizing fluid balance, rehydrating without circulatory overload, monitoring urine output, evaluating electrolytes, providing oral care, maintaining skin integrity, preventing infection, and educating patients and families.** Because nurses simultaneously monitor several system functions, collect multiple laboratory values, and provide various interventions, an accurately maintained flow sheet is essential.

Normalizing blood glucose

Blood glucose tests are performed hourly at the bedside throughout the insulin therapy. Both patient response and laboratory data are assessed for changes related to glucose levels. Recognizing the clinical signs of hypoglycemia is important.

Rehydrating without circulatory overload

Dehydrated patients are tachycardic and have low blood pressure, low CVP, low pulmonary artery pressures (PAP), and low cardiac output. During the acute rehydration phase, nurses continuously monitor specific vital signs, including pulse rate, blood pressure, and hemodynamics. Evidence that fluid replacement is effective includes a change from a rapid, weak, thready pulse to a pulse that is strong and full. Systolic blood pressure above 90 mm Hg and an increase in CVP, PAP, and cardiac output also suggest effective fluid replacement. Rapid volume expansion places patients with DKA at risk for circulatory overload. This complication is most frequently seen in patients with a compromised cardiac or renal system, or both. Dyspnea, decreased oxygen saturation (SaO_2), increased respiratory rate, increased heart

---

B O X   2 2 - 2

 NURSING DIAGNOSIS PRIORITIES

DIABETIC KETOACIDOSIS

Fluid Volume Deficit related to osmotic diuresis secondary to hyperglycemia, p. 504

Decreased Cardiac Output related to decreased preload secondary to fluid volume deficit, p. 476

Altered Nutrition: less than body-protein calorie requirements related to organ dysfunction, p. 506

Anxiety related to threat to biologic, psychologic, and/or social integrity, p. 464

Knowledge Deficit: Self-Care of Diabetes Mellitus related to lack of previous exposure to information, p. 455

rate, elevated CVP and PAP, lung crackles, and neck vein engorgement signal circulatory overload. Nurses prevent fluid overload by slowing the rate of the intravenous infusions as vital signs normalize. If hypervolemia has already developed, nursing interventions include reducing the rate and volume of infusion, elevating the head of the bed, and administering oxygen.

Monitoring urine output

Measuring hourly urine output is mandatory when assessing renal output and adequacy of fluid replacement. Catheterizing alert patients remains controversial because of the risk for secondary infection. Tests for urine glucose, ketones, and specific gravity are performed frequently at the bedside. Accurate intake and output measurements are maintained to record the body's use of fluid. Hourly measurement of urine output helps evaluate renal function and provide information to prevent overhydration or underhydration.

Assessing electrolytes

Electrolytes are measured at 1 to 4 hour intervals, depending on the degree of potassium shift from the serum into the cell. The electrolytes of acutely ill patients are measured at the bedside. Patients with DKA are often hyperkalemic during the acute acidotic phase and can develop severe hypokalemia as the infusion of insulin pushes the potassium back into the cells. Therefore continuous cardiac monitoring is required because potassium affects the heart's electrical condition and hypokalemia or hyperkalemia can lead to lethal cardiac dysrhythmias.

HYPERKALEMIA. Hyperkalemia is registered on a cardiac monitor by a large, peaked T wave; flattened P wave; and broad, slurred QRS complex. Ventricular fibrillation can follow. Additional changes related to increased potassium levels include bradycardia, increased gastrointestinal motility (with nausea and diarrhea), and oliguria. Neuromuscular signs of hyperkalemia include weakness, impaired muscle activity, and flaccid paralysis.

HYPOKALEMIA. Hypokalemia is depicted on the cardiac monitor by a prolonged QT interval, flattened or depressed T wave, and depressed ST segments. Physical signs of hypokalemia include muscle weakness, decreased gastrointestinal motility (evidenced by abdominal distention or paralytic ileus), hypotension, and weak pulse. Respiratory arrest can occur as a result of severe hypokalemia.

OTHER LABORATORY TESTS. Other laboratory tests for evaluation of renal function include daily measurement of serum osmolality, BUN, and creatinine.

Providing oral care

Unconscious, dehydrated patients with DKA require careful oral care. Lip balm and a moist sponge or gauze sticks are used to moisten oral membranes. Mouth care is necessary to displace the bacteria that collect when saliva, which has a bacteriostatic action, is curtailed by dehydration. For conscious patients, ice chips are used to keep the mouth moist, and bacteria removed by frequent tooth brushing and oral rinsing.

Maintaining skin integrity

Skin care takes on new dimensions for patients with DKA. Dehydration, hypovolemia, and hypophosphatemia interfere with oxygen delivery at the cell site and contribute to inadequate perfusion and tissue breakdown. Patients must be repositioned at least every 2 hours to relieve capillary pressure and promote adequate perfusion to body tissues. A circulating air cushion bed may be helpful. Typically, patients with type I diabetes are either of normal weight or underweight. Bony prominences are assessed and circulation promoted with massage before position change. Irritation of skin from shearing force and detergents is to be avoided.

Preventing infection

Strict sterile technique is used to maintain all intravenous systems. All venipuncture sites are checked every 4 hours for signs of inflammation, phlebitis, or infiltration. Strict surgical asepsis is maintained for all invasive procedures. If catheterization is necessary to obtain urine samples for testing, careful sterile technique is essential.

Educating patients and families

Throughout patients' hospitalization, nurses explain the precipitating causes of the DKA with patients and families. For patients whose diabetes is newly diagnosed, information about the disease process and self-care is provided. Comprehensive instruction for patients and families involves various health care personnel, including nurses, certified diabetes educators, dietitians, and physicians. During the acute phase, emphasis is placed on reducing the anxiety associated with the critical care unit environment. Patients previously diagnosed with diabetes should be assessed for knowledge level and compliance history. Learning objectives include the pathophysiologic process of DKA, definition of hyperglycemia, causes of DKA, harmful effects, and symptoms. Additional information includes a discussion of ketoacidosis and its causes, symptoms, and harmful consequences. Patients and families are taught the principles of diabetes management during illness. They also are expected to know warning signs to report to their health care practitioner.

Hyperglycemic Hyperosmolar Nonketotic Coma

Description and Etiology

A frequently lethal complication of diabetes mellitus, HHNC occurs when the pancreas produces a relatively insufficient amount of insulin for the high levels of glucose that flood the bloodstream (Box 22-3). The hallmarks of HHNC are extremely high levels of plasma glucose with resulting serum hyperosmolality and os-

ETIOLOGY OF HHNC

INSUFFICIENT INSULIN

Diabetes mellitus
Pancreatic disease
Pancreatectomy
Pharmacologic
    Phenytoin
    Thiazide/sulfonamide diuretics

INCREASED ENDOGENOUS GLUCOSE

Acute stress
    Extensive burns
    Myocardial infarction
    Infection
Pharmacologic
    Glucocorticoids
    Steroids
    Sympathomimetics
    Thyroid preparations

INCREASED EXOGENOUS GLUCOSE

Hyperalimentation (total parenteral nutrition)
High-calorie enteral feedings
Hemodialysis
Peritoneal dialysis

---

motic diuresis. Inability to replace fluids lost through diuresis, vomiting, and severe diarrhea leads to profound dehydration and changes in level of consciousness. HHNC has a mortality rate greater than 40%.[5] The severity of symptoms with minimal or absent ketosis distinguishes HHNC from DKA (Table 22-2). The disorder occurs mainly although not exclusively in older, obese people with underlying conditions that require medical treatment. Patients may have type II non–insulin-dependent diabetes that is treated with diet and oral hypoglycemic agents. HHNC can also occur in people with previously undiagnosed and therefore untreated diabetes.

Pathophysiology

The syndrome of HHNC represents both (1) a deficit of insulin and (2) an excess of glucagon. The pathophysiology of HHNC is outlined below and shown in Fig. 22-2.

1. A reduced insulin level prevents the movement of glucose into the cells. As a result, glucose accumulates in the plasma.
2. The release of glucagon is triggered by the decreased insulin level.
3. Hepatic glucose from glycogenolysis is poured into circulation.
4. Hyperglycemia causes an osmotic diuresis.
5. Serum osmolality increases as the numbers of particles increase in the blood. In an effort to decrease the hyperosmolality, fluid is drawn from the intracellular compartment into the vascular bed. Profound intracellular volume depletion occurs if this fluid is not replaced by oral or intravenous fluid intake.

Assessment and Diagnosis

HHNC has a slow, subtle onset. Initially the symptoms may be nonspecific, and clinicians may ignore them or attribute them to patients' concurrent disease processes.

Neurologic status

Before admission to the critical care unit, patients have experienced polyuria, polydipsia, and advancing weakness. These conditions cause progressive dehydration, leading to mental confusion, convulsions, and possible obtundation or coma. The alteration in level of consciousness is directly related to hyperglycemic osmotic diuresis and resulting intracellular dehydration.

Fluid balance

A profound fluid deficit is often present. Signs of severe dehydration include longitudinal wrinkles in the tongue, decreased salivation, and decreased CVP with tachycardia and hypotension. Kidney impairment resulting from the severe reduction in renal circulation is suggested by elevated BUN and creatinine levels. Metabolic acidosis is usually absent.

Laboratory studies

Serum glucose levels are strikingly elevated, often double the levels seen in DKA (2000 mg/dl). Serum osmolality, normally 285 to 295 mOsm/kg H_2O, may reach 350 mOsm/kg H_2O. Typical initial laboratory values seen with HHNC include blood glucose levels greater than 400 mg/dl and serum osmolality greater than 315 mOsm/Kg. In addition, elevated hematocrit and depleted potassium and phosphorus levels result from the osmotic diuresis.[7] Arterial blood gas testing is not required as often in HHNC as in DKA, but serum osmolality is measured more frequently in HHNC than in DKA.

Medical Management

The goals of medical management are to interrupt glycemic diuresis and prevent vascular collapse. The underlying cause of HHNC must then be identified. The same basic principles used to treat DKA are used for patients with HHNC:

1. Rehydration
2. Restoration of the insulin/glucagon ratio
3. Electrolyte replacement

TABLE 22-2
GENERAL COMPARISON OF DKA AND HHNC

	DIABETIC KETOACIDOSIS	HYPERGLYCEMIC HYPEROSMOLAR NONKETOTIC COMA
Cause	Insufficient exogenous insulin for glucose needs	Insufficient exogenous/endogenous insulin for glucose needs
Onset	Sudden (hours)	Slow, insidious (days, weeks)
Predisposing factors	Noncompliance to type I DM, illness, surgery, decreased activity	Older patients with recent acute illness; therapeutic procedures
Mortality	8% to 10%[1]	12% to 50%[2]
Population affected	Type I DM	Type II DM, age > 65 yr
Clinical manifestations	Dry mouth, polydipsia, polyuria, polyphagia, dehydration, dry skin, hypotension, weakness, mental confusion, tachycardia, changes in level of consciousness	Dry mouth, polydipsia, polyuria, polyphagia, dehydration, dry skin, hypotension, weakness, mental confusion, tachycardia, changes in level of consciousness
	Ketoacidosis: air hunger, acetone breath odor, respirations rapid and deep, nausea, vomiting	No ketosis, no breath odor, respirations rapid and shallow, usually mild nausea and vomiting
Laboratory tests		
Serum glucose	300-800 mg/dl	600-2000 mg/dl
Serum ketones	Strongly positive	Normal or mildly elevated
Serum pH	< 7.30	Normal
Serum osmolality	< 350 mOsm/L	> 350 mOsm/L
Serum sodium	Normal or low	Normal or elevated
Serum potassium	Low, normal, or elevated (total body K^+ is depleted)	Low, normal, or elevated
Serum bicarbonate	< 15 mEq/L	Normal
Serum phosphorus	Low, normal, or elevated (possibly decreasing after insulin therapy)	Low, normal, or elevated (possibly decreasing after insulin therapy)
Urine glucose*	3% to 4%	4% or highest concentration
Urine acetone	Strong	Absent or mild

DM, Diabetes mellitus.
*Clinitest, 2-drop method.

Rehydration

Because the fluid deficit may be as much as 150 ml/kg of body weight, rapid rehydration is the primary intervention. The average 150 lb adult may lose more than 10 L of fluid a day.[4] This volume deficit is replaced with 2 L of physiologic normal saline (0.9%) during the first hour of treatment,[4] especially for patients in a state of circulatory collapse.[6] Half-strength hypotonic saline (0.45%) can subsequently be used to reduce serum osmolality. Patients may need replacement of 6 to 10 L of fluid in the first 10 hours. Sodium input should not exceed that required to replace the losses. Careful monitoring for sodium and water balance is required to prevent hemolysis as hemoconcentration is reduced. Relative hypoglycemia is prevented by changing the hydrating solution to 5% dextrose in water, in 0.9% saline, or in 0.45% saline when the serum glucose levels fall within a 250 to 300 mg/dl range.

Restoration of insulin/glucagon ratio

Vigorous fluid therapy alone can reverse HHNC. However, intravenously administered insulin is also given to facilitate the cellular use of glucose and decrease the serum osmolality more rapidly.[6] An initial bolus of 10 to 15 U of regular insulin is given intravenously. Maintenance insulin at 0.1 U/kg/hr is infused to reduce hyperglycemia. This dose mimics the physiologic secretion of 5 to 10 U/hr and may be given until the glucose falls between 250 and 300 mg. Another treatment method provides a one-time insulin administration of 15 U subcutaneously.[4] Once glucose levels are at or below 250 mg/dl, insulin treatment is usually discontinued.

Electrolyte replacement

Serial laboratory tests keep clinicians apprised of the fluctuating serum electrolyte levels and provide a basis for electrolyte replacement. Intracellular potassium is

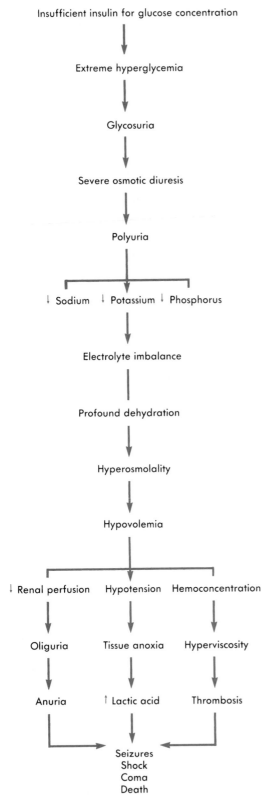

FIG. 22-2 Pathophysiology of hyperglycemic, hyperosmolar nonketotic coma (HHNC).

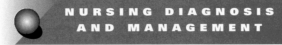

NURSING DIAGNOSIS AND MANAGEMENT

HHNC

- *Decreased Cardiac Output* related to decreased preload secondary to fluid volume deficit, p. 476
- *Altered Nutrition: Less than Body Requirements* related to organ dysfunction, p. 506
- *Anxiety* related to threat to biologic, psychologic, and/or social integrity, p. 464
- *Knowledge Deficit: Self Care of Diabetes Mellitus* related to previous lack of exposure to information, p. 455

usually depleted as a result of the HHNC dehydration. Potassium quickly reenters the cells when insulin is administered, and intravenous or oral potassium replacement is required. Phosphate levels are also carefully monitored and replaced.

Nursing Management

Nursing management of patients with HHNC incorporates a variety of nursing diagnoses (Box 22-4). **Nursing priorities are directed toward achieving optimal fluid balance; normalizing serum glucose, electrolytes, and osmolality; and educating patients and families.**

Achieving optimal fluid balance

Patients with HHNC have a severe fluid volume deficit. Hemodynamic monitoring is advisable during the acute rehydration phase. This includes monitoring CVP, pulmonary arterial wedge pressure, PAP, and cardiac output to evaluate the degree of dehydration and effectiveness of rehydration therapy. Because preexisting cardiopulmonary or renal problems often exist in older patients, the hemodynamic criteria are based on values normal for patients' age groups and current medical conditions. Nurses assess for clinical manifestations of fluid overload and vigorously rehydrate patients. Symptoms of circulatory overload include elevated CVP and pulmonary artery pressure, tachycardia, bounding pulse, dyspnea, tachypnea, lung crackles, and engorged neck veins.

Normalizing glucose, electrolytes, and osmolality

Blood glucose, sodium, potassium, hematocrit, and osmolality levels are monitored. In the acute period, bedside serum glucose is elevated every 30 to 60 minutes to determine effectiveness of treatment. Urine ketones are tested at the bedside to rule out the presence of ketoacidosis. A convenient formula used to identify the **serum**

osmolality on the basis of known laboratory values is the following:

$$2(Na^+ + K^+) + \frac{Glucose\ (mg/dl)}{18} + \frac{BUN\ (mg/dl)}{2.8}$$

Serum osmolality values in excess of 320 mOsm/kg H_2O indicate hyperosmolality.[1,3]

Educating patients and families

Because HHNC usually occurs in older persons, education for this age group is particularly important. Throughout the critical care period, nurses collect information to identify the precipitating cause of the HHNC and teach patients and families ways to prevent its recurrence. Patients receive information about the underlying medical condition that precipitated the HHNC and early clinical manifestations of HHNC. If the HHNC is the result of untreated diabetes, comprehensive instruction on diabetes is necessary.

Hypothalamic-Pituitary System

The posterior pituitary regulates secretion of antidiuretic hormone (ADH), which controls fluid balance within the body. Two disorders of ADH are frequently seen in critically ill patients: diabetes insipidus (DI) and syndrome of inappropriate antidiuretic hormone (SIADH).[8]

Diabetes Insipidus

Description and Etiology

Diabetes insipidus (DI) occurs when ADH is insufficient. ADH normally stimulates the kidney tubules to reabsorb filtered water when the body needs to increase fluid stores, either in response to an increase in particles in the blood plasma (rising osmolality) or falling blood pressure. Unrestricted serum hyperosmolality develops when ADH does not function adequately. Intense thirst and passage of excessively large quantities of very dilute urine are characteristics of the disease. DI is categorized into three types according to cause: central DI, nephrogenic DI, and psychogenic DI (Box 22-5).

Pathophysiology

Abnormal ADH function

ADH is the hormone directly responsible for maintaining fluid balance within the body. When ADH is absent, inefficient, or insufficient, the kidney tubules prevent the reabsorption of urinary substrate, and an excessive amount of water is lost to the body. This pathologic condition is known as *diabetes insipidus (DI)*. The pathophysiology of DI is summarized in the following list and in Fig. 22-3.

BOX 22-5

ETIOLOGY OF DI

CENTRAL DI

Occurs when there is an interruption in the synthesis and release of ADH, further divided into primary and secondary categories

PRIMARY DI

Occurs when structural abnormalities within the hypothalamus, infundibular stalk, and neurohypophysis prevent the release of ADH according to the body's inherent signals; primary DI that is possibly idiopathic, congenital, or result of an inherited familial disorder.

SECONDARY DI

Occurs as a result of trauma or pathologic condition that affects the pituitary-hypothalamus functioning unit

NEPHROGENIC DI

Results from the inability of the kidney nephrons to respond to circulating ADH

PSYCHOGENIC DI

A rare form of the disease that occurs with compulsive water drinking

---

1. A decreased amount of effective ADH decreases the kidney tubules' reabsorption of water and leads to excessive water excretion in the urine.
2. As free water is lost from the bloodstream, the serum osmolality rises and excessive sodium concentration (hypernatremia) in the vascular space stimulates thirst receptors.
3. Extremely dilute urine is excreted (polyuria). The body is depleted of the fluid necessary for hydration. Urine osmolality and urine specific gravity decrease.
4. Hypotension and hypovolemic shock may occur. Decreased cerebral perfusion and severe dehydration disrupt the neurologic system, causing seizures, loss of consciousness, and possibly death.

Normal ADH function

In a healthy body capable of balancing fluid losses, the rising serum osmolality triggers synthesis and release of ADH, which activates the kidney tubules to conserve water. This action returns fluid to the vascular space, thereby diluting or decreasing the osmolality. Consequently the concentration of electrolytes, especially sodium, returns to a balanced state. In people with the pathologic condition of decreased ADH secretion, this negative feed-

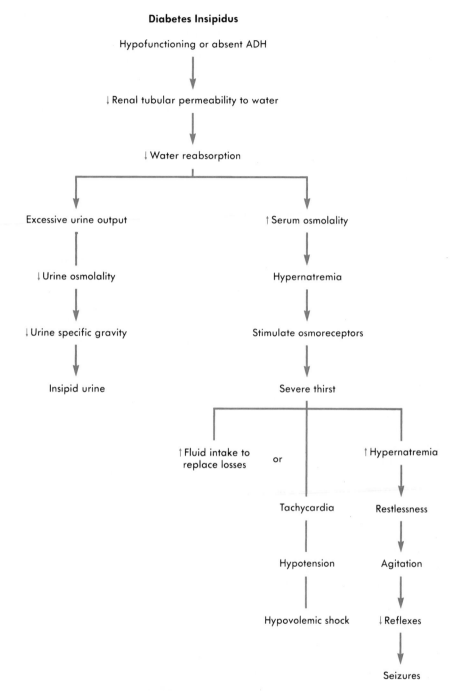

Diabetes Insipidus

Hypofunctioning or absent ADH

↓ Renal tubular permeability to water

↓ Water reabsorption

Excessive urine output   ↑ Serum osmolality

↓ Urine osmolality   Hypernatremia

↓ Urine specific gravity   Stimulate osmoreceptors

Insipid urine   Severe thirst

↑ Fluid intake to replace losses   or   ↑ Hypernatremia

Tachycardia   Restlessness

Hypotension   Agitation

Hypovolemic shock   ↓ Reflexes

Seizures

FIG. 22-3 Pathophysiology of diabetes insipidus (DI).

back system is interrupted and ADH is either not released or ineffective.

Assessment and Diagnosis

Clinical manifestations of DI may develop gradually or occur suddenly after a head injury or precipitating disease. Urine production always exceeds 3 L/24 hr, often exceeding 300 ml/hr.[9] The urine has a very low osmolality. The dilute urine in DI is "insipid" or odorless, as opposed to the sweet, honey *(mellitus)* urine associated with diabetes mellitus. Unless people with DI are able to replace the lost fluid, hypernatremia and severe dehydration result. Diagnostic tests used to establish the presence of DI evaluate the body's innate ability to balance fluid and electrolytes (see Chapter 21).

Fluid balance

Critical assessment of fluid status is critical for patients with DI, who usually have fluid volume deficit. Intake and output measurement, condition of buccal membranes, skin turgor, daily weights, and presence of thirst and temperature are major concerns for patients unable to regulate fluid needs and losses.

Medical Management

Medical management is based on (1) initial fluid volume replacement and (2) pharmacologic management of the underlying condition causing the lack of ADH.

Initial fluid volume replacement

Fluid replacement is provided in the initial phase of treatment to prevent circulatory collapse. Patients who are able to drink receive voluminous amounts of fluid orally to balance output. For those unable to take sufficient fluids orally, hypotonic intravenous solutions are rapidly infused and carefully monitored to restore hemodynamic balance.

Pharmacologic management

Medications play a major role in the management of DI. Patients with primary and secondary DI who are unable to synthesize ADH require exogenous ADH (vasopressin) replacement therapy.

PITRESSIN. One form of the ADH hormone available for short-term substitution is aqueous synthetic **Pitressin,** which is administered intramuscularly, subcutaneously, or topically to the nasal mucosa. The onset of antidiuresis (reduced urine output) is rapid and lasts up to 8 hours.

PITRESSIN TANNATE. Pitressin Tannate is a more potent pituitary extract used to treat chronic DI. The drug is given intramuscularly, never intravenously. The onset of antidiuresis is slow, with the peak activity occurring after 48 hours, and the effects of this drug last several days. Both Pitressin and Pitressin Tannate constrict smooth muscle and can elevate systemic blood pressure. Water intoxication can also occur if the dose is higher than the required therapeutic level.

DESMOPRESSIN ACETATE. Desmopressin acetate is another drug used for patients with mild forms of DI. A synthetic analog of vasopressin, desmopressin acetate is administered parenterally or via the nasal mucosa (not inhaled). The drug has fewer side effects than other vasopressin preparations. It has minimal effects on the smooth muscle tissue and does not cause hypertension.

VASOPRESSIN RELEASE. Various drugs stimulate the production and release of endogenous vasopressin for patients who have ADH in insufficient quantities. These drugs include carbamazepine (an anticonvulsive), clofibrate (a hypolipidemic), and chlorpropamide (an oral hypoglycemic agent).

INDOMETHACIN. Trial studies have shown indomethacin, a nonsteroidal antiinflammatory agent, to be therapeutic in the treatment of lithium-induced polyuria and polydipsia.

CHLORPROPAMIDE AND TOLBUTAMIDE. Nephrogenic DI does not respond to hormonal replacement treatment or anticonvulsive or hypolipidemic drugs. Chlorpropamide and tolbutamide are effective in increasing the responsiveness of the nephron site to circulating ADH.

THIAZIDE DIURETICS. Certain thiazide diuretics are used in the treatment of nephrogenic DI. Thiaziade diuretics are believed to induce a mild sodium diuresis, which encourages proximal tubular reabsorbtion of sodium and water and thereby decreases the amount of water reaching the distal tubule. However, because of untoward side effects, these drugs are used with extreme caution.

Nursing Management

Nursing management of patients with DI incorporates a variety of nursing diagnoses (Box 22-6). **Nursing priorities are directed toward correcting the fluid volume deficit and educating patients and families.**

Correcting fluid volume deficit

The nursing management of DI involves continual monitoring of patients' hydration status, hemodynamic response to fluid replacement, and response to medications used to replace or increase ADH availability. Effective treatment results in a urine output below 3 L/24 hr, a positive fluid balance that provides replacement of urinary losses, and increases in CVP and blood pressure to normal levels. Urine and blood specimens are simultaneously collected for osmolality studies. Bedside specific gravity analysis gives immediate information regarding variations in the kidney tubules' reabsorption of water.

Educating patients and families

Educating patients and families about the disease process and its effects on thirst, urination, and fluid balance encourages patients to become more involved in their health care. After discharge, patients with DI and their families are taught the signs and symptoms of dehydration and overhydration and conditions

---

B O X 2 2 - 6

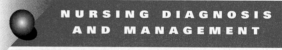

NURSING DIAGNOSIS AND MANAGEMENT

DIABETES INSIPIDUS

- *Fluid Volume Deficit* related to deceased secretion of ADH, p. 504
- *Decreased Cardiac Output* related to decreased preload secondary to fluid volume deficit, p. 476
- *Knowledge Deficit: Self-Care of Diabetes Insipidus* related to previous lack of exposure to information, p. 455

to report to their physicians. Nurses also teach the procedures for correct daily weight and urine specific gravity measurement and provide information about medications.

Syndrome of Inappropriate Antidiuretic Hormone

The opposite of DI is the **syndrome of inappropriate antidiuretic hormone (SIADH).** SIADH occurs when the release of ADH increases. The ADH secreted in the bloodstream exceeds the amount needed to maintain normal blood volume and serum osmolality.

Description and Etiology

Causes of SIADH are numerous in patients who are critically ill (Box 22-7).

Pathophysiology

In SIADH, ADH continues to be released into the bloodstream despite the feedback mechanism signaling

---

B O X   2 2 - 7

ETIOLOGY OF *SIADH*

Malignant disease associated with autonomous production of ADH
  Bronchogenic oat cell carcinoma
  Pancreatic adenocarcinoma
  Duodenal, bladder, ureter, prostatic carcinomas
  Lymphosarcoma, Ewing's sarcoma
  Acute leukemia, Hodgkin's disease
  Cerebral neoplasm, thymoma
Central nervous system diseases that interfere with the hypothalmic-hypophyseal system and increase the production and/or release of ADH
  Head injury
  Brain abscess
  Hydrocephalus
  Pituitary adenoma
  Subdural hematoma
  Subarachnoid hemorrhage
  Cerebral atrophy
  Guillain-Barré syndrome
  Tuberculous meningitis
  Purulent meningitis
  Herpes simplex encephalitis
  Acute intermittent porphyria
Neurogenic stimuli capable of increasing ADH
  Decreased glomerular filtration rate
  Physical and/or emotional stressors
    Pain
    Fear
    Trauma
    Surgery
  Myocardial infarction
  Acute infection
  Hypotension
  Hemorrhage
  Hypovolemia

Pulmonary diseases believed to stimulate the baroreceptors and increase ADH
  Pulmonary tuberculosis
  Viral and bacterial pneumonia
  Empyema
  Lung abscess
  Chronic obstructive lung disease
  Status asthmaticus
  Cystic fibrosis
Endocrine disturbances that hormonally influence ADH
  Myxedema
  Hypothyroidism
  Hypopituitarism
  Adrenal insufficiency—Addison's disease
Medications that mimic, increase the release of, or potentiate ADH
  Hypoglycemics
    Insulin
    Tolbutamide
    Chlorpropamide
  Potassium-depleting thiazide diuretics
  Tricyclic antidepressants
    Imipramine
    Amitriptyline
  Phenothiazine
    Fluphenazine
    Thioridazine
  Thioxanthenes
    Thiothixene
    Chlorprothixene
  Chemotherapeutic agents
    Vincristine
    Cyclophosphamide
  Narcotics
  Carbamazepine
  Clofibrate
  Acetaminophen
  Nicotine
  Oxytocin
  Vasopressin
  Anesthetics

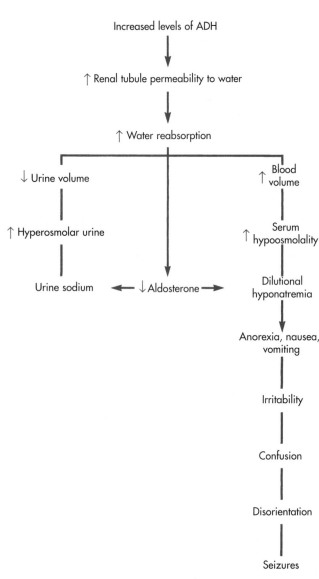

Increased levels of ADH

↓

↑ Renal tubule permeability to water

↓

↑ Water reabsorption

↓ Urine volume   ↑ Blood volume

↑ Hyperosmolar urine   ↑ Serum hypoosmolality

Urine sodium ← ↓ Aldosterone → Dilutional hyponatremia

Anorexia, nausea, vomiting

Irritability

Confusion

Disorientation

Seizures

FIG. 22-4 Pathophysiology of syndrome of inappropriate antidiuretic hormone (SIADH).

a normal serum osmolality and blood volume. Hypersecretion of ADH results in hyponatremia and hemodilution (Fig. 22-4).

Dilutional hyponatremia

The release of ADH increases the reabsorption of water by the kidney tubules, which increases circulating blood volume. Dilutional hyponatremia occurs as the expanded plasma volume dilutes the previously normal serum sodium levels. Serum hypoosmolality leads to a shift of fluid into the cells in an attempt to equalize osmotic pressure.

Assessment and Diagnosis

Fluid balance

Patients with SIADH develop water intoxication. The clinical manifestations of this condition relate to the ex-

cess fluid in the extracellular compartment and the proportionate dilution of the circulating sodium. Although edema is usually not present, slight weight gain may occur from the expanded extracellular fluid volume.

Neurologic status

The hyponatremia may initially be asymptomatic but later cause significant neurologic changes. Early clinical manifestations of dilutional hyponatremia include lethargy, anorexia, nausea, and vomiting. As the water and sodium imbalance progresses, neurologic signs of hyponatremia predominate. Inability to concentrate, mental confusion, apprehension, and seizures may lead to loss of consciousness and death.

Laboratory studies

Laboratory values display the clinical hallmarks of SIADH: hyponatremia, serum hypoosmolality, and urine osmolality greater than would be expected of hypotonic blood (Table 22-3). Characteristically, serum hypoosmolality is less than 250 mOsm/kg H_2O, with serum sodium levels below 120 mEq/L.

Medical Management

In the critical care unit, SIADH often occurs as a secondary disease. Ideally, recognition and treatment of the primary disease will reduce the production of ADH. If patients are receiving any of the chemical agents suspected of causing the disease, discontinuing the drug may return ADH levels to normal. Medical management includes restriction of fluids, correction of hyponatremia, diuresis, and use of drugs that decrease ADH secretion.

Fluid restriction

Along with treatment of the primary disease, the most successful medical therapy is simple reduction of fluid intake. Although fluid restrictions are calculated on the basis of individual needs and losses, a general criterion is to restrict fluids to 500 ml less than average daily output.[10]

Hyponatremia

Patients with severe hyponatremia (less than 115 mEq/L) or those with seizures receive infusions with 3% to 5% hypertonic saline[11] for rapid but temporary correction of the hemodilution caused by the retention of fluid at the renal tubules and severe sodium loss. Hypertonic saline solution is administered very slowly and cautiously until the serum sodium level increases to 125 mEq/L.[10] Treatment with a hypertonic solution is temporary because the sodium is continuously removed from the body through the urine.

Diuresis

Intravenous furosemide (Lasix) is added to stimulate diuresis and prevent risk of pulmonary edema related to the hypertonic saline solution.

T A B L E   2 2 - 3

LABORATORY VALUES AND INTAKE AND OUTPUT FOR PATIENTS WITH DI AND SIADH

VALUE	NORMAL	DIABETES INSIPIDUS	SYNDROME OF INAPPROPRIATE ANTIDIURETIC HORMONE
Serum ADH	1-5 pg/ml	↓ in central DI, possibly normal with nephrogenic or psychogenic DI	Elevated
Serum osmolality	285-300 mOsm/kg H$_2$O	> 300 mOsm/kg H$_2$O	< 250 mOsm/kg H$_2$O
Serum sodium	135-145 mEq/L	> 145 mEq/L	< 120 mEq/L
Urine osmolality	300-1400 mOsm/L	< 300 mOsm/L	Increased
Urine specific gravity	1.005-1.030	< 1.005	> 1.030
Urine output	1-1.5 L/24 hr	30-40 L/24 hr	Below normal
Fluid intake	1-1.5 L/24 hr	≥ 50 L/24 hr	Unchanged

Pharmacologic management

Narcotic agonists such as oxilorphan and butorphanol reduce the secretion of ADH in many patients with SIADH. These drugs, however, do not seem to be effective for patients with SIADH caused by lung malignancies. These patients are treated with demeclocycline hydrochloride, tetracycline (an antibiotic), and lithium carbonate (an alkali metal salt primarily used to alter psychogenic behavior). These drugs inhibit the tubular response to ADH and decrease water reabsorption at the renal tubules.

Nursing Management

Thorough, astute nursing assessments are required for patients with SIADH, especially during correction of the fluid and sodium imbalance. The systemic effects of hyponatremia occur rapidly and can be lethal. Nursing management of patients with SIADH incorporates a variety of nursing diagnoses (Box 22-8). **Nursing priorities are directed toward correcting fluid volume overload, normalizing serum sodium, preventing complications, evaluating neurologic status, monitoring gastrointestinal function, and educating patients and families.**

Correcting fluid volume overload

Patients with SIADH display symptoms of fluid volume overload. Accurate intake and output measurements are required to calculate fluid replacement and prevent fluid-related complications. Fluids are severely restricted to equal urine output. Patients are weighed every 24 hours to gauge fluid retention and loss. Weight gain signifies continual fluid retention, whereas weight loss indicates loss of body fluid. Hemodynamic parameters, including blood pressure, CVP, and pulmonary arterial wedge pressure (PAWP), are expected to be within patients' normal

B O X   2 2 - 8

NURSING DIAGNOSIS AND MANAGEMENT

SYNDROME OF INAPPROPRIATE ANTIDIURETIC HORMONE (SIADH)

- *Fluid Volume Excess* related to increased secretion of ADH secondary to SIADH, p. 508
- *Knowledge Deficit: Self-Care of SIADH* related to lack of previous exposure to information, p. 455

range. Elevations in blood pressure, CVP, and PAWP may indicate circulatory overload as a complication of fluid retention. Clinical manifestations of acute heart failure and pulmonary edema such as elevated blood pressure, PAWP, and CVP are reasons to discontinue the hypertonic saline infusion. Apprehension, abrupt change to an upright position to breathe, dyspnea, moist cough, and increased respiratory and pulse rates also indicate the inability of the cardiopulmonary system to accommodate the increased fluid load. Moistening the buccal membrane may relieve discomfort during fluid restriction.

Normalizing serum sodium

Hypertonic saline is infused very cautiously in the treatment of severe hyponatremia. A volumetric pump is used to deliver 0.1 mg/kg/min or set to deliver a flow rate determined by the serum sodium levels.[11] The saline infusion is usually discontinued when patients' serum sodium levels reach 125 mEq/L. Serial measurements of urine output, blood and urine sodium, urine specific gravity, and urine and blood osmolality are taken.

Preventing complications

A complication that must be avoided, hypertonic expansion occurs when the hypertonic solution is infused so rapidly that it creates an immediate hyperosmolality of the bloodstream. Fluid is drawn from the more dilute intracellular spaces to the bloodstream in an effort to equalize the concentration of particles. The isosmotic conditions or equality of the compartments is not achieved because additional hypertonic solution continues to be rapidly infused. The hypertonic solution is discontinued if signs or symptoms occur, such as increased serum sodium levels, bounding pulse, increased thirst, and hand veins taking longer than 5 seconds to empty when the hand is elevated.

Evaluating neurologic status

Seizure precautions for patients with SIADH are provided regardless of the degree of hyponatremia. Serum sodium levels may fluctuate rapidly, and neurologic impairment may occur with no apparent warning. An altered neurologic response may also be influenced by the acuity of the primary disease and not solely by low sodium levels. Seizure precautions are designed to protect patients from injury and include providing padded side rails on the bed, keeping the bed in low position when patients are unattended, turning patients' heads to the side without forcibly restraining them, and using oral airway and suction apparatus at patients' bedsides. Oxygen is administered as needed.

Monitoring gastrointestinal function

Constipation may occur from restricted fluid intake and inactivity. Cathartics or low-volume hypertonic enemas may be given to stimulate peristalsis. Tap water or hypotonic enemas are never administered because the water in the solution may be absorbed through the bowel and cause water intoxication.

Educating patients and families

Rapidly occurring changes in patients' neurologic status may frighten visiting family members. Nurses can demonstrate sensitivity to their concerns by speaking empathically and providing time for patients and families to communicate their feelings. Nurses also describe the course of the disease, its effect on water balance, the reason for fluid restrictions, and the role of family members in treating SIADH. For example, teaching patients and families to measure intake and output encourages independence and is a positive way to involve them in the plan of care.

Thyroid

Extreme hypersecretion or hyposecretion of thyroid hormones can cause significant symptoms that may require admission to a critical care unit.

Thyrotoxic Crisis

Thyrotoxicosis, also called *hyperthyroidism,* occurs when the thyroid gland produces thyroid hormone in excess of the body's need. Hyperthyroid conditions may also result from ingestion of excessive, exogenous thyroid-replacement drugs. Although rare, excess thyroid hormone may be produced by a neoplasm of ectopic thyroid tissue. An uncommon, life-threatening condition that occurs when the overactive thyroid has not been diagnosed or adequately treated, **thyrotoxic crisis** is a critical stage of hyperthyroidism. Thyrotoxic crisis is often precipitated by a major stressor such as an acute infection or severe trauma. (Box 22-9 lists conditions known to precipitate thyrotoxic crisis.) The signs and symptoms of thyrotoxicosis are exaggerated in the crisis stage, and death occurs if emergency treatment is not provided.

Description and Etiology

Excessive circulating thyroid hormone causes cellular dysfunction in the body, regardless of the underlying etiologic factors causing hypersecretion. The effects of hyperthyroidism are the following:

1. Increased metabolic activity
2. Stimulation of the beta-adrenergic receptors, which results in a heightened sympathetic nervous system response
3. Increased number of epinephrine-binding sites that hyperactivate cardiac tissue, nervous tissue, smooth muscle tissue metabolism, and heat production

Pathophysiology

Thyroid hormone increases cellular oxygen consumption in almost all metabolically active cells. Energy in the form of heat is lost rather than used by the cells. Cellular oxygen demands are increased, causing the heart to pump blood more rapidly to deliver oxygen and expel

---

BOX 22-9

CONDITIONS PRECIPITATING THYROTOXIC CRISIS

Systemic infections
Diabetes out of control
Trauma
Myocardial infarction
Thyroid medication overdose
Thyroid ablations (surgical or radioiodine)
Surgery
Childbirth in patients with poorly controlled hyperthyroidism

carbon dioxide. The oxygen demands in the hypermetabolic state are so great that the cardiac system cannot compensate adequately. Fatigue and tachydysrhythmias ensue, along with a critically high fever.

Hypermetabolism

In hyperthyroidism, patients' appetites increase to meet metabolic demands. Generally, patients are unable to take in enough food to meet the demands and prevent mobilization of carbohydrates, fats, and protein for energy sources. As a result of rapidly broken-down nutrients, nitrogen and uric acid excretion are increased and metabolic acidosis is a potential problem. Intestinal peristalsis increases, often resulting in diarrhea, nausea, and vomiting. These conditions all lead to dehydration and compound the problem of malnutrition and weight loss. Excess metabolism generates heat, and the body temperature may rise as high as 41° C (106° F). Hypersensitivity at the adrenergic-binding sites potentiates cardiovascular and nervous system responses to the hypermetabolic state. Tachydysrhythmias often progress to pulmonary edema and acute heart failure. Increased beta-adrenergic activity manifests in emotional lability, fine muscular tremors, and delirium.

Assessment and Diagnosis

Thyrotoxic crisis is a potentially lethal complication of thyrotoxicosis. Metabolic pathways are accelerated, thermoregulation is impaired, and hyperactivity of the nervous and cardiovascular systems can lead to cardiac collapse and death. Clinical manifestations are listed in Box 22-10.

Hyperpyrexia and hydration

An elevated temperature is expected secondary to the hypermetabolic state. The production of increased body heat is evident by patient complaints of sweating and heat intolerance, and dehydration often results. Nurses should then perform a hydration assessment.

Neurologic status

Patients are anxious, nervous, and sometimes delirious in advanced thyrotoxic crisis. Restlessness and fine muscle tremors are common.

Cardiac dysrhythmias

Patients describe palpitations. These may be diagnosed as supraventricular atrial dysrhythmias or life-threatening ventricular dysrhythmias diagnosed by ECG monitoring. In advanced stages of crisis or in patients with underlying cardiac disease, acute heart failure occurs.

Laboratory studies

Clinical manifestations of thyrotoxicosis are exaggerated in thyrotoxic crisis. An important exception, however, is that the laboratory values of patients with thyrotoxic crisis will not show any sudden changes as a result of thyrotoxicosis. Serum triiodothyronine (T_3) and thyroxine (T_4) remain at their elevated thyrotoxic levels. No diagnostic test is available to differentiate thyrotoxic crisis from its predecessor, thyrotoxicosis.[10]

Medical Management

The medical management of thyrotoxicosis is of an acute, emergent nature. If left untreated, various abnormal processes occurring in the body can quickly lead to coma and death from acute heart failure. The goal of intense management of thyrotoxic crisis is to reduce thyroid hormone levels within 24 to 48 hours. During this time the life-threatening symptoms of hyperpyrexia, cardiac excitation, and nervous system dysfunction are controlled. Goals of treatment are to (1) decrease hyperthermia and (2) achieve pharmacologic control of the hypermetabolism by preventing thyroid hormone production and decreasing conversion of T_4 to the more active, potent T_3.

Hyperthermia

Pyrexia is treated with hypothermia treatment measures such as cooling blankets and acetaminophen. Aspirin is avoided because it is believed to free the thyroid hormone from its protein-bound state, thus rendering it more active. Intravenous infusion of dantrolene (used to prevent or treat malignant hyperthermia) has been used successfully in the management of pyrexia from thyrotoxic crisis.[12] Dantrolene appears to block the calcium release in select myocytes and inhibit the intense catabolism in these muscle cells. Preventing rapid breakdown of metabolites within the cells prevents the production of heat, which is believed to stimulate the critical rise in body temperature.[13] Vigorous fluid replacement is implemented to treat or prevent dehydration.

Pharmacologic management of hypermetabolism

The body's heightened sensitivity to the increased adrenergic and catecholamine receptors must be suppressed. Cardiac irregularities must be controlled and progression of acute heart failure halted. Table 22-4 lists the most commonly used medications for patients in thyrotoxic crisis. The goals of pharmacologic therapy are the following:

1. Block synthesis of thyroid hormone
2. Inhibit the conversion of T_4 to T_3
3. Inhibit release of thyroid hormone into the circulation
4. Decrease the body's sensitivity to sympathetic adrenergic receptor stimulation

DRUGS THAT BLOCK SYNTHESIS OF THYROID HORMONE. Antithyroid thioamide drugs block the synthesis of thyroid hormone. These drugs include propylthiouracil (PTU) and methimazole (Tapazole). Neither drug is

---

BOX 22-10

CLINICAL MANIFESTATIONS OF THYROTOXIC CRISIS

CARDIOVASCULAR

Prompted by increased number and affinity of beta-adrenergic receptors in the heart

Tachycardia
Systolic murmur
Increased stroke volume
Increased cardiac output
Increased systolic blood pressure
Decreased diastolic blood pressure
Extra systoles
Paroxysmal atrial tachycardia
Premature ventricular contraction
Palpitations
Chest pain
Increased cardiac contractility
Congestive heart failure
Pulmonary edema
Cardiogenic shock

CENTRAL NERVOUS SYSTEM

Resulting from an increased catecholamine response

Hyperkinesis
Nervousness
Muscle weakness
Confusion
Convulsions
Heat intolerance
Fine tremor
Emotional lability
Frank psychosis
Apathy
Stupor
Diaphoresis

GASTROINTESTINAL

Nausea
Vomiting
Diarrhea
Liver enlargement
Abdominal pain
Weight loss
Increased appetite

INTEGUMENTARY

Pruritus
Hyperpigmentation of skin
Fine, straight hair
Alopecia

THERMOREGULATORY

Hyperthermia
Heat dissipation
Diaphoresis

SERUM/URINE

Hypercalcemia
Hyperglycemia
Hypoalbuminemia
Hypoprothrombinemia
Hypocholesterolemia
Creatinuria

---

available in parenteral form and must be given by mouth or via a nasogastric tube. Methimazole has a slower action rate but is more potent than PTU. Antithyroid drugs do not block the release of previously synthesized thyroid hormone; therefore in a crisis state they are given with iodide preparations.

DRUGS THAT INHIBIT CONVERSION OF T_4 TO T_3. PTU is an especially therapeutic drug because it blocks the conversion of T_4 to the more active T_3 in addition to blocking thyroid hormone production.

DRUGS THAT INHIBIT THYROID HORMONE RELEASE. Iodides and dexamethasone, a glucocorticoid, reduce the release of thyroid hormone into circulation.

IODIDES. Rapid-acting drugs with a short duration, iodides are given 1 hour after the administration of antithyroid drugs to prevent the iodide from being used for thyroid hormone and possibly worsening the clinical state. Iodides maintain and increase the levels of protein-bound thyroid hormone, thereby decreasing the levels of free, active thyroid. The iodide most frequently used for thyrotoxic crisis is sodium iodide. Potassium iodide, saturated solution of potassium iodide, and strong iodide solution may also be used. Patients who cannot take iodides because of allergies may be given lithium carbonate, which inhibits release of the thyroid hormone.

DEXAMETHASONE. Dexamethasone is a powerful glucocorticoid that suppresses the release of thyroid hormone.[12]

DRUGS THAT DECREASE SYMPATHETIC ADRENERGIC RESPONSE. Beta blockers are used to decrease the catecholamine effects of excessive thyroid hormone. Propranolol, used in thyrotoxic crisis, has no effect on the thyroid hormone but protects the heart by reducing myocardial stimulation, decreasing myocardial contractile force, and slowing atrioventricular conduction. Doses vary among patients, but typically higher doses are required to affect the number of receptor sites active in the crisis. Esmolol, a short-acting beta blocker specifically used for short-

T A B L E   2 2 - 4
MEDICATIONS AND NURSING IMPLICATIONS FOR THYROTOXIC CRISIS

DRUG	DOSAGE/ FREQUENCY	ROUTE	ACTION	NURSING IMPLICATIONS	SIDE EFFECTS
ANTITHYROID THIOAMIDES					
Propylthiouracil	Loading dose: 800–1200 mg Maintenance: 100–400 mg q 4–6 hr	PO or gavage	Blocks synthesis of thyroid hormone Blocks conversion of T_4 to T_3	Monitor thyrotoxic response (e.g., heart rate, nervousness, fever, diarrhea, diaphoresis) Observe for sudden conversion to hypothyroidism: headache, sluggish responses Assess for skin rash Administer with meals to reduce GI effects	Rash, nausea, vomiting Agranulocytosis Skin hyperpigmentation Prothrombin deficiency
Methimazole	10–20 mg q 6–8 hr	PO or gavage	Blocks synthesis of thyroid hormone	Be aware that drug is more toxic than propylthiouracil Be aware that presence of rash may be reason to discontinue drug Monitor signs listed for propylthiouracil	Rash Agranulocytosis
IODIDES					
Sodium iodide	1 g/L q 12 hr	IV		Give iodide 1 hr after propylthiouracil or methimazole	Toxic iodinism/poisoning: edema
Potassium iodide	2–5 gtt q 8 hr	PO		Discontinue if rash appears	Mucosal hemorrhage/ stomatitis
Saturated solution of potassium iodide (SSKI)	10 gtt q 8 hr	PO	Suppresses release of thyroid hormone	Protect with covered container	Metallic taste Skin lesions
Strong iodine solution— Lugol's solution	6 gtt q 8 hr	PO		Give through a straw to prevent teeth discoloration Mix with juice or milk to lessen GI upset	Severe GI upset

Continued.

TABLE 22-4—cont'd
MEDICATIONS AND NURSING IMPLICATIONS FOR THYROTOXIC CRISIS

DRUG	DOSAGE/ FREQUENCY	ROUTE	ACTION	NURSING IMPLICATIONS	SIDE EFFECTS
GLUCOCORTICOIDS					
Dexamethasone	2 mg q 6 hr, variable	IV	Suppresses thyroid hormone release	Monitor intake and output; monitor serum glucose levels	Hypertension, nausea, vomiting, anorexia Increased susceptibility to infection
BETA BLOCKERS					
Propranolol hydrochloride	1-3 mg q 1-4 hr 40-80 mg q 4-6 hr	IV PO	Blocks beta-adrenergic response	Monitor cardiac activity CVP, PAWP Be alert for bradycardia, hypotension Hold if heart rate < 50 beats/min Have atropine available	Bradycardia Acute heart failure Edema Hypotension GI upset Fatigue Weakness
Esmolol hydrochloride	500 µg/kg/min for first minute, then 50 µg/kg/min for 4 min	IV	Blocks beta-adrenergic response	Monitor for bradycardia, orthostatic hypotension, dysrhythmia Measure and record intake and output	Edema Hypotension Diarrhea Dizziness Diaphoresis
ADRENERGIC NEURONAL BLOCKERS					
Reserpine	1.0-2.5 mg q 24 hr	PO	Depletes storage of catecholamine in sympathetic nerve endings	Monitor BP, heart rate changes in hyperthyroid conditions	Bradycardia Drowsiness GI bleeding Diarrhea
Guanethidine sulfate	50-150 mg q 24 hr	PO	Inhibits norepinephrine release in response to sympathetic nerve stimulation	Monitor BP for orthostatic hypotension Measure and record intake and output Monitor diarrhea	Drowsiness Edema Fatigue Orthostatic hypotension GI upset

term, rapid control of atrial fibrillation, can also be used. Clinicians are hesitant to use beta blockers for patients with overt heart failure because of the risk of worsening cardiac function. Calcium channel blockers such as verapamil are effective in controlling heart rate in patients for whom beta blockers are contraindicated. Alternative antihypertensive drugs include reserpine and guanethidine. These drugs, used infrequently because of the numerous side effects, deplete or inhibit norepinephrine release at the adrenergic nerve endings.

INCREASED DOSAGES. Medication doses are increased to achieve the desired effect and compensate for the rapid metabolism and clearance of chemicals from the body during thyrotoxic crisis. Digitalis and diuretics may be required to treat symptoms of acute heart failure, with dosages increased if necessary to achieve the desired effect.

Nursing Management

Patients with a hyperactive thyroid complain of increased body temperature, anxiety, restlessness, tremulousness, increased appetite, palpitations, sweating, and intolerance to heat. Also present are dysrhythmias and tachypnea. Patients who are hospitalized for a major illness with either undiagnosed or previously controlled thyrotoxicosis are at greatest risk for thyrotoxic crisis, which may be precipitated by the stress of a critical illness. Nursing management of patients in thyroid crisis incorporates a variety of nursing diagnoses (Box 22-11). **Nursing priorities are directed toward controlling hyperthermia, monitoring laboratory values, preventing dehydration, preventing fluid volume overload, evaluating cardiovascular dysfunction, assessing neurologic status, preventing sleep deprivation, maintaining oxygenation, and educating patients and families.**

Controlling hyperthermia

In thyrotoxic crisis, patients have hyperthermia related to a hypermetabolic state as evidenced by critically high body temperature—often above 106° F—diaphoresis; hot, flushed skin; intolerance to heat; tachycardia; and tachypnea. Temperature is assessed every 15 minutes and frequency gradually tapered after the temperature reaches a safe level and stabilizes. Core temperature is identified most accurately with an invasive pulmonary artery catheter. If a catheter is not used to monitor temperature, the second choice is a tympanic membrane core temperature sensor. The tympanic sensor provides a more accurate reading of body temperature than other noninvasive methods, including the rectal thermometer probe attached to a hypothermia cooling blanket. The accuracy of the tympanic sensor is determined by the fact that the eardrum (against which the sensor is held) shares the same blood supply and is near the hypothalamus, the body's "thermostat." A reading is available in less than 3 seconds. Measures to provide comfort while patients are intolerant to heat include maintaining a cool room temperature and air circulation and providing lightweight bed coverings and comfortable, nonrestrictive bed clothes. A tepid sponge bath helps reduce heat by evaporation, and ice application to the groin and axilla increases heat loss at major blood vessels through conduction.

Monitoring laboratory values

No diagnostic tests specific to thyrotoxic crisis are currently available. Standard laboratory tests are inconclusive. The results of thyroid function tests such as those that measure T_4 and T_3 show elevated levels caused by thyrotoxicosis but do not reflect the gross increases expected with the extreme hypermetabolic state seen in a crisis condition.[12]

Preventing dehydration

Hyperthermia, tachypnea, diaphoresis, vomiting, and diarrhea all predispose patients to a fluid volume deficit. Fluids and electrolytes are as vigorously replaced as the decompensated cardiovascular system can manage. The CVP, PAP, and hourly urine output are closely monitored. Hyponatremia from active fluid loss is prevented or treated with appropriate sodium concentrations of intravenous fluids. Glucose solutions are given to replace depleted glycogen stores.

Preventing fluid volume overload

A serious complication of rehydration, circulatory overload is signaled by increased CVP, increased PAWP, moist lung sounds, neck vein engorgement, and dyspnea without exertion. Reduction in fluid volume infusion, elevation of the head of the bed, and administration of diuretics and oxygen may be necessary to support breathing and alleviate increased fluid load. Intake and output measurements include estimating diaphoretic fluid loss through the number of gown and linen changes, check-

---

BOX 22-11

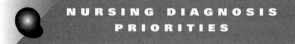

NURSING DIAGNOSIS PRIORITIES

THYROTOXIC CRISIS

- *Altered Nutrition: Less Than Body Protein-Calorie Requirements* related to lack of exogenous nutrients and increased metabolic demand, p. 506
- *Decreased Cardiac Output* related to ventricular tachycardia, p. 477
- *Fluid Volume Deficit* related to hypermetabolism, p. 504
- *Knowledge Deficit: Self-Care of Hyperthyroidism* related to lack of previous exposure to information, p. 455

ing buccal membranes for moisture, and recording daily weights.

Evaluating cardiovascular dysfunction

Changes in cardiac functioning relate to high metabolic activity and adrenergic response. The resulting tachydysrhythmia and heart failure, coupled with the hyperthermia, eventually cause death. Cardiovascular assessment includes heart rate, rhythm irregularities, blood pressure changes, pulse pressure variances, decrease in quality of peripheral pulses, and patient reports of chest pain and palpitations. Hemodynamic monitoring includes arterial blood pressure, CVP, PAWP, and cardiac output readings. High-output cardiac failure may occur as the demands of the hypermetabolic activity within the body far exceed the ability of the myocardium to pump oxygenated blood. Heart failure ensues as the catecholamine-driven receptors produce abnormal conduction patterns and weakening, rapid contractions. The rapid heart rate allows little time for the coronary arteries to fill and supply oxygen to the cardiac tissue.

Assessing neurologic status

Because patients in thyrotoxic crisis are agitated, anxious, and unable to rest, they require intensive care that is quiet, calm, and restful. Gradually the antithyroid medications and beta-adrenergic blocking drugs decrease neurologic symptoms related to the catecholamine sensitivity. Medications given for sedation include phenobarbital, which will also reduce T_4 levels in the bloodstream.[12] Patients are reassured that this extreme agitation is the result of the disease process and that the medications will help control the nonstop fidgeting and tremors. Frequent reassurance and clear, simple explanations help decrease fear brought on by the strange surroundings.

Preventing sleep deprivation

Providing adequate rest and sleep for patients experiencing intense neuroexcitation is a challenge for critical care nurses. All members of the health care team are encouraged to respect the need of these patients for uninterrupted blocks of rest time.

Maintaining oxygenation

Excess thyroid hormone increases cellular oxygen consumption in almost all metabolically active cells. Supplemental oxygen is provided to maintain an SaO_2 level above 92% to reduce patients' work of breathing. Oxygen titration is based on pulse oximeter readings or arterial blood gas values obtained to determine the presence of metabolic acidosis.

Educating patients and families

The reasons for the hypermetabolism, anxiety, and cardiac dysrhythmias are explained to patients and families. Before being discharged from the hospital, patients should receive information on their medications and symptoms that must be reported to their physicians.

References

1. Sikes PJ: Endocrine responses to the stress of critical illness, *AACN Clin Issues Crit Care* 3(2):379-390, 1992.
2. Siconolfi LA: The forgotten system: endocrine dysfunction during multiple system organ dysfunction, *Crit Care Nurs Q* 16(4):16-26, 1994.
3. Suave DO, Kessler CA: Hyperglycemic emergencies, *AACN Clin Issues Crit Care* 3(2):350-360, 1992.
4. Rifkin H, Porte D, editors: *Ellenberg and Rifkin's diabetes mellitus: theory and practice*, ed 4, New York, 1990, Elsevier.
5. Kelley W: *Textbook of internal medicine*, vol 2, ed 2, Philadelphia, 1992, JB Lippincott.
6. Wilson JD and others: *Harrison's principles of internal medicine*, ed 12, New York, 1991, McGraw-Hill.
7. American Diabetes Association: Clinical practice recommendations, Hospital Admission guidelines for diabetes mellitus, *Diabetes Care* 18(S1):35, 1995.
8. Batcheller J: Disorders of antidiuretic hormone secretion, *AACN Clin Issues Crit Care* 3(2):370-378, 1992.
9. Coroll A: *Primary care medicine*, ed 3, 1995, JB Lippincott.
10. Becker K: *Principles and practices of endocrinology and metabolism*, Philadelphia, 1992, JB Lippincott.
11. Sox HC: *Common diagnostic tests: use and interpretation*, ed 2, Philadelphia, 1990, American College of Physicians.
12. West JB: *Best and Taylor's physiological basis of medical practice*, ed 12, Baltimore, 1991, Williams & Wilkins.
13. Isley WL: Thyroid disorders, *Crit Care Nurs Q* 13(3):39, 1990.

Multisystem Alterations

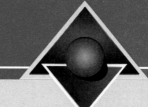

23

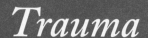

Trauma

KAREN JOHNSON

Over the past few decades major advances have been made in the management of patients with traumatic injuries, and significant improvements have been made in their care in both prehospital and emergency department settings. These improvements have affected the critical care setting in that patients with complex, multisystem trauma are admitted to critical care units. These patients require complex nursing care. This chapter reviews nursing management of patients with traumatic injuries, particularly in the critical care setting.

Mechanisms of Injury

Trauma occurs when an external force of energy strikes the body and causes structural or physiologic alterations, or "injuries." External forces can be radiation, electrical, thermal, chemical, or mechanical forms of energy. This chapter focuses on trauma from mechanical energy. Mechanical energy can produce either blunt or penetrating traumatic injuries. Knowledge of the mechanism of injury helps health care providers anticipate and predict potential internal injuries.

Blunt Trauma

Blunt trauma is usually seen with motor vehicle accidents (MVAs), contact sports, crush injuries, or falls. Injuries occur because of the forces sustained during a rapid change in velocity (deceleration). To estimate the amount of force a person would sustain in an MVA, nurses may multiply the person's weight by miles per hour of speed.[1] A 130-pound woman traveling at 60 miles per hour who hits a brick wall, for example, would sustain 7800 pounds of force within milliseconds. As the body stops suddenly, tissues and organs continue to move forward. This sudden change in velocity causes injuries that result in lacerations or crush injuries of internal body structures.

Penetrating Trauma

Penetrating injuries occur with stabbings, use of firearms, or impalement of foreign objects, which penetrate the skin and result in damage to internal structures along the path of penetration. Penetrating injuries can be misleading because the outside of the wound does not determine the extent of internal injury. High-velocity bullets can create internal cavities up to 10 times the diameter of the bullet.[2]

Several factors determine the extent of damage sustained as a result of penetrating trauma. Different weapons cause different types of injuries. The severity of a gunshot wound depends on the type of gun, type of ammunition used, and distance and angle from which the gun was fired. Pellets from a shotgun blast expand on impact and cause multiple injuries to internal structures. Handgun bullets, on the other hand, usually damage what is directly in the bullet's path. Once inside the body, the bullet can ricochet off bone and create further damage along its pathway. With penetrating stab wounds, factors that determine the extent of injury include type and length of object used as well as the angle of insertion.

Phases of Trauma Care

Prehospital Resuscitation

The goal of prehospital care is immediate stabilization and transportation. Stabilization is accomplished through assessments and interventions related to airway, breathing, and circulation (ABCs). Once stabilized at the scene, patients are transported to an appropriate medical facility by ground or air transport.

Emergency Department Resuscitation

Primary survey

After trauma patients are brought to the emergency department, the primary survey is initiated. During this assessment, life-threatening injuries are discovered and treated. The five steps in the primary survey comprise the ABCs, plus D (disability: minineurologic examination) and E (exposure: removal of clothes) (Table 23-1). **The cervical spine must be immobilized in all trauma patients until a cervical spinal cord injury has been definitively ruled out.** If the airway is obstructed, foreign bodies are removed. In the presence of ineffective airway clearance, ventilation is used for patients with a loss of consciousness, ineffective breathing patterns, or both. Cardiac monitoring is initiated to assess for rhythm disturbances. Life-threatening dysrhythmias are treated according to ACLS protocols. Military antishock trousers or a pneumatic antishock garment may be used to raise the systolic blood pressure. Both devices encompass the lower extremities and abdomen. When inflated, these garments increase systolic blood pressure by increasing peripheral vascular resistance and myocardial afterload. Use of these garments, however, is controversial.

Resuscitation phase

After the primary survey the resuscitation phase begins. Hypovolemic shock is the most common type of shock that occurs in trauma patients.[3] Hemorrhage must be identified and treated rapidly. Vigorous intravenous (IV) fluid replacement is initiated. Large-bore peripheral IV catheters (14 to 16 gauge) or a central venous catheter should be inserted. Restoration of volume is accomplished through administration of crystalloid (lactated Ringer's solution or 0.9% saline solution), colloid (plasma or albumin), and blood products. During the initiation of IV lines, blood samples for laboratory analysis should be drawn. High-flow fluid warmers may be used to deliver warmed IV solutions at rates up to 1000 ml/min. Transfusion of autologous salvaged blood (autotransfusion) may also be used to replace intravascular volume and provide oxygen-carrying capacity.

Gastric and urinary catheters are placed, unless contraindicated. Adequate resuscitation is assessed by monitoring for improvement in vital signs, arterial blood gas levels, and urinary output.

Secondary survey

After resuscitative measures, a rapid but thorough head-to-toe assessment of all systems is made.[4] The history is one of the most important aspects of the secondary survey. Specific information that should be elicited pertaining to the mechanism of injury is summarized in Box 23-1. This information can help predict internal injuries

TABLE 23-1
PRIMARY SURVEY OF THE TRAUMA PATIENT

SURVEY COMPONENT	NURSING DIAGNOSIS	NURSING ASSESSMENT/CARE
Airway	Airway clearance: Ineffective related to obstruction or actual injury	Look, listen, and feel Immobilize C-spine Position victim/patient: Supine Sitting Log roll Clear airway: Jaw thrust Chin lift Finger sweep Suctioning Use airway devices: Oropharyngeal Nasopharyngeal Endotracheal tube Cricothyrotomy
Breathing	Breathing pattern: Ineffective related to actual injury Gas exchange: Impaired related to actual injury or disrupted tissue perfusion	Assess for: Spontaneous breathing Respiratory rate, depth, and symmetry Chest wall integrity Administer high-flow oxygen Correct absent breathing: Intubate Positive-pressure ventilation Correct ineffective breathing: Assess and treat life-threatening conditions (e.g., tension pneumothorax, flail chest)
Circulation	Cardiac output, alteration in: Decreased related to actual injury Tissue perfusion, alteration in: Related to actual injury or shock Fluid volume deficit: Related to actual loss of circulating volume	Assess pulse: Quality Rate Treat absent pulse: Initiate BCLS Initiate ACLS Treat ineffective pulse: Assess and treat life-threatening conditions (e.g., uncontrolled bleeding, shock) Two large-bore (14- or 16-gauge) IVs Fluid replacement ECG monitoring
Disability	Injury, risk for: Trauma to spinal cord and brain related to actual injury	Perform brief neurologic examination Eye opening Verbal response Motor response Pupils Use Glasgow coma scale
Exposure	N/A	Remove all clothing to visualize entire body for inspection

Modified from Beaver BM: *Nurs Clin North Am* 25(1):13, 1990.

BOX 23-1

HISTORY OF MECHANISM OF INJURY

PENETRATING TRAUMA

Weapon used (handgun, shotgun, rifle, knife)
Caliber of weapon
Number of shots fired
Gender of assailant
Position of victim and assailant when injury occurred

BLUNT TRAUMA

Length of fall
MVA extrication time
Ejection
Location in automobile (passenger, driver; front seat, back seat)
Restraint status (lapbelt, shoulder harness, or combination; unrestrained)
Speed of automobile(s)
Occupants (number and morbidity status)

BOX 23-2

FACTORS THAT CONTRIBUTE TO TISSUE HYPOXIA IN TRAUMA PATIENTS

- Shifts to the left of the oxyhemoglobin dissociation curve (can be secondary to infusion of large volumes of banked blood, hypocarbia or alkalosis, or hypothermia)
- Reduced hemoglobin (secondary to hemorrhage)
- Reduced cardiac output (in the presence of cardiovascular insults)
- Impaired cellular oxygen consumption (associated with metabolic alterations of sepsis)
- Increased metabolic demands (associated with the stress response to injury)

and facilitate rapid intervention. **During the secondary survey, nurses ensure the completion of an electrocardiogram and radiographic studies (chest, cervical spine, thorax, and pelvis). Throughout this survey, nurses continuously monitor patients' vital signs and responses to medical therapies. Providing emotional support to patients and families is also imperative.**[5,6]

Definitive Care/Operative Phase

Once the secondary survey has been completed, specific injuries have usually been diagnosed. Definitive care related to specific injuries is described throughout this chapter. Trauma, often referred to as a *surgical disease* because of the nature and extent of the injuries, often requires operative management of injuries. After surgery, depending on patients' status, a transfer to the critical care unit may be indicated.

Critical Care Phase

Critically ill trauma patients are admitted into the critical care unit as a direct transfer from the emergency department or operating room. If surgery is required, trauma patients should be directly admitted to the critical care unit from the operating room.[7,8] **Priority nursing care during the critical care phase includes ongoing physical assessments and monitoring the patient's response to medical therapies. One of the most important nursing roles is assessment of the balance between oxygen delivery and oxygen demand. Oxygen delivery must be optimized to prevent further system**

damage.[9] **Assessment of circulatory status includes the use of noninvasive and invasive techniques.**

Tissue hypoxemia, which is a threat to trauma patients, results from a variety of factors. Box 23-2 lists these factors, as summarized by Von Reuden.[10] Prevention and treatment of hypoxemia depend on accurate assessment of the adequacy of pulmonary gas exchange, oxygen transport, and cellular oxygen use. Nursing interventions must promote adequate tissue oxygenation.

Head Injuries

At least 2 million persons incur head injuries each year in the United States, and more than 400,000 patients with head injuries are admitted to hospitals, approximately half of whom were involved in MVAs.[11] Head injuries account for 25% of all trauma deaths and 50% to 60% of all deaths as a result of motor vehicle trauma.[11]

Mechanism of Injury

Head injuries occur when mechanical forces are transmitted to brain tissue. Mechanisms of injury include penetrating and blunt trauma to the head. Penetrating trauma can result from the penetration of a foreign object (e.g., bullet) that causes direct damage to cerebral tissue.[12] Blunt trauma can be the result of deceleration, acceleration, or rotational forces. Deceleration causes the brain to crash against the skull after it has hit something (e.g., the dashboard of a car). Acceleration injuries occur when the brain has been hit by something (e.g., a baseball bat). In many instances, head injury can be caused by both acceleration and deceleration. Acceleration injuries occur when the skull is hit by a force that causes the brain to move forward to the point of impact, and then as the brain reverses direction and hits the other side of the skull, deceleration injuries occur.

Pathophysiology

The pathophysiology of head injury can be divided into two categories: primary injury (that which occurs on impact) and secondary injury (that which occurs secondarily in response to the original trauma).

Primary injury

The primary injury occurs at the time of impact as a result of the dynamic forces of acceleration/deceleration or rotation. Primary injuries include contusion, laceration, shearing injuries, and hemorrhage. Primary injury may be mild, with little or no neurologic damage, or severe, with major tissue damage.

Secondary injury

Secondary injury can be caused by further physiologic events that occur after the primary injury. Secondary injury can be caused by hypoxia, hypercapnia, hypotension, cerebral edema, and sustained hypertension. Beyond causing injury to tissue, each of these factors also contributes to significant increases in intracranial pressure (ICP).

Classification

Injuries of the brain are described by the functional changes or losses that occur. Some of the major functional abnormalities seen in head injury are described here.

Skull fractures

Skull fractures are common, but they do not by themselves cause neurologic deficits. Skull fractures can be classified as open (dura is torn) or closed (dura is not torn), or they can be classified as those of the vault or those of the base. Common vault fractures occur in the parietal and temporal regions. Basilar skull fractures are not usually visible on conventional skull films. Assessment findings may include cerebral spinal fluid (CSF), otorrhea or rhinorrhea, Battle's sign (ecchymosis overlying the mastoid process), or "raccoon eyes" (subconjunctival and periorbital ecchymosis).

All patients with skull fractures are hospitalized for observation.[3] Open skull fractures require surgical intervention to remove bony fragments and close the dura. The major complications of basilar skull fractures are cranial nerve injury and leakage of CSF. CSF leakage may result in a fistula, which increases the possibility of bacterial contamination and resultant meningitis. Because fistula formation may be delayed, patients with a basilar skull fracture are admitted to the hospital for observation and possible surgical intervention.

Concussion

A concussion is a brain injury accompanied by a brief loss of neurologic function, especially loss of consciousness.[3] Loss of consciousness may last for seconds to an hour. The neurologic dysfunctions present as confusion, disorientation, and sometimes a period of posttraumatic amnesia. Other clinical manifestations that occur after concussion are headache, dizziness, irritability, inability to concentrate, impaired memory, and fatigue. The work-up for concussion is probably responsible for more emergency department visits, x-ray films, and admissions to the hospital than any other type of brain injury. The diagnosis of concussion is based on the loss of consciousness inasmuch as the brain remains structurally intact despite functional impairment. Patients with a history of 5 or more minutes of loss of consciousness are usually admitted to the hospital for a 24-hour observation period.[3]

Contusion

Contusion, or bruising of the brain, is usually related to acceleration/deceleration injuries, which result in hemorrhage into the superficial parenchyma, often the frontal and temporal lobes. Frontal or temporal contusions can be seen in a coup-contrecoup mechanism of injury (Fig. 23-1). Coup injury affects the cerebral tissue directly under the point of impact. Contrecoup injury occurs in a line directly opposite the point of impact.

The clinical manifestations of contusion are related to the location of the contusion, degree of contusion, and presence of associated lesions. Contusions can be small, in which localized areas of dysfunction result in a focal neurologic deficit. Larger contusions can evolve over 2 to 3 days after injury as a result of edema and further hemorrhaging. A large contusion can produce a mass effect that can cause a significant increase in ICP.

Diagnosis of contusion is made by computed tomography (CT) scan. If the CT scan indicates contusion, especially in the temporal area, nurses must pay particular attention to neurologic assessments and look for subtle changes in pupillary signs or vital signs, irrespective of a stable ICP.

Medical management of cerebral contusions may consist of medical or surgical therapies. Because a contusion can progress over 3 to 5 days after injury, secondary injury may occur. If contusions are small, focal, or multiple, they are treated medically with serial neurologic assessments and possibly ICP monitoring. Increased ICP is usually managed medically as described in Chapter 16. Larger contusions that produce considerable mass effect require surgical intervention to prevent the increased edema and ICP as the contusion matures.[3] Outcome of cerebral contusion varies, depending on the location and degree of contusion. These injuries are often complicated by posttraumatic epilepsy.[13]

Hematomas

Hematomas resulting from head injury form a mass lesion and lead to increased ICP. Three types of hematomas are discussed here (Fig. 23-2).

EPIDURAL HEMATOMA. **Epidural hematoma (EDH),** which is a collection of blood between the inner table of the skull and the outermost layer of the dura, is usually associated with skull fractures and middle meningeal ar-

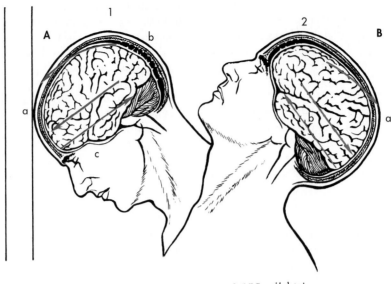

G.J. Wassilchenko

FIG. 23-1 Coup and contrecoup head injury after blunt trauma. **A,** Coup injury: impact against object. *a,* Site of impact and direct trauma to brain; *b,* shearing of subdural veins; *c,* Trauma to base of brain. **B,** Contrecoup injury: impact within skull. *a,* Site of impact from brain hitting opposite side of skull; *b,* Shearing forces throughout brain. These injuries occur in one continuous motion—the head strikes the wall (coup) and then rebounds (contrecoup).

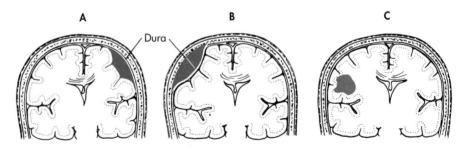

FIG. 23-2 Types of cerebral hematomas. **A,** Epidural hematoma. **B,** Subdural hematoma. **C,** Intracerebral hematoma.

tery laceration. A blow to the head that causes a linear skull fracture on the lateral surface of the head may tear the middle meningeal artery. As the artery bleeds, it pulls the dura away from the skull, creating a pouch that expands into the intracranial space.

The incidence of EDH is relatively low. This type of injury accounts for 1% to 3% of all head trauma but makes up at least 8% of severely injured patients.[13] EDH can occur as a result of low-impact injuries (such as falls) or high-impact injuries (such as MVAs). EDH occurs from trauma to the skull and meninges rather than the acceleration/deceleration forces seen in other head trauma.

The classic clinical manifestations of EDH include brief loss of consciousness followed by a period of lucidity that may last up to 12 hours. This lucid period is followed by a progressive deterioration in level of consciousness, dilation of the pupil on the same side of the hema-

toma (ipsilateral), and onset of abnormal flexion (decorticate) or abnormal extension (decerebrate). Diagnosis of EDH is based on clinical symptoms and evidence of a collection of epidural blood identified on CT scan. Treatment of EDH involves surgical intervention to remove the blood and cauterize the bleeding vessels. With early surgical intervention the prognosis is excellent.[3] Outcome varies from excellent, with no neurologic sequelae, to a persistent vegetative state or death. Outcome can depend on the timing of surgical intervention.

SUBDURAL HEMATOMA. Subdural hematoma (SDH), which is the accumulation of blood between the dura and underlying arachnoid membrane, is most often related to a rupture in the bridging veins between the brain and dura. Acceleration/deceleration and rotational forces are the major causes of SDH, which is often associated with cerebral contusions and intracerebral hemorrhage.

TABLE 23-2
CLASSIFICATION OF SUBDURAL HEMATOMAS (SDH)

TIME INTERVAL	SYMPTOMS
ACUTE Within 48 hr	Headache, drowsiness, agitation, confusion, deterioration in LOC, fixed and ipsilateral pupil dilation, contralateral hemiparesis *or* Profound coma
SUBACUTE 2 days to 2 wk	Similar to acute SDH except that symptoms appear more slowly
CHRONIC 2 wk to months	Progressive lethargy, absent-mindedness, headache, vomiting, seizures, ipsilateral pupil dilation, or contralateral hemiparesis

LOC, Level of consciousness.

The three types of SDH are based on the time frame from injury to clinical symptoms: acute, subacute, and chronic. Table 23-2 summarizes the time interval and presentation for each type of SDH.[14] Surgical intervention may require craniectomy, craniotomy, or burr hole evacuation. SDH has a mortality rate of 22%, which rises to 50% with injuries to other body systems.[14]

INTRACEREBRAL HEMATOMA. **Intracerebral hematoma (ICH)** results from bleeding within cerebral tissue. Traumatic causes of ICH include depressed skull fractures, penetrating injuries (bullet, knife), and sudden acceleration/deceleration motion. The ICH acts as a rapidly expanding lesion, and the mortality rate is high[14]; however, late ICH into the necrotic center of a contused area is also possible. Sudden clinical deterioration of patients 6 to 10 days after trauma may be the result of ICH.

Medical management of ICH may include surgical or nonsurgical management. Generally it is believed that hemorrhages not causing significant ICP problems should be treated nonsurgically. Over time the hemorrhage may be reabsorbed. If significant problems with ICP occur as a result of the ICH producing a mass effect, surgical removal is necessary. Outcome from ICH depends greatly on the location of the hemorrhage. Size, mass effect, and displacement of other intracranial structures also affect the outcome. ICH has a mortality rate between 25% and 72%.[15]

Missile injuries

Missile injuries are caused by objects that penetrate the skull to produce a significant focal damage but little acceleration/deceleration or rotational injury. The injury may be depressed, penetrating, or perforating (Fig. 23-3). Depressed injuries are caused by fractures of the skull with penetration of bone into cerebral tissue. Penetrating injury is caused by a missile that enters the cranial cavity but does not exit. A low-velocity penetrating injury (knife) may involve only focal damage and no loss of consciousness. A high-velocity missile (bullet) can produce shock waves that are transmitted throughout the brain in addition to injury caused by the bullet. Perforating injuries are missile injuries that enter and then exit the brain. Perforating injuries have much less ricochet effect but are still responsible for significant injury.

Diffuse axonal injury

Diffuse axonal injury (DAI) covers a wide range of brain dysfunction caused by acceleration/deceleration and rotational forces. This diagnosis is usually reserved for severe dysfunction. Cerebral concussion is the least severe form of diffuse axonal injury. *DAI* describes prolonged coma from the time of injury that does not result from mass lesions or ischemia.

The pathophysiology of DAI is related to the stretching and tearing of axons as a result of movement of the brain inside the cranium at the time of impact. The stretching and tearing of axons result in microscopic lesions throughout the brain but especially deep within cerebral tissue and the base of the cerebrum. Disruption of axonal transmission of impulses results in loss of consciousness. Unless surrounding tissue areas are significantly injured, causing small hemorrhages, DAI is not visible on CT scan. Patients remain in a deep coma, often with decerebrate or decorticate posturing and autonomic dysfunction, including hyperthermia, hypertension, and diaphoresis.

Treatment of DAI includes support of vital functions and maintenance of ICP within normal limits. The outcome after severe DAI is poor because of the extensive dysfunction of cerebral pathways. DAI occurs in 44% of all coma-producing head injuries, with an overall mortality rate of 33%. However, in its most severe form, the mortality rate can be 50%.[3]

Assessment

Rapid assessment and triage of patients with head injury are critical to a favorable prognosis.[16] Head injuries are divided into three descriptive categories on the basis of patients' Glasgow Coma Scale (GCS) and length of the unconscious state. This classification is useful during initial assessment.

Degree of injury

MILD INJURY. Mild head injury is associated with a GCS score of 13 to 15 and loss of consciousness that

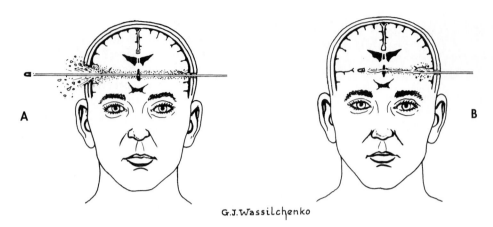

G.J.Wassilchenko

FIG. 23-3 Bullet wounds of the head. A bullet wound or other penetrating missile will cause an open (compound) skull fracture and damage to brain tissue. Shock wave effects are transmitted throughout the brain. **A,** Perforating injury. **B,** Penetrating injury.

lasts up to 15 minutes. Patients with mild injury are often seen in the emergency department and discharged home with family members who are instructed to evaluate patients routinely and bring them back to the hospital if any further neurologic symptoms appear.

MODERATE INJURY. Moderate head injury is associated with a GCS score of 9 to 12 and a loss of consciousness for up to 6 hours. Patients with this type of head injury are usually hospitalized. Because these patients are at risk for deterioration from increasing cerebral edema and ICP, serial clinical assessments are an important function of nurses. Hemodynamic and ICP monitoring and ventilatory support are often not required in this group unless other systemic injuries make them necessary. A CT scan is usually performed on admission. Repeat CT scans are indicated if patients' neurologic status deteriorates.

SEVERE INJURY. Severe head injury is associated with a GCS score of 3 to 8 and loss of consciousness for longer than 6 hours. Patients with severe head injury often receive ventilatory support along with ICP and hemodynamic monitoring. A CT scan is performed to rule out any mass lesions that can be surgically removed. Patients are placed in a critical care setting for continual assessment, monitoring, and management.

Diagnostic procedures

The advent of CT scanning has greatly improved the diagnosis and management of patients with head trauma. The CT scan is a rapid, noninvasive procedure that can provide invaluable information about the presence of mass lesions and cerebral edema. Electrophysiology studies can aid in ongoing assessments of neurologic function. Evoked potentials and electroencephalograph (EEG) are becoming widely used in the diagnosis of head injuries. (These studies are discussed in detail in Chapter 14.)

Medical Management

Surgical management

If a lesion identified by CT scan is causing a shift of intracranial contents or increasing ICP, surgical intervention is necessary. A craniotomy is performed to remove the EDH, SDH, or large ICH. Occasionally, if an area of contusion is large, hemorrhagic, and associated with an elevated ICP, a craniotomy for removal of the contused area may be performed to relieve pressure and prevent herniation.

Nonsurgical management

Nonsurgical management includes management of ICP, maintenance of vital sign parameters, and treatment of any complications such as pneumonia and infection. Medical management can include drainage of CSF through a ventricular catheter, use of diuretics, and administration of high-dose barbiturate therapy.[17,18] (For review of these treatments for increased ICP and complications, see Chapter 16.)

Nursing Management

Priority nursing goals include stabilization of vital signs, prevention of further injury, and reduction of increased ICP.[19] Ongoing nursing assessments are the cornerstone of care for patients with head injuries. Such assessments are the primary mechanism for determining secondary brain injury from cerebral edema and increased ICP. In addition to astute neurologic assessments, monitoring ventilatory support, fluid and electrolyte balance, and nutrition is critical. (For a more extensive discussion of nursing management of intracranial pressure, see Chapter 16.)

Spinal Cord Injuries

Spinal cord injury (SCI) occurs mostly in males. Most victims are between the ages of 15 and 30 years and sustain SCI as a result of vehicular accidents, assaults, falls, and sports-related injuries.[20]

Mechanism of Injury

The type of injury sustained depends on the mechanism of injury. Mechanisms of injury can include hyperflexion, hyperextension, rotation, axial loading (vertical compression), and missile or penetrating injuries.

Hyperflexion

Hyperflexion injury is usually seen in the cervical area, especially at the level of C5 to C6 because this is the most mobile portion of the cervical spine. This type of injury is caused most frequently by sudden deceleration motion, as in head-on collisions. Injury occurs from compression of the cord as a result of fracture fragments or dislocation of the vertebral bodies. Instability of the spinal column occurs because of the rupture or tearing of the posterior muscles and ligaments.

Hyperextension

Hyperextension injuries involve backward and downward motion of the head. With this injury, often seen in rear-end collisions and diving accidents, the spinal cord itself is stretched and distorted. Neurologic deficits associated with this injury are often caused by contusion and ischemia of the cord without significant bony involvement. A mild form of hyperextension is the whiplash injury.

Rotation

Rotation injuries often occur in conjunction with a flexion or extension injury. Severe rotation of the neck or body results in tearing of the posterior ligaments and displacement (rotation) of the spinal column.

Axial loading

Axial loading, or vertical compression injuries, occur from vertical force along the spinal cord. This is most commonly seen when people land on their feet or buttocks after falling from a height. Compression injuries cause burst fractures of the vertebral body that often send bony fragments into the spinal canal or directly into the spinal cord.

Penetrating injuries

Penetrating injury to the spinal cord can be caused by a bullet, knife, or any other object that penetrates the cord. These types of injury cause permanent damage by anatomically transecting the spinal cord.

Pathophysiology

SCIs are the result of a mechanical force that disrupts neurologic tissue, its vascular supply, or both. Much like head injuries, a primary injury causes a chain of secondary events in response to the injury. Spinal cord damage appears to be the result of these secondary events, which include hemorrhage, vascular damage, structural changes, and subsequent biochemical alterations.[21]

Vascular damage and hemorrhage occur as perfusion to the damaged area drops significantly. Decreased perfusion results in decreased oxygenation, ischemia, and necrosis of the spinal cord. The spinal cord becomes edematous, causing small hemorrhagic areas in the gray and white matter. Structural changes of the white and gray matter cause an opening of the tight vascular endothelial junction. This leads to an electrophysiologic alteration in neuronal conduction. Biochemical reactions to trauma result in vasoconstriction and a partial derangement in metabolism, with the release of vasoactive mediators (norepinephrine, serotonin, and histamines). These mediators generate free radicals that disrupt neuronal membranes and lead to ischemic hypoxia and rapid tissue destruction.[22] Because of the damage produced by these secondary events, neuronal conduction can no longer occur. Current medical and nursing management of patients with SCIs is directed toward arresting or reversing these secondary events.

Functional injury of the spinal cord

Functional injury of the spinal cord refers to the degree of disruption of normal spinal cord function. SCIs are first classified as complete or incomplete.

COMPLETE INJURY. Complete SCI results in a total loss of sensory and motor function below the level of injury. Regardless of the mechanism of injury, the result is a complete dissection of the spinal cord and its neurochemical pathways, resulting in one of two conditions: quadriplegia or paraplegia.

QUADRIPLEGIA. Injuries in the cervical spine region result in quadriplegia. Residual muscle function depends on the specific cervical segments involved. Cervical injuries that occur above C6 result in complete quadriplegia, whereas injuries below C6 produce incomplete quadriplegia with some potential for independence in activities of daily living.[20]

PARAPLEGIA. A complete injury in the thoracolumbar region results in paraplegia. Thoracic L1 and L2 injuries produce paraplegia with variable innervation to intercostal and abdominal muscles.

INCOMPLETE INJURY. Incomplete SCI results in a mixed loss of voluntary motor activity and sensation below the level of the lesion. Incomplete SCI exists if any function remains below the level of injury. Incomplete injuries can result in one of a variety of syndromes, which are classified according to the degree of motor and sensory loss below the level of injury.

SPINAL SHOCK. **Spinal shock** is a condition that occurs immediately after traumatic injury to the spinal cord. Spinal shock is the complete loss of all normal reflex activity below the level of injury, including loss of motor, sensory, reflex, and autonomic functions.[21] Flaccid paralysis below the level of injury occurs in addition to bowel and bladder retention. The duration of this shock state can last several weeks after injury. The intensity of this shock is influenced by the level of injury. Spinal shock ends when spastic paralysis replaces flaccid paralysis.

NEUROGENIC SHOCK. **Neurogenic shock** is a second shock state that can occur after an SCI above the T6 level. Injuries above this level disrupt sympathetic nervous system fibers. The parasympathetic pathway becomes predominant in spinal shock. Predominant parasympathetic innervation results in vasodilation and decreased heart rate. Vasodilation results in decreased blood pressure as a result of decreased venous return. All these events produce the classic signs of neurogenic shock: hypotension, hypothermia, and bradycardia.

Assessment

Assessment of patients with a known or suspected SCI must include stabilization of the spinal cord. *All* trauma patients should be protected from further spinal cord damage until presence of spinal cord injury is ruled out. The cervical spinal column must remain stabilized through the use of a cervical collar, backboard, or tape to prevent motion of the spine. Moving patients, especially turning them, requires the use of the log-roll technique. One person maintains the patient's head and neck alignment while others assist with turning. Patients are turned in straight alignment.

Assessment of breathing patterns and gas exchange is made after an airway has been secured. The level of injury dictates the degree of altered breathing patterns and gas exchange. Because complete injuries above the C3 level result in paralysis of the diaphragm,[23] these patients require ventilatory assistance. Kocan[23] described the effects of SCI on the respiratory process (Table 23-3), which affects almost all patients with SCI.

Patients with SCI are at risk for developing alterations in cardiac output and tissue perfusion because the cardiovascular system is subjected to a variety of serious and potential physiologic alterations, including dysrhythmias,

cardiac arrest, orthostatic hypotension, emboli, and thrombophlebitis.[20] In spinal shock the cardiovascular regulatory mechanisms are lost. Patients with SCI above T5 may have profound spinal shock as a result of interruption of the sympathetic nervous system and loss of vasoconstrictor response below the level of the injury.[20] Cardiac monitoring is required to detect bradycardia and other dysrhythmias that result from loss of vasomotor tone.

Diagnostic procedures

Diagnostic radiographic evaluations can identify the severity of damage to the spinal cord. Initial evaluation includes anteroposterior and lateral views for all areas of the spinal cord. Films of all seven cervical vertebrae and the top of T1 must be obtained to rule out cervicothoracic junction injury.[24] Flexion and extension views can identify subtle ligamentous injuries. CT scan, tomograms, myelography, and magnetic resonance imaging may also be used in the diagnostic process. (For a more detailed discussion of these procedures, see Chapter 14.)

Medical Management

After assessment and diagnosis of the SCI, medical management begins. The primary treatment goal is to preserve remaining neurologic function. Medical interventions are divided into pharmacologic, surgical, and nonsurgical interventions.

Pharmacologic management

The use of high-dose methylprednisolone has been incorporated into the care of patients with acute SCI.[25,26] Although research has demonstrated that steroids have a beneficial effect on injured spinal cords, the mechanism for action is less clearly understood. Proposed mechanisms of action include (1) facilitation of spinal cord impulse generation, (2) enhancement of spinal cord blood flow, and (3) decreased free radical action on the neuronal membrane.[22] Key points of administration of IV methylprednisolone[25] are summarized in Box 23-3.

TABLE 23-3
EFFECTS OF SPINAL CORD INJURY ON VENTILATORY FUNCTION

INJURY LEVEL	RESPIRATORY FUNCTION	COMMENTS
Complete above C3	Paralysis of diaphragm	Inability to sustain ventilation without mechanical assistance
C3 to C5	Varying degrees of diaphragm dysfunction	Ability to be weaned from mechanical ventilation in most cases
C6 to T11	Intercostal muscles lost or impaired Abdominal muscles lost or impaired	Reduced inspiratory ability Paradoxic breathing patterns Diminished chest mobility Ineffective cough
Below T12	Ventilation not affected	

BOX 23-3

ADMINISTRATION OF IV METHYLPREDNISOLONE FOR SPINAL CORD INJURY

1. Give bolus of 30 mg/kg IV over 15 minutes.
2. Pause for 45 minutes. (Administer IV fluid to keep vein open.)
3. Begin maintenance dosage of 5.4 mg/kg/hr intravenously for 23 hours.
4. Discontinue drug administration 24 hours after the last bolus dose.

Surgical management

Surgical intervention provides spinal column stability in the presence of an unstable injury. Unstable injuries include disrupted ligaments and tendons as well as a vertebral column that cannot maintain normal alignment. Identification and immobilization of unstable injuries are particularly important for patients with incomplete neurologic deficit. Without adequate stabilization, movement and dislocation of the vertebral column could cause a complete neurologic deficit. A variety of surgical procedures may be performed to achieve decompression and stabilization.

LAMINECTOMY. In a laminectomy the lamina of the vertebral ring is removed to allow decompression and removal of bony fragments or disk material from the spinal canal.

SPINAL FUSION. Spinal fusion entails the surgical fusion of two to six vertebral elements to provide stability and prevent motion. Fusion is accomplished through the use of bone parts, bone chips taken from the iliac crest, wire, or acrylic glue.

RODDING. Rodding stabilizes and realigns larger segments of the spinal column by means of a variety of rodding procedures, such as Harrington rods. The rods are attached by screws and glue to the posterior elements of the spinal column. These types of procedures are usually performed to stabilize the thoracolumbar area.

Nonsurgical management

If the injury to the spinal cord is stable, nonsurgical management is the treatment of choice. Nonsurgical management for cervical and thoracolumbar injuries is discussed separately.

CERVICAL INJURY. Management of cervical injuries involves the immobilization of the fracture site and realignment of any dislocation. This is accomplished through skeletal traction that involves the use of two-point tongs inserted into the skull through shallow burr holes and connected to traction weights. Several types of cervical tongs are used. Gardner-Wells and Crutchfield tongs are the most common. These tongs can be applied at the bedside with the use of a local anesthetic.

After the procedure, patients can be immobilized on a kinetic therapy or regular bed. The kinetic therapy bed is the most popular method of cervical immobilization because it maintains spinal column alignment while providing constant turning motion to reduce pulmonary and skin breakdown. Use of cervical skeletal traction on a regular bed makes it difficult to provide adequate care to the pulmonary system and skin because of the extensive degree of immobility.

After adequate realignment of the spinal column has occurred through skeletal traction, a halo traction brace is often applied. The halo vest consists of a metal ring secured to the skull with two occipital and two temporal screws. Steel bars anchor the screws to the vest to provide cervical immobilization. The halo traction brace immobilizes the cervical spine, which allows patients to ambulate and participate in self-care.

THORACOLUMBAR INJURY. Nonsurgical management of patients with a thoracolumbar injury also involves immobilization. Skeletal traction may be used in high thoracic injury. For the most part, misalignment of the spinal canal does not occur in stable injuries of the thoracolumbar spine. Bed rest (with bed flat) and the use of a plastic or fiberglass jacket, a body cast, or a brace immobilize patients so that fractures can heal.

Nursing Management

The goal during the critical care phase is to prevent life-threatening complications while maximizing the functioning of all organ systems. Nursing interventions are aimed at preventing secondary damage to the spinal cord and managing the cardiovascular and respiratory complications of the neurologic deficit.[21] Because almost all body systems are affected by SCI, nursing management should also include interventions that optimize nutrition, elimination, skin integrity, and mobility. Prevention of complications that can delay patients' rehabilitation is a goal of critical care.[21] In addition, patients with SCI have complex psychosocial needs that require a great deal of emotional support from critical care nurses.

Thoracic Injuries

Thoracic injuries involve trauma to the chest wall, lungs, heart, great vessels, and esophagus. Injuries resulting from thoracic trauma account for 25% of all trauma deaths in the United States.[27] Most deaths caused by pulmonary trauma occur after patients reach the hospital. Thoracic trauma is usually the result of a violent crime or an MVA.

Mechanism of Injury

Blunt thoracic trauma

Blunt trauma to the chest is usually caused by MVAs or falls. The underlying mechanism of injury tends to be a combination of acceleration/deceleration injury and direct transfer mechanics such as a crush injury. Varying mechanisms of blunt trauma are associated with specific injury patterns. After head-on collisions, drivers come in contact with the steering assembly and therefore have a higher frequency of injury than back-seat passengers. Severe thoracic injuries are frequently seen in patients who are unrestrained. Falls from greater than 20 feet are associated with thoracic injury.

Penetrating thoracic injuries

The penetrating object determines the damage sustained from penetrating thoracic trauma. Low-velocity weapons (.22-caliber gun, knife) usually damage only what is in the weapon's direct path. Of particular concern, however, are stab wounds that involve the anterior chest wall between the midclavicular lines, Louis' angle, and the epigastric region because these wounds are likely to affect the mediastinum, heart, and the great vessels.[28] High-velocity weapons (rifle, shotgun, and .38 caliber) produce more serious injuries. These weapons are associated with massive energy transfer and tissue destruction. Pellets from a shotgun blast cause further damage by expanding and causing multiple injuries.

Specific Thoracic Traumatic Injuries

Chest wall injuries

RIB FRACTURES. Interruption of a single rib is the most minor and common chest wall injury associated with blunt thoracic trauma.[27] Fractures of certain ribs or multiple ribs can be more serious. Fractures of certain ribs are associated with more underlying life-threatening injuries. Fractures of the first and second ribs are associated with intrathoracic vascular injuries (brachial plexus, great vessels). Fractures of the seventh through tenth ribs are associated with liver and spleen injuries. The pain of rib fractures can be aggravated by movement associated with respiratory excursion. As a result, patients often splint, take shallow breaths, and refuse to cough, which can result in atelectasis and pneumonia.

FLAIL CHEST. Flail chest, caused by blunt trauma, disrupts the continuity of chest wall structures. A **flail chest** occurs when three or more ribs are fractured in two or more places and are no longer attached to the thoracic cage. This results in a free-floating segment of the chest wall that moves independently from the rest of the thorax and results in paradoxic chest wall movement during the respiratory cycle (Fig. 23-4). During inspiration the intact portion of the chest wall expands while the injured part is sucked in. During expiration the chest wall moves in and the flail segment moves out. Hemorrhage and edema initially occur at the site of injury, followed by an accumulation of interstitial fluid and a decrease in alveolar membrane diffusion, which leads to increased pulmonary vascular resistance, decreased pulmonary blood flow, and hypoxemia.[29]

RUPTURED DIAPHRAGM. Diaphragmatic rupture is a frequently missed diagnosis in trauma patients because of the subtle and nonspecific symptoms this injury produces. The mechanism of injury appears to be a rapid rise in intraabdominal pressure as a result of compression force applied to the lower part of the chest or upper region of the abdomen. This injury can occur when people are thrown forward over the tip of the steering wheel in a high-speed deceleration accident. The force can cause the diaphragm, which offers little resistance, to rupture or tear. Abdominal viscera can then gradually enter the thoracic cavity, moving from the positive pressure of the abdomen to the negative pressure of the thorax. The stomach and colon are the most commonly herniated viscera.[30] Diaphragmatic rupture can be life threatening. Massive herniation of abdominal contents

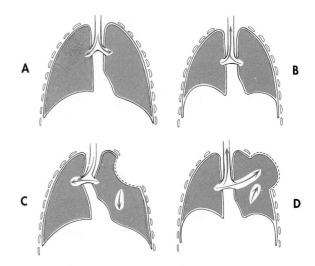

FIG. 23-4 Flail chest. **A,** Normal inspiration. **B,** Normal expiration. **C,** Inspiration: area of lung underlying unstable chest wall sucks in on inspiration. **D,** Same area balloons out on expiration. Note movement of mediastinum toward opposite lung on inspiration. (From Long BC, Phipps WJ, Cassmeyer VL: *Medical-surgical nursing: a nursing process approach,* ed 3, St Louis, 1992, Mosby.)

into the thoracic cavity can compress the lungs and mediastinum, which then hampers venous return and leads to decreased cardiac output. In addition, herniated bowel can become strangulated and perforate.

Pulmonary injuries

PULMONARY CONTUSION. Pulmonary contusion is frequently associated with blunt deceleration/acceleration injuries. These forces can produce bruises, tears, and lacerations under the area of blunt trauma. The pathophysiology of pulmonary contusions begins with initial hemorrhage and interstitial and alveolar edema at the contusion site, which then spreads to surrounding areas and results in general inflammation.[31] Damaged or closed alveolar capillaries result in increased pulmonary vascular resistance, reduced lung compliance, reduced pulmonary blood flow, and ventilation/perfusion imbalance.[32] Pulmonary contusion can interfere with oxygenation (saturation of hemoglobin in pulmonary blood) and ventilation (removal of carbon dioxide from pulmonary blood).

Clinical manifestations of pulmonary contusion may take up to 24 to 48 hours to develop.[31] Inspections of the chest wall may reveal ecchymosis at the site of impact. Moist rales may be noted in the contused lung. A cough may be present with blood-tinged sputum. Abnormal lung function can be detected by systemic arterial hypoxemia. A chest film taken within 6 hours after injury may reveal patchy areas of density that reflect intraalveolar hemorrhage.[31] Small pulmonary parenchymal tears and lacerations can be detected by CT scan.

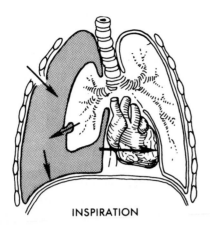
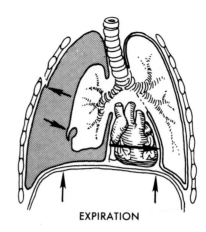

INSPIRATION   EXPIRATION

FIG. 23-5 A tension pneumothorax is usually caused by an injury that perforates the chest wall or pleural space. Air flows into the pleural space with inspiration and becomes trapped. As pressure in the pleural space increases, the lung on the injured side collapses and causes the mediastinum to shift to the opposite side. (From Rosen P and others: *Emergency medicine: concepts and clinical practice,* ed 3, St Louis, 1992, Mosby.)

TENSION PNEUMOTHORAX. A tension pneumothorax is usually caused by an injury that perforates the chest wall or pleural space. Air flows into the pleural space during inspiration and becomes trapped. As pressure in the pleural space increases, the lung on the injured side collapses and causes the mediastinum to shift to the opposite side (Fig. 23-5). As pressure continues to build, the shift exerts pressure on the heart and thoracic aorta, which results in decreased venous return and decreased cardiac output. Tissue perfusion with oxygenated blood is further hampered because the collapsed lung cannot participate in ventilation.

OPEN PNEUMOTHORAX. An open pneumothorax, or "sucking chest wound," is usually caused by penetrating trauma. Open communication between the atmosphere and intrathoracic pressure results in immediate lung deflation. Air moves in and out of the hole in the chest, producing a sucking sound during inspiration.

HEMOTHORAX. Blunt or penetrating thoracic trauma can cause bleeding into the pleural space to produce a hemothorax (Fig. 23-6). A massive hemothorax can cause a blood loss of more than 1500 ml.[32] The source of bleeding may be the intercostal or internal mammary arteries, lungs, heart, or great vessels. Increasing intrapleural pressure results in a decrease in vital capacity. Increasing vascular blood loss into the pleural space causes decreased venous return and decreased cardiac output.

Cardiac injuries

PENETRATING CARDIAC INJURIES. Penetrating cardiac trauma can occur from mechanical injuries as a result of bullets, knives, and impalements. The chest wall offers little protection to the heart from penetrating trauma. The most common site of injury is the right ventricle because of its anterior position. Mortality rates from penetrating trauma to the heart are high. The prehospital

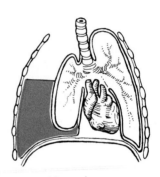

Hemothorax

FIG. 23-6 Blunt or penetrating thoracic trauma can cause bleeding into the pleural space to form a hemothorax.

mortality rate for penetrating cardiac injuries is 75%, and most deaths occur within 4 or 5 minutes after injury as a result of exsanguination or tamponade.[33]

CARDIAC TAMPONADE. Cardiac tamponade is the progressive accumulation of blood in the pericardial sac (Fig. 23-7). With cardiac tamponade a progressive accumulation of blood, 120 to 150 ml, increases the intracardial pressure and compresses the atria and ventricles. Increased intracardial pressures lead to decreased venous return and decreased filling pressure, followed by decreased cardiac output, myocardial hypoxia, cardiac failure, and cardiogenic shock.

BLUNT CARDIAC INJURIES. The most common causes of blunt cardiac trauma include high-speed MVAs, direct blows to the chest, and falls. The heart, because of its mobility and its location between the sternum and thoracic vertebrae, is susceptible to blunt traumatic injury. Sudden acceleration (as from contact with the steering wheel) can cause the heart to be thrown against the sternum. Sudden deceleration can cause the heart to be thrown against the thoracic vertebrae by a direct blow to

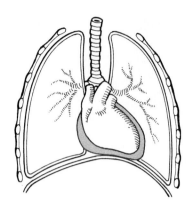

FIG. 23-7 Cardiac tamponade is the progressive accumulation of blood in the pericardial sac.

the chest (baseball, animal kick, fall). Myocardial contusion is one of the most common injuries sustained as a result of blunt cardiac trauma.

MYOCARDIAL CONTUSION. Myocardial cell injury results from the contusion. Histologically the contused myocardium is similar to an infarcted myocardium. In a contused myocardium, however, a well-demarcated zone exists between normal and contused myocardium.[34] If the contusion is large enough and has resulted in a large area of myonecrosis, patients may experience complications identical to those of an acute myocardial infarction. The right ventricle is most often affected because of its proximity to the sternum.

Abdominal Injuries

Abdominal injury accounts for 10% of trauma fatalities in the United States.[35] Most persons who are injured and suffer abdominal trauma are younger than 50 years of age.[36] Frequently associated with multisystem trauma, injuries to the abdomen result from blunt or penetrating trauma. Two major life-threatening conditions that occur after abdominal trauma are hemorrhage and hollow viscus perforation with its associated peritonitis.

Mechanism of Injury

Blunt trauma

Blunt abdominal injuries are common and usually result from MVAs, falls, and assaults. The spleen is the most commonly injured organ in blunt trauma and ranks second to the liver as the source of life-threatening abdominal injury.[37] In MVAs, abdominal injury is more likely to occur when a vehicle is struck from the side. In the passenger position of the front seat, hepatic injury is likely when the point of impact is on the same side as the passenger. A driver is likely to sustain injury to the spleen when the impact is on the driver's side. Seat belts, which substantially reduce morbidity and mortality risks, are also associated with causing bladder and bowel rupture.[35] Pedestrians hit by motor vehicles are at risk for serious abdominal injuries. Blunt trauma to the thorax

can produce injuries to the liver, spleen, and diaphragm. In SCI, large abdominal arteries and veins can be injured. Deceleration and direct forces can produce retroperitoneal hematomas. Blunt abdominal injuries are often hidden and more likely to be fatal than penetrating abdominal injuries.

Penetrating trauma

Penetrating abdominal trauma is generally caused by knives or bullets. The danger of penetrating abdominal trauma is that the outside appearance of the wound does not determine the extent of internal injury. The most commonly injured organs from knife wounds are liver, spleen, diaphragm, and colon.[38] Gunshot wounds to the abdomen are usually more serious than stab wounds because a bullet destroys tissue along its path. Once inside the abdomen, a bullet can travel in erratic paths and ricochet off bone. Death from penetrating injuries depends on the injury to major vascular structures and resultant intraabdominal hemorrhage.

Assessment

Physical assessment

The location of entry and exit sites associated with penetrating trauma should be assessed and documented. Inspection of the abdomen may reveal purplish discoloration of the flanks or umbilicus (Cullen's sign), which indicates blood in the abdominal wall. Ecchymosis in the flank area (Grey Turner's sign) may indicate retroperitoneal bleeding or a possible fracture of the pancreas. A hematoma in the flank area suggests renal injury. A distended abdomen may indicate the accumulation of blood, fluid, or gas secondary to a perforated organ or ruptured blood vessel. The increase of abdominal girth by 1 inch can indicate intraabdominal accumulation of 500 to 1000 ml of blood.[31] Auscultation of the abdomen may reveal friction rubs over the liver and spleen and may indicate rupture. Presence of rebound or tenderness and rigidity of the abdomen indicates peritoneal inflammation. Referred pain to the left shoulder (Kehr's sign) may indicate a ruptured spleen or irritation of the diaphragm from bile or other material in the peritoneum. Subcutaneous emphysema palpated on the abdomen suggests free air caused by a ruptured bowel.

Diagnostic procedures

Laboratory test results may be nonspecific for patients with abdominal trauma. A serum amylase determination can detect pancreatic injuries. Initial leukocytosis can suggest splenic or hepatic injury. Because of hemoconcentration, hemoglobin and hematocrit results may not reflect actual values. Serial values are more valuable in diagnosing abdominal injuries.

Diagnostic peritoneal lavage (DPL) can accurately exclude or confirm the presence of intraabdominal injury. After patients empty their bladders, physicians make a small incision in the abdomen through the skin and into the peritoneum and insert a small catheter. If frank blood is encountered, intraabdominal injury is obvious and patients are taken immediately to the operating room. If gross blood is not initially evident, 1 L of fluid (lactated Ringer's or 0.9% normal saline) is infused through the catheter into the abdomen. The IV bag is then placed in a dependent position and allowed to drain. The drainage fluid is sent to the laboratory for analysis. Positive DPL results signal intraabdominal trauma and usually necessitate surgical intervention.

Abdominal CT scanning can detect retroperitoneal hemorrhage, localize specific sites of abdominal injury, and determine the relative severity of intraperitoneal or retroperitoneal hemorrhage.[39]

Specific Organ Injuries

Liver injuries

The liver is the primary organ injured in penetrating trauma and the second most commonly injured organ in blunt trauma. Detection of liver injury, as with all intraabdominal injury, is accomplished through the use of physical assessment and DPL or CT scan. Surgical intervention can usually correct the defect. Resection of the devitalized tissue is required for massive injuries. Hemorrhage is common with liver injuries, and intraoperative ligation of the hepatic arteries or veins may be required to control hemorrhage.

Spleen injuries

The spleen is the organ most commonly injured by blunt abdominal trauma and is second to the liver as a source of life-threatening hemorrhage. Spleen injuries, like liver injuries, are graded for determining the amount of trauma sustained, care required, and possible outcomes. The treatment of an injured spleen is controversial because of the spleen's importance in preventing infection. Patients who are hemodynamically stable may be monitored in the critical care unit by means of serial hematocrit values and vital signs. Progressive deterioration may indicate the need for operative management. Patients who are hemodynamically unstable require operative intervention with splenectomy, partial splenectomy, or splenorraphy.

Intestinal injuries

Intestinal injuries can result from blunt or penetrating trauma. Regardless of mechanism of injury, intestinal contents (bile, stool, enzymes, bacteria) leak into the peritoneum and cause peritonitis, which requires surgical resection and repair. Patients' postoperative course is dictated by the amount of intestinal contents spilled.

Pancreatic injuries

Pancreatic injury rarely occurs alone. Death is related directly to the number of associated injuries. Penetrating wounds that cause injury to the pancreas require immediate surgical intervention. Diagnosing pancreatic injury that results from blunt trauma is difficult. Elevated serum amylase levels may not occur for 24 hours or more after injury. Diagnostic CT findings of pancreatic edema and fluid may not develop for 24 to 48 hours after injury. Surgical intervention is required if the possibility of pancreatic injury exists.

Genitourinary Injuries

Trauma to the genitourinary (GU) tract seldom occurs as an isolated injury. An associated GU injury should be suspected in patients with trauma to the chest, flank, abdomen, pelvis, perineum, and genitalia.[40]

Mechanism of Injury

Like all other traumatic injuries, GU injuries can result from blunt or penetrating trauma. Blunt GU trauma can be caused by deceleration injuries, and penetrating injuries can occur with stabbings or gunshot wounds to the abdomen or back.

Specific Genitourinary Injuries

Renal trauma

Blunt renal trauma produces 80% of all renal injuries.[40] Blunt trauma to the flank causes the twelfth rib to compress the kidney against the lumbar spine, resulting in a contusion or laceration of the kidney. Of all renal trauma, 80% to 90% involves contusions or minor lacerations without urinary extravasation.[39] Intravenous pyelography is used in the diagnosis of renal trauma because it can outline the collection system and establish the presence and function of both kidneys. Abdominal CT scan can define parenchymal lacerations, urinary extravasation, and perirenal hematoma.

Conditions that require surgical intervention for renal trauma include expanding hematoma, pulsatile hematoma, penetrating trauma with urinary extravasation, vascular injury, and evidence of continued hemorrhage after patients have received 3 U of blood.[40]

Bladder trauma

Most bladder injuries result from blunt trauma. The type of injury that occurs depends on not only the location and strength of the blunt force but also the volume of urine in the bladder at the time of injury.[39] Trauma to the bladder may result in a contusion or rupture. Urinary extravasation is the hallmark sign of a ruptured bladder. Definitive diagnosis of bladder rupture is made by means of cystographic examination.

Complications of Trauma

Ongoing nursing assessments are imperative for early detection of complications frequently associated with traumatic injuries (Box 23-4). Infection remains a major cause of mortality and morbidity in critical care units.

B O X   2 3 - 4

COMPLICATIONS OF TRAUMA

Infection
Sepsis
Pulmonary complications
    Respiratory failure
    Fat embolism syndrome (FES)
Gastrointestinal complications
    Hemorrhage
    Acalculous cholecystitis
Renal complications
    Renal failure
    Myoglobinuria
Vascular complications
    Compartment syndrome
Missed injury
Multiple organ dysfunction syndrome (MODS)

Of trauma patients who survive longer than 3 days, infection is a frequent cause of death.[41] Trauma patients are at risk for infection because of contaminated wounds, invasive therapeutic and diagnostic catheters, intubation and mechanical ventilation, host susceptibility, and iatrogenic factors in the critical care environment. Patients with multiple injuries are especially at risk for overwhelming infections and sepsis. The source of sepsis in trauma patients can be invasive therapeutic and diagnostic catheters or wound contamination with exogenous or endogenous bacteria.

Trauma to the pulmonary system is likely to result in complications through respiratory failure, particularly when patients were involved in a high-speed MVA, suffered major blunt trauma, experienced a mean arterial pressure of less than 60 mm Hg for a period of time, had 20% or more of blood volume replaced, or experienced a decrease in level of consciousness.[42] Respiratory insufficiency is one of the most common complications after multiple trauma.

Fat embolism syndrome (FES) can occur as a complication of orthopedic trauma. Characterized by pulmonary system dysfunction, FES appears to develop as a result of fat droplets that leak from fractured bone and embolize to the lungs. The droplets are broken down into free fatty acids that are toxic to the pulmonary microvascular membranes. Damage of these membranes results in edema, inactivation of surfactant, and atelectasis. Fat droplets further activate a coagulation cascade that results in thrombocytopenia. The lung becomes highly edematous and hemorrhagic. The clinical presentation is almost indistinguishable from that of acute respiratory disease syndrome (ARDS).

Life-threatening gastrointestinal bleeding as a result of stress ulcerations is infrequent but associated with high mortality rates. Patients with multiple traumatic injuries are particularly at risk for developing this complication. Risk factors associated with the development of stress ulcerations include sepsis, multiple trauma, hepatic failure, ARDS, renal failure, and major surgical procedures.[43]

Prolonged critical illness predisposes patients to bile stasis, biliary sludge development, and eventual cystic duct obstruction. *Acalculous cholecystitis* refers to inflammation of the gallbladder without evidence of gallstones. Several risk factors for acalculous cholecystitis are present in patients with traumatic injuries: volume depletion, prolonged gastrointestinal rest, morphine administration, ventilatory support, multiple transfusions, and infected wounds.[44]

Assessment and ongoing monitoring of renal function are critical to the survival of trauma patients. Prolonged hypoperfusion, hypoxia, or both, is the most common cause of renal failure in patients with multiple traumatic injuries.

Patients with a crush injury are susceptible to the development of myoglobinuria, with subsequent secondary renal failure. Crush injuries can result in arterial trauma. Loss of arterial blood flow, particularly to the extremities, results in the loss of oxygen transport to distal tissues and ischemia. This initiates a cascade of events that leads to the necrosis of skeletal muscle cells. As cells die, intracellular contents—particularly potassium and myoglobin—are released. Myoglobin, which is the muscular pigment, is a large molecule that causes acute renal tubular blockade and subsequent renal failure as it circulates in the cardiovascular system. Myoglobinuria frequently develops within 6 hours after injury.

Compartment syndrome is a condition in which increased pressure within a limited space compromises circulation, resulting in ischemia and necrosis of tissues within that space. Among those at risk for the development of compartment syndrome are patients with lower extremity trauma, including fractures, penetrating trauma, vascular ruptures, massive tissue injuries, and venous obstruction. Compartment syndrome is thought to be caused by the accumulation of interstitial fluid in a closed compartment. As fluid accumulates in a closed space, decreased tissue perfusion occurs as arteries and veins become obstructed.

Nursing assessment of the multiply injured patients in the critical care unit may reveal missed diseases or missed injuries. Missed diseases may include preexisting undiagnosed medical illnesses, such as endocrine disorders (diabetes, hypothyroidism), myocardial infarction, hypertension, respiratory insufficiency, renal insufficiency, and malnutrition.

Occasionally injuries may not be diagnosed in the precritical care phases. Injuries can be subtle or masked, preventing accurate diagnosis. In the critical care unit, a missed injury may be suspected if patients fail to show appropriate response to medical or surgical intervention.

Multiple organ dysfunction syndrome (MODS) represents the culmination of progressive organ system dysfunction. Patients with multiple injuries are particularly

BOX 23-5

NURSING DIAGNOSIS PRIORITIES

Trauma

- *Altered Cerebral Tissue Perfusion* related to increased intracranial pressure secondary to brain trauma, p. 492
- *Decreased Cardiac Output* related to vasodilation and bradycardia secondary to sympathetic blockade of neurogenic (spinal) shock after spinal cord injury above T6 level, p. 478
- *Ineffective Breathing Pattern* related to decreased lung expansion secondary to thoracic trauma (ruptured diaphragm, pneumothorax, hemothorax, rib fractures, pulmonary contusion, flail chest, penetrating and blunt cardiac injuries), p. 485
- *Risk for Infection* (risk factors: invasive monitoring devices), p. 482
- *Body Image Disturbance* related to actual change in body structure, function, or appearance, p. 458
- *Ineffective Individual Coping* related to situational crisis and personal vulnerability, p. 462

at risk for MODS because it can develop as a result of multiple system/organ trauma, major/emergency surgery, intraabdominal sepsis, ARDS, and renal failure. (MODS is described at length in Chapter 25.)

Nursing Management of Trauma Patients

Trauma patients present unique challenges to critical care nurses. Often, multiple organs or body systems are affected, which necessitates continuous monitoring and assessment of various potential problems. Priorities for nursing management of trauma patients are listed in Box 23-5.

References

1. Robertson L: Motor vehicles, *Pediatr Clin North Am* 32:87, 1985.
2. Martin K: Reducing complications of thoracic gunshot wounds, *Dimens Crit Care Nurs* 8(5):280, 1989.
3. American College of Surgeons, Committee on Trauma: *Advanced trauma life support instructor manual,* Chicago, 1989, The College.
4. Jarosz D and others: The tertiary nursing survey in the assessment of trauma patients: an important addendum to survival, *Crit Care Nurs* 14(4):98, 1994.
5. Cope D, Wolfson B: Crisis intervention with the family in the trauma setting, *J Head Trauma Rehabil* 9(1):67, 1994.
6. Hopkins A: The trauma nurse's role with families in crisis, *Crit Care Nurs* 14(4):35, 1994.
7. Boggs RL: Multiple system trauma: nursing implications, *J Adv Med Surg Nurs* 2(1):1, 1989.
8. Meyer AA, Trunkey DD: Critical care as an integral part of trauma care, *Crit Care Clin North Am* 2(4):673, 1986.
9. Whitehorne M, Cacciola R, Quinn ME: Multiple trauma: survival after the golden hour, *J Adv Med Surg Nurs* 2(1):27, 1989.
10. Von Reuden KT: Cardiopulmonary assessment of the critically ill trauma patient, *Crit Care Nurs Clin North Am* 1(1):33, 1989.
11. Gennarelli TA: *Triage of head injured patients.* In Trunkey DD, Lewis FR, editors: *Current therapy of trauma,* ed 3, Philadelphia, 1991, BC Decker.
12. Ward and others: Penetrating head injury, *Crit Care Nurs Q* 17(1):79, 1994.
13. Gress DR: Treatment of head and spine trauma, *Emerg Care Q* 5(2):15, 1989.
14. Ammons AM: Cerebral injuries and intracranial hemorrhages as a result of trauma, *Nurs Clin North Am* 25(1):23, 1990.
15. Stand PE: Diagnostic and therapeutic concerns in head injured patient, *J Am Acad Phys Assist* 1(2):112, 1988.
16. Sullivan TE and others: Closed head injury assessment and research methodology, *J Neurosci Nurs* 26(1):24, 1994.
17. Palter M and others: Intensive care management of severe head injury, *J Head Trauma Rehabil* 9(1):20, 1994.
18. Prendergast V: Current trends in research and treatment of intracranial hypertension, *Crit Care Nurs Q* 17(1):1, 1994.
19. Rising C: The relationship of selected nursing activities to ICP, *J Neurosci Nurs* 25(5):302, 1993.
20. Hughes MC: Critical care nursing for the patient with a spinal cord injury, *Crit Care Nurs Clin North Am* 2(1):33, 1990.
21. Walleck CA: Neurologic considerations in the critical care phase, *Crit Care Nurs Clin North Am* 2(3):357, 1990.
22. Hilton G, Frei J: High-dose methylprednisolone in the treatment of spinal cord injuries, *Heart Lung* 20(6):675, 1991.
23. Kocan MJ: Pulmonary considerations in the critical care phase, *Crit Care Nurs Clin North Am* 2(3):369, 1990.
24. Richmond TS: Spinal cord injury, *Nurs Clin North Am* 25(1):57, 1990.
25. Nayduch D, Lee A, Butler D: High-dose methylprednisolone after acute spinal cord injury, *Crit Care Nurs* 14(4):69, 1994.
26. Nolan S: Current trends in the management of acute spinal cord injury, *Crit Care Nurs Q* 17(1):64, 1994.
27. Hammond SG: Chest injuries in the trauma patient, *Nurs Clin North Am* 25(1):35, 1990.
28. Ross SE, Cernaianu AC: Epidemiology of thoracic injuries: mechanisms of injury and pathophysiology, *Top Emerg Med* 12(1):1, 1990.
29. Gough JE, Allison EJ, Raju VP: Flail chest: management and implications for emergency nurses, *J Emerg Nurs* 13(6):330, 1987.
30. Andrew L: Difficult diagnoses in blunt thoraco-abdominal trauma, *J Emerg Nurs* 15(5):399, 1989.
31. Ruth-Sahd L: Pulmonary contusion: the hidden danger in blunt chest trauma, *Crit Care Nurs* 11(6):46, 1990.
32. Hefti D: Chest trauma, *RN* 54:28, 1991.
33. Feliciano DV, Mattox KL: *The heart.* In Trunkey DD, Lewis FR, editors: *Current therapy of trauma,* ed 3, Philadelphia, 1991, BC Decker.
34. Bartlett R: Myocardial contusion, *Dimens Crit Care Nurs* 10(3):133, 1991.
35. Merrill CR, Sparger G: Current thoughts on blunt abdominal trauma, *Top Emerg Med* 12(2):21, 1990.
36. Semonin-Holleran R: Critical nursing care for abdominal trauma, *Crit Care Nurs* 8(3):48, 1988.
37. Carrico CJ: *The spleen.* In Trunkey DD, Lewis FR, editors: *Current therapy of trauma,* ed 3, Philadelphia, 1991, BC Decker.
38. Wagner MM: The patient with abdominal injuries, *Nurs Clin North Am* 25(1):45, 1990.

39. Kidd PS: Genitourinary trauma patients, *Top Emerg Med* 9(3):71, 1987.
40. Frevele G: Urinary tract injuries due to blunt abdominal trauma, *Phys Assist* 13(2):123, 1989.
41. Martin MT: Wound management and infection control after trauma: implications for the intensive care setting, *Crit Care Nurs Q* 11(2):43, 1988.
42. Thompson J, Dains J: Indices of injury: development and status, *Nurs Clin North Am* 12:655, 1986.
43. Konopad E, Noseworthy T: Stress ulceration: a serious complication in critically ill patients, *Heart Lung* 17(4):339, 1988.
44. Langdale L, Schecter WP: Critical care complications in the trauma patient, *Crit Care Clin North Am* 2(4):839, 1986.

Burns

LINDA VALENTINO

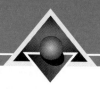

Pathophysiology and Etiology of Burn Injury

A burn is an injury resulting in tissue loss or damage. Injury to tissue can be caused by exposure to thermal, electrical, chemical, and radiation sources. Injury to the tissue is determined by the temperature or causticity of the burning agent and duration of tissue contact with the source.

At the cellular level the burning agent produces a dilation of the capillaries and small vessels, thus increasing the capillary permeability. Plasma seeps out into the surrounding tissue, producing blisters and edema. The type, duration, and intensity of the burn affect the amount and extent of fluid loss. This progressive fluid loss in major burns results in significant intravascular fluid volume deficit. The pathophysiologic response to injury is twofold. Early postinjury organ hypoperfusion develops as a result of low cardiac output as well as increased peripheral vascular resistance because of the normal neurohormonal response to trauma. With adequate volume repletion, hemodynamic functions improve, and as plasma volume increases, cardiac output rises, which results in a hypermetabolic response and overall increase in organ perfusion.

The clinical course of a burn injury comprises three phases: the resuscitative phase, acute care phase, and rehabilitative phase. The resuscitative phase begins with the initial hemodynamic response to injury and lasts until capillary integrity is restored and the repletion of plasma volume by fluid replacement occurs. The acute phase begins with the onset of diuresis of fluid mobilized from the interstitial space and ends with the closure of the burn wound. The rehabilitative phase often commences on patients' admission, and correction of functional deficits and scar management are major considerations. The rehabilitative phase may last from months to years depending on the severity of injury.

Classification of Burn Injuries

Burns are classified primarily according to the size and depth of the injury. The type and location of the burn, as well as patients' age and medical history, however, are significant considerations. Recognition of the magnitude of burn injury, which is based on the depth, size, and prior health of the host, is of crucial importance in the overall care plan.[1] Decisions concerning complete patient management are based on this assessment. Age and burn size are the cardinal determinants of survival.[2,3]

Size of Injury

Several different methods can be used to estimate the size of the burn area. A quick and easy method is the **rule of nines,** which is often used in the prehospital setting for initial triage of burn patients (Fig. 24-1). With this method the adult body is divided into surface areas of 9%. This method is modified in infants and very small children. The head and the anterior and the posterior surfaces of the trunk are each 18%, each arm is 9%, each leg is 14%, and the perineum is 1%.

Small and scattered areas of burns can be calculated with use of the principle that the palmar surface of the victim's hand represents 1% of the total body surface area (TBSA).

Depth of Injury

Traditionally, burn depth has been classified in degrees of injury based on the amount of injured epidermis or dermis, or both—that is, first-, second-, or third-degree burns (Fig. 24-2). These terms, however, are not descriptive of the burn surface.

Currently, burns are classified as partial thickness and full thickness. This description is based on the surface

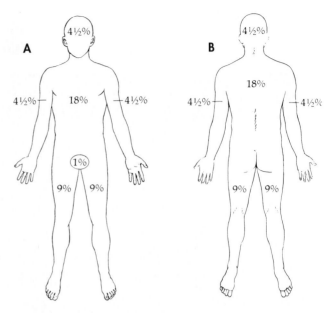

FIG. 24-1 Estimation of adult burn injury: rule of nines. **A,** Anterior view. **B,** Posterior view. (From Dains JE: *Integumentary system.* In Thompson JM and others: *Mosby's clinical nursing,* ed 3, St Louis, 1993, Mosby.)

appearance of the wound. Partial thickness includes first and second degree. Full thickness includes third degree. Partial-thickness burns are further classified as superficial, moderate, and deep dermal partial-thickness. Wound assessment involves recognition of the depth of injury and size of burn.

A superficial partial-thickness burn **(first-degree burn)** involves only the first two or three of the five layers of the epidermis. Superficial partial-thickness wounds are characterized by erythema and mild discomfort. Pain, the chief symptom, usually resolves in 48 to 72 hours. Common examples of these burn injuries are sunburns and minor steam burns that occur during cooking. Generally these wounds heal in 5 to 7 days and do not require medical intervention aside from pain relief and oral fluids.

A moderate partial-thickness burn **(second-degree burn)** involves the upper third of the dermis. These burns are usually caused by brief contact with flames or hot liquid or exposure to dilute chemicals. Superficial second-degree burns are characterized by a light- to bright-red or mottled appearance. These wounds may appear wet and weeping, may contain bullae, and are extremely painful and sensitive to air currents. The microvessels that perfuse this area are injured, and permeability is increased, resulting in the leakage of large amounts of plasma into the interstitium. This fluid, in turn, lifts off the thin, damaged epidermis, causing blister formation. Despite the loss of the entire basal layer of the epidermis, a burn of this depth will heal in 7 to 21 days. Minimal scarring can be expected. Moderately deep partial-thickness wounds frequently take 4 to 6 weeks to heal.

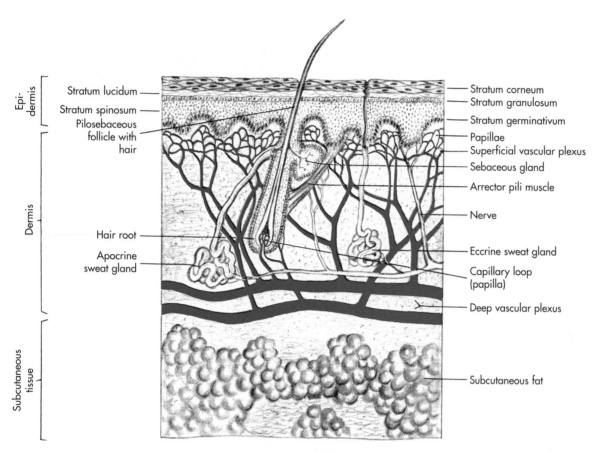

FIG. 24-2 Anatomy of the skin. (From Dains JE: *Integumentary system.* In Thompson JM and others: *Mosby's clinical nursing,* ed 3, St Louis, 1993, Mosby.)

A deep dermal partial-thickness burn (second degree) involves the entire epidermal layer and part of the dermis (Fig. 24-3). These burns often result from contact with hot liquids, solids, and intense radiant energy. A deep dermal partial-thickness burn is not generally characterized by blister formation. Only a modest plasma surface leakage occurs because of severe impairment in blood supply. The wound surface is usually red, with white areas in deeper parts, and blanching follows capillary refill. The appearance of the deep dermal wound changes over time. Dermal necrosis, along with surface coagulated protein, turns the wound white to yellow. These wounds have a prolonged healing time. They can heal spontaneously as the epidermal elements germinate and migrate until the epidermal surface is restored. This process of healing by epithelialization can take up to 6 weeks. Left untreated, these wounds can heal primarily with unstable epithelium, late hypertrophic scarring, and marked contracture formation. The treatment of choice is surgical excision and skin grafting. Partial-thickness injuries can become full-thickness injuries if they become infected, blood supply is diminished, or further trauma occurs to the site.

A full-thickness burn **(third-degree burn)** involves destruction of all the layers of the skin down to and including the subcutaneous tissue (Fig. 24-4). Composed of adipose tissue, the subcutaneous tissue includes the hair follicles and sweat glands and is poorly vascularized. A full-thickness burn appears pale white or charred, red or brown, and leathery. At first a full-thickness burn may resemble a partial-thickness burn. The surface of the burn may be dry, and if the skin is broken, fat may be exposed. Full-thickness burns are usually painless and insensitive to palpation. All epithelial elements are destroyed; therefore the wound will not heal by reepithelialization. Wound closure of small full-thickness burns (less than a 4 cm area) can be achieved with healing by contraction. All other full-thickness wounds require skin grafting for closure. Extensive full-thickness wounds leave patients extremely susceptible to infections, fluid and electrolyte imbalances, alterations in thermoregulation, and metabolic disturbances.

The exact depth of many burn wounds cannot be clearly defined on the first inspection. A major difficulty is distinguishing deep-dermal from full-thickness injury. Burn wounds may evolve over time and require frequent reassessment. Special consideration must always be given to very young and older patients because of their thin dermal layer. Burn injuries in these age groups may be more severe than they initially appear.

At the same time wound assessment for depth occurs, the total percentage, or TBSA, of the burn should be cal-

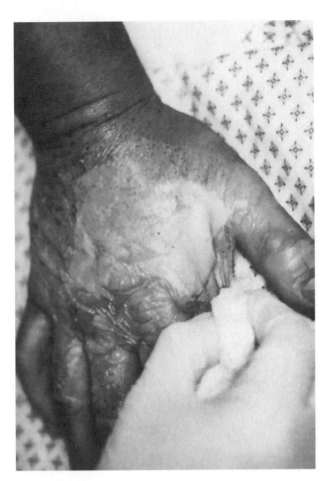

FIG. 24-3 Second-degree burn (deep partial thickness injury to dorsum of hand). (Courtesy Intermountain Burn Center, University of Utah Health Sciences Center.)

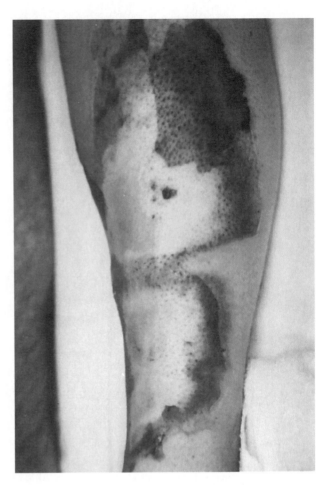

FIG. 24-4 Third-degree burn (marked color change). (Courtesy Intermountain Burn Center, University of Utah Health Sciences Center.)

culated. This calculation provides the basis for determining the amount of fluid that will be required for treatment.

Zones of Injury

Thermal burns are additionally classified into three concentric zones of injury—the central zone being most severe and the peripheral zone being least damaged. The outermost zone is termed the **zone of hyperemia** and is analogous to a first-degree burn. Next to the zone of hyperemia is the zone of stasis, in which tissue perfusion is compromised. The innermost zone is the **zone of coagulation**. This zone had most direct contact with the heat source. Cellular death occurs in this zone.[4]

Types of Injury

Thermal burns

The most common burns are thermal burns caused by steam, scalds, contact, and fire injuries. The most common age groups involved are toddlers (2 to 4 years), for whom scalds are the most common cause, and young

adults (17 to 25 years), usually male, for whom the most common cause is flammable liquid. Structural fires account for fewer than 5% of hospital admissions but are responsible for more than 45% of burn-related deaths.[3]

Electrical burns

Electrical and lightning injuries result in 1000 deaths per year in the United States. The incidence of electrical burn injury is 17 times greater in males. Electrical burns can be caused by low-voltage (alternating) current or high-voltage (alternating or direct) current. Common situations that may increase the risk for electrical injuries include occupational exposure and accidents involving household current. Lightning causes death in approximately 25% of those injured, and permanent sequelae in about 75%.[5]

Chemical burns

Chemical burns are caused by acids and alkalies. Alkalies frequently result in more severe injuries than acid burns. Acids and alkali agents are found in household substances such as drain cleaner and occupational substances such as liquid concrete. The concentration of the

TRIAGE CRITERIA FOR BURN PATIENTS

Minor burn injury: can be treated initially on outpatient basis
1. Second-degree burn
    a. Less than 15% of body surface in adult
    b. Less than 10% of body surface in child
2. Third-degree burn
    a. Less than 2% of body surface

Moderate uncomplicated burn injury: usually requires hospitalization (general hospital) with experience in burn care or specialized burn treatment facility
1. Second-degree burn
    a. 15%-20% of body surface in adult
    b. 10%-20% of body surface in child
2. Third-degree burn
    a. 2%-10% of body surface

Major burn injury: requires hospitalization in a specialized burn treatment facility
1. Second-degree burn
    a. More than 25% of body surface in adult
    b. More than 20% of body surface in child
2. Third-degree burn
    a. More than 10% of body surface
3. Smaller burns with complicating features
    a. Extremes of age: less than 5 or more than 60 years
    b. Burns of hands, face, perineum, feet
    c. Chronic alcoholism or drug addiction
    d. Inhalation injury
    e. Significant preexisting disease (e.g., diabetes mellitus)
    f. Associated trauma
    g. Unreliable home environment for small children
    h. Child abuse

From Shires GT: *Principles of trauma care,* New York, 1985, McGraw-Hill.

chemical agent and duration of exposure are the key factors that determine the extent and depth of damage. Time should not be wasted in looking for specific neutralizing agents because the injury is related directly to the concentration of the chemical and the duration of the exposure; also, the heat of neutralization can extend the injury.[6] Tar and asphalt burns are serious and rather common injuries. Approximately 70% of these burns occur to the hands.

Location of Injury

Location of injury can determine whether a burn is major or minor. According to triage criteria (Box 24-1), burns on the face, hands, feet, and perineum are considered major burns. These involve functional areas of the body and often require specialized intervention. Injuries to these areas can result in significant long-term morbidity, both from impaired function and altered appearance.

Patient Age and History

Age and history are significant determinants of survival. Patients considered most at risk are younger than 2 years of age and older than 65 years. History of inhalation injury, electrical burns, and all burns complicated by trauma and fractures significantly increase the risk of mortality and are considered major burns. Obtaining a past medical history is important, particularly relating to cardiac, pulmonary, and renal disorders as well as diabetes and central nervous system disorders.

Initial Emergency Burn Management

The goals of acute care of patients with thermal injuries are to save lives, minimize disabilities, and prepare patients for definitive care. The burn injury may involve multiple organ systems, and the approach to injured patients must be expeditious and methodic in identifying problems and establishing priorities of care.[9]

The resuscitation phase begins immediately after the burn insult has occurred; therefore nurses are concerned with patient management at the scene until admission to an appropriate medical facility and preparation for care of the burn injury can occur. As with any major trauma the first hour is crucial, but the first 24 to 36 hours are also vitally important in burn patient management. This time interval has a major impact on patients' survival and ultimate rehabilitation.

Obtaining a history of the nature of the injury is extremely valuable in management. Water heater, propane gas, grain elevator, and other types of explosions frequently throw patients some distance and may result in concomitant orthopedic, neurologic, and internal trauma. Knowing the specific agents involved in chemical burns is valuable. Nurses should also ask the names of substances burned or inhaled and the length of time patients were exposed to superheated air.

Airway Management

The first priority of emergency burn care is to secure and protect the airway. For patients with facial burns, exposure to an enclosed space fire, or both, a high index of suspicion exists for inhalation injury. Carbon monoxide poisoning or intoxication is associated with high mortality at the scene. Carboxyhemoglobin levels are obtained, and oxygen therapy is continued until levels are no longer toxic. All patients with major burns or suspected inhalation injury are initially administered 100% oxygen.[7] Nurses should continue to observe patients for clinical manifestations of impaired oxygenation such as tachypnea, agitation, anxiety, and upper airway obstruction—for example, hoarseness, stridor, and wheezing.

Endotracheal intubation may be necessary. Immobilization of the cervical spine should be maintained until full evaluation is completed. Cross-table lateral films, however, may not be possible to obtain before intubation. A detailed patient history is important, including the mechanism of injury; age; location and size of burn; type and amount of fluid already administered; known allergies; status of tetanus immunization; and significant past medical history. All rings, watches, and jewelry should be removed from injured limbs to avoid a tourniquet effect when edema occurs because of fluid shifts and fluid resuscitation.

Circulatory Management

At this point the extent and depth of the burn are assessed. The extent or TBSA of the burn is calculated by means of one of the formulas for estimation of fluid resuscitation requirements. The Parkland formula is the most widely used. Depth is assessed according to the percentage of partial- and full-thickness wounds present. Burn shock results from loss of fluid from the vascular compartment into the area of injury. Therefore the larger the percentage of burn, the greater the potential for shock. Lactated Ringer's solution is infused via large-bore cannula in a peripheral vein. Lactated Ringer's solution, an isotonic crystalloid, is the most popular resuscitation fluid. Lactated Ringer's solution given in large amounts can restore cardiac output toward normal in most patients. Because it most closely matches extracellular fluid, it is preferred to normal saline. Because isotonic salt solutions generate no difference in osmotic pressure between plasma and interstitial space, the entire extracellular space must be expanded to replace intravascular losses. The Parkland formula is as follows:

4 ml lactated Ringer's solution per body weight in kg/% body surface area of burn = the 24-hour fluid requirement

In the first 8 hours after injury, half the calculated amount is administered to patients, 25% is given in the second 8 hours, and 25% in the third 8 hours. **Nurses must remember that calculated fluid requirements are guidelines. The quantity of crystalloid needed depends on patients' responses to treatment and is determined by monitoring the volume of urine output. Meticulous attention to detail is taken to ensure that patients are neither underresuscitated nor overresuscitated.** Underresuscitation may result in inadequate organ perfusion and potential for wound conversion from partial- to full-thickness. Overresuscitation may lead to severe pulmonary edema, excessive wound edema causing a decrease in perfusion of unburned tissue in the distal portions of the extremities, and edema impeding perfusion of the zone of stasis, causing wound conversion.

Renal Management

If fluid resuscitation is inadequate, acute renal failure may occur. **A Foley catheter is placed to monitor renal per-** fusion and effectiveness of fluid resuscitation. Nurses should measure urine output hourly. For thermal injuries, adequate urine output is 30 to 50 ml/hr.[8]

Gastrointestinal Management

Patients with burns of more than 20% body surface area (BSA) are prone to gastric dilation as a result of paralytic ileus. Nasogastric tubes are placed in these patients to prevent abdominal distention, emesis, and potential aspiration. This decrease in gastrointestinal function is caused by a combination of the effect of hypovolemia and the neurologic and endocrine response to injury. Gastrointestinal activity usually returns in 24 to 48 hours.

Curling's ulcer is the major gastrointestinal complication. Its incidence varies widely. In a clinical survey of 2700 patients, the incidence is reported to be as low as 0.3%. In postmortem studies the incidence is approximately 25%, and the clinical incidence is about 10%.[9]

With the advent of histamine H_2-receptor antagonists and improved management of the early shock period, including early enteral feedings, the incidence of Curling's ulcer has been decreasing over the last decade.

Because an ulceration can occur as early as 96 hours after the burn, attempts to reduce the acidity of gastric contents should be implemented during the resuscitation period. The placement of a nasogastric tube is necessary. Antacids such as magnesium and aluminum hydroxides (Maalox) are administered every 2 to 6 hours, to maintain the pH of gastric aspirate above 4, and the rate of administration can be increased if the pH level is not maintained. An excessive amount of Maalox may form a bezoar and cause obstruction. In unintubated patients who can eat, the nasogastric tube should be removed as soon as bowel function is regained. Enteral tube feeding is effective in maintaining gastric pH above 5. Stress ulcers in patients with more than 50% TBSA are caused by the stress of the burn itself, but stress ulcers in patients with less than 50% TBSA are caused predominantly by sepsis.[10]

Pain Management

Pain is assessed frequently. Morphine sulphate is indicated for pain management; however, narcotics should be administered intravenously only in small doses. Changes in fluid volume and fluid shifts make the absorption of any drug given intramuscularly or subcutaneously unpredictable.

Extremity Pulse Assessment

In cases of circumferential extremity burns, arterial blood flow must be assessed frequently. Edema that develops beneath the eschar initially obstructs venous return. If this is not corrected, arterial flow is reduced to a level resulting in ischemia, necrosis, and eventually gangrene. Early signs include numbness and pain in the extremity. When venous return is interrupted, an escharotomy, or surgical incision into burned tissue to relieve pressure, is indicated. Nurses assess blood flow with an ultrasonic Doppler device.

Laboratory Assessment

Initial laboratory studies are performed, including determination of levels of hematocrit, electrolytes, and blood urea nitrogen; urinalysis; and chest roentgenogram. Special situations warrant arterial blood gas, carboxyhemoglobin, and alcohol and drug screens. An electrocardiogram (ECG) is obtained for all patients with electrical burns or preexisting cardiac problems.

Wound Care

Once the wounds have been assessed during emergency care, topical antimicrobial therapy is not a priority. **The wounds should be covered with clean, dry dressings or sheets. Every attempt should be made to keep patients warm because of the high risk for hypothermia.**

Special Management Considerations

Inhalation Injury

Inhalation injury can occur in the presence or absence of cutaneous injury. Inhalation injuries are usually associated with burns sustained in a closed space. Smoke inhalation accounts for 20% to 30% of burn center admissions and 60% to 70% of burn center fatalities.[7] Inhalation injury appears in three basic forms, alone or in combination: carbon monoxide poisoning, direct heat injury, and chemical damage. In the strict sense, carbon monoxide poisoning is not an injury but an intoxication.[7] Three distinguishable types of inhalation injury exist: carbon monoxide poisoning, upper airway injury, and lower airway injury. Immediate measures to save the lives of burn patients include management of the airway. Burn patients may present few if any signs of airway distress; however, thermal injury to the airway should be anticipated if patients exhibit facial burns, singed eyebrows and nasal hair, carbon deposits in the oropharynx, and carbonaceous sputum or if the history suggests confinement in a burning environment. Any of these findings indicates acute inhalation injury and requires immediate and definitive care. The use of early intubation and respiratory support should be considered before tracheal edema occurs to prevent the necessity of tracheostomy or cricothyrotomy.

Carbon monoxide poisoning

Persons found dead at the scene of a fire often have little or no cutaneous thermal injury but have died of carbon monoxide poisoning. Carbon monoxide is a colorless, odorless, and tasteless gas. It binds with hemoglobin at the expense of hemoglobin's oxygen-carrying capacity, and the affinity of hemoglobin molecules for carbon monoxide is approximately 200 times that for oxygen. Carboxyhemoglobin binds poorly with oxygen, reducing the oxygen-carrying capacity of blood and causing hypoxia. The major clinical manifestations of severe carbon monoxide poisoning are related to the central nervous system and the heart. Measurement of arterial oxygen tension is of no value because oxygen tension may be quite high in the presence of a dangerously low oxygen content of carbon monoxide–saturated hemoglobin. The most reliable treatment of carbon monoxide poisoning consists of 100% oxygen administration by a tight-fitting mask or endotracheal tube if patients are unresponsive. Carboxyhemoglobin levels of 40% to 60% frequently produce unresponsiveness or obtundation; levels of 15% to 40% may manifest central nervous system dysfunction of varying degrees, and levels of less than 15% are often found in cigarette smokers and are rarely symptomatic.[7]

Upper airway injury

Burns of the upper respiratory tract include those involving the pharynx, larynx, glottis, trachea, and larger bronchi. Injuries are caused by either direct heat or chemical inflammation and necrosis. Except for rare events, respiratory injury is confined to the upper airway. The heat exchange capability is so efficient that most heat absorption and damage occur in the pharynx and larynx above the true vocal cords.

Heat damage is often severe enough to cause upper airway destruction, which may also cause destruction at any time during the resuscitation. Caution is taken for patients with severe hypovolemia because supraglottic edema may be delayed until fluid resuscitation is underway. Patients should be monitored for hoarseness, stridor, audible air-flow turbulence, and the production of carbonaceous sputum.

Lower airway injury

Heated air rarely causes lower airway injury. If it does, it is usually associated with death at the scene. Lower airway injuries may also be caused by chemical damage to mucosal surfaces. Tracheobronchitis with severe spasm and wheezing may occur in the first minutes to hours after injury. The most accurate method of documenting lower airway injury is the xenon–ventilation-perfusion lung scan. Prolonged retention or asymmetry of washout of the radioisotope indicates pulmonary parenchymal injury on the side of the retained emissions.[11] Treatment is largely symptomatic. The fiberoptic bronchoscope is used in the diagnosis and management of inhalation injury associated with complications. The burn surgeon diagnoses inhalation injury by bronchoscopic examination. The onset of symptoms is so unpredictable with possible smoke inhalation that patients at risk must be closely observed for at least 24 to 48 hours.

Nonthermal Burns

Chemical burns

In the past the irrigation of acid, alkali, and organic compound burns with neutralizing solutions was recommended to limit the extent and depth of chemical burns.

Neutralizing agents, however, may cause reactions that are exothermic—that is, heat producing—thereby increasing the extent and depth of the burn. The neutralizing agent may not be immediately known or available. Therefore the use of large amounts of water to flush the area is recommended. Alkali burns of the eyes require continuous irrigation for many hours after the injury. Once the chemical agent has been diluted, more individualized treatment can be initiated to reduce systemic absorption of the toxin.

Phenol burns are first diluted, and then the skin is wiped quickly with polyethylene glycol or vegetable oil to decrease the severity of the burn. Areas exposed to hydrofluoric acid should also be copiously irrigated with water; the burned area can then be treated with 2.5% calcium gluconate gel. Patients may need calcium gluconate replacements because the fluoride ion precipitates serum calcium, causing hypocalcemia. White phosphorous can

ignite if kept dry; therefore wounds must be covered with moist dressings.[6]

After a tar or asphalt injury, the removal of tar and asphalt is best accomplished with the use of bacitracin or Neosporin ointment. The tar should not be peeled off because of potential damage to the involved hair and skin.

Daily wound care, consisting of débridement of loose skin and tar, followed by application of an antibiotic-containing emollient, is preferable. All chemical wounds are treated with appropriate topical therapy once the chemical has been diluted, neutralized, or removed.

Electrical burns

In electrical burns the type and voltage of the circuit, resistance, pathway of transmission through the body, and duration of contact should be considered in determining the amount of damage sustained. Frequently in these

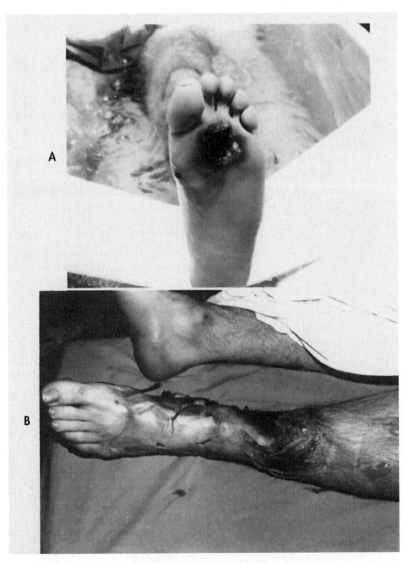

FIG. 24-5 A, Exit site of electrical burn on sole of foot. **B,** Same leg several days later, illustrating extension of tissue damage after the injury.

situations, rescuers may also sustain injuries if they become part of the electrical circuit. Rescuers must disconnect the electrical source to break the circuit or must know the way not to become part of the circuit. The use of appropriately insulated equipment that diverts the circuit elsewhere is essential. Extreme caution should be used in the rescue of victims.

Electricity always travels toward the ground. It travels most quickly through the circulatory system and through nerves, muscles, the integumentary system, and finally bone. Electrical burns are frequently much more serious than their surface appearance suggests. As the electrical current passes through the body, it damages the inner tissues and may leave little evidence of a burn on the skin surface (Fig. 24-5).

The electrical burn process can result in a profound alteration in acid-base balance and the production of myoglobinuria, which poses a serious threat to renal functioning. Fluid resuscitation does not correlate with the Parkland formula, and the fluid is adjusted according to urine output. If hemochromogen is present in the urine, a urine output of 100 to 150 ml/hr is established until the urine clears of all gross pigment. Myoglobin is a normal constituent of muscle; with extensive muscle destruction, it is released into the circulatory system and filtered by the kidney. It can be highly toxic and can lead to intrinsic renal failure.

The immediate management of an electrical burn includes placement of a large-bore intravenous (IV) line and Foley catheter to monitor kidney function. In the presence of hemoglobinuria, nurses must assume that myoglobinuria and acidosis are present. Sodium bicarbonate may be administered to bring the pH into normal range, correct a documented acidosis, and alkalize urine to promote myoglobin excretion. Mannitol may also be administered intravenously until the qualitative myoglobinuria disappears. A baseline ECG and cardiac enzyme levels are obtained while patients are in the emergency department.

Burn Management

Management of patients with burn injuries can be divided into three phases: resuscitation, acute care, and rehabilitation. Each phase is unique and has its own set of actual and potential problems. (Specific priority interventions for each phase are listed in Box 24-2. Nursing diagnosis priorities for burn injury are found in Box 24-3).

Resuscitation Phase

The resuscitation phase, or shock phase, of burn injury is characterized by cardiopulmonary instability, life-threatening airway and breathing problems, and hypovolemia. Every organ is involved in the physiologic response that occurs with thermal injury. The magnitude of this pathophysiologic response is proportional to the extent of cutaneous injury, which is maximal when approximately 60% of the total BSA is burned.[12]

After thermal injury, a marked increase in capillary hydrostatic pressure occurs in the injured tissue early in the postinjury phase. Later an increase in capillary permeability occurs, which returns toward normal during the latter half of the first 24 hours. A marked increase in pe-

---

BOX 24-2

PRIORITY INTERVENTIONS FOR THE SHOCK, ACUTE, AND REHABILITATIVE PHASES OF BURN MANAGEMENT

SHOCK PHASE

Treatment for inhalation injury
Airway management
Fluid resuscitation
Maintenance of tissue perfusion: renal, cerebral, peripheral, gastrointestinal
Thermoregulation

ACUTE PHASE

Early wound excision and skin graft procedures
Local wound care
Nutritional support
Infection control
Pain management
Emotional support

REHABILITATIVE PHASE

Physical remobilization
Continued wound care
Reconstructive surgery
Resocialization into lifestyle

BOX 24-3

NURSING DIAGNOSIS PRIORITIES

BURN INJURY

- *Impaired Gas Exchange* related to ventilation/perfusion mismatch secondary to inhalation injury, p. 488
- *Fluid Volume Deficit* related to active plasma loss and fluid shift into interstitium secondary to burns, p. 505
- *Risk for Infection* risk factors: invasive lines, immunodeficiencies, p. 482
- *Sensory/Perceptual Alterations* related to sensory overload, sensory deprivation, sleep pattern disturbance, p. 466
- *Body Image Disturbance* related to actual change in body structure, function, or appearance, p. 458

ripheral vascular resistance, accompanied by a decrease in cardiac output, is one of the earliest manifestations of the systemic effects of thermal injury. Organ hypoperfusion develops as a result of low cardiac output and increased peripheral vascular resistance caused by the normal neurohormonal response to trauma. With adequate volume repletion, hemodynamic functions improve, and as plasma volume increases, cardiac output rises, resulting in a hyperdynamic state and overall increase in organ perfusion.

These initial changes appear to be unrelated to hypovolemia and have been attributed to neurogenic and humoral effects.[1] These alterations result in the formation of edema within the wound. This progressive loss of fluid may result in significant intravascular fluid volume deficit. With adequate volume repletion, hemodynamic performance improves, and as plasma volume increases during the second 24 hours, cardiac output increases to supernormal levels, characteristic of the hypermetabolic response to injury.

Acute Care Phase

The acute care phase of burn management begins after resuscitation and lasts until complete wound closure is achieved. The early postresuscitation phase is a period of transition from the shock phase to the hypermetabolic phase. Major cardiopulmonary and wound changes occur that substantially alter the manner of patient care from that during resuscitation. In general, cardiopulmonary stability is optimal during this period because wound inflammation and infection have not developed. Hypermetabolic changes, however, may become complicated with the onset of wound infection and sepsis. Early wound excision and skin grafting procedures, local wound care, nutritional support, and infection control characterize this phase.

Inflammatory phase

The inflammatory phase begins immediately after injury. This period is characterized by vascular changes and cellular activity. Cooper[13] explains that changes in the severed vessels occur in an attempt to wall the wound off from the external environment. Platelets, activated as a result of vessel wall injury, aggregate; blood coagulation is initiated; and in larger vessels, smooth muscle tissue contraction occurs, resulting in reduction in the diameter of the vessel lumen. These brief but important compensatory mechanisms protect the entire organism from excessive blood loss and increased exposure to bacterial contamination.[13] As vasodilation occurs, vascular permeability and blood supply to the wound site increase. As extravascular volume increases, signs of erythema, edema, and tenderness become apparent. Granulocytes invade the wound within 24 hours and initiate the phagocytosis of necrotic tissue and bacteria. Fibroblasts migrate to the wound and multiply, producing a bed of collagen. This

phase of healing lasts from the moment of injury to 3 or 4 days after the traumatic event.

Proliferative phase

This phase of healing occurs approximately 4 to 20 days after injury. The key cell in this phase of healing, the fibroblast, rapidly synthesizes collagen. Collagen synthesis provides the needed strength for a healing wound. Epithelial cells migrate across the wound bed. Once these cells contact each other, the wound is covered. This process is known as *epithelialization*. Myofibroblasts also play a role in healing by pulling down the wound edge toward the center in an effort to close the wound; this process is known as *wound contraction*.

Maturation phase

This phase of healing occurs from approximately 20 days after injury to longer than 1 year after injury. During this period the wound develops tensile strength as collagen deposits form scar tissue. Regardless of how well collagen realigns itself, the tissue of the wound will never regain the degree of strength or intactness inherent in uninjured tissue. Over time, scar tissue matures and becomes smaller and less bulky, and pigmentation returns.

Rehabilitation Phase

The rehabilitation phase is one of recuperation and healing, both physically and emotionally. Patients are not acutely ill but may not be ready for discharge. This phase can last several years. Patients may require extensive reconstructive surgery. Psychologically, patients focus on attaining specific personal goals related to achieving as much preburn function as possible.[14] Nurses should praise minor and major accomplishments. The rehabilitation phase is characterized by scar management techniques and physical and occupational therapy. The burn team helps patients prepare themselves for the transition to the outside world. Group therapy is a valuable tool used at many burn centers. Patients, family members, and health care providers express ideas and feelings. Many times, burn patients establish priorities and make realistic decisions about their lives. Staff intervention during this phase is primarily supportive.

References

1. Demling RH, LaLonde C: *Burn trauma*, ed 9, New York, 1989, Thieme Medical Publishers.
2. Feller I, Crane KL, Flanders S: Baseline data on the mortality of burn patients, *QRB* 5:4, 1979.
3. Feller I, Jones CA: The National Burn Information Exchange, *Surg Clin North Am* 67:167, 1987.
4. Moncrief JA: *The body's response to heat*. In Artz CP, Moncrief JA, Pruitt BA Jr, editors: *Burns: a team approach*, Philadelphia, 1979, WB Saunders.
5. Finkelstein JL and others: Management of electrical injuries, *Inf Surg* 10: 43, 1990.

6. Madden MR and others: The acute management and surgical treatment of the burned patient. I. *Surg Rounds* 6:41-49, 1990.

7. Madden MR, Finkelstein JL, Goodwin CW Jr: Respiratory care of the burn patient, *Clin Plast Surg* 13(1):29, 1986.

8. Nebraska Burn Institute: *Advanced burn life support (ABLS) course* (first rev), Lincoln, 1990, Nebraska Burn Institute.

9. McConnell CM, Hummel RP: Perforating Curling's ulcer: a rare but lethal complication, *Burns* 7:203-207, 1980.

10. Martyn JAJ: *Acute management of the burned patient*, Philadelphia, 1990, WB Saunders.

11. Agee RN and others: Use of 133-xenon in early diagnosis of inhalation injury, *J Trauma* 16:218, 1976.

12. Pruitt BA Jr: The universal trauma model, *Bull Am Coll Surg* 70:2, 1985.

13. Cooper D: Optimizing wound healing: a practice within nursing domain, *Nurs Clin North Am* 25(1):165, 1990.

14. Watkins PN, Cook EL, May SR: A method for facilitating psychological recovery of burn victims, *J Burn Care Rehabil* 9:376, 1986.

Shock and Multiple Organ Dysfunction Syndrome

KATHLEEN M. STACY & LORRAINE FITZSIMMONS

CHAPTER OBJECTIVES

- Describe the generalized shock response.
- List the etiologies of hypovolemic, cardiogenic, anaphylactic, neurogenic, and septic shock and multiple organ dysfunction syndrome.
- Explain the pathophysiology of hypovolemic, cardiogenic, anaphylactic, neurogenic, and septic shock and multiple organ dysfunction syndrome.
- Identify the clinical manifestations of hypovolemic, cardiogenic, anaphylactic, neurogenic, and septic shock and multiple organ dysfunction syndrome.

- Outline the important aspects of the medical management of hypovolemic, cardiogenic, anaphylactic, neurogenic, and septic shock and multiple organ dysfunction syndrome.
- Summarize the nursing management of patients with hypovolemic, cardiogenic, anaphylactic, neurogenic, and septic shock and multiple organ dysfunction syndrome.

KEY TERMS

Shock is an acute, widespread process of impaired tissue perfusion that results in cellular, metabolic, and hemodynamic derangements. Impaired tissue perfusion occurs when an imbalance develops between cellular oxygen supply and cellular oxygen demand. This imbalance can occur for a variety of reasons and eventually results in cellular dysfunction and multiple organ dysfunction syndrome (MODS). This chapter presents an overview of the general shock response, or shock syndrome, followed by a discussion of the different shock states and MODS.

Shock Syndrome

Description and Etiology

Shock is a complex pathophysiologic process that often results in MODS and death. All types of shock eventually result in impaired tissue perfusion and the development of acute circulatory failure, or shock syndrome. Shock syndrome is a generalized systemic response to inadequate tissue perfusion.[1,2] It consists of four different stages: initial, compensatory, progressive, and refractory.[3] Progression through each stage varies depending on patients' prior conditions, duration of initiating events, responses to therapy, and correction of underlying cause.[4]

Shock can be classified as hypovolemic, cardiogenic, or distributive, depending on the pathophysiologic cause. Hypovolemic shock results from a loss of circulating or intravascular volume. Cardiogenic shock results from the impaired ability of the heart to pump. Distributive shock results from maldistribution of circulating blood volume and can be further classified as septic, anaphylactic, and neurogenic. Septic shock is the result of microorganisms entering the body. Anaphylactic shock is the result of a severe antibody-antigen reaction. Neurogenic shock is caused by loss of sympathetic tone.[5,6]

Pathophysiology

During the **initial stage,** cardiac output (CO) is decreased and tissue perfusion is impaired. As the blood supply to the cells decreases, the cells' energy source changes from aerobic to anaerobic metabolism. Anaerobic metabolism produces small amounts of energy but large amounts of lactic acid. Lactic acidemia quickly develops and causes more cellular damage.[3,7]

During the **compensatory stage,** the body's homeostatic mechanisms attempt to improve tissue perfusion. The compensatory mechanisms are mediated by the sympathetic nervous system (SNS) and consist of neural, hormonal, and chemical responses. Neural compensation includes an increase in heart rate (HR) and contractility, arterial and venous vasoconstriction, and shunting of blood to the vital organs. Hormonal compensation includes activation of the renin response and stimulation of the anterior pituitary and adrenal medulla. Activation of the renin response results in the production of angio-

tensin II, which causes vasoconstriction and the release of aldosterone and antidiuretic hormone (ADH), leading to sodium and water retention. Stimulation of the anterior pituitary results in the secretion of adrenocorticotropic hormone (ACTH), which stimulates the adrenal cortex to produce glucocorticoids, causing a rise in blood glucose levels. Stimulation of the adrenal medulla causes the release of epinephrine and norepinephrine, which further enhances the compensatory mechanisms. Chemical compensation includes hyperventilation to neutralize lactic acidosis.[3,4,7]

During the **progressive stage,** the compensatory mechanisms start to fail and the shock cycle is perpetuated. At the cellular level, the small amount of energy created by anaerobic metabolism is not enough to keep the cell functional, and irreversible damage begins to occur. The sodium-potassium pump in the cell membrane fails, causing the cell and its organelles to swell. Cellular energy production comes to a complete halt as the mitochondria swell and rupture. At this point the problem becomes one of oxygen utilization instead of oxygen delivery. Even if the cell were to receive more oxygen, it would be unable to use it because of damage to the mitochondria. The cell's digestive organelles swell, resulting in leakage of destructive enzymes into the cell. Autodigestion occurs with ensuing cell death.[7] Every system in the body is affected by this process.

During the **refractory stage,** shock becomes unresponsive to therapy and is considered irreversible. As the individual organ systems die, *MODS,* defined as failure of two or more body systems, occurs. Death is the final outcome.[3] Regardless of etiologic factors, death occurs from impaired tissue perfusion because of the failure of circulation to meet the oxygen needs of the cell.[1,2]

Assessment and Diagnosis

Clinical manifestations differ according to etiologic factors and the stage of the shock. They are related to both the cause of the shock and patients' general responses to shock.[8] (See sections on individual shock states for a discussion of clinical assessment and diagnosis of patients in shock.)

Medical Management

The major focus of the treatment of shock is improvement and preservation of tissue perfusion. Adequate tissue perfusion depends on an adequate supply of oxygen being transported to the tissues and on the cell's ability to use it. Pulmonary gas exchange, CO, and hemoglobin level influence oxygen transport. Oxygen utilization is influenced by the internal metabolic environment. Management of patients in shock focuses on supporting oxygen transport and oxygen utilization.[1,2]

Adequate pulmonary gas exchange is critical to oxygen transport. Establishing and maintaining an adequate airway are the first steps in ensuring adequate oxygenation. Once the airway is patent, emphasis is placed on improving ventilation and oxygenation. Therapies include administration of supplemental oxygen and mechanical ventilation.[7,9]

An adequate CO and hemoglobin level are crucial to oxygen transport. CO depends on HR, preload, afterload, and contractility. A variety of fluids and drugs are used to manipulate these parameters. The types of fluids used include both crystalloids and colloids. The categories of drugs used include vasoconstrictors, vasodilators, positive inotropes, and antidysrhythmic agents.[7]

Indicated for decreased preload related to intravascular volume depletion, fluid administration can be accomplished by use of either a crystalloid or colloid solution, or both. Crystalloids are balanced electrolyte solutions that may be hypotonic, isotonic, or hypertonic. Examples of crystalloid solutions are normal saline, lactated Ringer's solution, and 5% dextrose in water. Colloids are protein- or starch-containing solutions. Examples of colloid solutions are blood and blood components and pharmaceutic plasma expanders such as hetastarch, dextran, and mannitol. The choice of fluid depends on the situation. Advantages of colloids include faster restoration of intravascular volume and effectiveness with smaller amounts. Colloids stay in the intravascular space, unlike crystalloids, which readily leak into the extravascular space. Disadvantages include expense, allergic reactions, and difficulties in typing and crossmatching blood. Colloids can also leak out of damaged capillaries and cause a variety of additional problems, particularly in the lungs.[7,9-12] Blood should be used to augment oxygen transport if patients' hemoglobin levels are low.[1]

Vasoconstrictor agents are used to increase afterload by increasing the systemic vascular resistance (SVR) and improving blood pressure level. Vasodilator agents are used to decrease preload, afterload, or both by decreasing venous return and SVR. Positive inotropic agents are used to increase contractility. Antidysrhythmic agents are used to influence HR. Box 25-1 provides examples of each of these agents.[7,9,13]

An optimal metabolic environment is important to oxygen utilization. Once the oxygen is delivered to the cells, they must be able to use it. The major metabolic derangement seen in shock is lactic acidosis. Interventions to correct lactic acidosis include correcting the cause, reestablishing perfusion, inducing hyperventilation, and in severe cases, administering sodium bicarbonate.[14] The role of sodium bicarbonate in the treatment of acidosis is controversial and usually reserved for severe cases that are refractory to other treatments because of some associated risks. These risks include rebound increase in lactic acid production, development of hyperosmolar state, and fluid overload resulting from excessive sodium, shifting of the oxyhemoglobin curve to the left, and rapid cellular electrolyte shifts.[15] Patients should also begin nutritional support therapy. The type of nutritional supplementation varies according to the cause of shock and should be tailored to patients' needs as indicated by underlying conditions and laboratory data.

B O X   2 5 - 1

EXAMPLES OF THE DIFFERENT AGENTS USED IN THE TREATMENT OF SHOCK

VASOCONSTRICTORS

Epinephrine (Adrenalin)
Norepinephrine (Levophed)
Alpha-range dopamine (Intropin)
Metaraminol (Aramine)
Phenylephrine (Neo-Synephrine)
Ephedrine

VASODILATORS

Nitroprusside (Nipride, Nitropress)
Nitroglycerine (Nitrol, Tridil)
Hydralazine (Apresoline)
Labetalol (Normodyne, Trandate)

INOTROPES

Beta-range dopamine (Intropin)
Dobutamine (Dobutrex)
Amrinone (Inocor)
Epinephrine (Adrenalin)
Isuproterenol (Isuprel)
Norepinephrine (Levephed)
Digoxin (Lanoxin)

ANTIDYSRHYTHMICS

Lidocaine (Xylocaine)
Bretylium (Bretylol)
Procainamide (Pronestyl)
Labetalol (Normodyne, Trandate)
Verapamil (Calan, Isoptin)
Esmolol (Brevibloc)
Diltiazem (Cardizem)

The enteral route is generally preferred over the parenteral.[16]

Nursing Management

Nursing management of patients in shock is a complex and challenging responsibility. It requires an in-depth understanding of the pathophysiology of the disease and anticipated effects of each intervention as well as a solid understanding of the nursing process.[17] (Sections on individual shock states contain separate discussions of specific interventions for patients in shock.)

Hypovolemic Shock

Description and Etiology

Hypovolemic shock occurs from inadequate fluid volume in the intravascular space. The lack of adequate circulating volume leads to decreased tissue perfusion and ini-

Etiologic Factors in Hypovolemic Shock

ABSOLUTE

Loss of whole blood
  Trauma
  Surgery
  Gastrointestinal bleeding
Loss of plasma
  Thermal injuries
  Large lesions
Loss of other body fluids
  Severe vomiting
  Severe diarrhea
  Massive diuresis

RELATIVE

Loss of intravascular integrity
  Ruptured spleen
  Long bone or pelvic fractures
  Hemorrhagic pancreatitis
  Hemothorax or hemoperitoneum
  Arterial dissection
Increased capillary membrane permeability
  Sepsis
  Anaphylaxis
  Thermal injuries
Decreased colloidal osmotic pressure
  Severe sodium depletion
  Hypopituitarism
  Cirrhosis
  Intestinal obstruction

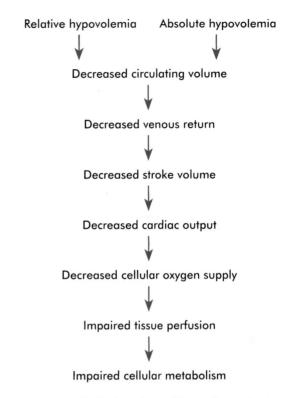

FIG. 25-1 Pathophysiology of hypovolemic shock.

tiation of the general shock response. Hypovolemic shock is the most commonly occurring form of shock.[3,12]

Hypovolemic shock can result from either absolute or relative hypovolemia. Absolute hypovolemia occurs when there is an external loss of fluid from the body, including losses of whole blood, plasma, or any other body fluid. Relative hypovolemia occurs when there is an internal shifting of fluid from the intravascular space to the extravascular space. This can result from a loss in intravascular integrity, increased capillary membrane permeability, or decreased colloidal osmotic pressure (Box 25-2).[3,12]

Pathophysiology

Hypovolemia results in a loss of circulating fluid volume. A decrease in circulating volume leads to a decrease in venous return, which results in decreased end-diastolic volume or preload. Preload is a major determinant of stroke volume (SV) and CO. A decrease in preload results in a decrease in SV and CO. The decrease in CO leads to inadequate cellular oxygen supply and impaired tissue perfusion (Fig. 25-1).[3,12]

Assessment and Diagnosis

The clinical manifestations of hypovolemic shock vary depending on the severity of fluid loss and patients' ability to compensate for it. The first, or initial, stage occurs with a fluid volume loss up to 15% or an actual volume loss up to 750 ml. Compensatory mechanisms maintain CO, and patients appear symptom free.[6,10,12]

The second, or compensatory, stage occurs with a fluid volume loss of 15% to 30% or an actual volume loss of 750 to 1500 ml.[10] CO falls, resulting in the initiation of a variety of compensatory responses. The HR increases in response to increased SNS stimulation. The pulse pressure narrows as the diastolic blood pressure increases because of vasoconstriction. Respiratory rate and depth increase in an attempt to improve oxygenation. Arterial blood gas (ABG) specimens drawn during this phase reveal respiratory alkalosis and hypoxemia, as evidenced by a low $PaCO_2$ and a low PaO_2, respectively. Urine output starts to decline as renal perfusion decreases. Urine sodium decreases while urine osmolarity and specific gravity increase as the kidneys start to conserve sodium and water. Patients' skin becomes pale and cool, with delayed capillary refill because of peripheral vasoconstriction. Jugular veins appear flat as a result of decreased venous return. Decreased cerebral perfusion causes a change in level of sensorium. Patients may appear disoriented, confused, restless, anxious, and irritable.[8,10,12]

The third, or progressive, stage occurs with a fluid volume loss of 30% to 40% or an actual volume loss of 1500 to 2000 ml.[10,12] The compensatory mechanisms become overwhelmed, and impaired tissue perfusion develops. The HR continues to increase, and dysrhythmias develop as myocardial ischemia ensues. Respiratory distress occurs as the pulmonary system deteriorates. ABG values during this phase reveal respiratory and metabolic acidosis and hypoxemia, as evidenced by a high $Paco_2$, low bicarbonate (HCO_3^-), and low Pao_2, respectively. Decreased renal perfusion results in the development of oliguria. Blood urea nitrogen and serum creatinine levels start to rise as the kidneys begin to fail. Patients' skin becomes ashen, cold, and clammy, with a marked delay in capillary refill. Patients appear lethargic as cerebral perfusion decreases and their level of consciousness continues to deteriorate.[8,10,12]

The fourth, or refractory, stage occurs with a fluid volume loss of greater than 40% or an actual volume loss of more than 2000 ml.[10] The compensatory mechanisms completely deteriorate, and organ failure occurs. Severe tachycardia and hypotension ensue. Peripheral pulses are absent, and because of marked peripheral vasoconstriction, capillary refill does not occur. The skin appears cyanotic, mottled, and extremely diaphoretic. Patients become unresponsive, and a variety of clinical manifestations associated with failure of the different body systems develop.[10,12]

Assessment of the hemodynamic parameters of patients in hypovolemic shock reveals a decreased CO and cardiac index (CI). Loss of circulation volume leads to a decrease in venous return to the heart, which results in a decrease in the preload of the right and left ventricles. This is evidenced by a decline in the right atrial pressure (RAP) and pulmonary artery wedge pressure (PAWP). Vasoconstriction of the arterial system results in an increase in the afterload of the heart, as evidenced by an increase in the SVR.[8,12]

Medical Management

The major goals of therapy are to correct the cause of the hypovolemia and restore tissue perfusion. This approach includes identifying and stopping the source of fluid loss and vigorously administering fluid to replace circulating volume. Fluids are administered with use of either a crystalloid or colloid solution or a combination of both. The type of solution used usually depends on the type of fluid lost.[9-12]

Two other therapies available for assisting with resuscitation of patients in hypovolemic shock are autotransfusion and the pneumatic antishock garment (PASG). Particularly useful in managing patients with hypovolemic shock caused by chest trauma and hemorrhage,[18] autotransfusion is the collection and administration of patients' own blood. PASG, also known as *military antishock trousers,* is a one-piece suit with three individually controlled compartments: one for the abdomen and one for each leg. When inflated, the PASG acts as a vaso-

---

BOX 25-3

NURSING DIAGNOSIS PRIORITIES

HYPOVOLEMIC SHOCK

- *Fluid Volume Deficit* related to active blood loss, p. 503
- *Decreased Cardiac Output* related to decreased preload, p. 476
- *Anxiety* related to threat to biologic, psychologic, and/or social integrity, p. 464

---

constrictor to improve blood pressure and augments venous return to improve preload.[19]

Nursing Management

Preventive measures include the identification of patients at risk and constant assessment of patients' fluid balance. Accurate monitoring of intake, output, and daily weights are essential components of preventive nursing care. Early identification and treatment result in decreased mortality rates.[20]

Patients with hypovolemic shock may have any number of nursing diagnoses, depending on the progression of the process (Box 25-3). **Nursing priorities are directed toward minimizing fluid loss, enhancing volume replacement, and monitoring patients' responses to care.** Measures to minimize fluid loss include limiting blood sampling, observing lines for accidental disconnection, and applying direct pressure to bleeding sites. Measures to enhance volume replacement include insertion of large-diameter peripheral intravenous catheters, rapid administration of prescribed fluids, and positioning of patients with their legs elevated, trunk flat, and head and shoulders above the chest. In addition, monitoring patients for clinical manifestations of fluid overload is critical to preventing further problems.[20]

Cardiogenic Shock

Description and Etiology

Cardiogenic shock occurs when the heart fails to pump blood forward effectively. It can occur with dysfunction of the right or left ventricle, or both. The lack of adequate pumping function leads to decreased tissue perfusion and initiation of the general shock response.[5,21,22] Cardiogenic shock occurs in approximately 15% of patients with an acute myocardial infarction (MI), and the mortality rate is 75% to 95%.[6]

Cardiogenic shock can result from primary ventricular ischemia, structural problems, and dysrhythmias. The most common cause is acute MI resulting in the loss of 40% or more of the functional myocardium. Damage to the myocardium may occur after one massive MI or may

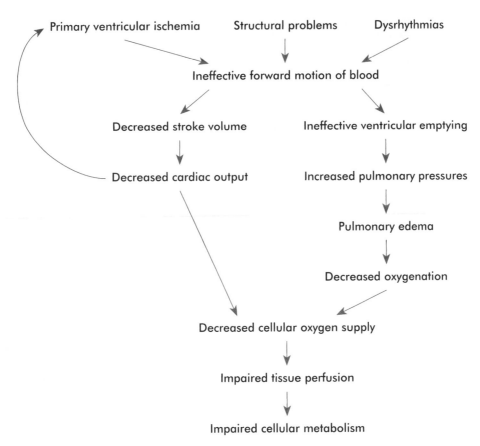

FIG. 25-2   Pathophysiology of cardiogenic shock.

BOX 25-4

ETIOLOGIC FACTORS IN CARDIOGENIC SHOCK

Primary ventricular ischemia
  Acute myocardial infarction
  Cardiopulmonary arrest
  Open heart surgery
Structural problems
  Septal rupture
  Papillary muscle rupture
  Free wall rupture
  Ventricular aneurysm
  Cardiomyopathies
    Congestive
    Hypertrophic
    Restrictive
  Intracardiac tumor
  Pulmonary embolus
  Atrial thrombus
  Valvular dysfunction
  Acute myocarditis
  Cardiac tamponade
  Myocardial contusion
Dysrhythmias
  Bradydysrhythmias
  Tachydysrhythmias

---

be the cumulative result of several smaller MIs.[5,21,23] Structural problems of the cardiopulmonary system and dysrhythmias may also cause cardiogenic shock if they disrupt the forward motion of the blood through the heart (Box 25-4).[3,22,23]

Pathophysiology

Cardiogenic shock results from the impaired ability of the ventricle to pump blood forward, which leads to a decrease in SV and an increase in the blood left in the ventricle at the end of systole. The decrease in SV results in a decrease in CO, which leads to decreased cellular oxygen supply and impaired tissue perfusion. When the underlying problem involves the left ventricle, the increase in end-systolic volume results in the backup of blood into the pulmonary system and the subsequent development of pulmonary edema. Pulmonary edema causes impaired gas exchange and decreased oxygenation of the arterial blood, which further impairs tissue perfusion (Fig. 25-2). Death may result from cardiopulmonary collapse.[5,21-23]

Assessment and Diagnosis

A variety of clinical manifestations occur when patients experience cardiogenic shock depending on etiologic factors in pump failure, patients' underlying medical status,

BOX 25-5

CLINICAL MANIFESTATIONS OF CARDIOGENIC SHOCK

Systolic blood pressure <90 mm Hg
HR >100 beats/min
Weak, thready pulse
Diminished heart sounds
Change in sensorium
Cool, pale, moist skin
UO <30 ml/hr
Chest pain
Dysrhythmias
Tachypnea
Crackles
Decreased CO
CI <1.8 L/m/m^2
Increased PAWP
Increased RAP
Increased SVR

and the severity of the shock state. Some clinical manifestations are caused by failure of the heart as a pump, whereas many relate to the overall shock response (Box 25-5).

Initially the clinical manifestations relate to the decline in CO. These signs and symptoms include systolic blood pressure less than 90 mm Hg; decreased sensorium; cool, pale, moist skin; and urinary output less than 30 ml/hr. Patients may also complain of chest pain. Once the compensatory mechanisms are activated, tachycardia develops to compensate for the fall in CO. A weak, thready pulse develops, and heart sounds may reveal a diminished S_1 and S_2 because of the decrease in contractility. Respiratory rate increases to improve oxygenation. ABG values at this time indicate respiratory alkalosis, as evidenced by a decrease in $Paco_2$. Urinalysis findings demonstrate a decrease in urine sodium and an increase in urine osmolarity and specific gravity as the kidneys start to conserve sodium and water. Patients may also experience a variety of dysrhythmias depending on the underlying problem.[8,21,22]

In patients with left ventricular failure a variety of additional clinical manifestations may be seen. Auscultation of the lungs may disclose crackles and wheezes, indicating the development of pulmonary edema. Hypoxemia occurs, as evidenced by a fall in Pao_2 as measured by ABG values. Heart sounds may reveal an S_3 and S_4. If right-sided failure occurs, jugular venous distention may become evident.[21,22]

Once the compensatory mechanisms become overwhelmed and impaired tissue perfusion develops, a variety of other clinical manifestations appear. Myocardial ischemia progresses, as evidenced by continued increases in HR, dysrhythmias, and chest pain. The pulmonary system starts to deteriorate, which leads to respiratory distress. ABG values during this phase reveal respiratory and metabolic acidosis and hypoxemia as indicated by a high $Paco_2$, low HCO_3^-, and low Pao_2, respectively.[21]

Assessment of the hemodynamic parameters of patients in cardiogenic shock reveals a decreased CO and a CI less than 1.8 L/min/m.[2,21] Inadequate pumping action leads to a decrease in SV, which results in an increase in the left ventricular end-diastolic pressure. This is reflected in an increase in the PAWP. Compensatory vasoconstriction results in an increase in the afterload of the heart, as evidenced by an increase in the SVR. If right ventricular failure is present, the RAP also will be increased.[8,22,23]

Medical Management

The major goals of therapy are to treat the underlying cause, enhance the effectiveness of the pump, and improve tissue perfusion. This approach includes identifying the etiologic factors of pump failure and administering pharmacologic agents to enhance CO. Inotropic agents are used to increase contractility, whereas vasodilating agents and diuretics are used for afterload and preload reduction, respectively. Antidysrhythmic agents should be used to suppress or control dysrhythmias that can affect CO.[9,21-23]

Once the cause of pump failure has been identified, measures should be taken to correct the problem if possible. If the problem is related to an acute MI, measures should be taken to increase myocardial oxygen supply and decrease myocardial oxygen demand. Therapies to increase myocardial oxygen supply include supplemental oxygen, intubation and mechanical ventilation, and coronary artery vasodilator agents such as nitroglycerine. Therapies to decrease myocardial demand include activity restrictions, pain medications, and sedatives. If these measures fail, coronary angioplasty or coronary artery bypass surgery may be used to help improve myocardial oxygen supply.[9,23]

Two other therapies available to improve the effectiveness of the pumping action of the heart are the intraaortic balloon pump (IABP) and the ventricular assist device (VAD). The IABP is a temporary measure to decrease myocardial workload by improving myocardial supply and decreasing myocardial demand. It achieves this goal by improving coronary artery perfusion and reducing left ventricular afterload.[24] The VAD is a temporary external pump that takes the place of the ventricle and allows it to heal.[9]

Nursing Management

Preventive measures include the identification of patients at risk and constant assessment of patients' cardiopulmonary status.[21,22] Patients who require IABP therapy need to be observed frequently for complications. Complications include emboli formation, infection, rupture of the

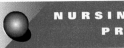

NURSING DIAGNOSIS PRIORITIES

CARDIOGENIC SHOCK

- *Decreased Cardiac Output* related to relative excess of preload and afterload, p. 473
- *Impaired Gas Exchange* related to ventilation/perfusion mismatching and/or intrapulmonary shunting, p. 488
- *Anxiety* related to threat to biologic, psychologic, and/or social integrity, p. 464

BOX 25-7

ETIOLOGIC FACTORS IN ANAPHYLACTIC SHOCK

Foods
  Eggs and milk
  Fish and shellfish
  Nuts and seeds
  Legumes and cereals
  Citrus fruits
  Chocolate
  Strawberries
  Tomatoes
  Other
Food additives
  Food coloring
  Preservatives
Diagnostic agents
  Iodinated contrast dye
  Sulfobromophthalein (Bromsulphalein) (BSP)
  Dehydrocholic acid (Decholin)
  Iopanoic acid (Telepaque)
Biologic agents
  Blood and blood components
  Insulin and other hormones
  Gamma globulin
  Seminal plasma
  Enzymes
  Vaccines and antitoxins
Environmental agents
  Pollens, molds, and spores
  Sunlight
  Animal hair
Drugs
  Antibiotics
  Aspirin
  Narcotics
  Dextran
  Vitamins
  Local anesthetic agents
  Muscle relaxants
  Barbiturates
  Other
Venoms
  Bees and wasps
  Snakes
  Jellyfish
  Spiders
  Deer flies
  Fire ants

aorta, thrombocytopenia, improper balloon placement, bleeding, improper timing of the balloon, balloon rupture, and circulatory compromise of the cannulated extremity.[24]

Patients in cardiogenic shock may have any number of nursing diagnoses depending on the progression of the process (Box 25-6). **Nursing priorities are directed toward limiting myocardial oxygen consumption, enhancing myocardial oxygen supply, and monitoring patients' responses to care.** Measures to limit myocardial oxygen consumption include administering pain medications and sedatives, positioning patients for comfort, limiting activities, offering support to reduce anxiety, providing a calm and quiet environment, and teaching patients about their conditions. Measures to enhance oxygen myocardial supply include administering supplemental oxygen, monitoring respiratory status, and administering prescribed medications.[20]

Anaphylactic Shock

Description and Etiology

A type of distributive shock, anaphylactic shock results from an immediate hypersensitivity reaction. It is a life-threatening event that requires prompt intervention. The severe antibody-antigen response leads to decreased tissue perfusion and initiation of the general shock response.[5,25-27]

Almost any substance can cause a hypersensitivity reaction. These substances, known as *antigens,* can be introduced by injection or ingestion or through the skin or respiratory tract. A number of antigens have been identified that can cause reactions in hypersensitive people. This list includes foods, food additives, diagnostic agents, biologic agents, environmental agents, drugs, and venoms (Box 25-7).[5,26,27]

Pathophysiology

The antibody-antigen response (immunologic stimulation) or the direct triggering (nonimmunologic activation) of the mast cells results in the release of biochemical **mediators.** These mediators include histamine, eosinophilic chemotactic factor of anaphylaxis (ECF-A), neutrophilic chemotactic factor of anaphylaxis (NCF-A), proteinases, heparin, serotonin, leukotrienes (formerly known as "slow-reacting substance of anaphylaxis"), prostaglandins, and platelet-activating factor. The activation of the biochemical mediators causes vasodilation, increased capillary permeability, bronchoconstriction, excessive mucus secretion, coronary vasoconstriction, inflammation, cutaneous reactions, and constriction of the smooth muscle in the intestinal wall, bladder, and uterus. Coronary vasoconstriction causes severe myocardial depression. Cutaneous reactions cause stimulation of nerve endings followed by itching and pain.

ECF-A promotes chemotaxis of eosinophils, thus facilitating the movement of eosinophils into the area. During allergic reactions, eosinophils phagocytose the antibody-antigen complex and other inflammatory debris and release enzymes that inhibit vasoactive mediators such as histamine and leukotrienes. In addition, secondary mediators are produced that either enhance or inhibit the already released biochemical mediators. Bradykinin, a secondary mediator, increases capillary permeability, facilitates vasodilation, and constricts smooth muscles.

Peripheral vasodilation results in decreased venous return. Increased capillary membrane permeability results in the loss of intravascular volume and the development of relative hypovolemia. Decreased venous return results in decreased end-diastolic volume and SV. The decline in SV leads to a fall in CO and impaired tissue perfusion. Death may result from airway obstruction, cardiovascular collapse, or both[5,25-27] (Fig. 25-3).

Assessment and Diagnosis

Anaphylactic shock is a severe systemic reaction that can affect any number of organ systems. A variety of clinical manifestations occur in patients experiencing anaphylactic shock depending on the extent of multisystem involvement. The symptoms usually start to appear within 20 minutes of exposure to the antigen. The severity of the reaction is directly related to the timing of the onset of clinical manifestations. The earlier they appear, the more severe the reaction (Box 25-8).[8]

The cutaneous effects usually appear first and include pruritus, generalized erythema, urticaria, and angioedema. Commonly seen on the face and in the oral cavity and lower pharynx, angioedema develops as a result of

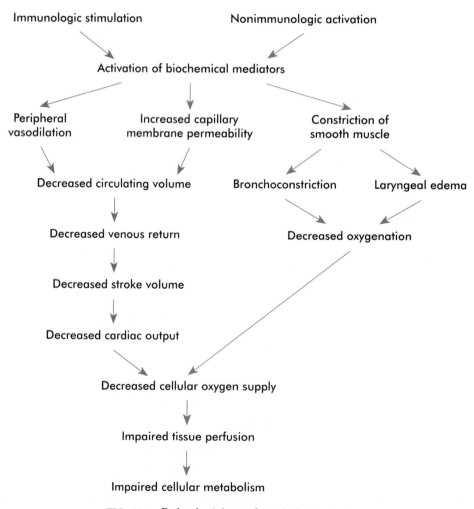

FIG. 25-3 Pathophysiology of anaphylactic shock.

fluid leaking into the interstitial space. Patients may appear restless, uneasy, apprehensive, and anxious and complain of being warm. The effects on the respiratory system include the development of laryngeal edema, bronchoconstriction, and mucus plugs. Clinical manifestations of laryngeal edema include inspiratory stridor, hoarseness, a sensation of fullness or a lump in the throat, and dysphagia. Bronchoconstriction causes dyspnea, wheezing, and chest tightness.[8,25-27] In addition, gastrointestinal and genitourinary manifestations may develop as a result of smooth muscle contraction. These manifestations include vomiting, diarrhea, cramping, abdominal pain, urinary incontinence, and vaginal bleeding.[25-27]

As the anaphylactic reaction progresses, hypotension and reflex tachycardia develop. This occurs in response to massive vasodilation and loss of circulating volume. Jugular veins appear flat as right ventricular end-diastolic volume is decreased. The eventual outcome is circulatory failure and shock.[8,25-27] Pulmonary edema may also result from fluid leaking into the lungs, as evidenced by the development of crackles and wheezes.[26] Patients' levels of consciousness may deteriorate to unresponsiveness.[8]

Assessment of the hemodynamic parameters of patients in anaphylactic shock reveals decreased CO and CI. Venous vasodilation and massive volume loss lead to a decrease in preload, which results in a decline in the RAP and PAWP. Vasodilation of the arterial system results in a decrease in the afterload of the heart, as evidenced by a decrease in the SVR.[8]

Medical Management

The goals of therapy are to remove the offending antigen, reverse the effects of the biochemical mediators, and promote adequate tissue perfusion. When the hypersensitivity reaction occurs as a result of medications, dye, blood, or blood products, the infusion should be immediately discontinued. Removing the antigen is often impossible because it is unknown or has already entered patients' systems.

Reversal of the effects of biochemical mediators involves the preservation and support of patients' airways, ventilation, and circulation through intubation, oxygen therapy, mechanical ventilation, and administration of drugs and fluids. Epinephrine is given to promote bronchodilation and vasoconstriction and inhibit further release of biochemical mediators. Aminophylline may also be administered in cases of severe bronchospasm. Diphenhydramine (Benadryl) is used to block the histamine response. Corticosteroids such as methylprednisolone (Solu-Medrol) may be given with the goal of preventing a delayed reaction and stabilizing capillary membranes. Fluids are replaced by use of either a crystalloid or colloid solution. In addition, positive inotropic agents and vasoconstrictor agents may be necessary to reverse the effects of myocardial depression and vasodilation.[9,25-27]

Nursing Management

Preventive measures include the identification of patients at risk and cautious assessment of patients' responses to the administration of drugs, blood, and blood products. A complete and accurate history of patients' allergies is an essential component of preventive nursing care. In addition to a list of the allergies, a detailed description of the type of response for each should be obtained.[20]

Patients in anaphylactic shock may have any number of nursing diagnoses depending on the progression of the

---

BOX 25-8

CLINICAL MANIFESTATIONS OF ANAPHYLACTIC SHOCK

Cardiovascular
  Hypotension
  Tachycardia
Respiratory
  Lump in throat
  Dysphagia
  Hoarseness
  Stridor
  Wheezing
  Rales and rhonchi
Cutaneous
  Pruritus
  Erythema
  Urticaria
  Angioedema
Neurologic
  Restlessness
  Uneasiness
  Apprehension
  Anxiety
  Decreased level of consciousness
Gastrointestinal
  Nausea
  Vomiting
  Diarrhea
Genitourinary
  Incontinence
  Vaginal bleeding
Subjective complaints
  Sensation of warmth
  Dyspnea
  Abdominal cramping and pain
  Itching
Hemodynamic parameters
  Decreased CO
  Decreased CI
  Decreased RAP
  Decreased PAWP
  Decreased SVR

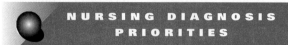

BOX 25-9

NURSING DIAGNOSIS PRIORITIES

ANAPHYLACTIC SHOCK

- *Decreased Cardiac Output* related to decreased preload, p. 474
- *Impaired Gas Exchange* related to alveolar hypoventilation, p. 488
- *Anxiety* related to threat to biologic, psychologic, and/or social integrity, p. 464

process (Box 25-9). **Nursing priorities are directed toward facilitating ventilation, enhancing volume replacement, promoting comfort, and monitoring patients' responses to care.** Measures to facilitate ventilation include positioning patients to assist with breathing and instructing them to breathe slowly and deeply. Measures to enhance volume replacement include inserting large-diameter peripheral intravenous catheters, rapidly administering prescribed fluids, and positioning patients with legs elevated, trunk flat, and head and shoulders above the chest. Measures to promote comfort include administering medications to relieve itching, applying warm soaks to skin, and if necessary, covering patients' hands to discourage scratching. In addition, observing patients for clinical manifestations of a delayed reaction is critical to prevent further problems.[26]

Neurogenic Shock

Description and Etiology

Neurogenic shock, a type of distributive shock, is the result of the loss or suppression of sympathetic tone. Its onset is within minutes, and it may last for days, weeks, or months depending on the cause.[28] The lack of sympathetic tone leads to decreased tissue perfusion and initiation of the general shock response. Neurogenic shock is the rarest form of shock and can be caused by anything that disrupts the SNS. The problem can occur as the result of interrupted impulse transmission or blockage of sympathetic outflow from the vasomotor center in the brain.[5,29] The most common cause is a spinal cord injury above the level of T6.[28] Other causes are spinal anesthesia, drugs, emotional stress, pain, and central nervous system dysfunction.[5]

Pathophysiology

Loss of sympathetic tone results in massive peripheral vasodilation, inhibition of the baroreceptor response, and

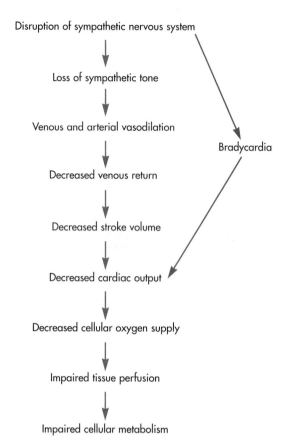

FIG. 25-4 Pathophysiology of neurogenic shock.

impaired thermoregulation. Arterial vasodilation leads to a decrease in SVR and a fall in blood pressure. Venous vasodilation leads to decreased venous return because of pooling of blood in the venous circuit. A decreased venous return results in a decrease in end-diastolic volume or preload. A decrease in preload results in a decrease in SV and CO, and relative hypovolemia develops. The fall in blood pressure and CO leads to inadequate or impaired tissue perfusion.[1,28] Inhibition of the arterial baroreceptor response results in loss of compensatory reflex tachycardia. The HR does not increase to compensate for the fall in CO, which further compromises tissue perfusion.[39] Impaired thermoregulation occurs because of loss of vasomotor tone in the cutaneous blood vessels that dilate and constrict to maintain body temperature. Patients become poikilothermic, or dependent on the environment for temperature regulation (Fig. 25-4).[28,30]

Assessment and Diagnosis

Patients in neurogenic shock usually have initial symptoms such as hypotension, bradycardia, hypothermia, and warm, dry skin. The decreased blood pressure results from massive peripheral vasodilation. The decreased HR is caused by inhibition of the baroreceptor response and unopposed parasympathetic control of the heart. Hypothermia occurs from uncontrolled heat loss peripherally. The warm, dry skin is a consequence of pooling of blood in the extremities and loss of vasomotor control in surface vessels of the skin that control heat loss.[28,30]

Assessment of the hemodynamic parameters of patients in neurogenic shock reveals a decreased CO and CI. Venous vasodilation leads to a decrease in preload, which results in a decline in the RAP and PAWP. Vasodilation of the arterial system causes a decrease in the afterload of the heart, as evidenced by a decrease in the SVR.[29]

Medical Management

The goals of therapy are to treat or remove the cause, prevent cardiovascular instability, and promote optimal tissue perfusion. Cardiovascular instability can occur from hypovolemia, hypothermia, hypoxia, and dysrhythmias. Specific treatments are aimed at preventing or correcting these problems as they occur.

Hypovolemia is treated with careful fluid resuscitation. The minimum amount of fluid is administered to ensure adequate tissue perfusion. Volume replacement is initiated for systolic blood pressure lower than 90 mm Hg, urine output less than 30 ml/hr, or changes in mental status that indicate decreased cerebral tissue perfusion. Patients are carefully observed for evidence of fluid overload.[28] Vasopressors may be used as necessary to maintain blood pressure and organ perfusion.[29] Hypothermia is treated with warming measures and environmental temperature regulation. The goal is to maintain normothermia and avoid large swings in body temperature. The treatment of hypoxia varies with the underlying cause. Chest wall paralysis, retained secretions, pulmonary edema, and suctioning contribute to the development of hypoxia. Management of this problem may include ventilatory support, vigorous pulmonary hygiene, and supplemental oxygen. The major dysrhythmia seen in neurogenic shock is bradycardia, which should be treated with atropine.[28,30]

Nursing Management

Preventive measures include the identification of patients at risk and constant assessment of the neurologic status. Vigilant immobilization of patients with spinal cord injuries and slight elevation of the heads of their beds after spinal anesthesia are essential components of preventive nursing care. Early identification allows for early treatment and decreased mortality rates.[20,28]

Patients with neurogenic shock may have any number of nursing diagnoses depending on the progression of the process (Box 25-10). **Nursing priorities are directed toward treating hypovolemia, maintaining normothermia, preventing hypoxia, observing for dysrhythmias, and monitoring patients' responses to care.**[28]

B O X   2 5 - 1 0

NURSING DIAGNOSIS PRIORITIES

NEUROGENIC SHOCK

- *Decreased Cardiac Output* related to Vasodilation and Bradycardia, p. 478.
- *Hypothermia* related to exposure to cold environment, trauma, or damage to the hypothalamus, p. 494
- *Anxiety* related to threat to biologic, psychologic, and/or social integrity, p. 464

Septic Shock

Description and Etiology

Septic shock, a form of distributive shock, occurs when microorganisms invade the body. The primary mechanism of this type of shock is the maldistribution of blood flow to the tissues, with overperfusion in some areas and underperfusion in others.[6,31]

A variety of terms such as *bacteremia, sepsis,* and *septic shock* may be used to describe the condition patients with an infection experience. *Bacteremia* simply refers to the presence of viable bacteria in the blood. *Sepsis* describes the systemic response to infection that manifests in two or more of the following conditions: temperature greater than 38°C or less than 36°C; HR greater than 90 beats/min; respiratory rate greater than 20 breaths/min or $PaCO_2$ less than 32 mm Hg; and white blood cell (WBC) count greater than 12,000 cells/mm^3, less than 4000 cells/mm^3, or greater than 10% bands. Septic shock is sepsis with hypotension, despite fluid resuscitation, combined with the presence of perfusion abnormalities such as altered cerebral function, acidosis, and oliguria.[32]

Sepsis and septic shock are caused by a wide variety of microorganisms, including gram-negative and gram-positive bacteria, fungi, viruses, and protozoa. The source of these microorganisms varies. Exogenous sources include the hospital environment and members of the health care team. Endogenous sources include patients' skin, gastrointestinal (GI) tract, respiratory tract, and genitourinary tract. Gram-negative bacteria are responsible for approximately two thirds of the cases of septic shock. Another one fourth of the cases result from a combination of microorganisms.[5,33-37]

Sepsis and septic shock are associated with a number of intrinsic and extrinsic precipitating factors (Box 25-11). All these factors interfere directly or indirectly with the body's anatomic and physiologic defense mechanisms. Several of the intrinsic factors are not modifiable or are very difficult to control. Several of the extrinsic factors may be required for diagnosis and management.

PRECIPITATING FACTORS ASSOCIATED WITH SEPTIC SHOCK

INTRINSIC FACTORS

Extremes of age
Coexisting diseases
  Malignancies
  Burns
  Acquired immunodeficiency syndrome (AIDS)
  Diabetes
  Substance abuse
  Dysfunction of one or more of the major body systems
Malnutrition

EXTRINSIC FACTORS

Invasive devices
Drug therapy
Fluid therapy
Surgical and traumatic wounds
Surgical and invasive diagnostic procedures
Immunosuppressive therapy

All critically ill patients are therefore at risk for the development of septic shock.[33-37]

Pathophysiology

A complex systemic response, septic shock is initiated when a microorganism enters the body and endotoxins or exotoxins are released. Endotoxins are liberated from the cell walls of gram-negative bacteria when the body's immune system destroys them. Exotoxins are released from gram-positive bacteria and other microorganisms while they are alive in the body.[5,33,35,38] Toxic shock syndrome is an example of gram-positive, or exotoxic, shock.[39]

Once a microorganism invades the body and releases the toxin, a variety of mechanisms occur, including activation of the immune mediators, damage to the endothelium, and activation of the central nervous and endocrine systems. Consequently a variety of physiologic and pathophysiologic events occur that affect capillary membrane permeability, clotting, distribution of blood flow to the tissues and organs, and the metabolic state of the body. A systemic imbalance between cellular oxygen supply and demand subsequently develops that results in cellular hypoxia, damage, and death (Fig. 25-5).[5,33,35,38]

The septic process is initiated by the activation of immune mediators that are part of the inflammatory process and are released in response to invading microorganisms. These humoral, cellular, and biochemical mediators initiate a chain of complex interactions controlled by numerous feedback mechanisms. Eventually the immune system is overwhelmed, the feedback mechanisms fail, and a process that was designed to protect the body actually harms it.[5,35,40]

The septic cascade is also initiated by damage to the endothelial cells caused by toxins released from invading microorganisms. Endothelial cell damage results in activation of the immune mediators, increased capillary membrane permeability, and formation of microemboli. These events lead to disruption of blood flow to the tissues, more endothelial cell damage, and further propagation of the septic process.[33,35]

Activation of the central nervous and endocrine systems also occurs as part of the primary response to invading microorganisms. This activation leads to stimulation of the SNS and the release of ACTH. These events trigger the release of epinephrine, norepinephrine, glucocorticoids, aldosterone, glucagon, and renin, which results in the development of a hypermetabolic state and further contributes to the vasoconstriction of the renal, pulmonary, and splanchnic beds. Activation of the central nervous system also causes the release of endogenous opiates that are believed to cause vasodilation and decrease myocardial contractility.[41]

Once the initial sequence of events is triggered, a series of pathophysiologic responses occurs that eventually culminates in the maldistribution of circulating blood volume. These responses include massive peripheral vasodilation, microemboli formation, selective vasoconstriction, and increased capillary membrane permeability. The maldistribution of circulating blood volume eventually results in decreased cellular oxygen supply.[31,33,35,38]

The hypermetabolic state also increases the cellular metabolic needs. Increased glucose requirements in conjunction with the high level of catabolic hormones result in the limited ability of the cells to use glucose as a substrate for energy production. This causes glucose intolerance, hyperglycemia, relative insulin resistance, and the use of fat for energy (lipolysis). The relative insulin resistance causes the body to produce more insulin, which inhibits the use of fat as an energy substrate. This promotes the use of protein as an energy substrate and catabolism of protein stores in the visceral organs and skeletal muscles.[38,42]

Assessment and Diagnosis

Patients in septic shock may exhibit a variety of clinical manifestations (Box 25-12). During the initial stage, massive vasodilation occurs in both the venous and arterial beds. Dilatation of the venous system leads to a decrease in venous return to the heart, which results in a decrease in the preload of the right and left ventricles. This is evidenced by a decline in the RAP and PAWP. Dilatation of the arterial system results in a decrease in the afterload of the heart, as evidenced by a decrease in the SVR. Patients' blood pressures fall in response to the reduction in preload and afterload. Their skin becomes

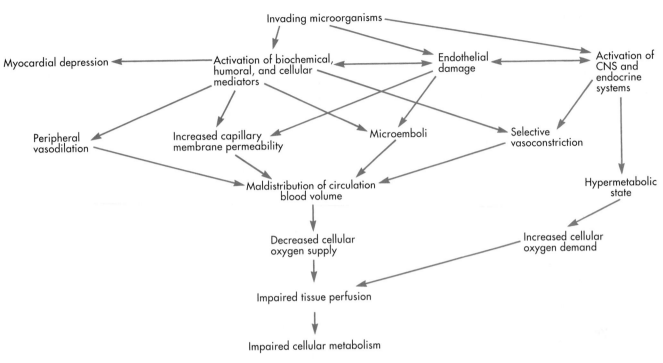

FIG. 25-5 Pathophysiology of septic shock.

pink, warm, and flushed as a result of the massive vaso-dilation.[8,35,43]

The HR rises to compensate for the hypotension and in response to increased metabolic, SNS, and adrenal gland stimulation. This results in a normal to high CO and CI. The pulse pressure widens as the diastolic blood pressure decreases because of the vasodilation, and the systolic blood pressure increases because of the elevated CO. A full, bounding pulse develops. Myocardial con-tractility is decreased, as evidenced by a decline in the left ventricular stroke work index, an effect of myocar-dial depression.[8,35,43]

In the lungs a ventilation/perfusion mismatch devel-ops as a result of pulmonary vasoconstriction and the for-mation of pulmonary microemboli. Hypoxemia occurs, and the respiratory rate increases to compensate for the lack of oxygen. Crackles develop as increased pulmonary capillary membrane permeability leads to pulmonary in-terstitial edema.[33]

Level of consciousness starts to change as a result of decreased cerebral perfusion, immune mediator activa-tion, hyperthermia, and lactic acidosis. Patients may appear disoriented, confused, combative, or lethargic. Urine output declines because of decreased perfusion of the kidneys. Temperature rises in response to pyro-gens released from the invading microorganisms, im-mune mediator activation, and increased metabolic ac-tivity.[8,33,38]

BOX 25-12

CLINICAL MANIFESTATIONS OF SEPTIC SHOCK

Increased HR
Decreased blood pressure
Wide pulse pressure
Full, bounding pulse
Pink, warm, flushed skin
Increased respiratory rate (early)/decreased respiratory rate (late)
Crackles
Change in sensorium
Decreased urine output
Increased temperature
Increased CO and CI
Decreased SVR
Decreased RAP
Decreased PAWP
Decreased left ventricular stroke work index
Decreased Pao_2
Decreased $Paco_2$ (early)/increased $Paco_2$ (late)
Decreased HCO_3^-
Increased mixed venous oxygen saturation (Svo_2)

ABG values during this phase reveal respiratory alkalosis, hypoxemia, and metabolic acidosis, which are demonstrated by a low Pa_{O_2}, low Pa_{CO_2}, and low HCO_3^- respectively. The respiratory alkalosis is caused by an increased respiratory rate. As patients become fatigued, the respiratory rate decreases and the Pa_{CO_2} increases, resulting in respiratory acidosis. The metabolic acidosis is caused by lack of oxygen to the cells and the development of lactic acidemia. The mixed venous oxygen saturation (Sv_{O_2}) is increased because of maldistribution of the circulating blood volume and impaired cellular metabolism.[33]

The WBC count is elevated as part of the immune response to the invading microorganisms. In addition, the white blood cell differential reveals an increase in immature neutrophils (shift to the left). This occurs because the body has to mobilize increasing numbers of WBCs to fight the infection.[35] Increased serum glucose also occurs as part of the hypermetabolic response and the development of insulin resistance.[41,42] As impaired tissue perfusion develops, a variety of other clinical manifestations appear indicating the development of MODS.

Medical Management

The goals of treatment are to control the infection, reverse the pathophysiologic responses, and promote metabolic support. This approach includes identifying and treating the infection, supporting the cardiovascular system and enhancing tissue perfusion, and initiating nutritional therapy. In addition, dysfunction of the individual organ systems must be prevented or treated.

One of the first measures taken in the treatment of septic shock is finding and eradicating the cause of the infection. Blood, urine, sputum, and wound cultures should be obtained to find the location of the infection. Antibiotic therapy should be initiated as soon as possible. If the microorganism is unknown, a broad-spectrum antibiotic should be administered. Once the microorganism is identified, an antibiotic more specific to the microorganism should be started. Administration of antibiotics can be particularly hazardous in gram-negative shock because more endotoxin is released from the cell walls when the microorganisms die.[35,36] This further aggravates the entire septic process. Surgical intervention to debride infected or necrotic tissue or drain abscesses may also be necessary to facilitate removal of the septic source.[9] Temperature control is also necessary to decrease the metabolic demands created by hyperthermia. Antipyretic agents and cooling measures are often used.

Another important measure in the treatment of septic shock is supporting the cardiovascular system and enhancing tissue perfusion. Specific interventions are aimed at increasing cellular oxygen supply and decreasing cellular oxygen demand. These treatments include administration of fluids, vasoactive agents, and positive inotropic agents as well as ventilatory support, temperature control, and reversal of acidosis.

Aggressive fluid administration to augment intravascular volume and increase preload is extremely important during the initial phase. Crystalloids or colloids may be used depending on patients' conditions. The amount of fluid that is administered may vary, but generally the goal is to restore PAWP to the 10 to 15 mm Hg range.[33,38]

The administration of vasoconstrictor agents is indicated to reverse the massive peripheral vasodilation. These agents help increase the SVR and augment blood pressure. Positive inotropic agents are used to increase contractility and treat myocardial depression. All these medications are titrated to patient response.[13,33,38]

The initiation of nutritional therapy is critical in the management of patients in septic shock. The goal of nutritional support is to improve overall nutritional status, enhance the immune system, and promote wound healing. Nutritional supplements for patients in septic shock should be high in protein because of the metabolic derangements that develop in the hypermetabolic state. The amount of protein calories given depends on nitrogen balance. In early sepsis the mix of nonprotein calories may be divided evenly between carbohydrates and fats. In the later stages of septic shock, significant alterations in fat metabolism occur, and the lipid content should be limited to 10% to 15% of the total nonprotein calories. The lipid emulsion should contain medium-chain triglycerides because they are easier to metabolize than long-chain triglycerides.[16]

Studies are now being conducted with drugs that are believed to block or alter the effects of the immune mediators or stimulate phagocytic cells. These include colony-stimulating factors, immunoglobins, antitumor necrosis factor, and interleukin-1 receptor antagonists. Although these therapies have demonstrated positive results in animals, their efficacy in humans requires more extensive testing.[44]

Nursing Management

Preventive measures include the identification of patients at risk and reduction of their exposure to invading microorganisms. Hand washing, aseptic technique, and an understanding of ways microorganisms can invade the body are essential components of preventive nursing care. Early identification allows for early treatment and decreased mortality.[20]

Patients with septic shock may have any number of nursing diagnoses depending on the progression of the process (Box 25-13). **Nursing priorities are directed toward administering prescribed antibiotics, fluids, and vasoactive agents; preventing the development of concomitant infections; observing for complications of nutritional therapy; and monitoring patients' responses to care.** Continual observation to detect subtle changes indicating the progression of the septic process is also very important.[20]

BOX 25-13

NURSING DIAGNOSIS PRIORITIES

Septic Shock

- *Decreased Cardiac Output* related to decreased preload, p. 477
- *Impaired Gas Exchange* related to ventilation/perfusion mismatching and intrapulmonary shunting, p. 488
- *Altered Nutrition: Less Than Body Requirements* related to increased metabolic demands and/or lack of exogenous nutrients, p. 506
- *Anxiety* related to threat to biologic, psychologic, and/or social integrity, p. 464

Multiple Organ Dysfunction Syndrome

Description and Etiology

MODS is a recently named clinical syndrome that results from progressive physiologic failure of several interdependent organ systems. The initial insult itself is often not the major threat to survival during critical illness. *MODS is defined as the "presence of altered organ function in an acutely ill patient such that homeostasis cannot be maintained without intervention."*[32]

Complex interrelationships exist among dysfunctional organ systems; failure or dysfunction of one organ potentially amplifies dysfunction in another. Organ dysfunction may be absolute or relative and can occur over varying times. MODS, which can provide the final common pathway that leads to the death of many critically ill patients, is a leading cause of late mortality after trauma.[45,46] Organ failure may be a direct consequence of the insult (primary MODS) or can manifest latently and involve organs not directly injured or involved in the initial insult (secondary MODS). Patients can experience both primary and secondary MODS.[32] Organ dysfunction must be recognized early so that organ-specific treatment modalities can be started.[32,47] Despite modern technology and intensive medical and nursing care, the mortality rate in hospitalized patients with organ dysfunction after an acute insult remains high.[48]

Although various patient populations are at risk for organ dysfunction, trauma patients are particularly vulnerable because they frequently experience prolonged episodes of circulatory shock, with tissue hypoxia, tissue injury, and infection.[49] Others at high risk include those who have experienced shock associated with a ruptured aneurysm, acute pancreatitis, sepsis, burns, and surgical complications.[49-51] Patients 65 years of age and older are at increased risk because of their decreased organ reserve.[49]

BOX 25-14

Clinical Conditions and Manifestations Associated with Systemic Inflammatory Response Syndrome (SIRS)

CLINICAL CONDITIONS

Infection
Infection of vascular structures (heart and lungs)
Pancreatitis
Ischemia
Multiple trauma with massive tissue injury
Hemorrhagic shock
Immune-mediated organ injury
Exogenous administration of tumor necrosis factor or other cytokines
Aspiration of gastric contents
Massive transfusion
Host defense abnormalities

CLINICAL MANIFESTATIONS

Temperature $<38°C$ or $>36°C$
Heart rate >90 beats/min
Respiratory rate >20 breaths/min or $Paco_2$ <32 torr
WBC $>12,000$ cells/mm^3 or <4000 cells/mm^3 or $>10\%$ immature (band) forms

Primary MODS is organ dysfunction that directly results from and occurs soon after a well-defined event. Direct insults initially cause localized inflammatory responses. Examples of primary MODS include pulmonary dysfunction after aspiration, pulmonary contusion, or inhalation lung injury and renal dysfunction after emergency aortic surgery or rhabdomyolysis.[32] Patients who develop primary MODS may either die soon after the initiating event, recover, or develop severe systemic inflammation that progresses to secondary MODS.[52] Manifestations of severe systemic inflammation following a well-defined event is termed *systemic inflammatory response syndrome (SIRS)*[32] (Box 25-14).

Secondary MODS is organ dysfunction that develops latently after clinical conditions such as septic shock, perfusion defects, inflammation, and the presence of dead or injured tissue.[32] These altered physiologic states evoke widespread, uncontrolled systemic inflammation and organ dysfunction from the excessive release of inflammatory mediators. (Box 25-15)[52] The lungs, kidneys, and liver are the organs most commonly affected. The impairment of organ systems such as the gastrointestinal organs and liver that normally have immunoregulatory function intensifies the systemic inflammatory response.[53-55] Secondary MODS is accompanied by persistent hypermetabolism, a metabolic consequence of sustained systemic inflammation and physiologic stress. Mortality rates from secondary MODS range from 70% to 100%.[52]

Sepsis is a common initiating event in the development of secondary MODS. Severe sepsis initiates a period of circulatory instability and relative physiologic shock that perpetuates systemic inflammation and resultant organ damage. Noninfectious stimuli (inflammation, perfusion deficit, or dead tissue) also effectively initiate similar cellular consequences. Physiologic shock may create a tissue oxygen debt that sets the stage for activation of the systemic inflammatory response.[56]

Currently the definitive clinical course of secondary MODS has not been completely identified. Clinical observations suggest that organ dysfunction may occur in a progressive pattern; however, organs may fail simultaneously.[45,49-51,57,58] Renal dysfunction, for example, may occur concurrently with hepatic dysfunction. In secondary MODS, organ dysfunction is latent.[32,47] The lungs are generally the first major organ affected. After the initial insult and resuscitation, a state of persistent hypermetabolism develops, most likely as a metabolic consequence of sustained systemic inflammation and physiologic stress, followed closely by lung dysfunction, manifested as adult respiratory distress syndrome (ARDS).

Hypermetabolism, which may not occur immediately after insult, may last for 14 to 21 days. During hypermetabolism, changes occur in cellular anabolic and catabolic function, resulting in autocatabolism. Autocatabolism manifests as a severe decrease in lean body mass, severe weight loss, anergy, and increased CO and volume of oxygen consumption (V_{O_2}).[48] Patients experience profound alterations in carbohydrate, protein, and fat metabolism (see Chapter 6). Concurrently, GI, hepatic, and immunologic dysfunction may occur, which intensifies the systemic inflammatory response. Clinical manifestations of cardiovascular instability and central nervous system dysfunction may be present. Ongoing perfusion deficits and septic foci continue to perpetuate the systemic inflammatory response. About 25% to 40% of patients die during hypermetabolism. The development of renal and hepatic failure may be preterminal events in secondary MODS. Death may occur in 21 to 28 days after the initial insult.[51] Clinical manifestations of organ dysfunction may occur earlier after an insult in patients with decreased physiologic organ reserve than in the normal patient population.[56] Patients who survive MODS often require prolonged, expensive rehabilitation because of generalized polyneuropathy and a chronic form of lung disease from ARDS.[48]

Pathophysiology

Secondary MODS results from altered regulation of patients' acute immune and inflammatory responses. This dysregulation or failure to control the normal inflammatory response leads to excessive production and activity of inflammatory cells and biochemical mediators that cause organ damage.[58] Mediators associated with MODS can be classified as inflammatory cells, biochemical mediators, and plasma protein systems (see Box 25-15). Complex interactions occur among these inflammatory cells and biochemicals that cause organ dysfunction. Activation of one mediator often leads to activation of another.

Neutrophils, macrophages, mast cells, platelets, and endothelial cells are inflammatory cells that mediate widespread systemic inflammation and organ dysfunction through their production of cytokines (biochemical mediators). In addition, neutrophils overreact systemically and damage normal cells, adhere to microvascular endothelium, and release cytotoxic inflammatory biochemicals that cause tissue damage, vascular injury, edema, thrombosis, and hemorrhage in multiple organ systems.[49,51,53,54,57] Macrophages cause organ injury by their production of toxic oxygen metabolites, interleukin-1, and tumor necrosis factor (TNF).[59-63] Lymphocytes adhere to and sequester in the microvascular endothelium. Stimulated T lymphocytes and B lymphocytes produce cytokines that activate other inflammatory cells.[59] Endothelial cells are common targets for leukocyte-derived mediators during the systemic inflammatory response and manufacture chemotactic agents that attract neutrophils to areas of inflammation and endothelial injury.[52] Widespread endothelial destruction leads to increased vascular permeability, a key element in sepsis and systemic inflammation.[52] Inflammatory mediators that damage the endothelium include endotoxin, TNF, interleukin-1, and platelet activating factor (PAF). Most of these mediators also recruit and activate neutrophils and activate complement. The result is sustained inflammation and continued destruction of the endothelium.[59] Healthy endothelial cells also produce and maintain a balance between endothelin (a vasoconstrictor) and endothelial-derived–relaxant factor (nitric oxide). Damage to endothelial cells leads to vascular instability and perfusion abnormalities. Endothelial cells also produce procoagulants such as PAF and plasminogen activating inhibitor, angiotensin II, and prostacyclin (AA metabolite), substances associated with systemic inflammation and organ dysfunction.[52,59]

TNF, interleukins, PAF, AA metabolites, and toxic oxygen metabolites are biochemical mediators that cause organ dysfunction. The excessive production of toxic oxygen metabolites causes lipid peroxidation, damage to the cell membrane and deoxyribonucleic acid, and activation of the complement and coagulation cascades.[64] Neutrophils produce toxic oxygen metabolites that cause tissue injury when combined with proteases. Oxygen metabolites can cause organ injury after reperfusion in the small intestines, liver, lungs, muscles, heart, brain, stomach, and skin.[64]

TNF, also known as *cachectin*, is a mononuclear phagocyte and T lymphocyte derived from cytokine that is produced in response to endotoxin, tissue injury, viral agents, and interleukins. When present in excessive amounts, TNF causes widespread destructive effects in most organ systems. TNF is responsible for the pathophysiologic changes in sepsis and gram-negative shock, including fever, hypotension, decreased organ perfusion, and increased capillary permeability. TNF may precipitate organ injury by causing generalized endothelial injury, fibrin deposition, and a procoagulant state. TNF causes disseminated intravascular coagulopathy (DIC), interstitial pneumonitis, acute renal tubular necrosis, and necrosis of the GI tract, liver, and adrenal glands. TNF stimulates AA metabolism, the clotting cascade, and production of PAF. Metabolically, excessive TNF causes hyperglycemia progressing to hypoglycemia and hypertriglyceridemia. The destructive effects of TNF are enhanced by AA metabolites and the stress hormones.[59,61-63,65]

Interleukins have similar biologic responses to those of TNF, and both work synergistically to cause organ dysfunction. However, the effects of TNF are more destructive. Interleukin-1 also causes vascular congestion, capillary leakage, and increased coagulation associated with sepsis. Like TNF, interleukin-1 has profound vascular endothelial effects. Interleukin-1 stimulates the production of procoagulants by endothelial cells, increases the production of acute-phase reactant proteins, increases catabolism of muscle tissue, and causes neutrophilia. Cardiovascular and inflammatory effects commonly include hypotension, fever, tachycardia, diarrhea,

acute lung injury, leukopenia, platelet aggregation, and intravascular coagulation.[52,59,62,66]

PAF is released by platelets, mast cells, monocytes/macrophages, neutrophils, and endothelial cells. PAF has widespread effects on the heart, vascular system, coagulation, platelets, and the lungs. PAF causes platelet aggregation, with resultant microvascular stasis and ischemia in the microvascular bed; platelet release of serotonin, which increases vascular permeability; and increased vasoconstriction from increased production of thromboxane A_2, an AA metabolite.[67-69]

AA metabolites (eicosanoids) such as prostaglandins, thromboxanes, and leukotrienes play a primary role in the pathogenesis of systemic inflammation and MODS by altering vascular reactivity and permeability and fostering the accumulation and activation of inflammatory cells.[69-72] Numerous stimuli, including hypoxia, ischemia, endotoxin, catecholamines, and tissue injury, stimulate AA metabolism. Select AA metabolites cause vascular instability and maldistribution of blood flow and alter leukocyte activity.

Proteases are proteolytic (protein-digesting) enzymes released from inflammatory cells that cause significant parenchmal damage. For example, neutrophils in the lung produce proteases that destroy lung tissue. In the gastrointestinal tract, protease-induced mucosal injuries are associated with acute ulcerative colitis, colitis associated with antibiotic treatment, and acute ischemic enteropathy.[55]

In summary, complex interactions occur among inflammatory cells, biochemical mediators, and plasma protein systems implicated in organ dysfunction after an insult. Organ dysfunction or failure results from (1) the adherence of neutrophils to vascular endothelial surfaces and the release of toxic mediators, (2) direct effects of mediators on organ parenchymal endothelial cells, (3) metabolic abnormalities, and (4) poor oxygen delivery and consumption by individual organs. The biologic activity of inflammatory cells, biochemical mediators, and plasma protein systems and ways they work in concert to cause MODS are not completely defined.

Assessment and Diagnosis

Secondary MODS is a systemic disease with organ-specific manifestations. Organ dysfunction may be present when laboratory measurement of organ function exceeds the normal range.[52] Organ dysfunction is influenced by numerous factors, including (1) organ host defense function, (2) response time to the injury, (3) metabolic requirements, (4) organ vasculature response to vasoactive drugs, and (5) organ sensitivity to damage and physiologic reserve. Discussion of the responses of the GI, hepatobiliary, cardiovascular, pulmonary, renal, and coagulation systems in organ dysfunction follow. Clinical manifestations of organ dysfunction are outlined in Box 25-16.

BOX 25-16

CLINICAL MANIFESTATIONS OF ORGAN DYSFUNCTION

GASTROINTESTINAL

Abdominal distention
Intolerance to enteral feedings
Paralytic illeus
Upper/lower GI bleeding
Diarrhea
Ischemic colitis
Mucosal ulceration
Decreased bowel sounds
Bacterial overgrowth in stool

LIVER

Jaundice
Increased serum bilirubin (hyperbilirubinemia)
Increased liver enzymes (AST, ALT, LDH, alkaline phosphatase)
Increased serum ammonia
Decreased serum albumin
Decreased serum transferrin

GALLBLADDER

Right upper quadrant tenderness/pain
Abdominal distention
Unexplained fever
Decreased bowel sounds

METABOLIC/NUTRITIONAL

Decreased lean body mass
Muscle wasting
Severe weight loss
Negative nitrogen balance
Hyperglycemia
Hypertriglyceridemia
Increased serum lactate
Decreased serum albumin, serum transferrin, prealbumin
Decreased retinol-binding protein

IMMUNE

Infection
Decreased lymphocyte count
Anergy

PULMONARY

Tachypnea
ARDS pattern of respiratory failure (dyspnea, patchy infiltrates, refractory hypoxemia, respiratory acidosis, abnormal O_2 indexes)
Pulmonary hypertension

RENAL

Increased serum creatinine, blood urea nitrogen levels
Oliguria, anuria, or polyuria consistent with prerenal azotemia or acute tubular necrosis
Urinary indexes consistent with prerenal azotemia or acute tubular necrosis

CARDIOVASCULAR

Hyperdynamic

Decreased pulmonary capillary wedge pressure
Decreased SVR
Decreased RAP
Decreased left ventricular stroke work index
Increased oxygen consumption
Increased CO, CI, HR

Hypodynamic

Increased SVR
Increased RAP
Increased left ventricular stroke work index
Decreased oxygen delivery and consumption
Decreased CO and CI

CENTRAL NERVOUS SYSTEM

Lethargy
Altered level of consciousness
Fever
Hepatic encephalopathy

COAGULATION/HEMATOLOGIC

Thrombocytopenia
DIC pattern

Gastrointestinal dysfunction

The GI tract plays an important role in secondary MODS. GI organs normally have immunoregulatory functions. GI dysfunction amplifies the systemic inflammatory response, and gut damage may lead to bacterial translocation and endogenous endotoxemia.[49,54,55,73]

Three specific mechanisms link the GI tract and latent organ dysfunction. First, hypoperfusion or shocklike states or both damage the normal mucosa barrier of the GI tract. The GI tract is extremely vulnerable to oxygen metabolite–induced reperfusion injury. Endothelial injury and GI lesions occur in response to mediator-induced tissue damage. In addition, the absence of enteral feedings can disrupt the normal metabolism of the gastric/intestinal lumen and the normal protective function of the gut barrier.[55] The low glycogen reserve of the gastric mucosa may require enteral feedings to maintain normal metabolism. Atrophy of the intestinal villi and ulceration may occur when patients do not receive enteral feedings.[55] Clinical manifestations of altered GI function may include abdominal distention, intolerance to enteral feedings, paralytic ileus, GI bleeding, diarrhea, and ischemic colitis.[55,73]

Second, the translocation of normal flora bacteria of the gut into the systemic circulation initiates and perpetuates an inflammatory focus (endogenous/endotoxemia). The GI tract harbors organisms that present an inflammatory focus in critically ill patients when translocated from the gut into the portal circulation and inadequately cleared by the liver. Hepatic macrophages respond to an increase in enteric organisms by producing tissue-damaging amounts of TNF. Bacterial translocation may be associated with paralytic ileus, antibiotics, antacids, and histamine blockers.[55]

The third mechanism linking the GI tract and organ dysfunction is colonization. The oropharynx of critically ill patients becomes colonized with potentially pathogenic organisms from the GI tract. Pulmonary aspiration of colonized sputum creates an inflammatory focus in critically ill patients. Antacids, histamine blockers, and antibiotics increase colonization of the upper GI tract.[55,73]

Hepatobiliary dysfunction

The liver plays a vital role in limiting the acute inflammatory response. Consequently, hepatic dysfunction after a critical insult may be a primary threat to survival. The liver normally controls the inflammatory response by several mechanisms. Kupffer's cells, which are hepatic macrophages, detoxify substances that might normally induce systemic inflammation as well as vasoactive substances that cause hemodynamic instability. Failure to detoxify gram-negative bacteria translocated from the intestinal tract causes endotoxemia, perpetuates the systemic inflammatory response, and may lead to organ dysfunction. In addition, the liver produces proteins and antiproteases to control the inflammatory response; however, hepatic dysfunction limits this response.[53,54]

The splanchnic organs, including the liver, pancreas, and gallbladder, are extremely susceptible to ischemic injury. Associated with centrilobular hepatocellular necrosis, ischemic hepatitis occurs after prolonged physiologic shock. The degree of hepatic damage is directly related to the severity and duration of the shock episode. Terms such as *shock liver* and *posttraumatic hepatic insufficiency* have been used to describe ischemic hepatitis. Both anoxic and reperfusion injury damage hepatocytes and the vascular endothelium.[74]

Patients at risk for ischemic hepatitis after a hypotensive event include those with a history of cardiac failure, cardiac dysrhythmias, or both. Clinical manifestations of hepatic insufficiency are evident 1 to 2 days after the insult. Jaundice and transient elevations in serum transaminase and bilirubin levels occur. Hyperbilirubinemia results from hepatocyte anoxic injury and increased production of bilirubin from hemoglobin catabolism. Ischemic hepatitis either resolves spontaneously or progresses to hepatic failure and hepatic encephalopathy. Although ischemic hepatitis is not a life-threatening complication, it can contribute to patient morbidity and mortality as a component of multiple organ dysfunction.[74]

Acalculous cholecystitis generally occurs 3 to 4 weeks after the initial insult. Its pathogenesis is unclear but may be related to ischemic reperfusion injury, narcotics, and cystic duct obstruction as a result of hyperviscous bile. Acalculous cholecystitis may be related to the release of thromboxanes and leukotrienes (vasoactive substances) into the microcirculation in response to a damaged endothelium, aggregated platelets, and neutrophils. Clinical manifestations of acalculous cholecystitis may mimic acute cholecystitis with gallstones. Patients may demonstrate vague symptoms, including right upper quadrant pain and tenderness. Critical to the detection of acalculous cholecystitis is the recognition of abdominal distention, unexplained fever, loss of bowel sounds, and a sudden deterioration in patients' conditions. About 50% of patients with acalculous cholecystitis have gallbladder gangrene, and 10% have gallbladder perforation. Consequently, surgical removal of the gallbladder may be performed. A high mortality rate is associated with acalculous cholecystitis because of the seriousness of the underlying disease process.[75]

Pulmonary dysfunction

The lungs are a frequent target organ for mediator-induced injury. Acute lung injury most frequently manifests as ARDS. This clinical syndrome, described in Chapter 12, is addressed here only briefly. Although MODS does not develop in all patients with ARDS, acute respiratory failure as a result of ARDS generally occurs in those with organ dysfunction. Patients with ARDS who experience persistent inflammation with sepsis concurrently with respiratory failure are at greatest risk for MODS.[50,52]

Clinical manifestations of mediator-induced pulmonary injury are consistent with ARDS. Damage to the pulmonary vascular endothelium and the alveolar epithelium from a multitude of mediators results in surfactant deficiency, pulmonary hypertension, increased lung water (noncardiogenic pulmonary edema) because of increased pulmonary capillary permeability, and hypoxemia. Pulmonary hypertension and hypoxic pulmonary vasoconstriction may be the result of loss of the vascular bed during the proliferative phase of ARDS. Pulmonary function is acutely disrupted, resulting in altered airway mechanics and bronchoconstriction. Patients exhibit a low-grade fever, tachycardia, dyspnea, and mental confusion. Diagnostic studies show patchy infiltrates on chest film, thrombocytopenia, and consumptive coagulopathy. Dyspnea and hypoxemia worsen, and intubation and mechanical ventilation are required. Mediators associated with acute lung injury include AA metabolites, toxic oxygen metabolites, proteases, TNF, and interleukins.[48,50]

Renal dysfunction

Acute renal failure is a frequent manifestation of both primary and secondary MODS. As discussed in Chapter 18, acute renal failure can result from renal hypoperfusion (prerenal cause) or direct damage to renal tubular cells (intrarenal cause). The kidney is highly vulnerable to reperfusion injury. Renal ischemic-reperfusion injury may be a major cause of renal failure in MODS. Patients may demonstrate oliguria secondary to decreased renal perfusion and relative hypovolemia. The condition may become refractory to diuretics, fluid challenges, and dopamine. Prerenal oliguria may progress to acute renal failure and require hemodialysis or other renal therapies. The frequent use of nephrotoxic drugs during critical illness also intensifies the risk of renal failure.[76]

Cardiovascular dysfunction

The initial cardiovascular response associated with systemic inflammation is characterized by cardiac excitation and altered vascular resistance during hypermetabolism. This response parallels the hyperdynamic response seen in patients undergoing septic shock and is characterized by decreased RAP and SVR as well as increased venous capacitance, V_{O_2}, CO, and HR. During this hyperdynamic phase, patients have increased volume requirements. The inability to increase CO in response to a low SVR, which may indicate myocardial failure or inadequate fluid resuscitation, is associated with increased mortality. V_{O_2} increases and may be flow dependent. Mediators implicated in the hyperdynamic response include bradykinin, vasodilator prostaglandins, PAF, endogenous opioids, and beta-adrenergic stimulators.[49,77-79]

As organ failure progresses and mediator effects become more deleterious, cardiac failure develops. Cardiac dysfunction is characterized by ventricular dilatation, decreased diastolic compliance, and decreased systolic contractile function. Cardiovascular function becomes vasopressor dependent. Cardiac failure may be caused by immune mediators, TNF, acidosis, or myocardial depressant factor, a substance thought to be secreted by the pancreas. TNF has a myocardial-depressant effect and is associated with myocardial depression during septic shock.[80] Myocardial depression is exacerbated by myocardial hypoperfusion from a low CO state and persistent lactic acidosis. Late cardiovascular responses include decreased CO and an increased SVR. Cardiogenic shock and biventricular failure occur and lead to death.

Coagulation system dysfunction

Failure of the coagulation system may manifest as DIC. DIC results in simultaneous microvascular clotting and hemorrhage in organ systems because of the depletion of clotting factors and excessive fibrinolysis. Cell injury and damage to the endothelium initiate the intrinsic or extrinsic coagulation pathways (Fig. 25-6). The endothelium is closely involved in DIC. Several relationships have been proposed. Endotoxins may roughen and expose the endothelial lining of blood vessels and consequently stimulate clotting. Low-flow states during hypotensive episodes may damage vessel endothelium and release tissue thromboplastin, with subsequent activation of the extrinsic pathway. A variety of clinical conditions such as trauma, burns, and radiographic procedures can also cause damage to the local endothelium and activation of the intrinsic coagulation pathway.[81,82]

An overstimulation of the normal coagulation process, DIC is a complex, consumptive coagulopathy that occurs in patients with a variety of disorders, including sepsis, tissue injury, and shock. Thrombosis and fibrinolysis are magnified to life-threatening proportions. The initial alteration in DIC is a generalized state of systemic hypercoagulation that produces organ ischemia. All organs, particularly the skin, lungs, and kidneys, are involved.[82,83] The thrombotic clinical manifestations of DIC are presented in Box 25-17.

Hemorrhage is the second pathophysiologic alteration in DIC. The lysis of clots (fibrinolysis) is normally initiated by the coagulation cascade. The intensity of the thrombosis in DIC enhances an equally intense lysis; however, clot lyse cannot effectively maintain blood vessel patency. The production of fibrin split products exerts further anticoagulant effects, and hemorrhage ensues (Fig. 25-6). Clotting factors, platelets, fibrinogen, and thrombin are consumed in large quantities during the thrombosis. Consequently, coagulation substances are depleted. The hemorrhagic signs and symptoms of DIC are presented in Box 25-17.

The abnormal clotting studies in patients with DIC may indicate thrombocytopenia, prolonged clotting times, depressed levels of clotting factors (particularly factor VII and fibrinogen/fibrin), and high levels of breakdown products of fibrinogen and fibrin (fibrin degradation products, D-dimer). Medical management of DIC includes immediate treatment of the underlying cause; transfusion of blood products such as red blood cells, platelets, and fresh frozen plasma to correct the clotting factor deficiencies; and cryoprecipitate to treat hypofibrinogenemia. The use of heparin therapy in DIC remains controversial. Heparin must be used with caution and is contraindicated in patients with bleeding in critical areas such as the cranium. Antifibrinolytic agents may be used concurrently with heparin therapy but are generally contraindicated because of the risk of thrombotic complications. Strict adherence to bleeding precautions is essential to minimize tissue and vascular trauma.[81-82]

Medical Management

The goals of therapy are control of the source of inflammation, maintenance of tissue oxygenation, nutritional/metabolic support, and support for individual organs.* Investigational drug therapies may be part of patients' clinical management.

---

*References 45, 49, 50, 52, 57, 83.

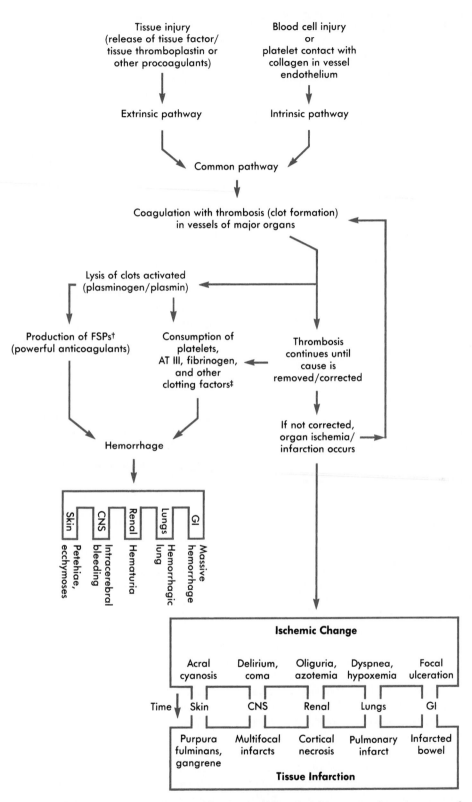

FIG. 25-6 Pathophysiology of DIC. Lysis of clots (fibrinolysis) is a natural consequence of and is activated by coagulation. It is intensified in patients with DIC. DIC is termed a *consumptive coagulopathy.* During thrombosis, clotting factors are used to form clots. During fibrinolysis, clotting factors are destroyed inside the clot. The end result is a depletion of coagulation substances. *FSP,* Fibrin split products or fibrin degradation products. (Modified from Carr M: *J Emerg Med* 5[4]:316, 1987.)

BOX 25-17

CLINICAL MANIFESTATIONS OF DISSEMINATED INTRAVASCULAR COAGULATION

THROMBOTIC CLINICAL MANIFESTATIONS

Skin involvement
Red, indurated areas along vessel wall
Purpura fulminans (diffuse skin infarction)
Acral cyanosis
Necrosis of fingers, toes, nose, and genitalia
Cool, pale extremities with mottling, cyanosis, or edema
Renal involvement
  Renal failure
Cerebral infarcts or hemorrhage
Focal neurologic deficits (e.g., hemiplegia, loss of vision)
Nonspecific changes (e.g., altered LOC, confusion, headache, seizures)
Bowel infarction
Melena, hematemesis, abdominal distention, or absent or hyperactive bowel sounds
Thrombophlebitis
Pulmonary embolism

HEMORRHAGIC CLINICAL MANIFESTATIONS

Spontaneous hemorrhage into body cavities and skin surfaces
Classic symptom of oozing or bleeding from invasive-line insertion sites or body orifices
Bleeding from body orifices such as the rectum, vagina, urethra, nose, and ears as well as from the lung and GI tract
Petechiae, purpura, or ecchymosis
Gingival, nasal, or scleral hemorrhage on physical examination
Hemorrhaging into all body cavities, including the abdomen, retroperitoneal space, cranium, and thorax

---

Elimination of the source of systemic inflammation or infection can reduce mortality.[52] Therefore surgical procedures such as control of bleeding, early fracture stabilization, removal of infected organs or tissue, and burn excision may limit the systemic inflammatory response and organ dysfunction. Appropriate antibiotics are needed if the focus cannot be removed surgically. Although steroids have been used in the past to suppress systemic inflammation, their use does not significantly decrease mortality rates in this patient population.[84]

Despite compliance with meticulous infection control practices, critically ill patients may "infect" themselves. As previously noted, bacterial contamination of the highly vulnerable respiratory tract and pneumonia can result from the colonization of GI tract bacteria. New approaches to infection control have been proposed, including selective decontamination of the GI tract with enteral antibiotics to prevent nosocomial infections, topical antibiotics in the oral pharynx to prevent colonization, monoclonal antibodies against endotoxin, and passive antibody protection.[51,61,73] Gut decontamination and prevention of oral pharyngeal colonization reduce the incidence of infection; however, the death rate from multiple organ dysfunction has not been significantly affected.[73]

New approaches to infection and inflammation control are currently being investigated, including immunotherapy. Based on the principle that antibodies directed against endotoxin can prevent the endotoxin from stimulating the systemic inflammatory response, immunotherapy is antibody therapy that lessens the systemic inflammatory response to microbes (antiinflammatory immunotherapy).[84]

Hypoperfusion and resultant organ hypoxemia frequently occur in patients at risk for MODS, subjecting essential organs to failure. Therefore effective fluid resuscitation and early recognition of flow-dependent Vo_2 is essential. Patients at risk for MODS require pulmonary artery catheterization, frequent measurements of oxygen delivery (Do_2) and Vo_2, and arterial lactate to guide therapy. Arterial lactate levels provide information regarding the severity of impaired perfusion and presence of lactic acidosis.[52] Failure to maintain adequate oxygenation to vital organs results in organ dysfunction. Despite adequate Do_2, Vo_2 may not meet the needs of the body during MODS. Normally under steady state conditions, Vo_2 is relatively constant and independent of Do_2 unless delivery becomes severely impaired.[69] Patients with systemic inflammatory responses such as ARDS and sepsis, however, may have an abnormality in which tissue Vo_2 becomes dependent on the amount of oxygen delivered. Patients are unable to use oxygen appropriately despite normal delivery.[77,78,85,86]

Interventions that decrease oxygen demand and increase oxygen delivery are essential. Decreasing oxygen demand may be accomplished by sedation, mechanical ventilation, temperature control, and rest. Do_2 may be increased by maintaining a normal hemoglobin and Pao_2, using positive end-expiratory pressure, increasing preload or myocardial contractility to enhance cardiac output, or reducing afterload to increase cardiac output. Recent evidence suggests that the maintenance of supranormal oxygen levels significantly decreases the incidence of organ failure in patients with trauma.[46]

Hypermetabolism in MODS results in profound weight loss, cachexia, and loss of organ function. The goal of nutritional support in MODS is the preservation of organ structure and function. Although nutritional support may not alter the course of organ dysfunction, it prevents generalized nutritional deficiencies and preserves gut integrity. The enteral route is preferable to parenteral support.[42,51,52] Enteral feedings should be given distal to the pylorus to prevent pulmonary aspiration. Early enteral feedings may limit bacterial translocation and hy-

EXPERIMENTAL PHARMACOLOGIC APPROACHES IN MODS

Neutrophil inhibitors (pentoxifylline, adenosine, amino-phylline, terbutaline, dibutyl-cAMP, caffeine, forskolin)
WBC adherence inhibitors
Antioxidants/oxygen radical scavengers
Arachidonic acid metabolite modulators
   Monoconal antibodies to phospholipase A$_2$
   Cyclooxygenase inhibitors (ibuprofen, indomethacin)
   Thromboxane synthetase inhibitors
   Thromboxane receptor blockers
   Lipooxygenase inhibitors
   Leukotrienes antagonists
PAF inhibitors
Monoconal antibodies to decrease adhesion of neutrophils to the endothelium
Protease inhibitors
Modulation of macrophage function (n-3 polyunsaturated fatty acids)
Stimulation of lymphocyte function (arginine, n-3 polyunsaturated fatty acids)
Antiendorphin therapy
Antihistamines
Glucocorticoids

NURSING DIAGNOSIS PRIORITIES

MULTIPLE ORGAN DYSFUNCTION SYNDROME

* *Risk for Infection* risk factors: malnutrition and immunodeficiencies, p. 507
* *Decreased Cardiac Output* related to excess preload and afterload, p. 473
* *Impaired Gas Exchange* related to ventilation/perfusion mismatching and intrapulmonary shunting, p. 488
* *Altered Nutrition: Less Than Body Requirements* related to lack of exogenous nutrients and increased metabolic demand, p. 506
* *Anxiety* related to threat to biologic, psychologic, and/or social integrity, p. 464

permetabolism.[52] In addition to early nutritional support the pharmacologic properties of newly developed enteral feeding formulas may have beneficial effects for patients with systemic inflammation and MODS. Supplementation of enteral feedings with glutamine and arginine may be beneficial.[42,87-89] Enteral feedings with omega-3 fatty acids may lessen the systemic inflammatory response in patients at risk for MODS.[88] (The advantages and disadvantages of enteral and parenteral nutrition are discussed in Chapter 6.)

Recent guidelines have been proposed regarding nutritional support during MODS. Patients should receive a total of 25 to 30 kcal/kg/day, with 3 to 5 g/kg/day as glucose. The respiratory quotient should be monitored and maintained under 0.9. Long chain polyunsaturated fatty acids (less than 1.5 g/kg/day) and amino acids (1.5 g/kg/day) should be given. Plasma transferrin and prealbumin levels should be used to monitor hepatic protein synthesis.[51] Efficient protein use should be assessed via nitrogen balance studies.

Organ-specific interventions have not been effective in improving survival rates in patients with multiple organ involvement. Although organ-specific therapies such as mechanical ventilation and hemodialysis are needed for immediate survival, future medical treatment must be aimed at targeting and controlling the destructive activity of mediators that cause cell and organ death. Studies with animal models continue to provide information regarding the efficacy of agents and drugs in preventing organ dysfunction. Numerous experimental drugs and agents are currently under investigation (Box 25-18).[52,60]

Additional therapies for this patient population include the use of subcutaneous heparin or pneumatic compression boots to prevent deep vein thrombosis and pulmonary embolism and histamine blockers or cytoprotective drugs to prevent stress gastritis.[52]

Nursing Management

Preventive measures include a multitude of assessment strategies to detect early organ manifestations of this syndrome. Initial identification of patients at risk for primary and secondary MODS involves an awareness of the complications related to the initial insult. Patients at risk for systemic inflammation (pancreatitis, burns, multitrauma and tissue injury, ischemia, hemorrhagic shock, and immune-mediated organ injury) should be continuously assessed for organ dysfunction. Currently, information about organ blood flow and oxygen delivery is generally not available at the bedside of most patients with MODS; nurses must therefore rely on systemic measures of oxygenation, including pulse oximetry and data concerning mixed venous oxygen saturation (SvO$_2$). New techniques such as gastric tonometry[90] may provide information regarding individual organ oxygenation in the future.

Patients with MODS may have any number of nursing diagnoses depending on the progression of the process (Box 25-19). **Nursing priorities are directed toward preventing the development of infections, facilitating tissue oxygen delivery and limiting tissue oxygen demand and energy expenditure, administering prescribed fluids and medications, observing for com-**

plications of metabolic/nutritional therapy, and monitoring patients' responses to care. Patients should be assessed closely for inflammation and infection. Subtle expressions of infection warrant investigation. Nursing measures include strict adherence to standards of practice to prevent infection as they relate to infection control in the use of invasive procedures such as hemodynamic monitoring, urinary catheterization, endotracheal intubation, intracranial pressure monitoring, total parenteral nutrition, and wound care. Meticulous oral care to limit the number of colonizing organisms is essential. Effective pain control reduces the stress response, promotes an environment for healing, and decreases patient anxiety.

References

1. Barone JE, Snyder AB: Treatment strategies in shock: use of oxygen transport measurement, *Heart Lung* 20:81, 1991.
2. Shoemaker WC: Pathophysiology, monitoring, outcome prediction, and therapy of shock states, *Crit Care Clin* 3:307, 1987.
3. Rice V: Shock, a clinical syndrome: an update. Part II. The stages of shock, *Crit Care Nurse* 11(5):74, 1991.
4. Perry AG: Shock complications: recognition and management, *Crit Care Nurs Q* 11(1):1, 1988.
5. Rice V: Shock, a clinical syndrome: an update. Part I. An overview of shock, *Crit Care Nurse* 11(4):20, 1991.
6. Houston MC: Pathophysiology of shock, *Crit Care Nurs Clin North Am* 2:143, 1990.
7. Astiz ME, Rackow EC, Weil MH: Pathophysiology and treatment of circulatory shock, *Crit Care Clin* 9:183, 1993.
8. Summers G: The clinical and hemodynamic presentation of the shock patient, *Crit Care Nurs Clin North Am* 2:161, 1990.
9. Rice V: Shock, a clinical syndrome: an update. Part III. Therapeutic management, *Crit Care Nurse* 11(6):34, 1991.
10. Sommers MS: Fluid resuscitation following multiple trauma, *Crit Care Nurse* 10(10):74, 1990.
11. Kuhn MM: Colloids vs crystalloids, *Crit Care Nurse* 11(5):37, 1991.
12. Daleiden A: Physiology and treatment of hemorrhagic shock during the early postoperative period, *Crit Care Nurs Q* 16:45, 1993.
13. Burns KM: Vasoactive drug therapy in shock, *Crit Care Nurs Clin North Am* 2:167, 1990.
14. Lorenz A: Lactic acidosis: a nursing challenge, *Crit Care Nurse* 9(4):64, 1989.
15. Arieff AI: Managing metabolic acidosis: update on the sodium bicarbonate controversy, *J Crit Illness* 8:224, 1993.
16. Kuhn MM: Nutritional support for the shock patient, *Crit Care Nurs Clin North Am* 2:201, 1990.
17. Lancaster LE, Rice V: Nursing care planning: overview and application to the patient in shock, *Crit Care Nurs Clin North Am* 2:279, 1990.
18. Blansfield J: Emergency autotransfusion in hypovolemia, *Crit Care Nurs Clin North Am* 2:195, 1990.
19. Frame SB, McSwain NE: Pneumatic antishock garments: where they stand today, *Emerg Care Q* 3(4):65, 1988.
20. Rice V: Shock, a clinical syndrome: an update. Part IV. Nursing care of the shock patient, *Crit Care Nurse* 11(7):28, 1991.
21. Roberts SL: Cardiogenic shock: decreased coronary artery tissue perfusion, *Dimens Crit Care Nurs* 7:196, 1988.
22. Jeffries PR, Whelan SK: Cardiogenic shock: current management, *Crit Care Nurs Q* 11(1):48, 1988.
23. Alpert JS, Becker RC: Mechanisms and management of cardiogenic shock, *Crit Care Clin* 9:205, 1993.
24. Schott KE: Intra-aortic balloon counterpulsation as a therapy for shock, *Crit Care Nurs Clin North Am* 2:187, 1990.
25. Crnkovich DJ, Carlson RW: Anaphylaxis: an organized approach to management and prevention, *J Crit Illness* 8:332, 1993.
26. Dickerson M: Anaphylaxis and anaphylactic shock, *Crit Care Nurs Q* 11(1):68, 1988.
27. Atkinson TP, Kaliner MA: Anaphylaxis, *Med Clin North Am* 9:205, 1993.
28. Schwenker D: Cardiovascular considerations in the critical care phase, *Crit Care Nurs Clin North Am* 2:363, 1990.
29. Walleck CA: Neurological considerations in the critical care phase, *Crit Care Nurs Clin North Am* 2:357, 1990.
30. Kidd PS: Emergency management of spinal cord injuries, *Crit Care Nurs Clin North Am* 2:349, 1990.
31. Vincent JL, Van Der Linden P: Septic shock: particular type of acute circulatory failure, *Crit Care Med* 18:S70, 1990.
32. American College of Chest Physicians/Society of Critical Care Medicine Consensus Conference Committee: Definitions for sepsis and organ failure and guidelines for the use of innovative therapies in sepsis, *Crit Care Med* 20:864, 1992.
33. Hazinski MF and others: Epidemiology, pathophysiology and clinical presentation of gram-negative sepsis, *Am J Crit Care* 2:224, 1993.
34. Hoyt NJ: Preventing septic shock: infection control in the intensive care unit, *Crit Care Nurs Clin North Am* 2:287, 1990.
35. Rackow EC, Astiz ME: Mechanisms and management of septic shock, *Crit Care Clin* 9:219, 1993.
36. Roach AC: Antibiotic therapy in septic shock, *Crit Care Nurs Clin North Am* 2:179, 1990.
37. Segreti J: Nosocomial infections and secondary infections in sepsis, *Crit Care Clin* 5:177, 1989.
38. Rackow EC, Astiz ME: Pathophysiology and treatment of septic shock, *JAMA* 266:548, 1991.
39. Broscious SK: Toxic shock syndrome and its potential complications, *Crit Care Nurse* 11(4):28, 1991.
40. Stroud M, Swindell B, Bernard GR: Cellular and humoral mediators of sepsis syndrome, *Crit Care Nurs Clin North Am* 2:151, 1990.
41. Kimbrell JD: *Alterations in metabolism.* In VB Huddleston, editor: *Multisystem organ failure: pathophysiology and clinical implications,* St Louis, 1992, Mosby.
42. Lehmann S: Nutritional support in the hypermetabolic patient, *Crit Care Nurs Clin North Am* 5:97, 1993.
43. Parrillo JE and others: Septic shock in humans: advances in the understanding of pathogensis, cardiovascular dysfunction, and therapy, *Ann Int Med* 113:227, 1990.
44. Mann HJ, Vance-Bryan K: Immunotherapy targets in critical care, *Crit Care Nurs Clin North Am* 5:333, 1993.
45. DeCamp MM, Demling RH: Posttraumatic multisystem organ failure, *JAMA* 260:530, 1988.
46. Bishop M and others: Prospective trial of supranormal values in severely traumatized patients, *Crit Care Med* 20:S93, 1992 (abstract).
47. Bone RC, Sprung CL, Sibbald WJ: Definitions for sepsis and organ failure, *Crit Care Med* 20:724, 1992.
48. Knaus WA, Wagner DP: Multiple systems organ failure: epidemiology and prognosis, *Crit Care Clin* 5:221, 1989.
49. Matuschak GM: *Multiple systems organ failure: clinical expression, pathogenesis, and therapy.* In Hall JB, Schmidt GA, Wood LD, editors: *Principles of critical care,* New York, 1992, McGraw-Hill.
50. Cerra FB: The multiple organ failure syndrome, *Hosp Pract* 1:69, 1990.

51. Cerra FB: *The syndrome of hypermetabolism and multiple systems organ failure.* In Hall JB, Schmidt GA, Wood LD, editors: *Principles of critical care,* New York, 1992, McGraw-Hill.

52. Cipolle MD, Pasquale MD, Cerra FB: Secondary organ dysfunction: from clinical perspectives to molecular mediators, *Crit Care Clin* 9:261, 1993.

53. Pinsky MR: Multiple systems organ failure: malignant intravascular inflammation, *Crit Care Clin* 5:195, 1989.

54. Pinsky MR, Matuschak GM: Multiple systems organ failure: failure of host defense homeostasis, *Crit Care Clin* 5:199, 1989.

55. Deitch EA: *Gut failure: its role in the multiple organ failure syndrome.* In Deitch EA, editor: *Multiple organ failure pathophysiology and basic concepts of therapy,* New York, 1990, Thieme Medical.

56. Waxman K: Postoperative multiple organ failure, *Crit Care Clin* 3:429, 1987.

57. Cerra FB: Hypermetabolism-organ failure syndrome: a metabolic response to injury, *Crit Care Clin* 5:289, 1989.

58. Cerra FB: Nutritional pharmacology: its role in the hypermetabolism-organ failure syndrome, *Crit Care Med* 18:S154, 1990.

59. Zimmerman JJ, Ringer TV: Inflammatory host responses in sepsis, *Crit Care Clin* 8:163, 1992.

60. Bone RC: Inhibitors of complement and neutrophils: a critical evaluation of their role in the treatment of sepsis, *Crit Care Med* 20:891, 1992.

61. Beutler B: Cachectin in tissue injury, shock, and related states, *Crit Care Clin* 5:353, 1989.

62. Damas P and others: Tumor necrosis factor and interleukin-1 serum levels during severe sepsis in human, *Crit Care Med* 17:975, 1989.

63. Demets JM and others: Plasma tumor necrosis factor and mortality in critically ill septic patients, *Crit Care Med* 17:489, 1989.

64. Nahum A, Sznajder JI: *Role of free radicals in critical illness.* In Hall JB, Schmidt GA, Wood LD, editors: *Principles of critical care,* New York, 1992, McGraw-Hill.

65. Streiter R, Kunkel SL, Bone RC: Role of tumor necrosis factor in disease states and inflammation, *Crit Care Med* 21(suppl):447, 1993.

66. Dinarello CA, Wolff SM: The role of interleukin-1 in disease, *N Eng J Med* 328:106, 1993.

67. Koltai M, Hosford D, Braquet PG: Platlet-activating factor in septic shock, *New Horiz* 1:87, 1993.

68. Shapiro L, Gelfand JA: Cytokines and sepsis: pathophysiology and therapy, *New Horiz* 1:13, 1993.

69. Bernard GR: Cyclooxygenase inhibition, *Crit Care Report* 1:193, 1990.

70. Bone RC: Phospholipids and their inhibitors: a critical evaluation of their role in the treatment of sepsis, *Crit Care Med* 20:884, 1992.

71. Petrak RA, Balk RA, Bone RC: Prostaglandins, cyclooxygenase inhibitors, and thromboxane synthetase inhibitors in the pathogenesis of multiple systems organ failure, *Crit Care Clin* 5:303, 1989.

72. Sprague RS and others: Proposed role of leukotrienes in the pathophysiology of multiple systems organ failure, *Crit Care Clin* 4:315, 1989.

73. van Saene HK, Stoutenbeek CC, Stoller JK: Selective decontamination of the digestive tract in the intensive care unit: current status and future prospects, *Crit Care Med* 20:691, 1992.

74. Vickers SM, Bailey RW, Bulkley GB: *Ischemic hepatitis.* In Marston A and others, editors: *Splanchnic ischemia and multiple organ failure,* St Louis, 1989, Mosby.

75. Haglund UH, Arvidsson D: *Acute acalculous cholecystitis.* In Marston A and others, editors: *Splanchnic ischemia and multiple organ failure,* St Louis, 1989, Mosby.

76. Gamelli RL, Silver GM: *Acute renal failure.* In Deitch EA, editor: *Multiple organ failure pathophysiology and basic concepts of therapy,* New York, 1990, Thieme Medical.

77. Berstern A, Sibbald WJ: Circulatory disturbances in multiple systems organ failure, *Crit Care Clin* 5:233, 1989.

78. Shoemaker WC, Kram HB, Appel PL: Therapy of shock based on pathophysiology, monitoring, and outcome prediction, *Crit Care Med* 18:S19, 1990.

79. Vincent JL, De Backer D: Initial management of circulatory shock as prevention of MSOF, *Crit Care Clin* 5:369, 1989.

80. Kumar A and others: Tumor necrosis factor produces depression of myocardial cell contraction in vitro, *Crit Care Med* 20:S52, 1992 (abstract).

81. Bell TN: Disseminated intravascular coagulation and shock, *Crit Care Nurs Clin* 2:255, 1990.

82. Guyton AC: *Textbook of medical physiology,* ed 8, Philadelphia, 1991, WB Saunders.

83. Macho JR, Luce JM: Rational approach to the management of multiple systems organ failure, *Crit Care Clin* 5:379, 1989.

84. Sheagren JN: Mechanism-oriented therapy for multiple systems organ failure, *Crit Care Clin* 5:393, 1989.

85. Feustel PJ and others: Oxygen delivery and consumption in head-injured and multiple trauma patients, *J Trauma* 30:30, 1990.

86. Edwards JD: Use of survivors' cardiopulmonary values as therapeutic goals in septic shock, *Crit Care Med* 17(11):1098, 1989.

87. Moore FA, Feliciano DV, Andrassy RJ: Early enteral feeding compared to parenteral reduces postoperative septic complications, *Ann Surg* 216:172, 1992.

88. Daly JM, Lieberman MD, Goldfine: Enteral nutrition with supplemental arginine, RNA and omega-3 fatty acids in patients after operation: immunologic, metabolic, and clinical outcome, *Surgery* 112:56, 1992.

89. Keithley J, Eisenberg P: The significance of enteral nutrition in the intensive care unit patient, *Crit Care Nurs Clin North Am* 5:23, 1993.

90. Clark CH, Guitiezzez G: Gastric intramucosal pH: a noninvasive method for the indirect measurement of tissue oxygenation, *Am J Crit Care* 1:53, 1992.

Nursing Management Plans of Care

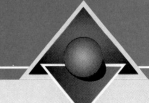

Nursing Management of Health Promotion

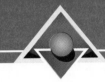

KNOWLEDGE DEFICIT

Definition
Absence or deficiency of cognitive information related to specific topic.

Knowledge Deficit (Specify) Related to Lack of Previous Exposure to Information

DEFINING CHARACTERISTICS

- Verbalized statement of inadequate knowledge or skills
- New diagnosis or health problem requiring self-management or care
- Lack of prior formal or informal education about the specific health problem
- Demonstration of inappropriate behaviors related to management of health problem

OUTCOME CRITERIA

- Patients verbalize adequate knowledge about or perform skills related to disease process, its causes, factors related to onset of symptoms, and self-management of disease or health problem.
- Patients actively participate in health behaviors required for performance of a procedure or in those behaviors enhancing recovery from illness and preventing recurrence or complications.

NURSING INTERVENTIONS AND *RATIONALE*

1. Continue to monitor the assessment parameters listed under "Defining Characteristics."
2. Determine existing level of knowledge or skill.
3. Assess factors affecting the knowledge deficit:
   Learning needs, including patients' priorities and the necessary knowledge and skills for safety

Learning ability of patients, including language skills, level of education, ability to read, preferred learning style

Physical ability to perform prescribed skills or procedures; consider effect of limitations imposed by treatment such as bedrest, restriction of movement by intravenous or other equipment, and effect of sedatives or analgesics

Psychologic effect of stage of adaptation to disease

Activity tolerance and ability to concentrate

Motivation to learn new skills or gain new knowledge

4. Reduce or limit barriers to learning:
   Provide consistent nurse-patient contact *to encourage development of trusting and therapeutic relationship.*
   Structure environment *to enhance learning;* control unnecessary noise, interruptions.
   Individualize teaching plan *to fit patients' current physical and psychologic status.*
   Delay teaching until patients are ready to learn.
   Conduct teaching sessions during period of day when patients are most alert and receptive.
   Meet patients' immediate learning needs as they arise, e.g., give brief explanation of procedures when they are performed.

Continued.

KNOWLEDGE DEFICIT CONT'D

NURSING INTERVENTIONS AND *RATIONALE* CONT'D

5. Promote active participation in the teaching plan by patients and families:
   Solicit input during development of plan.
   Develop mutually acceptable goals and outcomes.
   Solicit expression of feelings and emotions related to new responsibilities.
   Encourage questions.
6. Conduct teaching sessions, using the most appropriate teaching methods:
   Discussion
   Lecture
   Demonstration/return demonstration
   Use of audiovisual or printed educational materials

7. Repeat key principles and provide them in printed form *for reference at a later time.*
8. Give frequent feedback to patients when practicing new skills.
9. Use several teaching sessions when appropriate. *New information and skills should be reinforced several times after initial learning.*
10. Initiate referrals for follow-up if necessary:
    Health educators
    Home health care
    Rehabilitation programs
    Social services
11. Evaluate effectiveness of teaching plan, based on patients' abilities to meet preset goals and objectives, and determine need for further teaching.

Knowledge Deficit (Specify) Related to Cognitive/Perceptual Learning Limitations (e.g., sensory overload, sleep deprivation, medications, anxiety, sensory deficits, language barrier)

DEFINING CHARACTERISTICS

- Verbalized statement of inadequate knowledge of skills
- Verbalization of inadequate recall of information
- Verbalization of inadequate understanding of information
- Evidence of inaccurate follow-through of instructions
- Inadequate demonstration of a skill
- Lack of compliance with prescribed behavior

OUTCOME CRITERIA

- Patients participate actively in necessary and prescribed health behaviors.
- Patients verbalize adequate knowledge or demonstrate adequate skills.

NURSING INTERVENTIONS AND *RATIONALE*

1. Continue to monitor the assessment parameters listed under "Defining Characteristics."
2. Determine specific cause of patients' cognitive or perceptual limitation. (See also table of contents for Impaired Verbal Communication, Anxiety, Sleep Pattern Disturbances, Sensory/Perceptual Alterations.)

3. Provide uninterrupted rest period before teaching session *to decrease fatigue and encourage optimal state for learning and retention.*
4. Manipulate environment as much as possible *to provide quiet and uninterrupted learning sessions:*
   Ensure lights are bright enough to see teaching aids but not too bright.
   Close door if necessary *to provide quiet environment.*
   Schedule care and medications *to allow uninterrupted teaching periods.*
   Move patients to quiet, private room for teaching if possible.
5. Adapt teaching sessions and materials to patients' and families' levels of education and ability to understand:
   Provide printed material appropriate to reading level.
   Use terminology understood by patients.
   Provide printed materials in patients' primary language if possible.
   Use interpreters during teaching sessions when necessary.
6. Teach only present-tense focus during periods of sensory overload.

KNOWLEDGE DEFICIT CONT'D

NURSING INTERVENTIONS AND *RATIONALE* CONT'D

7. Determine potential effects of medications on ability to retain or recall information. Avoid teaching critical content while patients are taking sedatives, analgesics, or other medications affecting memory.

8. Reinforce new skills and information in several teaching sessions. Use several senses when possible in teaching session (e.g., see a film, hear a discussion, read printed information, and demonstrate skills related to self-injection of insulin).

9. Reduce patients' anxiety:

   Listen attentively and encourage verbalization of feelings.

   Answer questions as they arise in a clear and succinct manner.

Elicit patients' concerns and address those issues first.

Give only correct and relevant information.

Continually assess response to teaching session and discontinue if anxiety increases or physical condition becomes unstable.

Provide nonthreatening information before more anxiety-producing information is presented.

Plan for several teaching sessions so information can be divided into small, manageable packages.

Nursing Management of Psychosocial Alterations

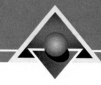

BODY IMAGE DISTURBANCE

Definition
Disruption in the way subjects perceive their body image.

Body Image Disturbance Related to Actual Change in Body Structure, Function, or Appearance

DEFINING CHARACTERISTICS

- Actual change in appearance, structure, or function
- Avoidance of looking at body part
- Avoidance of touching body part
- Hiding or overexposure of body part (intentional or unintentional)
- Trauma to nonfunctioning part
- Change in ability to estimate spatial relationship of body to environment
- Verbalization of the following:
  Fear of rejection or reaction by others
  Negative feelings about body
  Preoccupation with change or loss
  Refusal to participate in or accept responsibility for self-care of altered body part
- Personalization of part or loss with a name
- Depersonalization of part or loss by use of impersonal pronouns
- Refusal to verify actual change

OUTCOME CRITERIA

- Patients verbalize the specific meaning of the change to themselves
- Patients request appropriate information about self-care
- Patients complete personal hygiene and grooming daily with or without help
- Patients interact freely with family or other visitors
- Patients participate in the discussions related to planning their medical and nursing care in the critical care unit and transfer from the unit
- Patients talk about their loss at least twice with trained visitors (support group representatives)

NURSING INTERVENTIONS AND *RATIONALE*

1. Continue to monitor the assessment parameters listed under "Defining Characteristics." In addition, assess the patients' mental, physical, and emotional state and recognize assets, strengths, response to illness, coping mechanisms, past experience with stress, support systems, and coping mechanisms.
2. Appraise the response of the families and significant others. *Body image is derived from the "reflected appraisals" of family and significant others.*
3. Determine patients' goals and readiness for learning.
4. Provide the necessary information to help patients and families adapt to the change. Clarify misconceptions about future limitations.
5. Permit and encourage patients to express the significance of the loss or change. Note nonverbal behavioral responses.
6. Allow and encourage patients' expression of *Anxiety. Anxiety is the most predominant emotional response to a body image disturbance.*

NURSING INTERVENTIONS AND *RATIONALE* CONT'D

7. Recognize and accept the use of denial as an adaptive defense mechanism when used early and temporarily.
8. Recognize maladaptive denial as that interfering with patients' progress and/or alienating support systems. Use confrontation.
9. Provide an opportunity for patients to discuss sexual concerns.
10. Touch the affected body part *to provide patients with sensory information about altered body structure and/or function.*
11. Encourage and provide movement of the altered body part *to establish kinesthetic feedback, enabling persons to know their body as it now exists.*
12. Prepare patients to look at the body part. Call the body part by its anatomical name (e.g., stump, stoma, limb) as opposed to "it" or "she." *The use of impersonal pronouns increases a sense of fantasy and depersonalization of the body part.*
13. Allow patients to experience excellence in some aspect of physical functioning—walking, turning, deep breathing, healing, and self-care—and point out progress and accomplishment. *This intervention helps to balance patients' sense of dysfunction with function.*
14. Avoid false reassurance. Acknowledge the difficulty of incorporating the altered body part or function into patients' body image. *This intervention shows nurses' sensitivity and promotes trust.*
15. Talk with patients about their lives, generativity, and accomplishments. *Patients with disturbances in body image frequently see themselves in a distorted, narrow sense. Encouraging a wider focus of themselves and their lives reduces this distortion.*
16. Help patients explore realistic alternatives.
17. Recognize that incorporating a body change into patients' body image takes time. Avoid setting unrealistic expectations and *thereby inadvertently reinforcing a low self-esteem.*
18. Suggest the use of additional resources such as trained visitors who have mastered situations similar to those of patients. Refer patients to a psychiatric liaison nurse or psychiatrist if needed.

Body Image Disturbance Related to Functional Dependence on Life-Sustaining Technology
(ventilator, dialysis, IABP, halo traction)

DEFINING CHARACTERISTICS

- Actual change in function requiring permanent or temporary replacement
- Refusal to verify actual loss
- Verbalization of the following:
  Feelings of helplessness
  Hopelessness
  Powerlessness
  Fear of failure to wean from technology

OUTCOME CRITERIA

- Patients verify actual change in function
- Patients do not refuse or fight technologic intervention
- Patients verbalize acceptance of expected change in lifestyle

NURSING INTERVENTIONS AND *RATIONALE*

1. Continue to monitor the assessment parameters listed under "Defining Characteristics." In addition, assess patient's response to the technologic intervention.
2. Assess responses of the families and significant others. *Body image is derived from the "reflected appraisals" of family and significant others.*
3. Provide information needed by patients and families.
4. Promote trust, security, comfort, and privacy.
5. Recognize *Anxiety;* allow and encourage its expression. *Anxiety is the most predominant emotion accompanying body image alterations.*
6. Assist patients to recognize their own functioning and performance in the face of technology. For example, help patients distinguish spontaneous breaths from mechanically delivered breaths. *This activity will assist in weaning the patients from the ventilator when feasible. To establish realistic, accurate body boundaries, patients need help separating themselves from the technology that is supporting their functioning. Any participation or function on the part of patients during periods of dependency is helpful in preventing and/or resolving an alteration in body image.*
7. Plan for discontinuation of the treatment (e.g., weaning from ventilator). Explain the procedure that will be followed, and be present during its initiation.
8. Plan for patients' transfer from the critical care environment.
9. Document care, ensuring that an up-to-date care plan is available for all involved caregivers.

SELF-ESTEEM DISTURBANCE

▼

Definition

Negative self-evaluation/feelings about self or self-capabilities, which may be directly or indirectly expressed.

Self-Esteem Disturbance Related to Feelings of Guilt About Physical Deterioration

DEFINING CHARACTERISTICS

- Inability to accept positive reinforcement
- Lack of follow-through
- Nonparticipation in therapy
- Lack of responsibility for self-care (self-neglect)
- Self-destructive behavior
- Lack of eye contact

OUTCOME CRITERIA

- Patients verbalize feelings of self-worth
- Patients maintain positive relationships with significant others
- Patients manifest active interest in appearance by completing personal grooming daily

NURSING INTERVENTIONS AND *RATIONALE*

1. Continue to monitor the assessment parameters listed under "Defining Characteristics." In addition, assess the meaning of the health-related situation: How do patients feel about themselves, the diagnosis, and the treatment? How does the present fit into the larger context of life?
2. Assess patients' emotional levels, interpersonal relationships, and feelings about themselves. Recognize patients' uniqueness (e.g., how the hair is worn, preference for name used).
3. Help patients discover and verbalize feelings and understand the crisis by listening and providing information.

4. Assist patients to identify strengths and positive qualities that increase the sense of self-worth, focusing on past experiences of accomplishment and competency. Help patients with positive self-reinforcement and emphasize the obvious love and affection of family and significant others.
5. Assess coping techniques that have been helpful in the past. Help patients decide how to handle negative or incongruent feedback about the situation.
6. Encourage visits from family and significant others, facilitating interactions and ensuring privacy. Help family members entering the critical care unit by explaining what they will see. Increase visitors' comfort with resources: offer chairs and other courtesies.
7. Encourage patients to pursue interest in individual or social activities, even though such pursuits may be difficult in the critical care unit.
8. Reflect caring, concern, empathy, respect, and unconditional acceptance in nurse-patient relationships.
9. Remember that for patients, nurses are significant others who provide important appraisals and can facilitate the change process.
10. Help families support patients' self-esteem.
11. Provide for continuity of nurse assignment to ensure consistent contacts that can *facilitate support of patients' self-esteem.*

POWERLESSNESS

▼

Definition

Perception that one's own action will not significantly affect an outcome; a perceived lack of control over a current situation or immediate happening.

Powerlessness Related to Health Care Environment or Illness-Related Regimen

DEFINING CHARACTERISTICS
Severe

- Verbal expressions of having no control or influence over situation
- Verbal expressions of having no control or influence over outcome
- Verbal expressions of having no control over self-care
- Depression over physical deterioration that occurs despite patients' compliance with regimens
- Apathy

Moderate

- Nonparticipation in care or decision making when opportunities are provided
- Expressions of dissatisfaction and frustration about inability to perform previous tasks and/or activities
- Lack of progress monitoring
- Expressions of doubt about role performance
- Reluctance to express true feelings, fearing alienation from caregivers
- Passivity

POWERLESSNESS CONT'D

DEFINING CHARACTERISTICS CONT'D
Moderate cont'd

- Inability to seek information about care
- Dependence on others that may result in irritability, resentment, anger, and guilt
- No defense of self-care practices when challenged

Low

- Passivity

OUTCOME CRITERIA

- Patients verbalize increased control over situation by wanting to do things their way
- Patients actively participate in planning care
- Patients request needed information
- Patients choose to participate in self-care activities
- Patients monitor progress

NURSING INTERVENTIONS AND *RATIONALE*

1. Continue to monitor the assessment parameters listed under "Defining Characteristics." In addition, assess patients' feelings and perception of the reasons for lack of power and sense of helplessness.
2. Determine as far as possible patients' usual responses to limited control situations. Determine through ongoing assessment patients' usual locus of control (i.e., believe influence over their life is exerted by luck, fate, powerful persons [external locus of control], or believe influence is exerted through personal choices, self-effort, self-determination [internal locus of control]).
3. Support patients' physical control of the environment by involving them in care activities; knock before entering the room if appropriate; ask permission before moving personal belongings. Inform patients that although an activity may not be to their liking, it is necessary. *This intervention gives patients permission to express dissatisfaction with the environment and regimen.*
4. Personalize patients' care using their preferred name. *This intervention supports patients' psychologic control.*
5. Provide the therapeutic rationale for all patients are asked to do for themselves and for all that is being done for and with them. Reinforce the physician's explanations; clarify misconceptions about the illness situation and treatment plans. *This supports patients' cognitive control.*
6. Include patients in care planning by encouraging participation and allowing choices whenever possible (e.g., timing of personal care activities, deciding when pain medicines are needed). Point out situations in which no choices exist.
7. Provide opportunities for patients to exert influence over themselves, thereby affecting an outcome. For example, share with patients the nurses' assessment of their breath sounds and explain that improvement can be made by self-initiated deep breathing exercises. *Feedback that patients have been successful in helping clear their lungs reinforces the influence they retain.*
8. Encourage families to permit patients to do as much independently as possible *to foster perceptions of personal power.*
9. Assist patients to establish realistic short- and long-term goals. *Setting unrealistic or unattainable goals inadvertently reinforces patients' perception of powerlessness.*
10. Document care to provide for continuity *so that patients can maintain appropriate control over the environment.*
11. Assist patients to regain strength and activity tolerance as appropriate, *thus increasing a sense of control and self-reliance.*
12. Increase the sensitivity of the health team members and significant others to patients' sense of powerlessness. Use power over patients carefully. Use the words *must, should,* and *have to* with caution *because they communicate coercive power and imply that the objects of "musts" and "shoulds" are of benefit to nurses versus patients.*
13. Plan with patients for transfer from the critical care unit to the intermediate unit and eventually to home.

INEFFECTIVE INDIVIDUAL COPING

Definition
Impairment of adaptive behaviors and problem-solving abilities of a person in meeting life's demands and roles.

Ineffective Individual Coping Related to Situational Crisis and Personal Vulnerability

DEFINING CHARACTERISTICS

- Verbalization of inability to cope
  Sample statements:
  "I can't take this anymore."
  "I don't know how to deal with this."
- Ineffective problem solving (problem lumping)
  Examples:
  "I have to eliminate salt from my diet."
  "They tell me I can no longer mow the lawn."
  "This hospitalization is costing a mint."
  "What about my kids' future?"
  "Who's going to change the oil in the car?"
  "This is an incredible amount of time away from work."
- Ineffective use of coping mechanisms
  Projection: blames others for illness or pain
  Displacement: directs anger and/or aggression toward family.
  Examples:
  "Get out of here"
  "Leave me alone."
  Curses, shouts, or demands attention; strikes out or throws objects
  Denial of severity of illness and need for treatment
- Noncompliance
  Examples:
  Activity restriction
  Refusal to allow treatment or to take medications
- Suicidal thoughts (verbalizes desire to end life)
- Self-directed aggression
  Examples:
  Disconnects or attempts to disconnect life-sustaining equipment
  Deliberately tries to harm self
- Failure to progress from dependent to more independent state (refusal or resistance to care for self)

OUTCOME CRITERIA

- Patients verbalize beginning ability to cope with illness, pain, and hospitalization
  Sample statements:
  "I'm trying to do the best I can."
  "I want to help myself get better."
- Patients demonstrate effective problem solving (lists and prioritizes problems from most to least urgent)
- Patients use effective behavioral strategies to manage the stress of illness and care

- Patients demonstrate interest or involvement in illness or environment
  Examples:
  Request medications when anticipating pain
  Question course of treatment, progress, and prognosis
  Ask for clarification of environmental stimuli and events
  Seek out in their environment supportive individuals
  Use coping mechanisms and strategies more effectively to manage situational crisis
  Demonstrate significant reduction in impulsive, angry, or aggressive outbursts (projection, shouting, cursing) directed toward family
  Verbalize futuristic plans with cessation of self-directed aggressive acts and suicidal thoughts
  Willingly comply with treatment regimen
  Begin to participate in self-care

NURSING INTERVENTIONS AND *RATIONALE*

1. Continue to monitor the assessment parameters listed under "Defining Characteristics."
2. Listen and respond to patients' verbal and behavioral expressions. *Listening signifies unconditional respect for and acceptance of patients. Listening also builds trust and rapport, guides nurses toward problem areas, encourages patients to express concerns, and promotes compliance.*
3. Offer effective coping strategies to help patients better tolerate the stressors related to their illness and care. Give permission to vent feelings in a safe setting.
   Sample statements:
   "I don't blame you for feeling angry or frustrated."
   "Others who are ill like you have expressed similar feelings."
   "I will listen to anything you want to share with me."
   "We don't have to talk; I'd like to sit here with you."
   "It's perfectly okay to cry."
   Individuals who are provided with opportunities to express their feelings will be better able to release pent-up emotions and derive a greater sense of relief and comfort. Thus they are less likely to resort to overly impulsive, aggressive acts, which may harm themselves or others.

INEFFECTIVE INDIVIDUAL COPING CONT'D

NURSING INTERVENTIONS AND *RATIONALE* CONT'D

4. Inform families of patients' needs to displace anger occasionally but that the staff will be working with patients to help them release feelings in a more constructive, effective way. *Family members who are well-informed are better equipped to cope with their loved ones' emotional anguish and outbursts. They are less likely to waste energy on feelings of guilt, fear, anger, or despair and can use their strength to help patients in constructive ways. The knowledge that their loved ones are being cared for emotionally and physically offers family members a greater sense of comfort and understanding. They will feel nurtured and respected by nurses' attempts to include them in the process.*

5. With patients, list and number problems from most to least urgent. Assist the patients in finding immediate solutions for the most urgent problems, postpone those problems that can wait, delegate some problems to family members, and help patients acknowledge problems that are beyond their control. *Listing and numbering problems in an organized way help break them down into more manageable pieces so that patients are better able to identify solutions for those problems that are solvable and to suppress those that are less relevant or not amenable to interventions.*

6. Identify individuals in patients' environments who best help them to cope as well as those who do not. Validate your observations with the patients.
   Sample statements:
   "I notice you seemed more relaxed during your daughter's visit."
   "After the clergy left, you were able to sleep a bit longer than usual; would you like to see him more often?"
   "Your grandson was a bit upset today; I'll be glad to talk to him if you like."
   Supportive persons can invoke a calming effect on patients' physiologic and psychologic states. Conversely, well-meaning but nonsupportive individuals can have a deleterious effect on patients' abilities to cope and must be carefully screened and counseled by nurses.

7. Teach patients effective cognitive strategies to help them better manage the stress of critical illness and care. Help patients construct pleasant thoughts, situations, or images that can simultaneously inhibit unpleasant realities.
   Examples:
   A day at the beach
   A walk in the park
   Drinking a glass of wine

Being with a loved one
Pleasant thoughts or images constructed during critical illness and care tend to inhibit or reduce the intensity of the unpleasant, stressful effects of the experience.

8. Assist patients in using coping mechanisms more effectively so that they can better manage their situational crisis:
   Suppression of problems beyond patients' control
   Compensation for illness and its effects; focusing on patients' strengths, interests, family, and spiritual beliefs
   Adaptive displacement of anger, fear, or frustration through healthy, verbal expressions to staff
   Effective use of coping mechanisms helps assuage patients' painful feelings in a safe setting. Thus patients are strengthened and need not resort to the use of more ineffective defenses to eliminate anxiety.

9. Initiate a suicidal assessment if patients verbalize the desire to die, state that life is not worth living, or exhibit self-directed aggression.
   Sample statement:
   "We know this is a bad time for you. You're saying repeatedly that you want to die. Are you planning to harm yourself?"
   If the response is yes, remain with patients, alert staff members, and provide for psychiatric consultation as soon as possible. Continue to express concern to patients and protect them from harm. *Suicidal thoughts as a result of ineffective coping or exhaustion of coping devices are common occurrences in critically ill patients. If the mood is distressing enough, patients may seek relief by attempting a self-destructive act. Although patients may not imminently have the energy to succeed in their attempt, voicing specific plans signifies a depressed mood and a depletion of coping strategies. Thus immediate intervention is needed, because the attempt may be successful when patients' energy is restored.*

10. Encourage patients to participate in self-care activities and the treatment regimen in accordance with their level of progress. Offer praise for the patients' efforts toward self-care. *Patients who take an active role in their own treatment and progress are less apt to feel like helpless or powerless victims. This greater sense of control over illness and environment will guide patients more swiftly toward becoming as independent as possible.*

ANXIETY

Definition
A vague, uneasy feeling, the source of which is often nonspecific or unknown by the individual.

Anxiety Related to Threat to Biologic, Psychologic, and/or Social Integrity

DEFINING CHARACTERISTICS

Subjective

- Verbalizes increased muscle tension
- Expresses frequent sensation of tingling in hands and feet
- Relates continuous feeling of apprehension
- Expresses preoccupation with a sense of impending doom
- States difficulty in falling asleep
- Repeatedly expresses concerns about changes in health status and outcome of illness

Objective

- Psychomotor agitation (fidgeting, jitteriness, restlessness)
- Tightened, wrinkled brow
- Strained (worried) facial expression
- Hypervigilance (scans environment)
- Easily startled
- Distractibility
- Sweaty palms
- Fragmented sleep patterns
- Tachycardia
- Tachypnea

OUTCOME CRITERIA

- Patients effectively use learned relaxation strategies
- Patients demonstrate significant decrease in psychomotor agitation
- Patients verbalize reduction in tingling sensations in hands and feet
- Patients can focus on tasks at hand
- Patients express positive, futuristic plans to families and staff
- Patients' heart rates and rhythms remain within limits commensurate with physiologic status

NURSING INTERVENTIONS AND *RATIONALE*

1. Continue to monitor the assessment parameters listed under "Defining Characteristics."
2. Instruct the patient in the following simple, effective relaxation strategies:
   If not contraindicated cardiovascularly, tense and relax all muscles progressively from toes to head
   Perform slow, deep-breathing exercises
   Focus on a single object or person in the environment
   Listen to soothing music or relaxation tapes with eyes closed
   Progressive toe-to-head relaxation releases the muscular tension that may be a stress-related effect resulting from the threat or change in patients' health status and outcome of illness. Deep-breathing exercises provide slow, rhythmic, controlled breathing patterns that relax patients and distract them from the effects of their illness and hospitalization. Focusing on a single object or person helps patients dismiss the myriad of disorienting stimuli from their visual-perceptual field, which can have a dizzying, distorted effect. A clear sensorium allows patients to feel more in control of their environments. Music or words expressed in soft, low tones tend to produce soothing, relaxing effects that counteract or inhibit escalating anxiety and provide respites from patients' situational crises. Closed eyes eliminate distracting visual stimuli and promote a more restful environment.
3. Listen to and accept patients' concerns regarding the threats from their illness, outcome, and hospitalization. *Listening and unconditional acceptance validate patients as worthwhile individuals and give assurance that their concerns, no matter how great, will be addressed. Knowledge that patients have an avenue for ventilation will assuage anxiety.*
4. Help patients distinguish between realistic concerns and exaggerated fears through clear, simple explanations.
   Sample statements:
   "Your lab results show that you're doing okay right now."
   "The shortness of breath you're experiencing is not unusual."
   "The pain you described is expected, and this medication will relieve it."
   Patients who are informed about their progress and are reassured about expected symptoms and management of care will be better equipped to maintain a more realistic perspective of the illness and its outcome. Thus anxiety emanating from imagined or exaggerated fears will likely be assuaged or averted.
5. Provide simple clarification of environmental events and stimuli that are not related to patients' illness and care.
   Sample statement:
   "That loud noise is coming from a machine that is helping another patient."
   "The visitor behind the curtain is crying because she's had an upsetting day."
   "That gurney is here to bring another patient to x-ray."
   Clarification of events and stimuli that are unrelated to patients helps to disengage them from the extant

ANXIETY CONT'D

NURSING INTERVENTIONS AND *RATIONALE* CONT'D

anxiety-provoking situations surrounding them, thus avoiding further anxiety and apprehension.

6. Assist patients in focusing on building on prior coping strategies to deal with the effects of their illness and care.
   Sample statements:
   "What methods have helped you get through difficult times in the past?"
   "How can we help you use those methods now?"
   Use of previously successful coping strategies in conjunction with newly learned techniques arms patients with an arsenal of weapons against anxiety, providing them with greater control over their situational crises and decreased feelings of doom and despair.
   (See Ineffective Individual Coping care plan, p. 462, for interventions that assist patients to use coping strategies effectively.)

7. Give patients permission to deny or suppress the effects of their illness and hospitalization with which they cannot cope.
   Sample statements:
   "It's perfectly okay to ignore things you can't handle right now."
   "How can we help ease your mind during this time?"
   "What are some things or tasks that may help distract you?"
   Adaptive denial can be helpful in reducing feelings of anxiety in patients with life-threatening illness. Bigus reported that in studies of two groups of patients suffering from myocardial infarction, the group that used adaptive denial demonstrated significantly fewer symptoms of anxiety than those patients who failed to use it.

SENSORY/PERCEPTUAL ALTERATIONS

Definition
The state in which an individual experiences a change in the amount or patterning of incoming stimuli accompanied by a diminished, exaggerated, distorted, or impaired response to such stimuli.

Sensory/Perceptual Alterations Related to Sensory Overload, Sensory Deprivation, and Sleep Pattern Disturbance

DEFINING CHARACTERISTICS

- Hallucinations
- Delusions
- Illusions
- Disorientation
- Short-term memory deficits
- Impaired abstraction

OUTCOME CRITERIA

- Patients have no evidence of hallucinations, delusions, or illusions
- Results of reality testing are appropriate
- Short-term memory is intact
- Abstract reasoning is intact

NURSING INTERVENTIONS AND *RATIONALE*

1. Continue to monitor the assessment parameters listed under "Defining Characteristics." Determine and document patients' dominant spoken language, their literacy, and the language(s) in which they are literate. Determine and document patients' premorbid degree of orientation, cognitive capabilities, and any sensory-perceptual deficits. *Sometimes individuals are not literate in their spoken language or, less frequently, in their second language. These situations can result in unfortunate errors in the appraisal of patients' ability to communicate in writing and in estimating the extent of their orientation. Similarly, assuming that the patients were or were not fully oriented before critical care admission bases nurses' assessments on possibly erroneous assumptions.*

For sensory overload

1. Initiate nurse-patient encounters by calling patients by name and identifying yourself by name. *This intervention fosters reality orientation and assists patients in filtering irrelevant or impersonal conversation.*
2. Assess patients' immediate physical environments from their viewpoint, and explain any equipment, its sounds, and its therapeutic purpose. Demonstrate audible and visual alarms, and explain the possible alarm conditions. *This intervention decreases alienation of patients from the technologic environment and reduces the sense of fear and urgency accompanying alarm conditions.*
3. For each procedure performed, provide preparatory sensory information (i.e., explain procedures in relation to the sensations patients will experience, including duration of sensations). *Preparatory sensory information enhances learning and lessens anticipatory anxiety.*
4. Limit noise levels. Certainly audible alarms cannot and should not be silenced, and many critical, albeit noisy, activities must take place in the critical care area. However, noise levels produced by clinical personnel exceed those levels designated as "acceptable" and are often greater than those generated by technologic devices. Staff conversations should be kept soft enough that they are inaudible to patients whenever possible. Critical care personnel should assume that everything said at or around a patient's bedside is intended for that patient's awareness. *As in the discussion that follows, conversations about patients but not to them foster depersonalization and delusions of reference.*
5. Well-enforced noise limits should exist for nighttime.
6. Readjust alarm limits on physiologic monitoring devices as patients' conditions change (improve or deteriorate) *to lessen unnecessary alarm states.*
7. Consider the use of head phones and audio cassettes with patients' favorite and/or subliminal or classical music. *This intervention can effectively filter out assaultive noise of the critical care environment and supplant it with familiar, soothing sounds and rhythms.*
8. Modify lighting. Day-night cycles should be simulated with environmental lighting. At no time should overhead fluorescent lights be abruptly turned on without either warning patients, assisting them out of the supine position, and/or shielding their eyes with gauze or a face cloth. *Continuous bright lighting sustains Anxiety and promotes circadian rhythm desynchronization.*
9. Shield patients from viewing urgent and emergent events in the critical care unit to the extent possible. *Resuscitation efforts, albeit difficult to conceal, engender fear in patients and a sense of instability and vulnerability (e.g., "I'm next").* When such an event occurs, nurses should endeavor to elicit patients' cognitive and emotional reactions by sharing thoughts, impressions, and feelings and by clarifying misconceptions. A useful approach for nurses in this interchange is that of emphasizing the differences between the patient at hand and the one resuscitated (e.g., "He was considerably older," "more unstable," "had serious lung disease").

SENSORY/PERCEPTUAL ALTERATIONS CONT'D

NURSING INTERVENTIONS AND *RATIONALE* CONT'D
For sensory overload cont'd

10. Ensure patients' privacy, modesty, and, at the very least, dignity. Physical exposure and nudity, although seeming to pale in importance alongside such priorities as physiologic assessment and stabilization, are primal indignities in all individuals. Patients should be kept minimally exposed. When it becomes necessary to expose patients, nurses should first verbally apologize for this necessity. *To be naked is to feel vulnerable; to be vulnerable is to feel fearful. In this regard, fear is an emotion concomitant to critical care that is preventable through nursing intervention.*

For sensory deprivation

1. Provide reality orientation in four spheres (person, place, time, and situation) at more frequent intervals than when testing. Convey this information in the context of routine conversation.
   Sample statement:
   "Mr. Clark, this is Tuesday morning and you're in University Hospital. Your heart surgery was yesterday morning, and you're doing well. My name is Joe, and I'm your nurse today."
   Patients are made to feel patronized by repetitions such as, "Do you know where you are?" Given the effects of general anesthesia, narcotic analgesics, sedatives, and sleep, it is fully expected that some degree of disorientation will exist.

2. Ensure patients' visual access to a calendar. (The design of most state-of-the-art critical care units now reflects many of the principles of sensory stimulation. One such coronary care unit was designed with a large wall clock facing patients. A patient who had spent more than a week in this unit later reflected that one of the most "distressing, frustrating" aspects of his stay in the coronary care unit was the monotonous, inescapable attention to the clock and its painfully slow documentation of the passing of time.)

3. Apprise patients of daily news events and the weather.

4. Touch patients for the express purpose of communicating a caring attitude. Hold their hands, stroke their brows, rub the skin on their arms. *Touch is the universal language of caring. In the setting of critical care, in which considerable physical body manipulation is present, contrasting assaultive touch to comforting touch is useful and important.* Touch can be used as a technique for distraction from painful stimuli when used in conjunction with uncomfortable procedures.

5. Foster liberal visitation by family and significant others. Encourage significant others to touch patients as consistent with their individual comfort level and cultural norms.

6. Structure and identify opportunities for patients to exercise decision-making skills, however small. *Although not so designated, patients with sensory alterations experience a type of "cognitive deprivation" as well.*

7. Assist patients to find meaning in their experiences. Explain the therapeutic purpose of all that they are asked to do for themselves and all that is done with them and for them. Avoid statements such as, "Will you turn to that side for me?" or "I need you to swallow this medication." *These statements convey that the maneuver has some value for the nurses versus the patients. Similarly, use "thank you" judiciously. This simple salutation, when used indiscriminately, suggests something was done to benefit the nurses and not the patients. Patients need to find meaning and to identify their roles in the experience of critical illness and care. The sensations that constitute this experience and those that do not are made bearable and intelligible when attached to the larger picture of patients' conditions, treatment, and progress.*

For Sleep Pattern Disturbances. For management strategies of *Sleep Pattern Disturbance*, refer to Chapter 5.

For management of patients experiencing hallucinations

1. Approach patients with a calm, matter-of-fact demeanor. *The goal of this interaction is for nurses to demonstrate external control, helping to decrease the Anxiety and Fear that generally accompany hallucinations and allowing patients to feel safe. Anxiety is transferable.*

2. Address patients by name. *This interaction is a useful presentation of reality because self-identity is the last sphere of orientation to vanish.*

3. In responding to patients' descriptions of hallucinations, *do not* deny, argue, or attempt to disprove the existence of the perceived events. *Statements such as, "There are no voices coming from that air vent" or "Look, I'm brushing my hand across the wall, and there are no bugs" confuse patients further because the hallucination, although frightening, is their perceived reality.*

4. Express to patients that your experiences are dissimilar, and acknowledge how frightening theirs must be.
   Sample statement:
   "I don't hear (see) what you do, but I know how frightening such an experience must be to you. I'm Joe, your nurse, and I'm going to stay with you until the voices go away."

Continued.

NURSING INTERVENTIONS AND *RATIONALE* CONT'D
For management of patients experiencing hallucinations cont'd

Remain with any patient who is experiencing a hallucination. *Feelings of fear and anxiety often accelerate when patients are left alone. Patients need someone to represent a nonthreatening reality. In addition, validating patients' feelings demonstrates acceptance and sensitivity to the experience and promotes trust.*

5. *Do not* explore the content of hallucinations with patients by asking about its nature or character. *Nurses are patients' links with reality. Pursuit of a detailed description of a hallucination may signify to patients that nurses accept their sensory distortion as factual. This indication may further confuse patients and distance them more from reality.* Nurses can help bridge the gap between patients' misperceptions and reality by addressing the feelings (e.g., fear, anxiety) and/or meanings (e.g., danger, death) engendered by hallucinations. Determination of how misperceptions affect patients emotionally, acknowledgment of those feelings, and a calm, controlled, matter-of-fact approach will provide the trust and comfort patients need to tolerate these frightening experiences. In other words, deal with the intent more than the content of the hallucination. *The resultant decrease in anxiety will enable patients to focus more accurately on their immediate environments.*

6. Talk concretely with patients about things that are really happening.
   Sample statements:
   "How does your chest incision feel this afternoon, Mr. Clark?"
   "Your sister Kate was here to see you, but you were sleeping. She went down to the cafeteria and will be back."
   "Your secretions are a little easier for you to cough up today."
   Interpretation of reality-based stimuli by nurses encourages patients to focus on actual circumstances and discourages a preoccupation with sensory misperceptions.

7. Circumstances may exist in which it is appropriate for nurses simply to distract patients by changing the topic. This tactic is useful in situations of escalating anxiety and confusion or when all else fails. Topics should consist of basic themes that are universally understood and culturally congruent, such as music, food, or weather. Also appropriate are topics of special interest to patients, such as hobbies, crafts, or sports. Topics that evoke strong emotions, such as politics, religion, or sexuality, should be avoided with most patients. *This final point is especially true of patients with reality distortions; sometimes hallucinations and delusions are expressions of repressed conflicts associated with religious, sexual, or aggressive issues. Pursuit of such subjects could increase confusion and Anxiety.*

8. *Touch presents a nonthreatening external reality and can therefore be useful in the management of patients with sensory alterations. However, in instances of patients experiencing hallucinations (as well as delusions and illusions), touch can be readily misinterpreted as, for instance, aggression or Pain, or it can actually provide the basis for a tactile illusion. Therefore the use of touch as an intervention strategy should be avoided in any patient who evidences escalating Anxiety or paranoid, suspicious, or mistrustful thoughts.*

9. Types of hallucinations include the following: auditory—voices or running commentaries, with self-destructive messages; visual—persons or images that appear threatening; olfactory—smells that may be interpreted as poisonous gases; gustatory—tastes that seem peculiar or harmful; and tactile—touch that feels unusual or unnatural.

10. Specific management strategies for patients experiencing hallucinations include the following:
    • Auditory hallucinations
      a. Patient behaviors:
         Head cocked as if listening to an unseen presence
         Lips moving
      b. Therapeutic nurse responses:
         "Mr. Clark, you appear to be listening to something." If the patient acknowledges voices, reply, "I don't hear any voices, but I know this is troubling you. The voices will go away. Nothing is going to harm you. I'm Joe, your nurse, and I'll be here with you."
      c. Nontherapeutic nurse responses:
         "Tell me about your conversations with these voices."
         "To whom do the voices belong—anyone you know?"
    • Visual hallucinations
      a. Patient behaviors:
         Staring into space as if focused on an unseen object
         Startled movements and anxious facial expression
      b. Therapeutic nurse responses:
         "Mr. Clark, something seems to be troubling you. Tell me what it is." If patients state that they visualize people, images, or the devil and imply a sense of danger, respond, "There are only nurses and doctors here, Mr. Clark. I know this must be upsetting, but these

*Exceptions to this rule include instances in which the nurses suspect the patients are experiencing auditory hallucinations (i.e., hearing "voice commands." To ascertain that the voices are not telling patients to harm themselves, nurses should ask simply and concretely, "What are the voices saying?"

SENSORY/PERCEPTUAL ALTERATIONS CONT'D

NURSING INTERVENTIONS AND *RATIONALE* CONT'D
For management of patients experiencing hallucinations cont'd

images will go away. We're here with you in the hospital. Nothing will happen to you."
  c. Nontherapeutic nurse responses:
    "Describe the people you see. What are they wearing?"
    "What does the devil mean in your life? What about God?"

For management of patients experiencing delusions

1. Explain all unseen noises, voices, and activity simply and clearly. These elements readily feed a delusional system.
   Sample statements:
   "That is Dr. Smith. He's come to see you and other patients here in the hospital."
   "The voices and activity you hear are from the bedside of the patient behind this curtain. He's being helped by one of the nurses."
2. Avoid any negative challenge of the patients' delusion (e.g., "Nobody here stole your belongings" or "Doctors and nurses do not harm people"). Similarly, avoid defending the referents of patients' beliefs: "Nurses are good" and "Doctors mean well." *Remember, a delusion is a belief, albeit false, that cannot be changed with logic. To attempt this change is to challenge patients' belief systems and thereby escalate their Anxiety, further blurring the boundaries between reality and patients' internally based "logic."*
3. For patients with persecutory delusions who refuse food, fluids, or medications because of a belief that these things have been poisoned or tainted, permit the refusal unless it is a life-threatening event. Try again in 20 minutes; allow patients to choose an alternative selection of food or to read the label on the unit's medication. Coercion, show of force, or engaging in complicated, logical justifications will only heighten patients' suspiciousness and possibly reinforce delusional beliefs. *When patients feel more in control, they need not rely on the paradoxical quality of the delusion to equip them with a false sense of power. Instead, patients' power is derived from making reality-based decisions.*
4. Staff members should be particularly careful not to engage in unnecessary laughter or whispering within view of delusional patients. *Delusional patients are hypervigilant, scanning the environment for evidence to corroborate or confirm their belief that staff members are colluding against them; clearly,*

laughter and whispers easily encourage this delusion of reference. This rationale pertains to patients experiencing hallucinations and/or illusions as well.
5. Observe the principles detailed in the third intervention under "Management of Patients Experiencing Hallucinations."

For management of patients experiencing illusions

1. As with the management of delusions, nurses should simply and briefly interpret reality-based stimuli for patients in a calm, matter-of-fact manner. *Seen and unseen noises, voices, activity, and people can provide the stimulus for a sensory misinterpretation, an illusion.*
2. The immediate environments of patients should provide as low a level of stimulation as possible. Nursing interventions detailed previously under "Sensory Overload" are especially relevant here.
3. The theme of nurses' verbal approaches to patients experiencing illusions is similar to that outlined for hallucinations and delusions: address the feelings and meanings associated with the experience, not the content of the sensory misinterpretation.
   • Patient behaviors:
     Darting eyes
     Startled movements
     Frightened facial expression.
     "I know who you are. You're the devil come to take me to hell."
   • Therapeutic nurse responses:
     "I'm Joe, your nurse. I know this experience is troubling for you. You're in the hospital, and no one here will harm you."
   • Nontherapeutic nurse responses:
     "There are no such things as devils or angels."
     "Do you think the devil would be dressed in white?"
     The first nontherapeutic nurse response carries a parental tone (i.e., "you know better than that"), thus infantilizing patients and adding to their feelings of powerlessness over the environment. The second nontherapeutic response reflects obvious logic, which is not in patients' sensory domain; therefore the response cannot be processed and only adds to patients' confused state.
4. Observe the principles detailed under the fifth item in "Management of Patients Experiencing Hallucinations."

Nursing Management of Sleep Alterations

SLEEP PATTERN DISTURBANCE

Definition
Disruption of sleep time causes discomfort or interferes with desired lifestyle.

Sleep Pattern Disturbance Related to Fragmented Sleep

DEFINING CHARACTERISTICS

- Decreased sleep during one block of sleep time
- Daytime sleepiness
- Sleep deprivation
  Less than one half of normal sleep time
  Decreased slow wave, or REM, sleep
- Anxiety
- Fatigue
- Restlessness
- Disorientation and hallucinations
- Combativeness
- Frequent wakenings
- Decreased arousal threshold

OUTCOME CRITERIA

- Patients' total sleep times approximate patients' usual sleep times.
- Patients can complete sleep cycles of 90 minutes without interruption
- Patients have no delusions, hallucinations, illusions.
- Patients have reality-based thought content.
- Patients are oriented to four spheres.

NURSING INTERVENTIONS AND *RATIONALE*

1. Continue to monitor the assessment parameters listed under "Defining Characteristics."
2. Assess normal sleep pattern on admission and any history of sleep disturbance or chronic illness that may affect sleep or sedative/hypnotic use. Promote normal sleep activity while patients are in critical care unit. Assess sleep effectiveness by asking patients how sleep in the hospital compares with sleep at home.
3. Minimize awakenings *to allow for at least 90-minute sleep cycles.* Continually assess the need to awaken patients, particularly at night. Distinguish between essential and nonessential nursing tasks. Organize nursing care to allow for maximum amount of uninterrupted sleep while ensuring close monitoring of patients' condition. Whenever possible, monitor physiologic parameters without waking patients. Coordinate awakenings with other departments, such as respiratory therapy, laboratory, and x-ray, *to minimize sleep interruptions.*
4. Minimize noise, particularly that of the staff and noisy equipment. Reduce the level of environmental stimuli.
5. Plan nap times to assist in equilibrating the normal total sleep time. Discourage naps longer than 90 minutes at a time *because this may alter the stimulus for night sleep.* Early morning naps, however, may be beneficial in promoting REM sleep *because a greater proportion of early morning sleep is allocated to REM activity.*
6. Promote comfort, relaxation, and a sense of well-being. Treat pain. Eliminate stressful situations before bedtime. Use of relaxation techniques, imagery, backrubs, or warm blankets may be helpful. Other interventions may include increased privacy or a private room and providing patients with gar-

SLEEP PATTERN DISTURBANCE CONT'D

NURSING INTERVENTIONS AND *RATIONALE* CONT'D

ments or coverings brought from home. Individual patients may prefer quiet or the background noise of the television *to best promote sleep.*

7. Be aware of the effects of commonly used medications on sleep. *Many sedative and hypnotic medications decrease REM sleep.* Sedative and analgesic medications should not be withheld, but rather medications and routes of administration that minimally disrupt sleep should be used to complement comfort measures. Do not abruptly withdraw REM-suppressing medications, *because this can result in REM rebound.*

8. Foods containing tryptophan (e.g., milk, turkey) may be appropriate *because these promote sleep.*

9. Be aware that the best treatment for sleep deprivation is prevention.

10. Facilitate staff awareness that sleep is essential and health promoting. Assess the critical care unit for sleep-reducing stimuli and work to minimize them.

11. Document amount of uninterrupted sleep per shift, especially sleep episodes lasting longer than 2 hours. This can be effectively documented as part of the 24-hour flow sheet and reported routinely, shift to shift. *Sleep pattern disturbance is diagnosed, treated, and resolved more efficiently when formally documented in this manner.*

Sleep Pattern Disturbance Related to Circadian Desynchronization

DEFINING CHARACTERISTICS

- Sleep is occurring out of synchronization with biologic rhythms, resulting in sleeping during the day and awakening at night
- Anxiety and restlessness
- Decreased arousal threshold

OUTCOME CRITERIA

- Majority of patients' sleep time will fall during low cycle of the circadian rhythm (normally at night).

NURSING INTERVENTIONS AND *RATIONALE*

1. Continue to monitor the assessment parameters listed under "Defining Characteristics."

2. Assist patients to maintain normal day-night cycles by decreasing lighting, noise, and sensory stimulation at night and critically evaluating the need to awaken patients at night. Maintain a regular schedule for external time cues, such as mealtimes and favorite television shows.

3. Activity during the daytime should be increased to stimulate wakefulness. Increased physical activity until 2 hours before bedtime is useful in *promoting naturally induced sleep.* Limiting caffeine intake after early afternoon will promote sleep in the evening.

4. Do not schedule routine procedures at night.

5. Be aware that cardiac dysrhythmias can be precipitated by the decreased arousal threshold secondary to desynchronization.

6. If desynchronization occurs, plan for resynchronization by maintaining constancy in day-night pattern for at least 3 days (may require 5 to 12 days to re-acclimatize). Plan for activities during the day *to stimulate wakefulness* and use comfort measures (e.g., comfortable body position, warm blankets, backrub) *to promote sleep* at night. Resynchronization is characteristically associated with chronic fatigue, malaise, and a decreased ability to perform life tasks.

Nursing Management of Cardiovascular Alterations

DECREASED CARDIAC OUTPUT

Definition
The state in which the blood pumped by an individual's heart is sufficiently reduced to the extent that it is inadequate to meet the needs of the body's tissues.

Decreased Cardiac Output Related to Supraventricular Tachycardia

DEFINING CHARACTERISTICS

- Sudden drop in blood pressure
- Atrial and/or ventricular rate >100 bpm
- Decreased mentation
- Decreased urine output
- Chest pain
- Dyspnea

OUTCOME CRITERIA

- Systolic blood pressure (SBP) is >100 mm Hg.
- Mean arterial pressure (MAP) is >70 mm Hg.
- Ventricular heart rate is <100 bpm.
- Sensorium is intact.
- Urine output is >30 ml/hr.

NURSING INTERVENTIONS AND *RATIONALE*

1. Continue to monitor the assessment parameters listed under "Defining Characteristics."
2. Carefully distinguish supraventricular tachycardia from ventricular tachycardia. Monitoring patients in lead V_1 or MCL_1 *may assist in distinguishing ventricular ectopy for aberrancy.*
3. Follow critical care emergency standing orders regarding the administration of supraventricular antidysrhythmic agents such as verapamil, quinidine, procainamide, propranolol, digoxin, and adenosine.
4. Consider positioning patients supine *to increase preload.*

5. Identify precipitating factors when possible, such as emotional stress, caffeine, nicotine, and sympathomimetic drugs and intervene to reduce or eliminate their effect.
6. Assess apical-radial pulse *to identify deficits indicating nonperfused beats.* Monitor amplitude of peripheral pulses *to ascertain perfusion to extremities.*
7. Monitor arterial blood pressure *to determine symptomatic decompensation.*
8. With physician collaboration, consider carotid sinus massage or Valsalva maneuver, *thereby increasing vagal tone.*
9. Anticipate possibility of synchronized cardioversion or overdrive pacing.
10. For atrial fibrillation that is either spontaneously, pharmacologically, or electrically converted, monitor for signs of cerebral, pulmonary, and peripheral thromboembolization as a result of liberation of mural thrombi.
11. If patients are hypoxemic or if dysrhythmia is suspected to be a result of or exacerbated by ischemia, administer oxygen observing the following principles:
    - Without physician collaboration, liter flow should be no greater than 2 L/min via nasal prongs in patients whose pulmonary history either is unknown or reveals a pattern of chronic CO_2 retention. *Administration of oxygen at con-*

DECREASED CARDIAC OUTPUT CONT'D

▼

NURSING INTERVENTIONS AND *RATIONALE* CONT'D

centrations higher than 2 L/min via nasal prongs *may induce CO_2 narcosis in patients who chronically retain CO_2.*

- Oxygen should be administered with the goal of achieving *an oxygen saturation (SaO_2) above 92% when measured by pulse oximetry or ABGs.*

- Observe caution when administering oxygen at an FIO_2 greater than 40% *in view of the higher risk for oxygen toxicity.*

12. Assess serum electrolyte levels, especially potassium and calcium, *because increased or decreased electrolyte levels may exacerbate the dysrhythmia or impair treatment of the dysrhythmia.*

▼

Decreased Cardiac Output Related to Relative Excess of Preload and Afterload Secondary to Impaired Ventricular Contractility

DEFINING CHARACTERISTICS

- Systolic blood pressure (SBP) <100 mm Hg
- Mean arterial pressure (MAP <80 mm Hg
- Change in mentation
- Decreased urine output
- Cardiac index (CI <2.2 L/min/m^2
- Pulmonary artery wedge pressure (PAWP) >15 mm Hg
- Pulmonary artery diastolic pressure (PAD) >15 mm Hg
- Bibasilar fluid crackles
- Faint peripheral pulses
- Ventricular gallop rhythm (S_3)
- Skin cool, pale, moist
- Activity intolerance

OUTCOME CRITERIA

- Cardiac index is 2.2-4.0 L/min/m^2.
- SBP is >90 mm Hg.
- MAP is >80 mm Hg.
- PAWP and PAD are <15 mm Hg.

NURSING INTERVENTIONS AND *RATIONALE*
The Following Interventions Reduce Preload

1. Continue to monitor the assessment parameters listed under "Defining Characteristics."
2. Implement fluid restriction.
3. Double concentrate intravenous drug drips when possible *to decrease the amount of volume infused to patients.*

4. Position patients with extremities dependent *to pool blood in the extremities, thus decreasing preload.*
5. With physician collaboration, administer diuretics.
6. Titrate venous vasodilators and inotropic drips, per protocol, to desired SBP, MAP, PAWP, and/or PAD. Withhold and/or change drip rate when SBP, MAP, PAWP, and/or PAD begin to drop.

The Following Interventions Reduce Afterload

1. Intervene to reduce anxiety and *thereby limit catecholamine release:* administer intravenous MSO_4 per protocol and titrate to MAP or SBP, relaxation techniques, imagery.
2. Titrate arterial vasodilator drips to attain desired SBP, PAWP, and/or PAD. Change drip rate when SBP, PAWP, and/or PAD stabilize or begin to drop.
3. Anticipate possibility of intraaortic balloon pumping.

The Following Interventions Reduce Myocardial Oxygen Consumption

1. Absolute bed rest *to decrease metabolic demand.*
2. Consider slackening activity restrictions if such restrictions precipitate anxiety. *Anxiety stimulates the sympathetic outpouring of catecholamines and thereby increases myocardial oxygen consumption.*
3. Ensure that patients and families understand routine of critical care unit and explain all care given to patients *to increase patient comfort level and decrease catecholamine release associated with fear of being in an unknown environment.*

Relative excess of preload and afterload refers not to an actual increase in these volumes, but rather to the ability of the ventricle to handle normal volumes because of impaired ventricular function. Therefore the normal volumes become "excessive" to the poorly functioning ventricle.

DECREASED CARDIAC OUTPUT CONT'D

Decreased Cardiac Output Related to Decreased Preload Secondary to Mechanical Ventilation with or without PEEP

DEFINING CHARACTERISTICS

- Sudden drop in SBP, PAWP, or PAD corresponding to the application of mechanical ventilation or PEEP, or changes in tidal volume delivery or level of PEEP.

OUTCOME CRITERIA

- SBP is >90 mm Hg; MAP is >70 mm Hg.
- PAWP, PAD are >6 mm Hg.

NURSING INTERVENTIONS AND *RATIONALE*

1. Continue to monitor the assessment parameters listed under "Defining Characteristics."
2. Monitor vital organ perfusion (through assessment of urine output and mentation, for example) carefully *because some degree of reduction in cardiac output will coexist with the successful application of mechanical ventilation and/or PEEP.*
3. Position patients supine *to increase preload and therefore cardiac output.*
4. With physician collaboration, consider increasing the administration of parenteral fluids to achieve ideal preload. *(The ideal preload may be that which existed before the application of mechanical ventilation and/or PEEP.)*

Decreased Cardiac Output Related to Atrioventricular (AV) Heart Block

DEFINING CHARACTERISTICS

- Systolic blood pressure (SBP) <90 mm Hg
- Mean arterial pressure (MAP) <70 mm Hg
- Ventricular rate <60 bpm
- Decreased mentation or syncope
- Decreased urine output

OUTCOME CRITERIA

- Systolic blood pressure is >90 mm Hg.
- MAP is >70 mm Hg.
- Ventricular rate is >60 bpm.
- Patients are awake and responsive.
- Urine output is >30 ml/hr.

NURSING INTERVENTIONS AND *RATIONALE*
First-Degree AV Block

1. Continue to monitor the assessment parameters listed under "Defining Characteristics."
2. Monitor closely, measuring P-R intervals *to determine further prolongation, which would suggest progression of heart block.*
3. With physician collaboration, consider withholding supraventricular antidysrhythmic agents such as digitalis, quinidine, beta blocking agents, and calcium channel blockers.

Second-Degree AV Block—Mobitz I (Wenckebach Pattern)

1. Continue to monitor the assessment parameters listed under "Defining Characteristics."
2. Monitor for symptomatic decompensation resulting from slow ventricular rate (rare).
3. Position patients supine while symptomatic *to increase preload and therefore cardiac output.*
4. Monitor for progression to complete heart block.
5. With physician collaboration, consider withholding digitalis.
6. Eliminate sources of vagal stimulation. *Vagal stimulation increases the delay in conduction at the AV node.*

Second-Degree AV Block—Mobitz II

1. Continue to monitor the assessment parameters listed under "Defining Characteristics."
2. Monitor closely for symptomatic decompensation as a result of slow ventricular rate (common).
3. Position patients supine while symptomatic *to increase preload and therefore cardiac output.*
4. Monitor for progression of existing block, such as 2:1, 3:1, 4:1 conduction, and for progression to complete heart block.

DECREASED CARDIAC OUTPUT CONT'D

NURSING INTERVENTIONS AND *RATIONALE* CONT'D
Second-Degree AV Block—Mobitz II Cont'd

5. Follow critical care emergency standing orders regarding the administration of positive chronotropic agents such as atropine, or isoproterenol.
6. Anticipate possibility of temporary transvenous pacemaker insertion.

Third-Degree (Complete) AV Block

1. Continue to monitor the assessment parameters listed under "Defining Characteristics."

2. Monitor closely for symptomatic decompensation resulting from flow ventricular rate (common).
3. Position patients supine while symptomatic *to increase preload and therefore cardiac output*.
4. Follow critical care emergency standing orders regarding the administration of isoproterenol.
5. Anticipate the necessity of pacemaker insertion or use of external pacemaker.

Decreased Cardiac Output Related to Hemopericardium (Tamponade) Secondary to Open Heart Surgery

DEFINING CHARACTERISTICS

- Cardiac output (CO) <4.0 L/min
- Cardiac index (CI) <2.2 L/min/m^2
- Elevated PAWP, PAD, or CVP
- Narrowed pulse pressure
- Pulsus paradoxus
- Muffled heart sounds
- Distended neck veins
- Decreasing SBP or MAP
- Tachycardia
- Enlarged cardiac silhouette on chest film

OUTCOME CRITERIA

- Cardiac output is >4.0 L/min.
- Cardiac index is >2.2 L/min/m^2.
- PAWD, PAD, CVP are reduced to baseline.
- Crisp heart sounds are heard.

- SBP is >100 mm Hg; MAP is >70 mm Hg.
- Heart rate is reduced to baseline.
- Cardiac silhouette is reduced to baseline.

NURSING INTERVENTIONS AND *RATIONALE*

1. Continue to monitor the assessment parameters outlined under "Defining Characteristics."
2. Monitor mediastinal chest tube drainage for sudden cessation and/or increase. *Either event is to be considered highly suggestive of impending cardiac tamponade.*
3. Milk mediastinal chest tubes per protocol *to ensure continual patency.*
4. Titrate vasodilator drips *to keep SBP below level at which graft(s) or anastomoses may leak or tear (usually SBP kept <100 mm Hg).*
5. Anticipate the necessity of either bedside pericardiocentesis or return to surgery.

DECREASED CARDIAC OUTPUT CONT'D

Decreased Cardiac Output Related to Decreased Preload Secondary to Fluid Volume Deficit

DEFINING CHARACTERISTICS

- CO <4.0 L/min
- CI <2.2 L/min/m^2
- PAWP, PAD, CVP less than normal or less than baseline
- Tachycardia
- Narrowed pulse pressure
- SBP <90 mm Hg
- Mean arterial pressure (MAP) <70 mm Hg
- Urine is <30 ml/hr.
- Skin pale, cool, moist
- Apprehensiveness

OUTCOME CRITERIA

- CO is >4.0 L/min.
- CI is >2.2 L/min/m^2.
- PAWP, PAD, CVP are normal or back to baseline level.
- Pulse is normal or back to baseline.
- SBP is >90 mm Hg.
- MAP is >70 mm Hg.
- Urine is >30 ml/hr.

NURSING INTERVENTIONS AND *RATIONALE*
For Active Blood Loss

1. Continue to monitor the assessment parameters listed under "Defining Characteristics." In addition, a serum lactate level >3 mosm is believed to represent cellular perfusion failure at its earliest stage.
2. Secure airway and administer oxygen.
3. Position patients supine with legs elevated *to increase preload and therefore cardiac output.* Avoid Trendelenburg's position *because this position causes abdominal viscera to exert pressure against the diaphragm, thereby limiting diaphragmatic descent and inhalation.* Consider low Fowler's position with legs elevated for patients with head injury *to avoid increases in intracranial pressure.*
4. For fluid repletion use the 3:1 rule, replacing 3 parts of fluid for every unit of blood lost.
5. Administer solutions using the fluid challenge technique: infuse precise amounts of fluid (usually 5 to 20 ml/min) over 10-minutes periods and monitor cardiac loading pressures serially to determine successful challenging. If the PAWP or PAD elevates more than 7 mm Hg above beginning level, the infusion should be stopped. If the PAWP or PAD rises only to 3 mm Hg above baseline or falls, another fluid challenge should be given.
6. Assess for signs and symptoms of fluid overload once fluid replacement has begun. These may include elevations above normal of PAP or CVP levels, pulmonary crackles, or dyspnea.
7. Replace fluids first before considering use of vasopressors, *because vasopressors increase myocardial oxygen consumption out of proportion to the reestablishment of coronary perfusion in the early phases of treatment.*
8. When blood available or indicated, replace with fresh packed red cells and fresh-frozen plasma *to keep clotting factors intact.*
9. Move or reposition patients minimally *to decrease or limit tissue oxygen demands.*
10. Evaluate patients' anxiety levels and intervene via patient education or sedation *to decrease tissue oxygen demands.*
11. Be alert to the possibility of development of adult respiratory distress syndrome (ARDS) and disseminated intravascular coagulation (DIC) in the ensuing 72 hours.

For Dehydration

1. Continue to monitor the assessment parameters listed under "Defining Characteristics."
2. Position patients supine with legs elevated *to increase preload and therefore cardiac output.* Avoid Trendelenburg's position because this position causes abdominal viscera to exert pressure against the diaphragm, thereby limiting diaphragmatic descent and inhalation. Consider low Fowler's position with legs elevated for patients with head injury *to avoid increases in intracranial pressure.*
3. Calculate patients' 24-hour fluid requirements per BSA and replace with the appropriate electrolyte solution.
4. Administer solutions using the fluid challenge technique: infuse precise amounts of fluid (usually 5 to 20 ml/min) over 10-minute periods and monitor cardiac loading pressure serially to determine successful challenging. If the PAWP or PAD elevates more than 7 mm Hg above beginning level, the infusion should be stopped. If the PAWP or PAD rises only to 3 mm Hg above baseline or falls, another fluid challenge should be given.
5. Assess for signs and symptoms of fluid overload once fluid replacement has begun. These may include elevations of PAP or CVP to above normal levels, pulmonary crackles, and dyspnea.
6. Replace fluids first before considering use of vasopressors, *because vasopressors increase myocardial oxygen consumption out of proportion to the reestablishment of coronary perfusion in the early phases of treatment.*

DECREASED CARDIAC OUTPUT CONT'D

▼

Decreased Cardiac Output Related to Ventricular Tachycardia

DEFINING CHARACTERISTICS

- Sudden drop in blood pressure
- Syncope
- Loss of consciousness
- Faint or absent peripheral pulses

OUTCOME CRITERIA

- Systolic blood pressure (SBP) is >90 mm Hg.
- Mean arterial pressure (MAP) is >70 mm Hg.
- Patients are awake and responsive.
- Peripheral pulses are palpable.

NURSING INTERVENTIONS AND *RATIONALE*

1. Continue to monitor the assessment parameters listed under "Defining Characteristics."
2. Carefully distinguish ventricular tachycardia from supraventricular tachycardia. Monitoring patients in lead V_1 or MCL_1 *may assist in distinguishing ventricular ectopy from aberrancy.*
3. Monitor and treat the "warning dysrhythmias" (i.e., >6 premature ventricular contractions [PVCs] per minute, multifocal PVCs, R on T phenomenon, couplets, bursts of ventricular tachycardia, bigeminy, trigeminy).
4. Assess serum electrolyte levels (potassium/magnesium) and arterial blood gases (ABGs) *because altered electrolytes, acid–base imbalance, and hypoxemia may exacerbate the dysrhythmia or impair effectiveness of treatment.*

5. Follow critical care emergency standing orders regarding the administration of ventricular antidysrhythmic agents such as lidocaine, bretylium, and procainamide.
6. For asymptomatic ventricular tachycardia, treat with lidocaine. For symptomatic ventricular tachycardia, treat with synchronized cardioversion. For pulseless ventricular tachycardia, treat as ventricular fibrillation and defibrillate. (See ACLS algorithms in Appendix B.)
7. Position patients supine *to increase preload.*
8. Anticipate possibility that sporadic ventricular dysrhythmias may progress to ventricular tachycardia or ventricular fibrillation and be prepared to treat with implementation of synchronized cardioversion and defibrillation, respectively.
9. Anticipate possibility of cardiac standstill and activation of resuscitation protocol.
10. When safe rhythm is reestablished, carefully assess for femoral and carotid pulsations *to rule out electromechanical dissociation.*
11. Identify precipitating factors when possible, such as hypoxia, electrolyte abnormalities, drug toxicity (especially amrinone, digitalis, quinidine, disopyramide, procainamide, phenothiazines, tricyclic and tetracyclic antidepressants), and recent myocardial infarction and intervene to reduce or eliminate their effect.

▼

Decreased Cardiac Output Related to Decreased Preload Secondary to Septicemia

DEFINING CHARACTERISTICS

- Tachycardia >100 bpm
- Skin dry, warm, flushed (early stage); cold, clammy, cyanotic (late stage)
- CO, CI, elevated (early stage), CO, CI, decreased (late stage)
- PA pressures decreased (early stage); elevated (late stage)
- SBP, MAP less than normal or baseline (early); profound hypotension (late stage)
- Urine output <30 ml/hr

OUTCOME CRITERIA

- Heart rate is normal or back to baseline.
- CO is >4.0 L/min; CI is >2.2 L/min/m^2; SBP is >90 mm Hg; MAP is >70 mm Hg.
- Urine output >30 ml/hr.

NURSING INTERVENTIONS AND *RATIONALE*

1. Continue to monitor the assessment parameters listed under "Defining Characteristics." In addition, a serum lactate level >3 mosm is believed to represent cellular perfusion failure at its earliest stage.

NURSING INTERVENTIONS AND *RATIONALE* CONT'D

2. Secure airway and administer oxygen.
3. Position patients supine with legs elevated *to increase preload and therefore cardiac output in late-stage shock.*
4. Administer intravenous solutions as prescribed using the fluid challenge technique: infuse precise amounts of fluid (usually 5 to 20 ml/min) over 10-minute periods and monitor cardiac loading pressures serially to determine successful challenging. If the PAWP or PAD elevates more than 7 mm Hg above beginning levels, the infusion should be stopped. If the PAWP or PAD rises only to 3 mm Hg above baseline or falls, another fluid challenge should be given.

5. Assess for signs and symptoms of fluid overload once fluid replacement has begun. These may include elevations above normal of PAP or CVP levels, pulmonary crackles, and dyspnea.
6. With physician collaboration, administer intravenous antimicrobials and closely monitor their effectiveness and specific side effects. Carefully assess patients for hypersensitivity reaction to antimicrobials.
7. With physician collaboration, administer vasopressor agents and positive inotropic drugs *to maintain perfusion and cardiac output.*

Decreased Cardiac Output Related to Vasodilation and Bradycardia Secondary to Sympathetic Blockade

DEFINING CHARACTERISTICS

- Postural hypotension, such as turning from supine to prone
- SBP <90 mm Hg or below patients' norm
- Decreased PAP, PAD, and PAWP
- Decreased cardiac index
- Decreased SVR
- Bradycardia
- Cardiac dysrhythmias
- Decreased urinary output
- Hypothermia as a result of inability to retain body heat (See section on Neurologic Alterations for the assessment and treatment of other neurologic manifestations of spinal shock.)

OUTCOME CRITERIA

- SBP is >90 mm Hg or within patients' norm.
- Fainting/dizziness with position change is absent.
- <10 mm Hg DBP with position change.
- HR is 60-100 beats/min.
- <20 beats/min HR increase with position change.
- CVP is 4 to 6 mm Hg.
- PAWP is 4 to 12 mm Hg.
- PAD is 8 to 14 mm Hg.
- SVR is 950 to 1300 dynes/sec/cm^{-5}.
- Cardiac index (CI) is 2.2 to 4.0 L/min/m^2.
- Urinary output is >30 ml/hr.
- Body temperature is normal.

NURSING INTERVENTIONS AND *RATIONALE*

1. Continue to monitor the assessment parameters listed under "Defining Characteristics."
2. Implement measures *to prevent episodes of postural hypotension.*

- Change patients' positions slowly.
- Apply antiembolic stockings *to promote venous return.*
- Perform range-of-motion exercises every 2 hours *to prevent venous pooling.*
- Collaborate with physical therapy personnel regarding use of a tilt table *to progress patients from supine to upright position.*

3. Administer crystalloid intravenous fluids using fluid challenge technique: infuse precise amounts of fluid (usually 5 to 20 ml/min) over 10-minute periods; monitor cardiac loading pressures serially to determine successful challenging.
4. Anticipate the administration of colloids.
5. Anticipate administration of vasopressors if fluid challenges are ineffective.
6. Monitor cardiac rhythm. Be especially vigilant during vagal stimulating procedures such as suctioning *because serious bradycardia can result.*
7. Administer atropine per critical care emergency standing orders for symptomatic sinus bradycardia.
8. Maintain normothermia by increasing temperature in patients' rooms and applying blankets. Avoid use of electric warming devices *because of decreased peripheral blood flow and sensation.*

ALTERED TISSUE PERFUSION

▼

Definition
The state in which an individual experiences a decrease in nutrition and oxygenation at the cellular level due to a deficit in capillary blood supply.

Risk for Altered Peripheral Tissue Perfusion Risk Factor: High-Dose Vasopressor Therapy

RISK FACTORS
- Vasopressor therapy

DEFINING CHARACTERISTICS
- Pale or cyanotic digits
- Ischemic pain
- Delayed capillary refill
- Weak peripheral pulses

OUTCOME CRITERIA
- Digits are free from pallor or cyanosis.
- Ischemic pain is absent.
- Capillary refill is immediate.
- Peripheral pulses are full and equal.

NURSING INTERVENTIONS AND *RATIONALE*
1. Continue to monitor the assessment parameters listed under "Defining Characteristics."
2. Careful evaluation of the adequacy of peripheral perfusion is essential in patients receiving infusions of the following vasopressor drugs. In addition, *extravasation of these agents into tissues results in localized ischemic necrosis, and the drugs are therefore infused through central lines when possible.* Dopamine infusions: at dosages >10 mcg/kg/min, alpha adrenergic receptors are stimulated *producing moderate peripheral vasoconstriction;* at dosages >20 μg/kg/min, intense peripheral vasoconstriction results, *producing serious perfusion alterations.* Levarterenol bitartrate infusions: at all dosages alpha adrenergic receptors are stimulated *producing the potential for perfusion alterations.*
3. Avoid high-dose vasopressor therapy. Titrate vasopressor drips to achieve and maintain SBP of 90 mm Hg or MAP above 70 mm Hg. Further augmentation of SBP or MAP should be accomplished by means of other modalities.
4. Immediate physician notification is indicated at the earliest sign of peripheral perfusion alterations.

PERIPHERAL NEUROVASCULAR DYSFUNCTION

▼

Definition
A state in which an individual is at risk of experiencing a disruption in circulation, sensation, or motion of an extremity.

Risk for Peripheral Neurovascular Dysfunction Risk Factor

RISK FACTORS
- Peripheral vascular disease
- Orthopedic trauma
- Cannulation of femoral artery (leg)
- Cannulation of radial artery (hand)

DEFINING CHARACTERISTICS
- Absent, weak, and/or unequal peripheral pulses
- Delayed capillary refill
- Ischemic pain distal to injury/catheter
- Cool skin distal to injury/catheter
- Paresthesias

OUTCOME CRITERIA
- Peripheral pulses are full and equal bilaterally.
- Capillary refill is equal bilaterally.
- No ischemic pain distal to injury/catheter
- Equal skin temperature distal to injury/catheter
- Paresthesias are absent.

Continued.

PERIPHERAL NEUROVASCULAR DYSFUNCTION CONT'D

NURSING INTERVENTIONS AND *RATIONALE*

1. Continue to monitor the assessment parameters listed under "Defining Characteristics."
2. Maintain extremity at or above heart level *to promote venous return.*
3. Maintain patency of any wound drainage device *to prevent excessive interstitial swelling or blood accumulation.*
4. Assess dressings for fit and loosen if constrictive.
5. Maintain integrity of arterial catheter.

ALTERED TISSUE PERFUSION: MYOCARDIAL

Definition

The state in which an individual experiences a decrease in nutrition and oxygenation at the myocardial cellular level due to a deficit in capillary blood supply.

Altered Tissue Perfusion: Myocardial: Related to Acute Myocardial Ischemia Secondary to Coronary Artery Disease (CAD)

DEFINING CHARACTERISTICS

- Angina for more than 30 min but less than 6 hr
- ST segment elevation on 12-lead ECG
- Elevation of CK and CK-MB enzymes
- Apprehension

OUTCOME CRITERIA

- Systolic blood pressure (SBP) is >90 mm Hg.
- Mean arterial pressure (MAP) is >70 mm Hg.
- Ventricular heart rate is <100 bpm.
- PAP pressures are within normal limits or back to baseline.
- Cardiac index is 2.2 L/min/m^2
- Urine output is >30 ml/hr.
- 12-lead ECG is normalized without new q waves.
- Angina is absent.
- CK and CK-MB enzymes are within normal range.
- Patients and families are educated about coronary artery disease (CAD) risk factor modification.

NURSING INTERVENTIONS AND *RATIONALE*

Continue to monitor the assessment parameters listed under "Defining Characteristics."

The Following Interventions Control Pain

1. In collaboration with the physician, administer sublingual nitroglycerin (NTG) and start an intravenous (IV) NTG infusion. Titrate IV NTG *to control pain.* Maintain SBP >90 mm Hg.
2. Administer morphine sulfate IV.

The Following Interventions are to Lyse Clot in Coronary Artery

1. In collaboration with physician, if appropriate for patients, infuse thrombolytic agent of choice *to lyse clot in coronary artery.* Maintain SBP at >90 mm Hg.
2. Infuse IV heparin and assess coagulation studies (ACT or PTT) per hospital protocol *to prevent recurrent thrombosis.*
3. Administer low dose aspirin (80 mg to 325 mg) p.o.

Monitor Hemodynamic/Cardiac Rhythm Status

1. Monitor cardiac rhythm for presence of dysrhythmias. Assess serum electrolytes (potassium and magnesium) and arterial blood gases (ABGs). Correct any imbalance. Administer lidocaine IV (1 mg/kg body weight) if PVCs are >6/min.
2. In case of cardiac/respiratory arrest, follow ACLS/hospital protocols. Have cardioversion/defibrillation equipment nearby.
3. Monitor SBP *because many conditions (drugs, dysrhythmias, myocardial ischemia) may cause hypotension (SBP <90 mm Hg).*
4. *If clinical condition deteriorates, a pulmonary artery (PA) catheter may be required. Be prepared to assist with insertion of PA catheter and to assess hemodynamic profile (PA pressures, PAWP, CO, and CI).*
5. *In collaboration with the physician, if appropriate for patients titrate additional vasodilator medications (sodium nitroprusside) or inotropic medications (dopamine, dobutamine) to maintain SBP >90 mm Hg and CI >2.2 L/min/m^2.*

ACTIVITY INTOLERANCE

Definition
The state in which an individual has insufficient physiological or psychological energy to endure or complete required or desired daily activities.

Activity Intolerance Related to Postural Hypotension Secondary to Prolonged Immobility, Narcotics, Vasodilator Therapy

DEFINING CHARACTERISTICS

- SBP drop >20 mm Hg; heart rate increase >20 bpm on postural change
- Vertigo on postural change
- Syncope on postural change

OUTCOME CRITERIA

SBP drop is <10 mm Hg; heart rate increase is <10 bpm on postural change.

- Vertigo or syncope is absent on postural change.

NURSING INTERVENTIONS AND *RATIONALE*

1. Continue to monitor the assessment parameters listed under "Defining Characteristics."
2. *To increase muscular and vascular tone,* instruct and assist in the following bed exercises: straight leg raises, dorsiflexion/plantar flexion, and quadriceps setting and gluteal setting exercises.

3. Determine that patients are hydrated to 24-hour fluid requirement per BSA *to increase preload and thus stroke volume and cardiac output.* Hydrate accordingly if not contraindicated by cardiac or renal disorders.
4. Assist with postural changes accomplished in increments:
   - Head of bed to 45 degrees and hold until symptom free
   - Head of bed to 90 degrees and hold until symptom free
   - Dangle until symptom free
   - Stand until symptom free and ambulate
5. As soon as it is medically safe, assist patients to sit at bedside for meals.
6. When treating pain with narcotic analgesics, plan ambulation to occur well before peak action of drug.

Activity Intolerance Related to Knowledge Deficit of Energy-Saving Techniques

DEFINING CHARACTERISTICS

- Dyspnea on exertion
- Subjective fatigue on activity
- Heart rate elevations 30 bpm above baseline on activity; heart rate 15 bpm above baseline on activity for patients on beta blockers or calcium channel blockers

OUTCOME CRITERIA

- Patients have subjective tolerance of activity.
- Heart rate elevations are <20 bpm above baseline on activity and are <10 bpm above baseline on activity for patients on beta blockers or calcium channel blockers.

NURSING INTERVENTIONS AND *RATIONALE*

1. Continue to monitor the assessment parameters listed under "Defining Characteristics."
2. Teach and supervise energy-saving techniques based on the principle of performing work on exhalation, that is, standing up from a bed or chair, repositioning self in bed with or without help, reaching, washing face, brushing hair or teeth.
3. To the extent possible, have patients perform work while seated.
4. Teach and supervise muscle-toning exercises, *observing that a toned muscle uses less oxygen,* such as arm bends with elbows down, elbow bends with arms up, straight arm raises inward and outward, plantar flexion and dorsiflexion of the feet, straight leg raises.

ACTIVITY INTOLERANCE CONT'D

Activity Intolerance Related to Decreased Cardiac Output and/or Myocardial Tissue Perfusion Alterations

DEFINING CHARACTERISTICS

- Heart rate elevations 30 bpm above baseline on activity; heart rate elevations 15 bpm above baseline on activity for patients on beta blockers or calcium channel blockers
- Heart rate elevations above baseline 5 minutes after activity
- Ischemic pain on activity
- Electrocardiographic changes on activity
- Subjective fatigue on activity

OUTCOME CRITERIA

- Heart rate elevations are <20 bpm above baseline on activity and are <10 bpm above baseline on activity for patients on beta blockers or calcium channel blockers.
- Heart rate returns to baseline 5 minutes after activity.
- Ischemic pain is absent on activity.
- Patients have subjective tolerance to activity.

NURSING INTERVENTIONS AND *RATIONALE*

1. Continue to monitor the assessment parameters listed under "Defining Characteristics."
2. Encourage active or passive range-of-motion exercises while patients are in bed *to keep joints flexible and muscles stretched.* Teach patients to refrain from holding breath while performing exercises, *avoiding Valsalva maneuver.*
3. Encourage performance of muscle-toning exercises at least 3 times daily *because a toned muscle uses less oxygen when performing work than an untoned muscle.*
4. Progress ambulation.
5. Teach patients pulse taking *to determine activity tolerance:* take pulse for full minute before exercise, then for 10 seconds and multiply by 6 at exercise peak.

RISK FOR INFECTION

Definition
The state in which an individual is at increased risk for being invaded by pathogenic organisms.

Risk for Infection Risk Factor: Invasive Monitoring Devices

RISK FACTOR
- Invasive monitoring devices

DEFINING CHARACTERISTICS
- Fever of undetermined origin
- Tachycardia
- Elevated white blood cell count
- Reddened, inflamed catheter insertion sites
- Drainage from catheter insertion sites

OUTCOME CRITERIA
- Patients are afebrile.
- Heart rate is within range of baseline.
- Catheter insertion sites are clear and dry.

NURSING INTERVENTIONS AND *RATIONALE*

NOTE: *Based on national standards and supported with research, the rationale for each of the following interventions is the avoidance of contamination and colonization of invasive lines.*

1. Continue to monitor the assessment parameters listed under "Defining Characteristics."
2. Practice handwashing—consisting of 15 seconds using mechanical friction and soap and water—before drawing blood or any line manipulation in which the closed system is interrupted.
3. Secure catheters to prevent piston movement (in and out).
4. Maintain an occlusive, sterile dressing. Gauze dressings over arterial lines are recommended.
5. Eliminate all nonessential stopcocks.
6. A different anatomic site should be selected for each catheter inserted.
7. Use uniform, prepackaged, sterile transducer/pressure monitoring and flush assembly.

RISK FOR INFECTION CONT'D

NURSING INTERVENTIONS AND *RATIONALE* CONT'D

8. A sterile gown should be worn when inserting central lines. For skin preparation, clean the skin with iodofor. Wear gloves, mask, and cap and use sterile drapes.
9. Use sterile normal saline as the flush solution.
10. To the extent possible, limit blood drawing by obtaining all specimens at the same time.
11. After obtaining a sample of blood, the stopcock should be flushed with saline to clear. All ports should be capped when not in use.
12. Transparent, occlusive dressings should be changed every 72 hours or when integrity is disrupted.

Gauze dressings should be changed every 24 hours or sooner if soiled, saturated, or disrupted. Change IV tubing every 72 hours and IV fluids every 24 hours.
13. Catheters inserted in an emergency, without proper asepsis, should be removed and, if necessary, replaced under aseptic conditions.
14. At any sign of infection (localized pain, inflammation, sepsis, fever of undetermined origin), catheters should be removed and cultured.

Nursing Management of Pulmonary Alterations

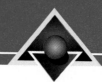

INEFFECTIVE AIRWAY CLEARANCE

Definition
The state in which an individual is unable to clear obstructions or secretions from the respiratory tract to maintain airway patency.

Ineffective Airway Clearance Related to Excessive Secretions or Abnormal Viscosity of Mucus

DEFINING CHARACTERISTICS
- Abnormal breath sounds (displaced normal sounds, adventitious sounds, diminished or absent sounds)
- Ineffective cough with or without sputum
- Tachypnea, dyspnea
- Verbal reports of inability to clear airway

OUTCOME CRITERIA
- Cough produces thin mucus.
- Lungs are clear to auscultation.
- Respiratory rate, depth, and rhythm return to baseline

NURSING INTERVENTIONS AND *RATIONALE*
1. Assess sputum for color, consistency, and amount.
2. Assess for clinical manifestations of pneumonia.
3. Provide for maximal thoracic expansion by repositioning, deep breathing, splinting, and pain management *to avoid hypoventilation and atelectasis.* If hypoventilation is present, implement "Ineffective Breathing Pattern Related to Decreased Thoracic Expansion" Management Plan.
4. Maintain adequate hydration by administering oral and intravenous fluids (as ordered) *to thin secretions and facilitate airway clearance.*
5. Provide humidification to airways via oxygen delivery device or artificial airway *to thin secretions and facilitate airway clearance.*

6. Administer bland aerosol every 4 hours *to facilitate expectoration of sputum.*
7. Collaborate with the physician regarding the administration of
   - Bronchodilators *to treat or prevent bronchospams and facilitate expectoration of mucus*
   - Mucolytics and expectorants *to enhance mobilization and removal of secretions*
   - Antibiotics *to treat infection*
8. Assist with coughing exercises *to facilitate expectoration of secretions.* If patients are unable to perform cascade cough, consider using huff cough (patients with hyperactive airways), end-expiratory cough (patients with secretions in distal airways), or augmented cough (patients with weakened abdominal muscles).
   - Cascade cough—Instruct patients to do the following:
     a. Take a deep breath and hold it for 1 to 3 seconds
     b. Cough out forcefully several times until all air is exhaled
     c. Inhale slowly through the nose
     d. Repeat once
     e. Rest and then repeat as necessary

NURSING INTERVENTIONS AND *RATIONALE* CONT'D

- Huff cough—Instruct patients to do the following:
  a. Take a deep breath and hold it for 1 to 3 seconds
  b. Say the word "Huff" while coughing out several times until air is exhaled
  c. Inhale slowly through the nose
  d. Repeat as necessary
- End-expiratory cough—Instruct patients to do the following:
  a. Take a deep breath and hold it for 1 to 3 seconds
  b. Exhale slowly
  c. At the end of exhalation, cough once
  d. Inhale slowly through the nose
  e. Repeat as necessary or follow with cascade cough
- Augmented cough—Instruct patients to do the following:
  a. Take a deep breath and hold it for 1 to 3 seconds
  b. Perform one or more of the following maneuvers to increase intraabdominal pressure
    1) Tighten knees and buttocks
    2) Bend forward at the waist
    3) Place a hand flat on the upper abdomen just under the xiphoid process and press in and up abruptly during coughing
    4) Keep hands on the chest wall and press inward with each cough
  c. Inhale slowly through the nose
  d. Rest and repeat as necessary
9. Suction nasotracheally or endotracheally as necessary *to assist with secretion removal.*
10. Reposition patients at least every 2 hours or use continuous lateral rotation therapy *to mobilize and prevent stasis of secretions.*
11. Consider chest physiotherapy (postural drainage and/or chest percussion) three to four times per day in patients with large amounts of sputum *to assist with the expulsion of retained secretions.*
12. Allow rest periods between coughing sessions, chest physiotherapy, suctioning, or any other demanding activities *to promote energy conservation.*

INEFFECTIVE BREATHING PATTERN

Definition
The state in which an individual's inhalation and/or exhalation pattern does not enable adequate pulmonary inflation or emptying.

Ineffective Breathing Pattern Related to Decreased Lung Expansion

DEFINING CHARACTERISTICS

- Abnormal respiratory patterns (hypoventilation, hyperventilation, tachypnea, bradypnea, obstructive breathing)
- Abnormal ABC values (increased Pa_{CO_2}, decreased pH)
- Unequal chest movement
- Shortness of breath, dyspnea

OUTCOME CRITERIA

- Respiratory rate, rhythm, and depth return to baseline.
- Minimal or absent use of accessory muscles
- Chest expands symmetrically
- ABG values return to baseline

NURSING INTERVENTIONS AND *RATIONALE*

1. Treat pain, if present, *to prevent hypoventilation and atelectasis.* Implement "Acute Pain Related to Transmission and Perception of Cutaneous, Visceral, Muscular, or Ischemic Impulses" Management Plan.
2. Position patients in high-Fowler's or semi-Fowler's position *to promote diaphragmatic descent and maximal inhalation.*
3. Assist with deep breathing exercises and incentive spirometry with sustained maximal inspiration 5 to 10 times/hr *to help reinflate collapsed portions of the lung.*
   - Deep breathing—Instruct patients to do the following:
     a. Sit up straight or lean forward slightly while sitting on edge of bed or chair (if possible)

Continued.

INEFFECTIVE BREATHING PATTERN CONT'D

NURSING INTERVENTIONS AND *RATIONALE* CONT'D

b. Take a slow, deep breath in
c. Pause slightly or hold breath for at least 3 seconds
d. Exhale slowly
e. Rest and repeat
- Incentive spirometry—Instruct patients to do the following:
  a. Exhale normally
  b. Place lips around the mouthpiece and close mouth tightly around it
  c. Inhale slowly and as deeply as possible, noting the maximum volume of air inspired
  d. Hold maximum inhalation for 3 seconds
  e. Take the mouthpiece out of mouth and slowly exhale
  f. Rest and repeat

4. Assist physician with intubation and initiation of mechanical ventilation as indicated.

Ineffective Breathing Pattern Related to Musculoskeletal or Neuromuscular Impairment

DEFINING CHARACTERISTICS

- Unequal chest movement
- Shortness of breath, dyspnea
- Use of accessory muscles
- Tachypnea
- Thoracoabdominal asynchrony
- Abnormal ABG values (increased $Paco_2$, decreased pH)
- Nasal flaring
- Assumption of 3-point position

OUTCOME CRITERIA

- Respiratory rate, rhythm, and depth return to baseline.
- Minimal or absent use of accessory muscles
- Chest expands symmetrically
- ABG values return to baseline

NURSING INTERVENTIONS AND *RATIONALE*

1. Prevent unnecessary exertion *to limit drain on patients' ventilatory reserve.*

2. Instruct patients in energy-saving techniques *to conserve patients' ventilatory reserve.*

3. Assist with pursed-lip and diaphragmatic breathing techniques *to facilitate diaphragmatic descent and improved ventilation.*
   - Diaphragmatic breathing—Instruct patients to do the following:
     a. Sit in the upright position
     b. Place one hand on the abdomen just above the waist and the other on the upper chest
     c. Breath in through the nose and feel the lower hand push out; the upper hand should not move
     d. Breathe out through pursed lips and feel the lower hand move in

4. Position patients in high-Fowler's or semi-Fowler's position *to promote diaphragmatic descent and maximal inhalation.*

5. Assist physician with intubation and initiation of mechanical ventilation as indicated.

INABILITY TO SUSTAIN SPONTANEOUS VENTILATION

Definition
A state in which the response pattern of decreased energy reserves results in an individual's ability to maintain breathing adequate to support life.

Inability to Sustain Spontaneous Ventilation Related to Respiratory Muscle Fatigue and Metabolic Factors

DEFINING CHARACTERISTICS

- Dyspnea and apprehension
- Increased metabolic rate
- Increased restlessness
- Increased use of accessory muscles
- Decreased tidal volume
- Increased heart rate
- Abnormal arterial blood gas values (decreased PaO_2, increased $PaCO_2$, decreased pH, decreased SaO_2)

OUTCOME CRITERIA

- Metabolic rate and heart rate are within patients' baseline
- Eupnea
- ABG values are within patients' baseline

NURSING INTERVENTIONS AND *RATIONALE*

1. Collaborate with the physician regarding the application of pressure support to the ventilator *to assist patients in overcoming the work of breathing imposed by the ventilator and endotracheal tube.*
2. Carefully snip excess length from the proximal end of the endotracheal tube *to decrease deadspace and thereby decrease the work of breathing.*
3. Collaborate with the physician and dietitian to ensure that at least 50% of the diet's nonprotein caloric source is in the form of fat versus carbohydrates *to prevent excess carbon dioxide production.*
4. Collaborate with the physician and respiratory therapist regarding the best method of weaning for individual patients *because each situation is different, and a variety of weaning options are available.*
5. Collaborate with the physician and physical therapist regarding a progressive ambulation and condi-

tioning plan *to promote overall muscle conditioning and respiratory muscle functioning.*
6. Determine the most effective means of communication for patients *to promote their independence and reduce their anxiety.*
7. Develop a daily schedule and post it in patients' rooms *to coordinate care and facilitate patients' involvement in the plan.*
8. Treat pain, if present, *to prevent respiratory splinting and hypoventilation.* Implement "Acute Pain Related to Transmission and Perception of Cutaneous, Visceral, Muscular, or Ischemic Impulses" Management Plan.
9. Ensure that patients receive at least 2 to 4 hour intervals of uninterrupted sleep in a quiet, dark room. Collaborate with the physician and respiratory therapist regarding the use of full ventilatory support at night *to provide respiratory muscle rest.*
10. Place patients in semi-Fowler's position or in a chair at the bedside *for best use of ventilatory muscles and to facilitate diaphragmatic descent.*
11. Explain the weaning procedure to patients before the initial trial *so patients will understand what to expect and how to participate.*
12. Monitor patients during the weaning trial for evidence of respiratory muscle fatigue *to avoid overtiring patients.*
13. Provide diversional activity during the weaning trial *to reduce patients' anxiety.*
14. Collaborate with physician and respiratory therapist regarding the removal of the ventilator and artificial airway when patients have been successfully weaned.

IMPAIRED GAS EXCHANGE

Definition
A state in which an individual experiences an imbalance between oxygen uptake and carbon dioxide elimination at the alveolar-capillary membrane gas exchange area.

Impaired Gas Exchange Related to Ventilation/Perfusion Mismatching and Intrapulmonary Shunting

DEFINING CHARACTERISTICS

- Abnormal ABG values (decreased Pa_{O_2}, decreased Sa_{O_2})
- Somnolence
- Neurobehavioral changes (restlessness, irritability, confusion)
- Central cyanosis

OUTCOME CRITERIA

- ABG values are within patients' baseline.
- Absence of central cyanosis

NURSING INTERVENTIONS AND *RATIONALE*

1. Initiate continuous pulse oximetry or monitor Sp_{O_2} every hour.
2. Collaborate with physician on the administration of oxygen to maintain an Sp_{O_2} >90%
   a. Administer supplemental oxygen via appropriate oxygen delivery device *to increase driving pressure of oxygen in the alveoli.*
   b. If supplemental oxygen alone is not effective, administer constant positive airway pressure or mechanical ventilation with positive end-expiratory pressure *to open collapsed alveoli and increase the surface area for gas exchange.*

3. Position patients to optimize ventilation/perfusion matching
   a. For patients with unilateral lung disease, position with the good lung down *because gravity will improve perfusion to this area, and this will best match ventilation with perfusion.*
   b. For patients with bilateral lung disease, position with the right lung down *because this lung is larger than the left and affords a greater area for ventilation and perfusion,* or change position every 2 hours, favoring those positions that improve oxygenation.
   c. Avoid any position that seriously compromises oxygenation status.
4. Perform procedures only as needed and provide adequate rest and recovery time in between *to prevent desaturation.*
5. Collaborate with the physician regarding the administration of
   - Sedatives *to decrease ventilator asynchrony and facilitate patients' sense of control*
   - Neuromuscular blocking agents *to prevent ventilator asynchrony and decrease oxygen demand*
   - Analgesics *to treat pain if present;* implement "Acute Pain Related to Transmission and Perception of Cutaneous, Visceral, Muscular, or Ischemic Impulses" Management Plan
6. If secretions are present, implement "Ineffective Airway Clearance Related to Excessive Secretions or Abnormal Viscosity of Mucus" Management Plan.

Impaired Gas Exchange Related to Alveolar Hypoventilation

DEFINING CHARACTERISTICS

- Abnormal ABG values (decreased Pa_{O_2}, increased Pa_{CO_2}, decreased pH, decreased Sa_{O_2})
- Somnolence
- Neurobehavioral changes (restlessness, irritability, confusion)
- Tachycardia or dysrhythmias
- Central cyanosis

OUTCOME CRITERIA

- ABG values within patients' baseline
- Absence of central cyanosis

NURSING INTERVENTIONS AND *RATIONALE*

1. Initiate continuous pulse oximetry or monitor SpO_2 every hour.
2. Collaborate with physician on the administration of oxygen to maintain an SpO_2 >90%
   a. Administer supplemental oxygen via appropriate oxygen delivery device *to increase driving pressure of oxygen in the alveoli.*
   b. If supplemental oxygen alone is not effective, administer constant positive airway pressure or mechanical ventilation with positive end-expiratory pressure *to open collapsed alveoli and increase the surface area for gas exchange.*

3. Prevent hypoventilation
   a. Position patients in high-Fowler's or semi-Fowler's position *to promote diaphragmatic descent and maximal inhalation.*
   b. Assist with deep breathing exercises and/or incentive spirometry with sustained maximal inspiration 5 to 10 times hr *to help reinflate collapsed portions of the lung.* See "Ineffective Breathing Pattern Related to Decreased Lung Expansion" Management Plan for further instructions.
   c. Treat pain, if present, *to prevent hypoventilation and atelectasis.* Implement "Acute Pain Related to Transmission and Perception of Cutaneous, Visceral, Muscular, or Ischemic Impulses" Management Plan.
4. Assist physician with intubation and initiation of mechanical ventilation as indicated.

RISK FOR ASPIRATION

Definition

A state in which an individual is at risk for entry of gastric secretions, oropharyngeal secretions, or exogenous food or fluids into tracheobronchial passages because of dysfunction of normal protective mechanisms.

Risk for Aspiration

RISK FACTORS

- Impaired laryngeal sensation or reflex
    Reduced level of consciousness
    Immediately post extubation
- Impaired pharyngeal peristalsis or tongue function
    Neuromuscular dysfunction
    Central nervous system dysfunction
    Head or neck surgery
- Impaired laryngeal closure or elevation
    Laryngeal nerve dysfunction
    Artificial airways
    Gastrointestinal tubes
- Increased gastric volume
    Delayed gastric emptying
    Enteral feedings
    Medication administration
- Increased intragastric pressure
    Upper abdominal surgery
    Obesity
    Pregnancy
    Ascites
- Decreased lower esophageal sphincter pressure
    Increased gastric acidity
    Gastrointestinal tubes
- Decreased antegrade esophageal propulsion
    Trendelenburg or supine position
    Esophageal dysmotility
    Esophageal structural defects or lesions

OUTCOME CRITERIA

- Normal breath sounds or no change in patients' baseline breath sounds.
- ABG values remain within patients' baseline.
- No evidence of gastric contents in lung secretions.

NURSING INTERVENTIONS AND *RATIONALE*

1. Assess gastrointestinal function *to rule out hypoactive peristalsis and abdominal distention.*
2. Position patients with head of bed elevated 30 degrees *to prevent gastric reflux through gravity.* If head elevation is contraindicated, position patients in right lateral decubitus position *to facilitate passage of gastric contents across the pylorus.*
3. Maintain patency and functioning of nasogastric suction apparatus *to prevent accumulation of gastric contents.*
4. Provide frequent and scrupulous mouth care *to prevent colonization of the oropharynx with bacteria and inoculation of the lower airways.*
5. Ensure that endotracheal/tracheostomy cuff is properly inflated *to limit aspiration of oropharyngeal secretions.*
6. Treat nausea promptly; collaborate with physician on an order for antiemetic *to prevent vomiting and resultant aspiration.*

RISK FOR ASPIRATION CONT'D

Additional Interventions for Patients Receiving Continuous or Intermittent Enteral Tube Feedings

1. Position patients with head of bed elevated 45 degrees *to prevent gastric reflux.* If a head-down position becomes necessary at any time, interrupt the feeding 30 minutes before the position change.
2. Check placements of feeding tube either by auscultation or radiographically at regular intervals (e.g., before administering intermittent feedings and after position changes, suctioning, coughing episodes, or vomiting) *to ensure proper placement of the tube.*
3. Instill blue food coloring to feeding solutions *to assist identification of gastric contents in pulmonary secretions.*
4. Monitor patients for signs of delayed gastric emptying *to decrease potential for vomiting and aspiration*
   a. For large-bore tubes, check residuals of tube feedings prior to intermittent feedings and every 4 hours during continuous feedings. Consider withholding feedings for residuals greater than 50% of the hourly rate (continuous feeding) or greater than 50% of the previous feeding (intermittent feeding).
   b. For small-bore tubes, observe abdomen for distention, palpate abdomen for hardness or tautness, and auscultate abdomen for bowel sounds.

Additional Interventions for Patients with Impaired Swallowing

1. Place patients in an upright position with their heads midline and their chins slightly down *to keep food in the anterior portion of the mouth and prevent it from falling over the base of the tongue into the open airway.*
2. Provide patients with single-textured soft foods (e.g., cream cereals) that maintain their shape *because these foods require minimal oral manipulation.*
3. Avoid particulate foods (e.g., hamburger) and foods containing more than one texture (e.g., stew) *because these foods require more chewing and oral manipulation.*
4. Provide patients with thick liquids (e.g., fruit nectar, yogurt) *because these liquids are more easily controlled in the mouth.*
5. Thicken thin liquids (e.g., water, juice) with a thickening preparation or avoid them *because these foods are easily aspirated.*
6. Place food in the uninvolved side of the mouth *because oral sensitivity and function is greatest in this area.*
7. Collaborate with physician and speech therapist regarding a swallowing evaluation and rehabilitation program *to decrease incidence of aspiration.*
8. Collaborate with physician and dietitian regarding a nutritional assessment and nutritional plan *to ensure that patients are receiving enough nutrition.*
9. Provide oral hygiene after meals *to clear food particles from the mouth that could be aspirated.*

Nursing Management of Neurologic Alterations

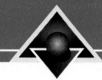

ALTERED TISSUE PERFUSION

Definition
The state in which an individual experiences a decrease in nutrition and oxygenation at the cellular level due to a deficit in arterial capillary blood supply.

Altered Cerebral Tissue Perfusion Related to Vasospasm or Hemorrhage

DEFINING CHARACTERISTICS
Hemorrhage

- Aneurysm grading system according to Hunt and Hess
  Grade I: minimal bleed
    Asymptomatic or minimal headache
    Slight nuchal rigidity
  Grade II; mild bleed
    Moderate-to-severe headache
    Nuchal rigidity
    Minimal neurologic deficit (for example, possible cranial nerve palsies—oculomotor [cranial nerve III] most common; unilateral pupillary dilation, ptosis, and dysconjugate gaze)
  Grade III: moderate bleed
    Drowsiness
    Confusion
    Nuchal rigidity
    Possible mild focal neurologic deficits
  Grade IV: moderate-to-severe bleed
    Extremely decreased level of consciousness, stupor
    Possible moderate-to-severe hemiparesis
    Possible early posturing (decorticate or decerebrate)
  Grade V: severe bleed
    Profound coma
    Posturing
    Moribund appearance

- Pathological reflexes resulting from meningeal irritation: Kernig's sign: resistance to full extension of the leg at the knee when the hip is flexed
- Brudzinski's sign: flexion of the hip and knee during passive neck flexion
- Photophobia
- Nausea and vomiting

Vasospasm

- Worsening headache
- Confusion and decreasing level of consciousness
- Focal motor deficits such as unilateral weakness of extremities
- Speech deficits such as slurring, receptive, or expressive aphasia
- Increasing BP

OUTCOME CRITERIA

- Patients are oriented to time, place, person, and situation.
- Pupils are equal and normoreactive.
- BP is within patients' norm.
- Motor function is bilaterally equal.
- Headache, nausea, and vomiting are absent.
- Patients verbalize importance of and displays compliance with reduced activity.

Continued.

491

ALTERED TISSUE PERFUSION CONT'D

NURSING INTERVENTIONS AND *RATIONALE*

1. Assess for indicators of increased ICP and brain herniation (see nursing management of Altered Cerebral Tissue Perfusion related to increased ICP). *ICP will increase during vasospasm only when caused by the edema resulting from brain infarction.*
2. If hypertensive-hypervolemic therapy is prescribed, administer crystalloid and colloid IV fluids and monitor pulmonary artery wedge pressure PAWP, pulmonary artery diastolic pressure (PAD), systemic vascular resistance (SVR), and BP to achieve and maintain prescribed parameters. Systolic blood pressure is usually maintained at 150-160 mm Hg.
3. Monitor lung sounds and chest x-ray reports because of *the risk of pulmonary edema associated with fluid overload.*
4. Anticipate administration of calcium channel blockers such as nifedipine *to decrease peripheral vascular resistance and cause vasodilation.*

5. Rebleeding is a potential complication of aneurysm rupture; to prevent rebleeding, the following interventions constitute subarachnoid precautions:
   - Ensure bed rest in a quiet environment *to lessen external stimuli.*
   - Maintain darkened room *to lessen symptoms of photophobia.*
   - Restrict visitors and instruct them to keep conversation as nonstressful as possible.
   - Administer prescribed sedatives as needed *to reduce anxiety and promote rest.*
   - Administer analgesics as prescribed *to relieve or lessen headache.*
   - Provide a soft, high-fiber diet and stool softeners *to prevent constipation, which can lead to straining and increased risk of rebleeding.*
   - Assist with activities of daily living (feeding, bathing, dressing, toileting).
   - Avoid any activity that could lead to increased ICP; ensure that patients do not flex their hips beyond 90 degrees and avoid neck hyperflexion, hyperextension, or lateral hyperrotation *that could impede jugular venous return.*

Altered Cerebral Tissue Perfusion Related to Increased Intracranial Pressure

DEFINING CHARACTERISTICS

- ICP >15 mm Hg, sustained for 15-30 minutes
- Headache
- Vomiting, with or without nausea
- Seizures
- Decrease in Glasgow Coma Scale of two or more points from baseline
- Alteration in level of consciousness, ranging from restlessness to coma
- Change in orientation: disoriented to time and/or place and/or person
- Difficulty or inability to follow simple commands
- Increasing systolic BP of more than 20 mm Hg with widening pulse pressure
- Bradycardia
- Irregular respiratory pattern (such as Cheyne-Stokes, central neurogenic hyperventilation, ataxic, apneustic)
- Change in response to painful stimuli (such as purposeful to inappropriate or absent response)

- Signs of impending brain herniation, which, in addition to the above, may include the following symptoms:
  - Hemiparesis or hemiplegia
  - Hemisensory changes
  - Unequal pupil size (1 mm or more difference)
  - Failure of pupil to react to light
  - Dysconjugate gaze and inability to move one eye beyond midline if third, fourth, or sixth cranial nerves involved
  - Loss of oculocephalic or oculovestibular reflexes
  - Possible decorticate or decerebrate posturing

OUTCOME CRITERIA

- ICP is ≤15 mm Hg.
- CPP is >60 mm Hg.
- Clinical signs of increased ICP as described above are absent.

ALTERED TISSUE PERFUSION CONT'D

NURSING INTERVENTIONS AND *RATIONALE*

1. Maintain adequate CPP.
   a. With physician's collaboration, maintain BP within patients' norm by administering volume expanders, vasopressors, or antihypertensives.
   b. Reduce ICP.
      - Elevate head of bed 30 to 45 degrees *to facilitate venous return.*
      - Maintain head and neck in neutral plane (avoid flexion, extension, or lateral rotation) *to enhance venous drainage from the head.*
      - Avoid extreme hip flexion.
      - With physician's collaboration, administer steroids, osmotic agents, and diuretics.
      - Drain CSF according to protocol if ventriculostomy in place.
      - Assist patients to turn and move self in bed (instruct patients to exhale while turning or pushing up in bed) *to avoid isometric contractions and Valsalva maneuver.*
2. Maintain patent airway and adequate ventilation and supply oxygen *to prevent hypoxemia and hypercarbia.*
3. Monitor arterial blood gas (ABG) values and maintain Pao_2 >80 mm Hg, $Paco_2$ at 25-35 mm Hg, and pH at 7.35-7.45.
4. Avoid suctioning beyond 10 seconds at a time; hyperoxygenate and hyperventilate before and after suctioning.
5. Plan patient care activities and nursing interventions around patients' ICP response. Avoid unnecessary additional disturbances and allow patients up to 1 hour of rest between activities as frequently as possible. *Studies have shown the direct correlation between nursing care activities and increases in ICP.*
6. Maintain normothermia with external cooling or heating measures as necessary. Wrap hands, feet, and male genitalia in soft towels before cooling measures *to prevent shivering and frostbite.*
7. With physician's collaboration, control seizures with prophylactic and as necessary (PRN) anticonvulsants. *Seizures can greatly increase the cerebral metabolic rate.*
8. With physician's collaboration, administer sedatives, barbiturates, or paralyzing agents *to reduce cerebral metabolic rate.*
9. Counsel family members to maintain calm atmosphere and avoid disturbing topics of conversation (such as patient condition, pain, prognosis, family crisis, financial difficulties).
10. If signs of impending brain herniation are present, do the following:
    - Notify physician at once.
    - Be sure head of bed is elevated 45 degrees and patients' heads are in neutral plane.
    - Slow mainline intravenous (IV) infusion to keep open rate.
    - If ventriculostomy catheter in place, drain CSF as ordered.
    - Prepare to administer osmotic agents and/or diuretics.
    - Prepare patients for emergency computed tomographic (CT) head scan and/or emergency surgery.

HYPOTHERMIA

Definition
The state in which an individual's body temperature is reduced below normal range.

Hypothermia Related to Exposure to Cold Environment, Trauma, or Damage to the Hypothalamus

DEFINING CHARACTERISTICS

- Core body temperature below 35° C (95° F)
- Skin cold to touch
- Slurred speech, incoordination
- At temperature below 33° C (91.4° F):
  - Cardiac dysrhythmias (atrial fibrillation, bradycardia)
  - Cyanosis
  - Respiratory alkalosis
- At temperatures below 32° C (89.5° F):
  - Shivering replaced by muscle rigidity
  - Hypotension
  - Dilated pupils
- At temperatures below 28°-29° C (82.4-84.2° F):
  - Absent deep tendon reflexes
  - Hypoventilation (3 to 4 breaths/min to apnea)
  - Ventricular fibrillation possible
- At temperatures below 26°-27° C (78.8-80.6° F):
  - Coma
  - Flaccid muscles
  - Fixed, dilated pupils
  - Ventricular fibrillation to cardiac standstill
  - Apnea

OUTCOME CRITERIA

- Core body temperature is greater than 35° C (95° F).
- Patients are alert and oriented.
- Cardiac dysrhythmias are absent.
- Acid-base balance is normal.
- Pupils are normoreactive.

NURSING INTERVENTIONS AND *RATIONALE*

1. Continuously monitor core body temperature with a low-reading thermometer.
2. Intubation and mechanical ventilation may be needed. Heated air or oxygen can be added *to help rewarm the body core*. Because carbon dioxide production is low, do not hyperventilate hypothermic patients because *this action may induce severe alkalosis and precipitate ventricular fibrillation*.
3. Apply cardiopulmonary resuscitation (CPR) and advanced cardiac life support until core body temperature is up to at least 29.5° C before determining that patients cannot be resuscitated.
   a. Electrical defibrillation is usually successful in terminating ventricular fibrillation if the temperature is greater than 28° C.
   b. Administer cardiac resuscitation drugs sparingly *because as the body warms, peripheral vasodilation occurs. Drugs that remain in the periphery are suddenly released, leading to a "bolus effect" that may cause fatal dysrhythmias.*
4. Monitor ABG values to direct further therapy, and be sure that the pH, PaO_2, and $PaCO_2$ are corrected for temperature.
5. For abrupt-onset hypothermia (for example, immersion in cold water, exposure to cold, wet climate, collapse in snow) rewarming can take place rapidly *because the pathophysiological changes associated with chronic hypothermia have not had time to evolve.*
   - Institute rapid, active rewarming by immersion in warm water (38°-43° C).
   - Apply thermal blanket at 36.6°-37.7° C. Some researchers suggest rewarming only the torso or trunk first, leaving the extremities exposed to room temperature. *This is to prevent early peripheral vasodilation with abrupt redistribution of intravascular volume. This also prevents colder blood trapped in the extremities from returning to the body core before the heart is rewarmed.*
   - Perform rapid core rewarming with heated (37°-43° C) IV infusion, hemodialysis, peritoneal dialysis, and colonic or gastric irrigation fluids.
6. Monitor peripheral circulation because *gangrene of the fingers and toes is a common complication of accidental hypothermia.*
7. For chronic hypothermia, the aggressiveness of treatment depends on the setting, underlying disease, and body temperature. Concurrent treatment of the underlying disease processes is indicated.
   - Core temperatures greater than 33° C may be rewarmed either slowly or rapidly.
   - Coma in patients with a temperature greater than 28° C is probably not caused by hypothermia. Look for other causes such as hypoglycemia, alcohol, narcotics, and head trauma and treat accordingly.
   - If patients are hyperglycemic, remember that insulin is ineffective at body temperatures below 30° C.
   - Restore intravascular volume cautiously *to avoid circulatory overloading of the hypothermic heart and to avoid precipitating pulmonary edema*. As circulation and a more normal temperature are restored, patients may require large volumes of crystalloid and colloid fluids *to refill the dilated vascular bed*.

UNILATERAL NEGLECT

Definition
The state in which an individual is perceptually unaware of and inattentive to one side of the body.

Unilateral Neglect Related to Perceptual Disruption

DEFINING CHARACTERISTICS
- Neglect of involved body parts and/or extrapersonal space
- Denial of the existence of the affected limb or side of body
- Denial of hemiplegia or other motor and sensory deficits
- Left homonymous hemianopsia
- Difficult with spatial-perceptual tasks
- Left hemiplegia

OUTCOME CRITERIA
- Patient is safe and free from injury.
- Patient is able to identify safety hazards in the environment.
- Patient recognizes disability and describes physical deficits present (for example, paralysis, weakness, numbness).
- Patient demonstrates ability to scan the visual field to compensate for loss of function or sensation in affected limb(s).

NURSING INTERVENTIONS AND *RATIONALE*
1. Adapt environment to patients' deficits *to maintain patient safety.*
   - Position patients' beds with the unaffected side facing the door.
   - Approach and speak to patients from the unaffected side. If patients must be approached from the affected side, announce your presence as soon as entering the room *to avoid startling patients.*
   - Position the call light, bedside stand, and personal items on patients' unaffected side.
   - If patients will be assisted out of bed, simplify the environment *to eliminate hazards* by removing unnecessary furniture and equipment.
   - Provide frequent reorientation of patients to the environment.
   - Observe patients closely and anticipate their needs. In spite of repeated explanations, patients may have difficulty retaining information about the deficits.
   - When patients are in bed, elevate their affected arm on a pillow *to prevent dependent edema and support the hand in a position of function.*
2. Assist patients to recognize the perceptual defect.
   - Encourage patients to wear any prescription corrective glasses or hearing aids *to facilitate communication.*
   - Instruct patients to turn the head past midline to view the environment on the affected side.

- Encourage patients to look at the affected side and to stroke the limbs with the unaffected hand. Encourage handling of the affected limbs *to reinforce awareness of the affected side.*
- Instruct patients to always look for the affected extremity or extremities when performing simple tasks *to know where it is at all times.*
- Have patients name the affected parts after pointing to them.
- Encourage patients to use self-exercises (for example, lifting the affected arm with the good hand).
- If patients are unable to discriminate between the concepts of "right" and "left," use descriptive adjectives such as "the weak arm," "the affected leg," or "the good arm" to refer to the body. Use gestures, not just words, to indicate right and left.
3. Collaborate with patients, physicians, and rehabilitation team *to design and implement a beginning rehabilitation program for use during critical care unit stay.*
   - Use adaptive equipment (braces, splints, slings) as appropriate.
   - Teach patients the individual components of any activity separately, then proceed to integrate the component parts into a completed activity.
   - Instruct patients to attend to the affected side, if able, and assist with the bath or other tasks.
   - Use tactile stimulation *to reintroduce the arm or leg to patients.* Rub the affected parts with different textured materials *to stimulate sensations (warm, cold, rough, soft).*
   - Encourage activities that require patients to turn their heads toward the affected side and retrain patients to scan the affected side and environment visually.
   - If patients are allowed out of bed, cue them with reminders to scan visually when ambulating. Assist and remain in constant attendance because *patients may have difficulty maintaining correct posture, balance, and locomotion.* There may be vertical-horizontal perceptual problems, with patients leaning to the affected side to align with the perceived vertical position. Provide sitting, standing, and balancing exercises before getting patients out of bed.
   - Feeding: see "Risk for Aspiration."
     a. Avoid giving patients any very hot food items that could cause injury.
     b. Place patients in an upright sitting position if possible.

Continued.

UNILATERAL NEGLECT CONT'D

▼

NURSING INTERVENTIONS AND *RATIONALE* CONT'D

c. Encourage patients to feed themselves; if necessary, guide patients' hand to the mouth.
d. If patients are able to feed themselves, place one dish at a time in front of them. When patients are finished with the first, add another dish. Tell patients what they are eating.
e. Initially place food in patients' visual field; then gradually move the food out of the field of vision and teach patients to scan the entire visual field.
f. When patients have learned to visually scan the environment, offer a tray of food with various dishes.
g. Instruct patients to take small bites of food and place the food in the unaffected side of the mouth.
h. Teach patients to sweep out pockets of food with the tongue after every bite *to eliminate retained food in the affected side of the mouth.*

i. After meals or oral medications, check patients' oral cavity for pockets of retained material.
4. Initiate patient and family health teaching.
  • Assess to ensure that patients and families understand the nature of the neurologic deficits and the purpose of the rehabilitation plan.
  • Teach the proper application and use of any adaptive equipment.
  • Teach the importance of maintaining a safe environment and point out potential environmental hazards.
  • Instruct family members how to facilitate relearning techniques (for example, cueing, scanning visual fields).

DYSREFLEXIA

▼

Definition
The state in which an individual with a spinal cord injury at T-7 or above experiences a life-threatening uninhibited sympathetic response of the nervous system to a noxious stimulus.

Dysreflexia Related to Excessive Autonomic Response to Certain Noxious Stimuli (i.e., Distended Bladder, Distended Bowel, Skin Irritation) Occurring in Patients With Cervical or High Thoracic (T-6 or Above) Spinal Cord Injury

DEFINING CHARACTERISTICS
• Paroxysmal hypertension (sudden periodic elevated BP in which systolic pressure is greater than 140 mm Hg and diastolic pressure is greater than 90 mm Hg); for many spinal cord injury patients, a normal BP may be only 90/60
• Bradycardia (most common; pulse rate <60 beats per minute) or tachycardia (pulse rate >100 beats per minute)
• Diaphoresis (above the injury)
• Facial flushing
• Pallor (below the injury)
• Headache (a diffuse pain in different portions of the head and not confined to any nerve distribution area)
• Nasal congestion
• Engorgement of temporal and neck vessels
• Conjunctival congestion
• Chills without fever
• Pilomotor erection (goose bumps)

• Blurred vision
• Chest pain
• Metallic taste in mouth
• Horner's syndrome (constriction of the pupil, partial ptosis of the eyelid, enophthalmos, and sometimes loss of sweating over the affected side of the face)

OUTCOME CRITERIA
• Systolic BP is <140 mm Hg, and diastolic blood pressure is <90 mm Hg (or within patients' norm).
• Pulse rate is >60 or <100 beats per minute (or within patients' norm).
• Headache is absent.
• Nasal stuffiness, sweating, and flushing above level of injury are absent.
• Chills, goose bumps, and pallor below level of injury are absent.
• Patients verbalize causes, prevention, symptoms, and treatment of condition.

DYSREFLEXIA CONT'D

NURSING INTERVENTIONS AND *RATIONALE*

1. Place on cardiac monitor and assess for bradycardia, tachycardia, and other dysrhythmias. *Disturbances of cardiac rate and rhythm can occur because of autonomic dysfunction associated with dysreflexia.*
2. Do not leave patients alone. One nurse monitors the blood pressure and patient status every 3 to 5 minutes while another provides treatment.
3. Place patients' head of bed to upright position *to decrease BP and promote cerebral venous return.*
4. Remove any support stockings or abdominal binders *to reduce venous return.*
5. Investigate for and remove offending cause of dysreflexia.
   a. Bladder
      • If catheter not in place, immediately catheterize patient.
      • Lubricate catheter with lidocaine jelly before insertion.
      • Drain 500 ml of urine and recheck BP.
      • If BP is still elevated, drain another 500 ml of urine.
      • If BP declines after the bladder is empty, serial BP should be monitored closely *because the bladder can go into severe contractions, causing hypertension to recur.* With physician's collaboration, instill 30 ml tetracaine through the catheter *to decrease the flow of impulses from the bladder.*
      • If indwelling catheter in place, check for kinks or granular sediment that may indicate occlusion.
      • If plugged catheter is suspected, irrigate it gently with no more than 30 ml of sterile normal saline solution. If the bladder is in tetany, fluid will go in but will not drain out.

      • If catheter cannot be irrigated, remove it, reinsert a new catheter, and proceed with its lubrication, drainage, and observation as stated above.
      • Atropine is sometimes administered *to relieve bladder tetany.*
   b. Bowel
      • Using glove lubricated with anesthetic ointment, check rectum for fecal impaction.
      • If impaction is felt, insert anesthetic ointment into rectum 10 minutes before manual removal of impaction *to decrease flow of impulses from bowel.*
      • A low, hypertonic enema or a suppository may be given *to assist bowel evacuation.*
   c. Skin
      • Loosen clothing or bed linens as indicated.
      • Inspect skin for pimples, boils, pressure sores, and ingrown toenails and treat as indicated.
6. If symptoms of dysreflexia do not subside, have available the IV solutions and antihypertensive drugs of the physician's choosing (for example, hydralazine, phentolamine, diazoxide, sodium nitroprusside). Administer medications and monitor their effectiveness. Assess BP, pulse, and subjective and objective signs and symptoms.
7. Instruct patients about causes, symptoms, treatment, and prevention of dysreflexia.
8. Encourage patients to carry informational card to present to medical personnel in the event dysreflexia may be developing.

IMPAIRED VERBAL COMMUNICATION

Definition
The state in which an individual experiences a decreased or absent ability to use or understand language in human interaction.

Impaired Verbal Communication: Aphasia Related to Cerebral Speech Center Injury

DEFINING CHARACTERISTICS
• Inappropriate or absent speech or responses to questions
• Inability to speak spontaneously
• Inability to understand spoken words

• Inability to follow commands appropriately through gestures
• Difficulty or inability to understand written language
• Difficulty or inability to express ideas in writing
• Difficulty or inability to name objects

Continued.

IMPAIRED VERBAL COMMUNICATION CONT'D

OUTCOME CRITERIA
• Patients are able to make basic needs known.

NURSING INTERVENTIONS AND *RATIONALE*

1. Consult with physician and speech pathologist *to determine the extent of patients' communication deficit (e.g., if fluent, nonfluent, or global aphasia is involved).*

2. Have the speech therapist post a list of appropriate ways to communicate with patients in patients' room *so that all nursing personnel can be consistent in their efforts.*

3. Assess patients' ability to comprehend, speak, read, and write.
   • Ask questions that can be answered with a "yes" or a "no." If patients answer "yes" to a question, ask the opposite (e.g., "Are you hot?" "Yes." "Are you cold?" "Yes.") *This may help determine if in fact patients understand what is being said.*
   • Ask simple, short questions and use gestures, pantomime, and facial expressions to give patients additional clues.
   • Stand in patients' line of vision, giving them a good view of your face and hands.
   • Have patients try to write with a pad and pencil. Offer pictures and alphabet letters at which to point.
   • Make flash cards with pictures or words depicting frequently used phrases (e.g., glass of water, bedpan).

4. Maintain an uncluttered environment and decrease external distractions *that could hinder communication.*

5. Maintain a relaxed and calm manner and explain all diagnostic, therapeutic, and comfort measures before initiating them.

6. Do not shout or speak in a loud voice. *Hearing loss is not a factor in aphasia, and shouting will not help.*

7. Have only one person talk at a time. *It is more difficult for patients to follow a multisided conversation.*

8. Use direct eye contact and speak directly to patients in unhurried, short phrases.

9. Give one-step commands and directions and provide cues through pictures or gestures.

10. Try to ask questions that can be answered with a "yes" or a "no" and avoid topics that are controversial, emotional, abstract, and lengthy.

11. Listen to patients in an unhurried manner and wait for their attempt to communicate.
    • Expect a time lag between your questions and patients' responses.
    • Accept patients' statement of essential words without expecting complete sentences.
    • Avoid finishing the sentence for patients if possible.
    • Wait approximately 30 seconds before providing the word patients may be attempting to find (except when patients are very frustrated and need something quickly, such as a bedpan).
    • Rephrase patients' messages aloud *to validate them.*
    • Do not pretend to understand patients' message if you do not.

12. Encourage patients to speak slowly in short phrases and say each word clearly.

13. Ask patients to write the message, if able, or draw pictures if only verbal communication is affected.

14. Observe patients' nonverbal clues for validation (e.g., answers "yes" but shakes head "no").

15. When handing an object to the patient, state what it is *because hearing language spoken is necessary to stimulate language development.*

16. Explain what has happened to patients and offer reassurance about the plan of care.

17. Verbally address the problem of frustration over inability to communicate and explain that patience is necessary for both nurses and the patients.

18. Maintain a calm, positive manner and offer reassurance (e.g., "I know this is very hard for you, but it will get better if we work on it together").

19. Talk to patients as adults. Be respectful and avoid talking down to patients.

20. Do not discuss patients' condition or hold conversations in patients' presence without including them in the discussion. *This tendency may be the reason some aphasic patients develop paranoid thoughts.*

21. Do not exhibit disapproval of emotional utterances or spontaneous use of profanity; instead, offer calm, quiet reassurance.

22. If patients make an error in speech, do not reprimand or scold but try to compliment them by saying, "That was a good try."

23. Delay conversation if patients are tired. *The symptoms of aphasia worsen with fatigue, anxiety, and emotional upset.*

24. Be prepared for emotional outbursts and tears in patients who have more difficulty in expressing themselves than with understanding. Patients may become depressed, refuse treatment and food, ignore relatives, and push objects away. Comfort patients with statements such as, "I know it's frustrating and you feel sad, but you are not alone. Other people who have had strokes have felt the way you do. We will be here to help you get through this."

ACUTE PAIN

Definition
The state in which an individual experiences and reports the presence of severe discomfort or an uncomfortable sensation.

Acute Pain Related to Transmission and Perception of Cutaneous, Visceral, Muscular, or Ischemic Impulses

DEFINING CHARACTERISTICS
- Patients verbalize presence of pain
- Patients rate pain on scale of 1 to 10
- Increase in BP, pulse, and respirations
- Pupillary dilation
- Diaphoresis, pallor
- Skeletal muscle reactions (grimacing, clenching fists, writhing, pacing, guarding or splinting affected part)
- Apprehensive, fearful appearance

OUTCOME CRITERIA
- Patients verbalize that pain is reduced to a tolerable level or is removed.
- Patients' pain rating on scale of 1 to 10 decreases every half hour after intervention.
- BP, heart rate, and respiratory rate return to baseline 5 minutes after administration of IV narcotic or 20 minutes after administration of intramuscular (IM) narcotic.

NURSING INTERVENTIONS AND *RATIONALE*
1. Monitor postural vital sign changes; determine hydration status and manage fluid volume deficit, if indicated, before administering narcotic analgesic.
2. Modify variables that heighten patients' experience of pain.
   - Explain to patients that frequent, detailed, and seemingly repetitive assessments will be conducted *to allow nurses to better understand patients' pain experience, not because the existence of pain is in question.*
   - Explain the factors responsible for pain production in the individual. Estimate the expected duration of the pain if possible.
   - Explain diagnostic and therapeutic procedures to patients in relation to sensations they should expect to feel. *Preparatory sensory information enhances learning and retention of knowledge and decreases anxiety.*
   - Reduce patients' fear of addiction by explaining the difference between drug tolerance and drug addiction. Drug tolerance is a physiological phenomenon in which a drug dose begins to lose effectiveness after repeated doses; drug dependence is a psychological phenomenon in which narcotics are used regularly for emotional, not medical reasons.
   - Instruct patients to ask for pain medication when pain is beginning and not to wait until it is intolerable.

- Explain that the physician will be consulted if pain relief is inadequate with the present medication.
- Instruct patients in the importance of adequate rest, especially when it reduces pain, *to maintain strength and coping abilities and reduce stress.*
3. Perform pharmacological interventions.
   - For postsurgical or posttraumatic cutaneous, muscular, or visceral pain, perform the following steps:
     a. Medicate with narcotic maximally to break the pain cycle as long as level of consciousness and HR and BP are stable: Check patient's previous response to similar dosage and narcotic.
     b. Continuous pain requires continuous analgesia.
        (1) Establish optimal analgesic dose that brings optimal pain relief.
        (2) Offer pain medication at prescribed regular intervals rather than making patients ask for it *to maintain steady blood levels.*
     c. If administering medication on prn basis, give it when pain is just beginning rather than at its peak. Advise patients to intercept pain, not endure it, or it may take several hours and higher doses of narcotics to relieve pain, leading to a cycle of undermedication and pain alternating with overmedication and drug toxicity.
     d. Perform rehabilitation exercises (turn, deep breathe, leg exercises, ambulate) shortly before peak of drug effect because *this will be the optimal time for* patients to increase activity with the least risk of increasing pain.
     e. In making the transition from IM or IV to by mouth (po) medications, use an equianalgesic chart.
     f. To assess effectiveness of pain medication, do the following steps:
        (1) Reevaluate pain 5 minutes after IV and 20 minutes after IM medication administration, observe patients' behavior, and ask patients to rate pain on scale of 1 to 10.
        (2) Collaborate with physician to add or delete other medications such as antiemetics, hypnotics, sedatives, or muscle relaxants that potentiate the action of analgesics.

Continued.

ACUTE PAIN CONT'D

NURSING INTERVENTIONS AND *RATIONALE* CONT'D

(3) Observe for indicators of undertreatment: report of pain not relieved; observed restlessness, sleeplessness, irritability, and anorexia; decreased activity level.

(4) Indicators of overtreatment: hypotension or bradycardia; respiratory rate <10/min; excessive sedation.

g. If IV patient-controlled analgesia (PCA) is used, perform the following steps:

(1) Instruct patients as follows: "When you have pain, instead of ringing for the nurse to receive pain medicine, push the button that activates the machine, and a small dose of pain medicine will be injected into your IV line. Give yourself only enough medicine to take care of your pain, but do not activate the machine for a dose if you start to feel sleepy. Try to balance the pain relief against sleepiness. If your pain medicine seems to stop working despite pushing the button several times, call the nurse to check your IV. If this is still a problem, the nurse will call your doctor."

(2) Monitor vital signs, especially BP and respiratory rate, every hour for the first 4 hours and assess postural heart rate and BP before initial ambulation.

(3) Monitor respirations every 2 hours while patients are on patient-controlled analgesia.

(4) If respirations decrease to <10/min or if patients are overly sedated, anticipate IV administration of naloxone.

h. If epidural narcotic analgesia is used, take the following actions:

(1) Keep patient's head elevated 30 to 45 degrees after injection *to prevent respiratory depressant effects.*

(2) Observe closely for respiratory depression up to 24 hours after injection. Monitor respiratory rate every 15 minutes for 1 hour, every 30 minutes for 7 hours, and every 1 hour for the remaining 16 hours.

(3) Assess for adequate cough reflex.

(4) Avoid use of other CNS depressants such as sedatives.

(5) Observe for reports of pruritis, nausea, or vomiting.

(6) Anticipate administration of naloxone for respiratory depression (and smaller doses of naloxone for pruritis).

(7) Assess for and treat urinary retention.

(8) Assess epidural catheter site for local infection. Keep catheter taped securely.

4. Perform nonpharmacologic interventions.
   • Treat contributing factors and provide explanations.
   • Apply comfort measures.

a. Use relaxation techniques such as back rubs, massage, warm baths. Use blankets and pillows *to support the painful part and reduce muscle tension.* Encourage slow, rhythmic breathing.

b. Encourage progressive muscle relaxation techniques.

(1) Instruct patients to inhale and tense (tighten) specific muscle groups, then relax the muscles as exhalation occurs.

(2) Suggest an order for performing the tension-relaxation cycle (for example, start with facial muscles and move down body, ending with toes).

c. Encourage guided imagery

(1) Ask patients to recall an image that is very pleasurable and relaxing and involves at least two senses.

(2) Have patients begin with rhythmic breathing and progressive relaxation, then travel mentally to the scene.

(3) Have patients slowly experience the scene—how it looks, sounds, smells, feels.

(4) Ask patients to practice this imagery in private.

(5) Instruct patients to end the imagery by counting to three and saying, "Now I'm relaxed." If patients do not end the imagery and fall asleep, the purpose of the technique is defeated.

d. If TENS unit is prescribed by physician, take the following actions.

(1) Take the TENS unit, patient pamphlet, and teaching electrodes to patients before surgery to explain the process.

(2) Apply electrodes to skin and instruct patients in proper use of unit. Let patients experience how the TENS unit should feel when activated. Refer to manufacturer's directions for proper application and operation of TENS unit.

(3) Electrodes are usually placed by the physician on the skin alongside the operative incision at the close of the surgical procedure in the operating room. The unit is usually used for 3 to 5 days as an adjunct to medications.

ACUTE PAIN CONT'D

NURSING INTERVENTIONS AND *RATIONALE* CONT'D

(4) When patients are awake and alert, readjust the amplitude or output of the TENS unit to patients' comfort as necessary. Keep the TENS unit on continuously unless ordered otherwise. Occasionally, percutaneous epidural nerve stimulation is used when more than one nerve root is involved in producing pain. Again, patients are able to control their pain by adjusting the rate and frequency of a millivoltage electrical current stimulator affixed externally.

e. Assist with biofeedback, which represents a wide range of behavioral techniques that provide patients with information about changes in body functions of which they are usually unaware. For example, information used to reduce muscle contraction is obtained by an electromyogram recorded from body surface electrodes. Changes in blood flow are produced by monitoring skin temperature changes. Patients using biofeedback try to change the display of information in the desired direction by actions such as reducing muscle tension or reducing or altering blood flow to a particular area.

Nursing Management of Renal Alterations

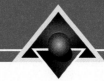

FLUID VOLUME DEFICIT

Definition
The state in which an individual experiences 1) vascular, cellular, or intracellular dehydration related to failure of regulatory mechanisms; or 2) vascular, cellular, or intracellular dehydration related to active loss.

Fluid Volume Deficit Related to Hyponatremia (Absolute Sodium Loss)

DEFINING CHARACTERISTICS
- Central nervous system (CNS) symptoms: headache, lethargy, confusion, muscular weakness
- Postural hypotension
- Tachycardia
- Gastrointestinal (GI) symptoms: nausea, diarrhea, cramping
- Diaphoresis, cold and clammy skin
- Loss of skin turgor and elasticity
- Serum sodium <135 mEq/L
- Urinary specific gravity <1.010
- Elevated red blood cell and plasma protein levels

OUTCOME CRITERIA
- CNS symptoms (e.g., headache, lethargy) are absent.
- Blood pressure and heart rate return to baseline.
- Skin turgor is normal.
- Serum sodium and urinary specific gravity levels are normal.

NURSING INTERVENTIONS AND *RATIONALE*

1. Continue to monitor the assessment parameters listed under "Defining Characteristics."
2. With physician's collaboration, replace fluid and sodium loss with normal saline solution or with hypertonic saline solution (3% or 5%).
3. Provide oral fluids that are high in sodium, such as juice or bouillon.
4. Avoid the use of diuretics, especially thiazide and loop diuretics *because they will further decrease sodium.*
5. If patients are ambulatory, protect from falls until CNS symptoms and/or postural hypotension clears.
6. If performing nasogastric suctioning, irrigate tube with normal saline solution, not water. In addition, carefully restrict ice chip intake; consider using iced saline solution chips. *Excessive intake of water dilutes serum sodium and can result in water intoxication.*

FLUID VOLUME DEFICIT CONT'D

Fluid Volume Deficit Related to Active Blood Loss

DEFINING CHARACTERISTICS
- Cardiac output <4.0 L/min
- Cardiac index <2.2 L/min
- Pulmonary capillary wedge pressure (PAWP), PAD, central venous pressure (CVP) less than normal or less than baseline (PAWP <6 mm Hg)
- Tachycardia
- Narrowed pulse pressure
- Systolic blood pressure <90 mm Hg
- Urinary output <30 ml/hour
- Pale, cool, moist skin
- Apprehensiveness

OUTCOME CRITERIA
- Patients' CO is >4.0 L/min, and CI is >2.2 L/min.
- Patients' PAWP, PAD, and CVP are normal or back to baseline level.
- Patients' pulse is normal or back to baseline.
- Patients' systolic blood pressure is >90.
- Patients' urinary output is >30 ml/hour.

NURSING INTERVENTIONS AND *RATIONALE*

1. Continue to monitor the assessment parameters listed under "Defining Characteristics." In addition, a serum lactate level >2 mOsm/L is believed to represent cellular perfusion failure at its earliest stage.
2. Secure airway and administer high flow oxygen.
3. Place patients in supine position with legs elevated *to increase preload.* Consider using low-Fowler's position with legs elevated for patients with head injury.
4. For fluid repletion use the 3:1 rule, replacing three parts of fluid for every unit of blood lost.
5. Administer crystalloid solutions using the fluid challenge technique: infuse precise aliquots of fluid (usually 5 to 20 ml/min) over 10-minute periods; monitor cardiac loading pressures serially *to determine successful challenging.* If the PAWP or PAD elevates more than 7 mm Hg above beginning level, the infusion should be stopped. If the PAWP or PAD rises only to 3 mm Hg above baseline or falls, another fluid challenge should be administered.
6. Replete fluids first before considering use of vasopressors, *which increase myocardial oxygen consumption out of proportion to the reestablishment of coronary perfusion in the early phases of treatment.*
7. When blood is available or its need is indicated, replace it with fresh packed red cells and fresh frozen plasma *to keep clotting factors intact.*
8. Move or reposition patients minimally *to decrease or limit tissue oxygen demands.*
9. Evaluate patients' anxiety level and intervene through patient education or sedation *to decrease tissue oxygen demands.*
10. Be alert for the possible development of adult respiratory distress syndrome (ARDS) in the ensuing 72 hours.

RISK FOR FLUID VOLUME EXCESS

Definition
The state in which an individual is at risk for experiencing increased fluid retention and edema.

Risk for Fluid Volume Excess

RISK FACTOR
- Renal failure

DEFINING CHARACTERISTICS
- Weight gain that occurs during a 24- to 48-hour period.
- Dependent pitting edema
- Ascites in severe cases
- Fluid crackles on lung auscultation
- Exertional dyspnea
- Oliguria or anuria
- Hypertension
- Engorged neck veins
- Decrease in urinary osmolality as renal failure progresses
- CVP >15 cm of H_2O
- PAWP 20-25 mm Hg

Continued.

RISK FOR FLUID VOLUME EXCESS CONT'D

OUTCOME CRITERIA

- Weight returns to baseline.
- Edema or ascites is absent or reduced to baseline.
- Lungs are clear to auscultation.
- Exertional dyspnea is absent.
- Blood pressure returns to baseline.
- Neck veins are flat.

NURSING INTERVENTIONS AND *RATIONALE*

1. Continue to monitor the assessment parameters listed under "Defining Characteristics."
2. Promote skin integrity of edematous areas by frequent repositioning and elevation of areas where possible. Avoid massaging pressure points or reddened areas of skin *because this results in further tissue trauma.*
3. Plan patient care to provide rest periods *to not heighten exertional dyspnea.*
4. Weigh patients daily at same time in same clothing, preferably with the same scale.
5. Instruct patients about the correlation between fluid intake and weight gain, using commonly understood fluid measurements (e.g., ingesting 4 cups [1000 ml] of fluid results in an approximate 2-pound weight gain in the anuric patient).

RISK FOR FLUID VOLUME DEFICIT

Definition
The state in which an individual is at risk for experiencing vascular, cellular, or intracellular dehydration.

Fluid Volume Deficit

DEFINING CHARACTERISTICS

- Dry mucous membranes and skin
- Weight loss in excess of 10%
- Acute thirst
- Hypotension
- Tachycardia
- Longitudinal wrinkling of the tongue
- Metabolic acidosis
- Serum electrolyte imbalances: hyperchloremia, hypokalemia
- Electrocardiogram (ECG) changes associated with hypokalemia

OUTCOME CRITERIA

- Mucous membranes are moist.
- Patients' weight returns to baseline.
- Patients' blood pressure returns to baseline.
- Patients' heart rate returns to baseline.
- Tongue is moist and nonwrinkled.
- The acid-base balance is normal.
- Serum electrolyte values are normal.

NURSING INTERVENTIONS

1. Continue to monitor the assessment parameters listed under "Defining Characteristics."
2. With physician's collaboration, replace base and electrolyte losses.
3. With physician's collaboration, replace fluid loss with intravenous isotonic saline solution or dextrose and one-half normal saline solution.
4. Provide oral fluids that are high in electrolytes, such as juices.
5. Provide oral potassium replacement according to serum potassium measurements as the metabolic acidosis is corrected.

RISK FOR FLUID VOLUME DEFICIT CONT'D

Fluid Volume Deficit Related to Active Plasma Loss and Fluid Shift into Interstitium Secondary to Burns

DEFINING CHARACTERISTICS
- PAWP, PAD, CVP less than normal or less than baseline
- Tachycardia
- Narrowed pulse pressure
- Systolic blood pressure <100 mm Hg
- Urinary output <30 ml/hour
- Increased hematocrit level

OUTCOME CRITERIA
- Patients' PAWP, PAD, and CVP are normal or back to baseline.
- Systolic blood pressure is >90 mm Hg.
- Urinary output is >30 ml/hour.
- Patients' hematocrit level is normal.

NURSING INTERVENTIONS AND *RATIONALE*
1. Continue to monitor the assessment parameters listed under "Defining Characteristics." In addition, inspect soft tissues *to determine the presence of edema.*
2. With physician's collaboration, administer intravenous (IV) fluid replacements (usually normal saline solution or lactated Ringer's solution) at a rate sufficient *to maintain urinary output >30 ml/hour.* Colloid solutions are avoided in the initial phases (but can be used later) because of the possibility of increased edema formation *as a result of the increased capillary permeability.*

Nursing Management of Gastrointestinal Alterations

ALTERED NUTRITION: LESS THAN BODY REQUIREMENTS

Definition
The state in which an individual experiences an intake of nutrients insufficient to meet metabolic needs.

Altered Nutrition: Less than Body Requirements Related to Lack of Exogenous Nutrients and Increased Metabolic Demand

DEFINING CHARACTERISTICS

- Unplanned weight loss of 20% of body weight within the past 6 months
- Serum albumin <3.5 g/dl
- Total lymphocytes <1500 mm^3
- Anergy
- Negative nitrogen balance
- Fatigue; lack of energy and endurance
- Nonhealing wounds
- Daily caloric intake less than estimated nutritional requirements
- Presence of factors known to increase nutritional requirements (e.g., sepsis, trauma, multiple organ dysfunction syndrome [MODS])
- Maintenance of NPO status for >7-10 days
- Long-term use of 5% dextrose intravenously
- Documentation of suboptimal calorie counts
- Drug or nutrient interaction that might decrease oral intake (e.g., chronic use of bronchodilators, laxatives, anticonvulsives, diuretics, antacids, narcotics)
- Physical problems with chewing, swallowing, choking, salivation, and presence of altered taste, anorexia, nausea, vomiting, diarrhea, or constipation

OUTCOME CRITERIA

- Patients exhibit stabilization of weight loss or weight gain of $^1/_2$ pound daily.

- Serum albumin is >3.5 g/dl.
- Total lymphocytes are >1500 mm^3.
- Patients have positive response to cutaneous skin antigen testing.
- Patients are in positive nitrogen balance.
- Wound healing is evident.
- Daily caloric intake equals estimated nutritional requirements.
- Increased ambulation and endurance are evident.

NURSING INTERVENTIONS AND *RATIONALE*

1. Monitor patients during physical care for signs of nutritional deficiencies.
2. Measure admission height and weight.
3. Weigh patients daily.
4. Ensure that specimens for biochemical tests of nutritional status are collected properly and on time.
5. Administer parenteral and enteral solutions as prescribed.
6. Control infusion rate of parenteral and enteral solutions through infusion control devices and check rate every hour.
7. Flush enteral feeding tubes every 4 hours *to maintain patency.*
8. Document oral intake through calorie counts.
9. Perform serial assessments of patients' strength, endurance, conditions of wounds.

RISK FOR INFECTION

Definition
The state in which an individual is at increased risk for being invaded by pathogenic organisms.

Risk for Infection

RISK FACTOR

- Inadequate primary defenses (broken skin, traumatized tissue, decreased ciliary action, stasis of body fluids, change in pH secretions, altered peristalsis).
- Inadequate secondary defenses (decreased hemoglobin, leukopenia, suppressed inflammatory response)
- Immunosuppression
- Inadequate acquired immunity
- Tissue destruction and increased environmental exposure
- Chronic disease
- Invasive procedures
- Malnutrition
- Pharmaceutical agents (antibiotics, steroids)

OUTCOME CRITERIA

- Total lymphocytes are >2000 mm.[3]
- White blood cell count is within normal limits.
- Temperature is within normal limits.
- Blood, urine, wound, and sputum cultures are negative.

NURSING INTERVENTIONS AND *RATIONALE*

1. Wash hands before and after patient care *to reduce the transmission of microorganisms.*
2. Use aseptic technique for insertion or manipulation of invasive monitoring devices, intravenous lines, and urinary drainage catheters *to maintain sterile environment.*
3. Use aseptic technique for dressing changes *to prevent contamination of wounds or insertion sites.*
4. Change any line placed under emergent conditions within 24 hours *because aseptic technique may have been breached during the emergency.*
5. Collaborate with the physician to change any dressing that is saturated with blood or drainage *because these are mediums for microorganism growth.*
6. Minimize use of stopcocks and maintain caps on all stopcock ports *to reduce the ports of entry for microorganisms.*
7. Avoid the use of nasogastric tubes, nasal endotracheal tubes, and nasopharyngeal suctioning in patients with suspected cerebrospinal fluid leaks *to decrease the incidence of central nervous system infection.*
8. Change respiratory equipment every 24 to 48 hours *to decrease incidence of pulmonary infections.*
9. Use disposable sterile scissors, forceps, and hemostats *to reduce the transmission of microorganisms.*
10. Maintain a closed urinary drainage system *to decrease incidence of urinary infections.*
11. Protect all access device sites from potential sources of contamination (NG reflux, draining wounds, ostomies, sputum).
12. Refrigerate compounded nutritional support solutions and open enteral formulas before use *to inhibit bacterial growth.*
13. Perform daily inspections of all invasive devices for signs of infection.

Nursing Management of Endocrine Alterations

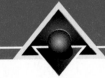

FLUID VOLUME EXCESS

Definition
The state in which an individual experiences increased fluid retention and edema.

Fluid Volume Excess Related to Increased Secretion of ADH

DEFINING CHARACTERISTICS

- Weight gain *without* edema
- Hyponatremia (dilutional)
- Decreased urinary output
- Urinary osmolality above normal, exceeding plasma osmolality
- Urinary specific gravity >1.030
- Evidence of water intoxication:
  Fatigue
  Headache
  Abdominal cramps
  Altered level of consciousness
  Diarrhea
  Seizures

OUTCOME CRITERIA

- Weight returns to baseline.
- Serum sodium is 135-145 mEq/L.
- Urinary output is >30 ml/hr.
- Urinary osmolality is 200-800 mOsm/kg.
- Urinary specific gravity is 1.005-1.030.
- Patients have no evidence of water intoxication.

NURSING INTERVENTIONS AND *RATIONALE*

1. Continue to monitor the assessment parameters listed under "Defining Characteristics." In addition, monitor patients closely for evidence of cardiac decompensation caused by excessive preload (i.e., elevated pulmonary artery diastolic pressure [PADP] or pulmonary capillary wedge pressure [PAWP], tachycardia, lung congestion).
2. Anticipate administration of demeclocycline, lithium carbonate, furosemide, and/or narcotic agonists.
3. With physician's collaboration, administer intravenous hypertonic sodium chloride *to temporarily correct hyponatremia.*
4. Weigh patients daily at same time in same clothing, preferably with same scale.
5. Maintain fluid restriction.
6. Monitor hydration status.
7. Initiate seizure precautions *because severe sodium deficit can result in seizures.*

FLUID VOLUME DEFICIT

Definition
The state in which an individual experiences vascular, cellular, or intracellular dehydration.

Fluid Volume Deficit Related to Decreased Secretion of ADH

DEFINING CHARACTERISTICS
- Polyuria (15 L per day)
- Serum sodium >145 mEq/L (particularly in patients who are not drinking to replace losses)
- Intense thirst
- Polydipsia (alert patients)
- Urinary specific gravity <1.005
- Urinary osmolality <300 mOsm/kg
- Plasma osmolality >300 mOsm/kg

OUTCOME CRITERIA
- Urinary volume, specific gravity, and osmolality are normal.
- Thirst is reduced.
- Plasma osmolality and serum sodium level are normal.

NURSING INTERVENTIONS AND *RATIONALE*

1. Continue to monitor the assessment parameters listed under "Defining Characteristics." Additionally, monitor for signs of critical volume deficits, i.e., hypotension, fall in pulmonary artery pressures, tachycardia.

2. With physician's collaboration, administer intravenous electrolyte replacement solutions *because critical electrolyte loss occurs along with water loss.* Replace losses milliliter for milliliter plus 50 ml/hr for insensible losses. Avoid replacement of losses with intravenous dextrose solutions *because of the risk of water intoxication.*

3. If patients are alert, encourage them to satisfy partially their replacement needs by drinking according to thirst. Caution should be observed regarding the excessive ingestion of water (typically, patients will crave iced water) *because of the risk of water intoxication.*

4. With physician's collaboration, administer vasopressin intravenously, intramuscularly, or per the nasal route.

5. For patients after hypophysectomy, teach the administration of vasopressin and its reportable side and toxic effects, the monitoring of intake and output measurement, and the documentation of daily weights.

A

Advanced Cardiac Life Support (ACLS) Guidelines

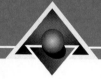

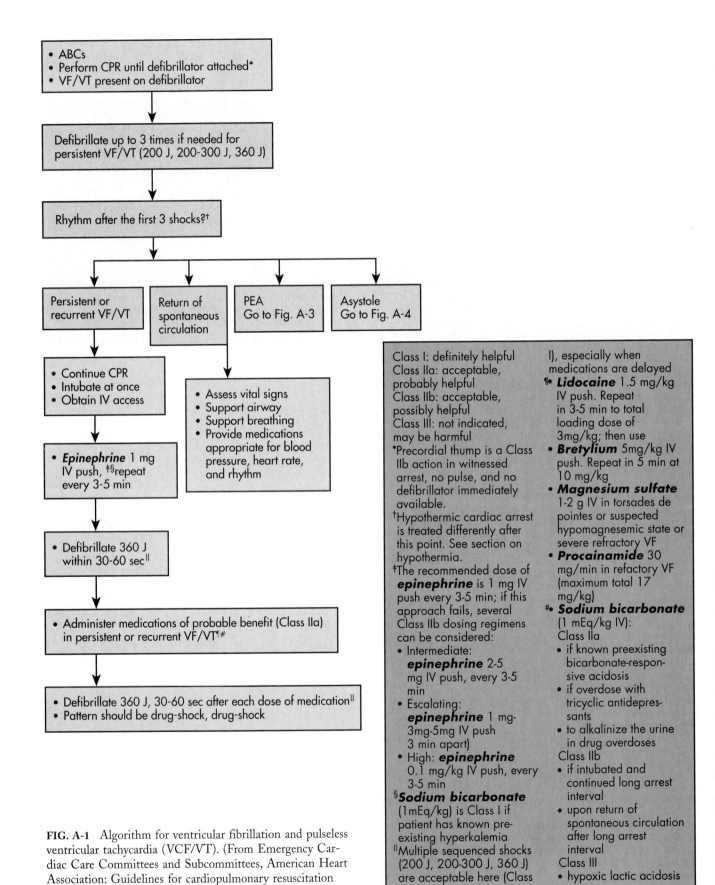

FIG. A-1 Algorithm for ventricular fibrillation and pulseless ventricular tachycardia (VCF/VT). (From Emergency Cardiac Care Committees and Subcommittees, American Heart Association: Guidelines for cardiopulmonary resuscitation and emergency care III: Adult advanced cardiac life support, *JAMA* 268(16):2217, 1992.)

PEA includes
- Electromechanical dissociation (EMD)
- Pseudo-EMD
- Idioventricular rhythms
- Ventricular escape rhythms
- Bradyasystolic rhythms
- Postdefibrillation idioventricular rhythms

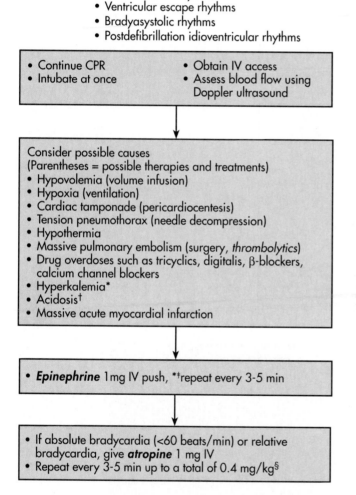

- Continue CPR
- Intubate at once
- Obtain IV access
- Assess blood flow using Doppler ultrasound

Consider possible causes
(Parentheses = possible therapies and treatments)
- Hypovolemia (volume infusion)
- Hypoxia (ventilation)
- Cardiac tamponade (pericardiocentesis)
- Tension pneumothorax (needle decompression)
- Hypothermia
- Massive pulmonary embolism (surgery, *thrombolytics*)
- Drug overdoses such as tricyclics, digitalis, β-blockers, calcium channel blockers
- Hyperkalemia*
- Acidosis†
- Massive acute myocardial infarction

- **Epinephrine** 1mg IV push, *†repeat every 3-5 min

- If absolute bradycardia (<60 beats/min) or relative bradycardia, give **atropine** 1 mg IV
- Repeat every 3-5 min up to a total of 0.4 mg/kg§

Class I: definitely helpful
Class IIa: acceptable, probably helpful
Class IIb: acceptable, possibly helpful
Class III: not indicated, may be harmful
***Sodium bicarbonate** 1 mEq/kg is Class I if patient has known preexisting hyperkalemia.
†**Sodium bicarbonate** 1mEq/kg:
Class IIa
- if known preexisting bicarbonate-responsive acidosis
- if overdose with tricyclic antidepressants
- to alkalinize the urine in drug overdoses
Class IIb
- if intubated and long arrest interval
- upon return of spontaneous circulation after long arrest interval
Class III
- hypoxic lactic acidosis
‡The recommended dose of **epinephrine** is 1 mg IV push every 3-5 min. If this approach fails, several Class IIb dosing regimens can be considered.
- Intermediate: **epinephrine** 2-5 mg IV push every 3-5 min
- Escalating: **epinephrine** 1mg-3 mg-5 mg IV push (3 min apart)
- High: **epinephrine** 0.1 mg/kg IV push every 3-5 min
§Shorter **atropine** dosing intervals are possibly helpful in cardiac arrest (Class IIb).

FIG. A-2 Algorithm for pulseless electrical activity (PEA) (electromechanical dissociation [EMD]). (From Emergency Cardiac Care Committees and Subcommittees, American Heart Association: Guidelines for cardiopulmonary resuscitation and emergency care III: Adult advanced cardiac life support, *JAMA* 268(16):2219, 1992.)

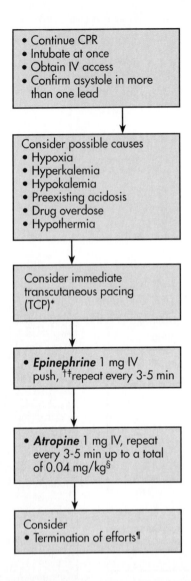

- Continue CPR
- Intubate at once
- Obtain IV access
- Confirm asystole in more than one lead

Consider possible causes
- Hypoxia
- Hyperkalemia
- Hypokalemia
- Preexisting acidosis
- Drug overdose
- Hypothermia

Consider immediate transcutaneous pacing (TCP)*

- *Epinephrine* 1 mg IV push, ††repeat every 3-5 min

- *Atropine* 1 mg IV, repeat every 3-5 min up to a total of 0.04 mg/kg§

Consider
- Termination of efforts¶

Class I: definitely helpful
Class IIa: acceptable, probably helpful
Class IIb: acceptable, possibly helpful
Class III: not indicated, may be harmful
*TCP is a Class IIb intervention. Lack of success may be due to delays in pacing. To be effective TCP must be performed early, simultaneously with drugs. Evidence does not support routine use of TCP for asystole.
†The recommended dose of *epinephrine* is 1mg IV push every 3-5 min. If this approach fails, several Class IIb dosing regimens can be considered:
- Intermediate: *epinephrine* 2-5 mg IV push every 3-5 min
- Escalating: *epinephrine* 1 mg-3 mg-5 mg IV push, (3 min apart)
- High: *epinephrine* 0.1 mg/kg IV push every 3-5 min
‡*Sodium bicarbonate* 1 mEq/kg is Class I if patient has known preexisting hyperkalemia.

§Shorter *atropine* dosing intervals are Class IIb in asystolic arrest.
Sodium bicarbonate 1 mEq/kg:
Class IIa
- if known preexisting bicarbonate-responsive acidosis
- if overdose with tricyclic antidepressants
- to alkalinize the urine in drug overdoses
Class IIb
- if intubated and continued long arrest interval
- upon return of spontaneous circulation after long arrest interval
Class III
- hypoxic lactic acidosis
¶If patient remains in asystole or other agonal rhythms after successful intubation and initial medications and no reversible causes are identified, consider termination of resuscitative efforts by a physician. Consider interval since arrest.

FIG. A-3 Asystole treatment algorithm. (From Emergency Cardiac Care Committees and Subcommittees, American Heart Association: Guidelines for cardiopulmonary resuscitation and emergency care III: Adult advanced cardiac life support, *JAMA* 268(16):2220, 1992.)

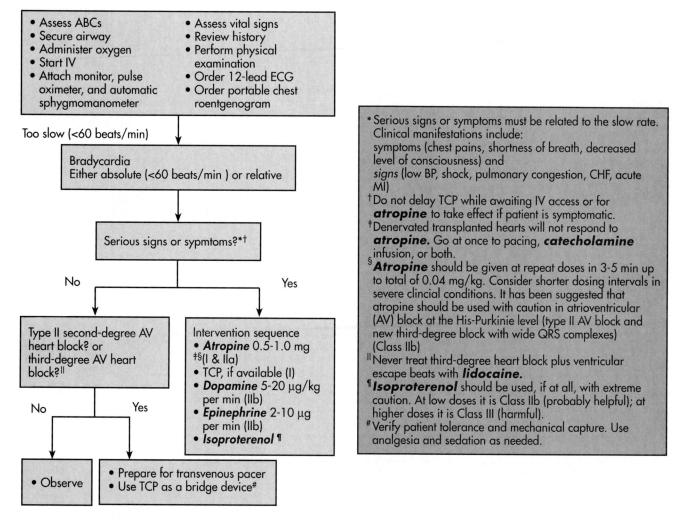

- Assess ABCs
- Secure airway
- Administer oxygen
- Start IV
- Attach monitor, pulse oximeter, and automatic sphygmomanometer

- Assess vital signs
- Review history
- Perform physical examination
- Order 12-lead ECG
- Order portable chest roentgenogram

Too slow (<60 beats/min)

Bradycardia
Either absolute (<60 beats/min) or relative

Serious signs or sypmtoms?*†

No

Yes

Type II second-degree AV heart block? or third-degree AV heart block?‖

Intervention sequence
- *Atropine* 0.5-1.0 mg ‡§(I & IIa)
- TCP, if available (I)
- *Dopamine* 5-20 μg/kg per min (IIb)
- *Epinephrine* 2-10 μg per min (IIb)
- *Isoproterenol* ¶

No

Yes

- Observe

- Prepare for transvenous pacer
- Use TCP as a bridge device#

* Serious signs or symptoms must be related to the slow rate. Clinical manifestations include:
symptoms (chest pains, shortness of breath, decreased level of consciousness) and
signs (low BP, shock, pulmonary congestion, CHF, acute MI)
† Do not delay TCP while awaiting IV access or for **atropine** to take effect if patient is symptomatic.
‡ Denervated transplanted hearts will not respond to **atropine.** Go at once to pacing, **catecholamine** infusion, or both.
§ **Atropine** should be given at repeat doses in 3-5 min up to total of 0.04 mg/kg. Consider shorter dosing intervals in severe clinical conditions. It has been suggested that atropine should be used with caution in atrioventricular (AV) block at the His-Purkinie level (type II AV block and new third-degree block with wide QRS complexes) (Class IIb)
‖ Never treat third-degree heart block plus ventricular escape beats with **lidocaine.**
¶ **Isoproterenol** should be used, if at all, with extreme caution. At low doses it is Class IIb (probably helpful); at higher doses it is Class III (harmful).
# Verify patient tolerance and mechanical capture. Use analgesia and sedation as needed.

FIG. A-4 Bradycardia algorithm (with the patient not in cardiac arrest). (From Emergency Cardiac Care Committees and Subcommittees, American Heart Association: Guidelines for cardiopulmonary resuscitation and emergency care III: Adult advanced cardiac life support, *JAMA* 268(16):2221, 1992.)

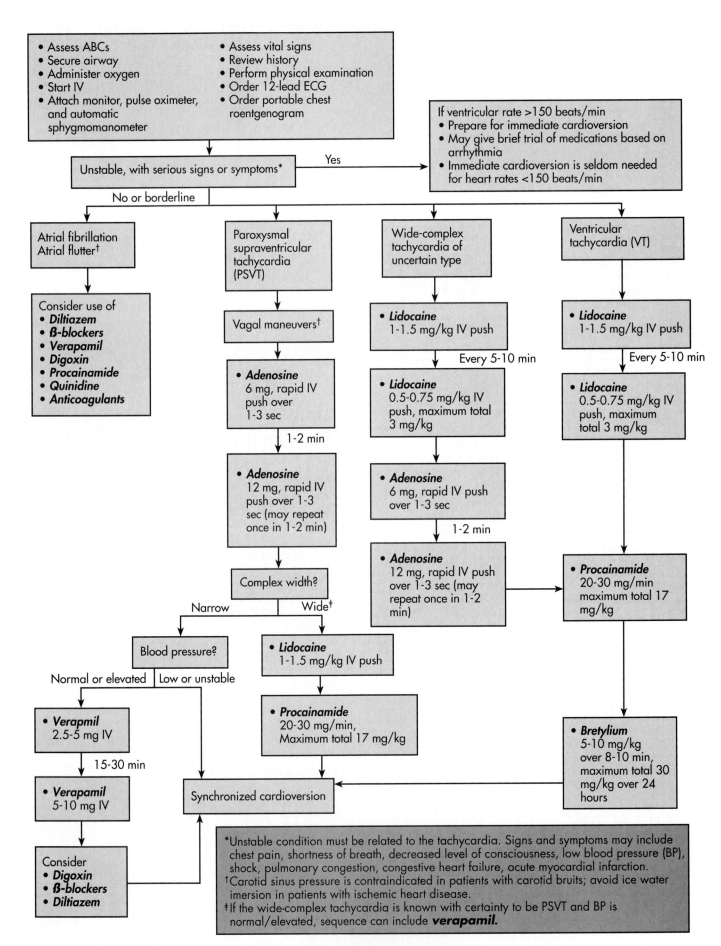

FIG. A-5 Tachycardia algorithm. (From Emergency Cardiac Care Committees and Sub-committees, American Heart Association: Guidelines for cardiopulmonary resuscitation and emergency care III: Adult advanced cardiac life support, *JAMA* 268(15):2223, 1992.)

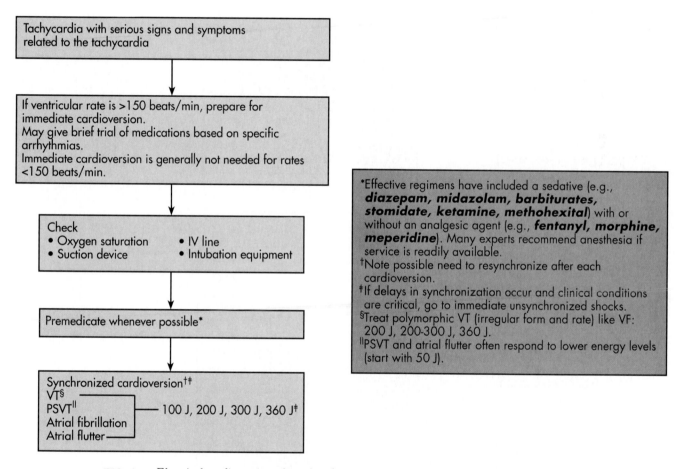

Tachycardia with serious signs and symptoms related to the tachycardia

If ventricular rate is >150 beats/min, prepare for immediate cardioversion.
May give brief trial of medications based on specific arrhythmias.
Immediate cardioversion is generally not needed for rates <150 beats/min.

Check
• Oxygen saturation
• Suction device
• IV line
• Intubation equipment

Premedicate whenever possible*

Synchronized cardioversion†‡
VT§
PSVT‖ —— 100 J, 200 J, 300 J, 360 J‡
Atrial fibrillation
Atrial flutter

*Effective regimens have included a sedative (e.g., **diazepam, midazolam, barbiturates, stomidate, ketamine, methohexital**) with or without an analgesic agent (e.g., **fentanyl, morphine, meperidine**). Many experts recommend anesthesia if service is readily available.
†Note possible need to resynchronize after each cardioversion.
‡If delays in synchronization occur and clinical conditions are critical, go to immediate unsynchronized shocks.
§Treat polymorphic VT (irregular form and rate) like VF: 200 J, 200-300 J, 360 J.
‖PSVT and atrial flutter often respond to lower energy levels (start with 50 J).

FIG. A-6 Electrical cardioversion algorithm (with the patient not in cardiac arrest). (From Emergency Cardiac Care Committees and Subcommittees, American Heart Association: Guidelines for cardiopulmonary resuscitation and emergency care III: Adult advanced cardiac life support, *JAMA* 268(16):2224, 1992.)

helan B-11

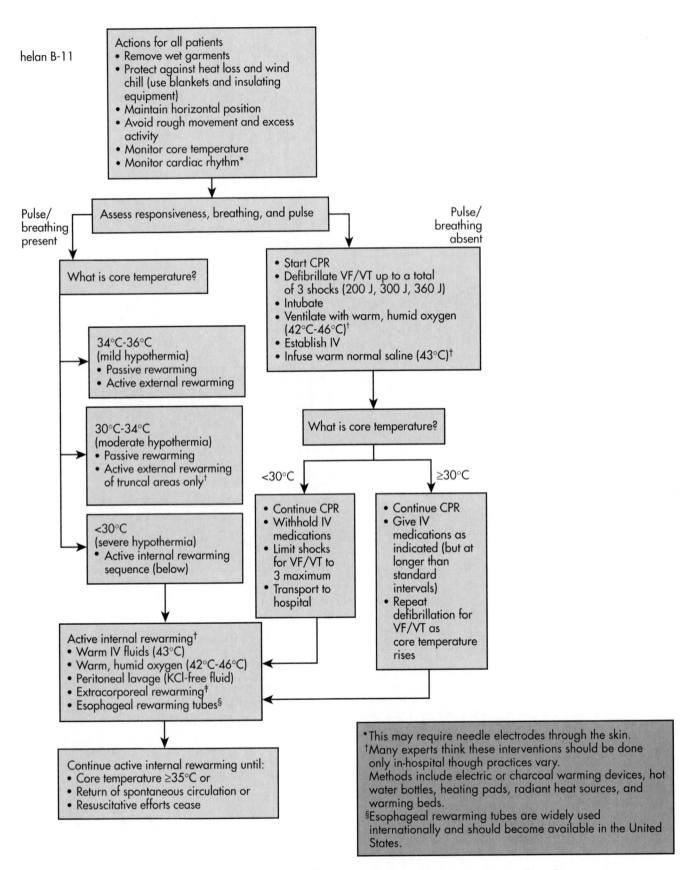

FIG. A-7 Algorithm for treatment of hypothermia. (From Emergency Cardiac Care Committees and Subcommittees, American Heart Association: Guidelines for cardiopulmonary resuscitation and emergency care IV: Special resuscitation situations, *JAMA* 268(16):2245, 1992.)

Physiologic Formulas for Critical Care

Hemodynamic Formulas

Mean (systemic) arterial pressure (MAP)

$$\frac{\text{(Systemic)}\ (\text{Diastolic} \times 2) + \text{(Systemic)}\ (\text{Systolic} \times 1)}{3}$$

Systemic vascular resistance (SVR)

$$\frac{\text{MAP} - \text{RAP}}{\text{CO}} = \begin{array}{l}\text{SVR in units}\\ \text{(Normal range 10-18 units)}\end{array}$$

$$\frac{\text{MAP} - \text{RAP}}{\text{CO}} \times 80 = \begin{array}{l}\text{SVR in dynes/sec/cm}^{-5}\\ \text{(Normal range 800-1400}\\ \text{dynes/sec/cm}^{-5})\end{array}$$

Systemic vascular resistance index (SVRI)

$$\frac{\text{MAP} - \text{RAP}}{\text{CI}} \times 80 = \begin{array}{l}\text{SVRI in dynes/sec cm}^{-5}/\text{m}^2\\ \text{(Normal range 2000-2400}\\ \text{dynes/sec/cm}^{-5}/\text{m}^2)\end{array}$$

Pulmonary vascular resistance (PVR)

$$\frac{\text{PAP mean} - \text{PAWP}}{\text{CO}} = \begin{array}{l}\text{PVR in units}\\ \text{(Normal range 1.2-3.0 units)}\end{array}$$

$$\frac{\text{PAP mean} - \text{PAWP}}{\text{CO}} \times 80 = \begin{array}{l}\text{PVR in dynes/sec/cm}^{-5}\\ \text{(Normal range 100-250 dynes/sec/cm}^{-5})\end{array}$$

Pulmonary vascular resistance index (PVRI)

$$\frac{\text{PAP Mean} - \text{PAWP}}{\text{CI}} \times 80 = \begin{array}{l}\text{PVRI in dynes/sec/cm}^{-5}/\text{m}^2\\ \text{(Normal range 225-315 dynes/sec/cm}^{-5}/\text{m}^2)\end{array}$$

Left cardiac work index (LCWI)

STEP **1.** MAP × CO × 0.0136 = LCW

STEP **2.** $\dfrac{\text{LCW}}{\text{BSA}} = \begin{array}{l}\text{LCWI}\\ \text{(Normal range 3.4-4.2 kg-m/m}^2)\end{array}$

Left ventricular stroke work index (LVSWI)

STEP **1.** MAP × SV × 0.0136 = LVSW

STEP **2.** $\dfrac{\text{LVSW}}{\text{BSA}} = \begin{array}{l}\text{LVSWI}\\ \text{(Normal range 50-62 g-m/m}^2)\end{array}$

Right cardiac work index (RCWI)

STEP **1.** PAP mean × CO × 0.0136 = RCW

STEP **2.** $\dfrac{\text{RCW}}{\text{BSA}} = \begin{array}{l}\text{RCWI}\\ \text{(Normal range 0.54-0.66 kg-m/m}^2)\end{array}$

RAP, Right atrial pressure; *CO,* cardiac output; *CI,* cardiac index; *SV,* stroke volume; *HR,* heart rate; *PAP* mean, pulmonary artery mean pressure; *PAWP,* pulmonary artery wedge pressure; *PB,* barometric pressure; Hgb, hemoglobin; Hbo_2, oxyhemoglobin; *Qs,* shunt flow; *Qt,* total blood flow; MAP, mean arterial pressure; ICP, intracranial pressure.

*pK = 6.1 is the dissociation constant of carbonic acid.

†$\text{Paco}_2 \times .03$ converts Paco_2 from mm Hg to mEq/L.

‡1.25 is a constant used to take into account the normal respiratory quotient.

§47 is a constant used to correct for the normal water vapor pressure of humidified gas.

‖.003 is a constant used because 0.003 ml of oxygen will dissolve in each 100 ml of blood.

¶1.34 is a constant used because each gram of hemoglobin will carry 1.34 ml oxygen. Actually, if the hemoglobin is chemically pure (rare), each gram is capable of carrying 1.39 ml of oxygen. Because most hemoglobin has impurities, 1.34 is the accepted constant.

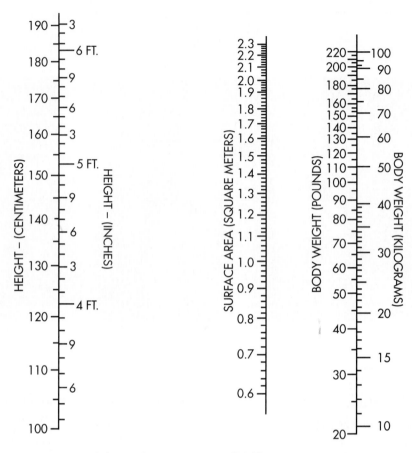

Fig. B-1   Body surface area (BSA) nomogram.

Right ventricular stroke work index (RVSWI)

STEP 1.   **PAP mean × SV × 0.0136 = RVSW**

STEP 2. $\dfrac{\text{RVSW}}{\text{BSA}}$ = **RVSWI**
(Normal range 7.9-9.7 g-m/m²)

Body surface area

Many hemodynamic formulas can be *indexed* or adjusted to body size by use of a body surface area (BSA) nomogram (Fig. B-1). To calculate BSA:

1. Obtain height and weight.
2. Mark height on the left scale and weight on the right scale.
3. Draw a straight line between the two points marked on the nomogram.

The number where the line crosses the middle scale is the BSA value.

Pulmonary Formulas

Henderson-Hasselbach equation (blood pH)

$$pH = pK^* + Log\,\frac{HCO_3^-\ mEq/L\ \text{(Base)}}{Paco_2\ mm\ Hg \times 0.3\dagger\ \text{(Acid)}}$$

$$pH = 6.1 = Log\,\frac{HCO_3^-\ mEq/L\ \text{(Base)}}{Paco_2\ mEq/L\ \text{(Acid)}}$$

Partial pressure of oxygen in the alveolus (Pao₂, expressed in mm Hg)

$$Pao_2 = Pio_2 - (Paco_2 \times 1.25)\ddagger$$

Partial pressure of inspired oxygen (PIo₂, expressed in mm Hg)

$$Pio_2 = Fio_2 \times (PB - 47)\S$$

Arterial oxygen saturation (Sao₂)

$$\frac{Hgbo_2}{(Hgb + Hgbo_2)} \times 100$$

Normal range > 92%

A-a gradient (also known as A-a Do₂)

A-a gradient = $PA_{O_2} - Pa_{O_2}$ (expressed in mm Hg; normal <10 mm Hg but normal increases with age and FI_{O_2})

Calculation of the arterial oxygen content (Cao₂)

Oxygen content is a measure of the total amount of oxygen carried in the blood—both the oxygen dissolved in plasma (Pa_{O_2}) and the oxygen bound to hemoglobin (Sa_{O_2}). Oxygen content is reported in ml/100 ml blood or as volume percent.

There are three steps in the Ca_{O_2} calculation.

STEP 1. Calculate the amount of oxygen dissolved in 100 ml of plasma:

$$Pa_{O_2} \times .003\| = ml\ O_2/100\ ml\ plasma$$

STEP 2. Calculate the amount of oxygen bound to hemoglobin:

$$Hgb \times 1.34\P \times Sa_{O_2} = ml\ of\ O_2\ bound\ to\ Hgb$$

STEP 3. Add the results of Steps 1 and 2 for the Ca_{O_2}.

EXAMPLE: PATIENT A

Pa_{O_2}	100 mm Hg
Sa_{O_2}	.97
Hgb	15 g%

STEP 1. $100 \times .003 = .3\ ml\ O_2$ in 100 ml plasma.
STEP 2. 15 g% $\times 1.34 \times .97 = 19.5$ ml O_2 bound to Hgb.
STEP 3. $0.3 + 19.5 = 19.8\ vol\%\ Ca_{O_2}$.

Calculation of venous oxygen content (Cvo₂)

Same steps as to calculate Ca_{O_2}, except that Pv_{O_2} and Sv_{O_2} are substituted into the equation in the place of the arterial values. Hgb remains the same.

Normal range 12-15 vol%

Tissue oxygen consumption (Vo₂)

$$(CO \times Ca_{O_2} \times 10) - (Co \times Cv_{O_2} \times 10)$$

Arterial − venous

Normal range 250 ml/min

Mixed venous oxygen saturation (Svo₂)

$$(CO \times Ca_{O_2} \times 10) - V_{O_2}$$

O_2 delivery − O_2 consumption

Normal range 60%-80%

Neurologic Formula
Cerebral perfusion pressure (CPP)

MAP − ICP

Normal range 80-100 mm Hg

Renal Formula

ANION GAP
$Na^+ - (Cl^- + HCO_3^-)$
Normal range is 10-12 mEq/L

Nutritional Formulas

ESTIMATING CALORIC NEEDS

$$= 2(Na^+ + K^+) + \frac{glucose\ mg/dl}{18} + \frac{BUN\ mg/dl}{2.8}$$

1. Calculate basal energy expenditure (BEE). This is the energy needed for basic life processes such as respiratory function and maintenance of body temperature.
   Women: BEE = $655 + (9.6 \times W) + (1.7 \times H) - (4.7 \times A)$
   Men: BEE = $66 + (13.7 \times W) + (5 \times H) - (6.8 \times A)$
   W = Current weight in kg; H = Height in cm; A = Age in yr
2. Multiply BEE by an appropriate activity factor.

LEVEL OF ACTIVITY	MULTIPLY BEE BY
Bed rest	1.2
Light (e.g., sedentary office work)	1.3
Moderate (e.g., nursing)	1.4
Strenuous (e.g., manual labor)	1.5 or more

3. Multiply by an appropriate stress factor to meet the needs of the ill or injured patient.

TYPE OF STRESS	MULTIPLY THE VALUE OBTAINED IN STEP 2 BY
Fever	1 + 0.13/° C elevation above normal (0r 0.07/° F)
Pneumonia	1.2
Major injury	1.3
Severe sepsis	1.5-1.6
Major burns	1.8-2.0

Continued.

Nutritional Formulas—cont'd.

ESTIMATING PROTEIN NEEDS

Protein needs vary with degree of malnutrition and stress.

CONDITION	MULTIPLY DESIRABLE BODY WEIGHT (kg) BY
Healthy individual or well-nourished elective surgery patient	0.8-1 g protein
Malnourished or catabolic state (e.g., sepsis, major injury, burns)	1.2-2+ g protein

EXAMPLE OF CALCULATION OF NEEDS

A 38-year-old male patient with pelvic, rib, and long-bone fractures; pneumothorax; and a ruptured spleen after a vehicle accident. Height 180 cm (5′11″), current weight 81.8 kg (180 lb), desirable weight 72.7 kg (160 lb).

Energy needs

1. BEE = 66 + (13.7 × 81.8) + (5 × 180) − (6.8 × 38) = 1829 calories/day
2. Energy needs for bed rest = 1829 calories × 1.2 = 2195 calories/day
3. Energy needs for injury = 2195 calories × 1.3 = 2853 calories/day

Protein needs = 72.7 kg × 1.5 g = 109 g/day

Index

A

Notes

Notes

Notes